HEALTH
ECONOMICS

The Addison-Wesley Series in Economics

Abel/Bernanke/Croushore
Macroeconomics*

Bade/Parkin
Foundations of Economics*

Bierman/Fernandez
Game Theory with Economic
Applications

Binger/Hoffman
Microeconomics with Calculus

Boyer
Principles of Transportation
Economics

Branson
Macroeconomic Theory and
Policy

Bruce
Public Finance and the
American Economy

Byrns/Stone
Economics

Carlton/Perloff
Modern Industrial
Organization

Caves/Frankel/Jones
World Trade and Payments: An
Introduction

Chapman
Environmental Economics:
Theory, Application, and Policy

Cooter/Ulen
Law & Economics

Downs
An Economic Theory of
Democracy

Ehrenberg/Smith
Modern Labor Economics

Ekelund/Ressler/Tollison
Economics*

Fusfeld
The Age of the Economist

Gerber
International Economics

Ghiara
Learning Economics

Gordon
Macroeconomics

Gregory
Essentials of Economics

Gregory/Stuart
Russian and Soviet Economic
Performance and Structure

Hartwick/Olewiler
The Economics of Natural
Resource Use

Hoffman/Averett
Women and the Economy:
Family, Work, and Pay

Holt
Markets, Games and Strategic
Behavior

Hubbard
Money, the Financial System,
and the Economy

Hughes/Cain
American Economic History

Husted/Melvin
International Economics

Jehle/Reny
Advanced Microeconomic
Theory

Johnson-Lans
A Health Economics Primer

Klein
Mathematical Methods for
Economics

Krugman/Obstfeld
International Economics:
Theory & Policy*

Laidler
The Demand for Money

Leeds/von Allmen
The Economics of Sports

Leeds/von Allmen/Schiming
Economics*

Lipsey/Ragan/Storer
Economics*

Melvin
International Money and
Finance

Miller
Economics Today*

Miller
Understanding Modern
Economics

Miller/Benjamin
The Economics of Macro Issues

Miller/Benjamin/North
The Economics of Public Issues

Mills/Hamilton
Urban Economics

Mishkin
The Economics of Money,
Banking, and Financial
Markets*

Mishkin
The Economics of Money,
Banking, and Financial Markets,
Business School Edition*

Murray
Econometrics: A Modern
Introduction

Parkin
Economics*

Perloff
Microeconomics*

Perloff
Microeconomics: Theory and
Applications with Calculus

**Perman/Common/McGilvray/
Ma**
Natural Resources and
Environmental Economics

Phelps
Health Economics

**Riddell/Shackelford/Stamos/
Schneider**
Economics: A Tool for
Critically Understanding
Society

Ritter/Silber/Udell
Principles of Money, Banking
& Financial Markets*

Rohlf
Introduction to Economic
Reasoning

Ruffin/Gregory
Principles of Economics

Sargent
Rational Expectations and
Inflation

Scherer
Industry Structure, Strategy,
and Public Policy

Sherman
Market Regulation

Stock/Watson
Introduction to Econometrics

Stock/Watson
Introduction to Econometrics,
Brief Edition

Studenmund
Using Econometrics: A
Practical Guide

Tietenberg/Lewis
Environmental and Natural
Resource Economics

Tietenberg
Environmental Economics and
Policy

Todaro/Smith
Economic Development

Waldman
Microeconomics

Waldman/Jensen
Industrial Organization:
Theory and Practice

Weil
Economic Growth

Williamson
Macroeconomics

* denotes **myeconlab** titles   **Log onto www.myeconlab.com to learn more**

FOURTH EDITION

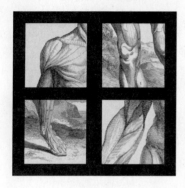

HEALTH
ECONOMICS

CHARLES E. PHELPS
University of Rochester

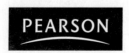

Boston   Columbus   Indianapolis   New York   San Francisco   Upper Saddle River
Amsterdam   Cape Town   Dubai   London   Madrid   Milan   Munich   Paris   Montreal   Toronto
Delhi   Mexico City   Sao Paulo   Sydney   Hong Kong   Seoul   Singapore   Taipei   Tokyo

Editor in Chief: Donna Battista
Acquisitions Editor: Noel Kamm Seibert
Assistant Editor: Mina Kim
Editorial Assistant: Gavin Broady
Managing Editor: Nancy H. Fenton
Senior Production Supervisor: Kathryn Dinovo
Executive Marketing Manager: Roxanne McCarley
Marketing Assistant: Kendra Bassi
Senior Author Support/Technology Specialist: Joe Vetere
Senior Prepress Supervisor: Caroline Fell
Permissions Project Manager: Shannon Barbe
Permissions Project Supervisor: Michael Joyce
Media Producer: Angela Lee
Senior Manufacturing Buyer: Carol Melville
Cover Designer: Jodi Notowitz
Production Coordination, Text Design, Illustrations, and Composition: Pine Tree
Composition/Laserwords

For permission to use copyrighted material, grateful acknowledgment is made to the copyright holders on pp. 623–624, which are hereby part of this copyright page.

If you purchased this book within the United States or Canada you should be aware that it has been wrongfully imported without the approval of the Publisher or the Author.

Copyright © 2010 Charles E. Phelps

All rights reserved. No part of this publication may be reproduced, stored in a retrieval system, or transmitted, in any form or by any means, electronic, mechanical, photocopying, recording, or otherwise, without the prior written permission of the publisher. Printed in the United States of America.

For information on obtaining permission for use of material in this work, please submit a written request to Pearson Education, Inc., Rights and Contracts Department, 501 Boylston Street, Suite 900, Boston, MA 02116, fax your request to 617-671-3447, or e-mail at http://www.pearsoned.com/legal/permissions.htm.

Many of the designations used by manufacturers and sellers to distinguish their products are claimed as trademarks. Where those designations appear in this book, and the publisher was aware of a trademark claim, the designations have been printed in initial caps or all caps.

1 2 3 4 5 6 7 8 9 10—CRW—13 12 11 10 09

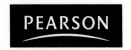

ISBN-10: 0-321-64290-2
ISBN-13: 978-0-321-64290-5

TO DALE—OUR TIME HAS JUST BEGUN.

CONTENTS

CHAPTER 5   Empirical Studies of Medical Care Demand and Applications   126

CHAPTER 6   The Physician and the Physician Firm   165

CHAPTER 7   Physicians in the Marketplace   197

CHAPTER 8   The Hospital as a Supplier of Medical Care   238

CHAPTER 9   Hospitals in the Marketplace   269

CHAPTER 10   The Demand for Health Insurance   300

CHAPTER 11   Health Insurance Supply and Managed Care   345

PREFACE

The study of health economics is becoming more important and more useful. The health care sector continues to grow in size, both in absolute dollars and as a portion of the overall economic activity of the United States. In terms of employment, now about one person of six in the country is employed in the health care sector.

At the same time, the ways in which we organize health care and its financing continue to have increasing importance. For example, the widespread reliance in the United States on employer-based financing of health care has placed domestic firms in an unenviable position of having a proportion of their costs rise steadily outside of the control of management, a situation in distinct contrast to the nations with which the United States competes in a globally open economy. In response to this cost pressure, health care finance organizations (both public and private) have tested an increasingly large and complicated array of cost-control and utilization-control mechanisms to keep total health insurance premium costs under control. These have been generally met with limited success here and abroad, often fueling consumer resistance when the control mechanisms actually impinge on patients' ability to acquire "necessary" health care. The U.S. government, through Medicare, Medicaid, and other federal programs, has in some sense led the way in devising cost-control measures, but the private sector has devised many as well, some of which Congressional mandate has placed "off limits" for federal programs. Both the public and private sectors will continue to learn from each others' triumphs and mistakes.

New approaches to studying health economics continue to unfold, including the introduction of cost-effectiveness analysis, more widespread use of game theory, and—perhaps most important of all—a much deeper understanding of the ways in which general human behavior (lifestyle choices) affect health outcomes. A parallel development comes from the world of genetics and molecular medicine, leading to a whole new array of diagnostic and therapeutic alternatives not previously available as well as a better understanding of how our genetic heritage may control our lifestyle choices. (For example some of us are genetically disposed to become addicted to nicotine.) These new findings from genetic medicine require rethinking not only diagnostic and therapeutic choices for physicians and their patients but also the structure of health insurance programs and (most importantly) how new technologies are introduced into the list of covered services. These same genetic findings alter the legal and ethical landscape in thinking about health care.

NEW TO THIS EDITION

Health Economics continues to bring new issues to the forefront with numerous substantive changes in the content and organization of the textbook in addition to utilizing the most current available data. The most significant changes include:

- Reorganization of Chapters 1 and 2 to provide a smoother introduction to the field with all data tables updated to most recent years available and projections to 2010.
- A new Chapter 2, Utility and Health, that combines previous material on the production of health using medical care and a greatly expanded section on how lifestyle choices affect health. The chapter includes discussions of the role of education on these lifestyle choices.
- New studies on the role of medical care in creating health including new estimates of health (mortality) with respect to medical care use specific to different age groups (Chapter 3).
- New insights into the importance of cross-elasticities of demand between prescription drugs and other medical care use (Chapter 5).
- New discussion on the economics of the production of a single physician visit: what actually happens when a patient visits a doctor (Chapter 6).
- Enhanced discussion about patient search when doctor quality varies (and is difficult to observe) (Chapter 7).
- A new state-preference approach to understanding demand for insurance (Chapter 10).
- New discussion of the role of preventive medical care in the demand for insurance (Chapter 10).
- Expanded discussion of managed care to include physician participation and reliance on managed care from the medical practice viewpoint (Chapter 11).
- New analysis of SCHIP, Medicare Advantage (Part C), Medicare prescription drug coverage (Part D), and the role of risk adjustment in Medicare Advantage programs (Chapter 12).
- Expansion of sections on externalities dealing with contagious diseases including issues of vaccine supply (Chapter 14).

- Discussion of additional shifts of regulation to emphasize its role in the introduction of new technologies (including discovery, patenting, distribution, and advertising to patients and coverage determination by health plans) (Chapter 15).
- Discussion of the benefits and costs of single payer systems in the analysis of universal health insurance (Chapter 16).

ADDITIONAL RESOURCES

Each chapter points readers to key chapters in the two-volume compendium *Handbook of Health Economics* edited by Anthony Culyer and Joseph P. Newhouse (2000). This two-volume series (part of an extended series of Handbooks in Economics edited by top scholars in their fields) contains summary articles from state-of-the-art researchers in topics spanning a wide array of the field of health economics. These articles, while "dated" to the 2000 publication year, still stand as a useful resource for scholars in this field and will do so for years to come.

The Companion Website for *Health Economics* (www.aw-bc.com/phelps) offers additional resources for students such as useful Web links, additional material on the role of genetics in obesity and the use of alcohol and tobacco, and self-study quizzes.

Instructors can download the Instructor's Manual from the Instructor's Resource Center (www.pearsonhighered.com/irc). This manual includes sample essay questions and project ideas as well as an extensive new set of "tricks of the trade" that I have acquired while teaching this course for a quarter of a century. The Instructor's Manual also includes information for peer-led student workshops, a powerful new learning method I recently have come to use. I have included resources for faculty to learn how to introduce this approach in their own setting and problems that can be used in these workshops or on exams.

ACKNOWLEDGMENTS

I wish to express my appreciation to the entire Addison-Wesley publication team for their excellent help and collaboration in preparing this fourth edition, beginning with the solicitation and collation of reviewers' comments, copy editing, manuscript management, production (many thanks to Bruce Hobart from Pine Tree Composition and Kathryn Dinovo), and all other steps leading to publication. I particularly wish to thank Noel Kamm Seibert and Mina Kim at Addison-Wesley for all of the "production" steps in the process and valued guidance in thinking about additions, modifications, and the inevitable deletions in the book.

Reviewers who provided valuable guidance in the revision process include the following:

Jeff DeSimone, *University of Texas at Arlington*
Ellen Magenheim, *Swarthmore College*
David Meltzer, *The University of Chicago*
Dana Mukamel, *University of California at Irvine—Center for Health Policy Research*
Reed Neil Olsen, *Missouri State University*
Jessica Wolpaw Reyes, *Amherst College*
Sara J. Solnick, *University of Vermont*
Shirley Svorny, *California State University, Northridge*

CHAPTER I

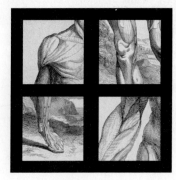

Why Health Economics?

Health care represents a collection of services, products, institutions, regulations, and people that in 2008, accounted for about 16 percent of our gross domestic product (GDP) growing at about 1 percent of GDP per decade in recent years. Projections for 2009 show that aggregate spending on medical care will surpass $2.6 trillion, of which $2.2 trillion represents "personal" health care (the remainder goes to administrative expenses, research, and construction). Thus, personal health care expenses average more than $8,500 annually for each of the 305 plus million people who live in the United States. About half of this comes from private spending, the other half from government spending (financed by taxation). This alone makes the study of health care a topic of potential importance.[1]

LEARNING GOALS

- Assess why the special study of health economics makes sense. Understand novel aspects of health care and ways to approach the issues.

- Identify how health care markets differ from others, particularly understanding the unique role of health insurance.

- Ascertain how medical spending has evolved over time (and why), dissecting changes over the years in medical spending.

---

[1] Annual data updates appear in numerous places on the Internet, most readily accessible at the Centers for Disease Control, www.cdc.gov/nchs/hus.htm They provide there an excellent data series, summarized in *Health 2008* (with annual revisions).

Almost every person has confronted the health care system at some point, often in situations of considerable importance or concern to the individual. Even the most casual contact with this part of the economy confirms that something is quite different about health care. Indeed, the differences are often so large that one wonders whether anything we have learned about economic systems and markets from other areas of the economy will apply, even partly, in the study of health care. Put most simply, does anybody behave as a "rational economic actor" in the health care market?

IMPORTANT (IF NOT UNIQUE) ASPECTS OF HEALTH CARE ECONOMICS

Although the health care sector shares many individual characteristics with other areas of the economy, the collection of unusual economic features that appears in health care markets seems particularly large. The unusual features include (1) the extent of government involvement; (2) the dominant presence of uncertainty at all levels of health care, ranging from the randomness of individuals' illnesses to the understanding of how well medical treatments work, and for whom; (3) the large difference in knowledge between doctors (and other providers) and their patients, the consumers of health care; and (4) externalities—behavior by individuals that imposes costs or creates benefits for others. Each of these is present in other areas of the economy as well, but seldom so much as in health care, and never in such broad combination. A brief discussion of each issue follows.

As background to each of these ideas, and indeed for the entire book, the student of health economics will be served by the following notion: Uncertainty looms everywhere. Uncertain events guide individual behavior in health care. This major uncertainty leads to the development of health insurance, which in turn controls and guides the use of resources throughout the economy. The presence of various forms of uncertainty also accounts for much of the role of government in health care. Thus, if all else fails, search for the role of uncertainty in understanding health care. Such a search will often prove fruitful, and will lead to a better understanding of why the health economy works the way it does and why the institutions in those markets exist.

Government Intervention

The government intrudes into many markets, but seldom as commonly or extensively as in health care. Licensure of health professionals, of course, is common. Many other professionals also require a license before they may practice, including barbers, beauticians, airplane pilots, attorneys, scuba divers, bicycle racers, and (ubiquitously) automobile drivers. But almost every specialist in health care has to pass a formal certification process before practicing, including physicians, nurses, technicians, pharmacists, opticians, dentists, dental hygienists, and a host of others. The certification processes include not only government licensure, but often private certification of competence as well. Why does our society so rigorously examine the competence of health care professionals?

The government also intrudes into health care markets in ways unheard of in other areas. For example, federal and state programs provide insurance or financial aid against health expenses for an extremely diverse set of people, including all elderly persons, the poor, military veterans, children with birth defects, persons with kidney disease, persons who are permanently disabled, people who are blind, migrant workers, families of military personnel, and schoolchildren of all stripes. In addition, a broad majority of people living in the United States can walk into a county hospital and claim the right to receive care for free if they have no obvious way of paying for the care. Probably only in public education do various levels of government touch as many individuals at any given time as in health care. Over a life cycle, nothing except for education comes close: Because Medicare has mandatory enrollment at age 65, every person who lives to that age will become affected by an important government health care program. By contrast, many individuals go through private schools and never see a public school. Why does the government involve itself so much in the financing of health care?

The government also controls the direct economic behavior of health care providers such as hospitals, nursing homes, and doctors, far more than in other sectors of the economy. We have seen economy-wide price controls sporadically in our country's history, and considerable regulation in various sectors such as petroleum, banking, and (by local governments) housing rental rates. After the Organization of Petroleum Exporting Countries (OPEC) raised the price of oil fourfold in 1973, petroleum regulations became a national phenomenon for several years, with such unintended consequences as gasoline shortages and hours-long queues to buy a tank of gas. However, such intervention pales in comparison to government involvement in prices in the health sector. At least in some form, the government has been controlling prices in the health care industry continually since 1971, and these controls, at least in terms of prices paid to physicians by government insurance programs, have become more rigorous and binding over time. During the same time, the government decontrolled prices in a broad array of industries, including airlines, trucking, telephones, and petroleum. Why do we spend so much effort controlling prices in health care in contrast to those in other industries?

For decades, the United States has also seen direct controls on the simple decision to enter the business of providing health care. Even ignoring licensure of professionals as an entry control, we have seen a broad set of regulations requiring such things as a "certificate of need" before a hospital can add so much as a single bed to its capacity. Similar laws control the purchase of expensive pieces of equipment such as diagnostic scanning devices. The reverse process also attracts considerable attention: If a hospital wants to close its doors, political chaos may ensue. What leads the government to intensively monitor and control the simple process of firms entering and exiting an industry?

Quite separately, both federal and state governments have commonly provided special assistance for providing education to people entering the health care field, through direct financial aid to professional schools and generous scholarships to students in those schools. This financial aid often directly benefits a group of persons (e.g., medical students) who will enter one of the highest paying professions in our society. Why do governments proffer this support for the medical education process?

Government research is also prominent in the health care sector. Although the government accounts for considerable research in other areas, most notably those involving national security (such as aircraft design, electronics, and computers), its concern with research in health care is unique. The campus of the National Institutes of Health (NIH) in Bethesda, Maryland (on the outskirts of Washington, D.C.) surpasses that of almost every major university in the country in health-related research and education. In no other nonmilitary area does the government directly undertake research at such a scale. How did biomedical research reach such a level of prominence?

Before any new drug reaches the market, it must undergo a rigorous series of hurdles—research requirements imposed by the government on pharmaceutical firms, drug testing, and reporting of potential side effects. New medical devices confront similar regulations now. By contrast, for example, no regulations exist to control the study of health economics—perhaps, you might argue, fortuitously for this textbook! Why does the government concern itself so much with the drugs we stuff into our mouths, and so little with the knowledge we stuff into our heads?

Other apparently minor aspects of the government can dramatically affect our lives through the health sector. A simple provision of the tax code makes employer-paid health insurance exempt from income taxation. Another tax provision [Section 501(c)3 of the Internal Revenue Code] grants corporate immunity from income taxes to most hospitals and to insurance plans that account for about half of the private health insurance in the United States. In turn, most states adopt this same tax treatment for state income and sales taxes, and most local governments exclude the same organizations from paying property taxes. Why does the health care sector receive these favored tax treatments, and how much has its size and shape been changed thereby?

These ideas touch only briefly on the extent of government involvement in health care, and indeed much of the remainder of this book refers continually to the presence and effects of the government. Astonishingly, though, the government's role in the health sector in the United States is much less than in almost all other countries. Chapter 16 describes how other nations have made choices to involve the government even more than in this country, and attempts to understand the consequences of such choices.

Uncertainty

Uncertainty lurks in every corner of the health care field. Many decisions to use health care begin because of seemingly random events—a broken arm, an inflamed appendix, an auto accident, or a heart attack. Most other medical events are initiated because an individual is concerned about the possibility of some illness—"Do I have cancer, Doctor?" "Am I crazy, Doctor?" "Why am I so tired, Doctor?"

Uncertainty may begin with the consumer-patient in health care, but it certainly doesn't end there. Providers also confront large uncertainty, although often they don't appear to recognize it individually. Yet, in similar situations, doctors often recommend treatment at vastly different rates, and often diverge greatly on which treatment they recommend. Therapies of choice change through time, often with little or no scientific basis for the decision. How can such medical confusion persist in a modern, scientific society?

The contrast between our approach to uncertainty in some areas of medical care (e.g., new drugs) and to similarly large uncertainty in other areas (e.g., the efficacy of a new surgical technique) also commands attention. In one case, we regulate the market intensively. In the other, we license the providers broadly, and then entrust them to make appropriate decisions. Thus, new therapies may sweep through the country with not so much as a single case-control study, let alone a true randomized controlled trial such as would be required for a new drug. Why do we behave so differently in these areas of uncertainty?

Asymmetric Knowledge

Symmetry exists when two objects are identical in size, shape, or power. When two people bargain in an economic exchange, and one holds far more relevant information than the other, the issues of asymmetric information arise. "Knowledge is power," so goes the old saying. This holds equally in international arms control negotiations and discussions between a doctor and patient. In the former case, however, both sides have similar opportunity and (presumably) similar skill in evaluating the positions and claims of the other. In health care, just the opposite holds true: One party (the doctor) generally has a considerably, possibly massively, greater level of knowledge than the other about the issues at hand, namely, the diagnosis and treatment of disease. Not only that, the incentives to reveal information differ. In the arms control case, the two parties hold similar incentives to reveal or hide information. In the doctor-patient case, the patient clearly wishes to reveal information to the doctor, but the doctor may be in a different position.[2] Professional duty, ethics, and personal responsibility make the doctor want to be open and honest. Conflicting with this, however, the simple profit motive can lead the doctor into different choices. Put most simply, if so desired, the doctor might be able to deceive the patient, and make more money doing so. In addition, the patient would have no way of telling when this was happening (if at all). Patients, after all, decide to consult with doctors because they want the doctors' advice.

As with many other facets of health care economics, this situation is not unique to health care. Most adults have confronted a similar circumstance in the most common setting imaginable—auto repair. There, the auto mechanic is in a position to do the same thing, that is, deceive the customer into believing that repairs are needed, and then possibly not even undertake them, because nothing really needed to be fixed.

We have evolved a variety of mechanisms to protect untutored consumers-patients in settings such as these, some applying with more force in health care than others. As Kenneth Arrow (1963) has discussed so well, one of the important reasons for "professions" to evolve, with a code of ethics and, commonly, professional licensure, is to provide an institutional mechanism to help balance transactions such as these.[3]

Arrow also emphasizes the importance of trust in ongoing relationships, and recent developments in the study of health care and other similar markets have formalized these ideas more completely: When two parties know

---

[2]Here, we ignore a common phenomenon that probably has more to do with psychology than economic behavior, namely that some patients "hide" symptoms and signs from their doctors. Most physicians and nurses who experience this feel that patients dread the prospect of a diagnosis (say) of cancer, and hence to not reveal symptoms to the doctor such as (say) coughing up blood that they (at least subconsciously) know are symptomatic of serious diseases.

[3]Every student of health care economics should read Kenneth Arrow's (1963) classic "Uncertainty and the Welfare Economics of Medical Care." Read it now, and also after you have completed your work with this book; you will get a lot more out of it the second time through. As with all citations in this book, the full reference for Arrow's essay appears in the bibliography at the end of the book.

that they will deal with one another for a long time—the classic "doctor-patient relationship"—their behavior can differ considerably from that in a one-time transaction.

The logic of this idea is quite simple: If a mechanic at a cross-country-route service station tells you that you need new shock absorbers in your car, pointing ominously to some oil dripping from one of your shock absorbers, the chances are a lot higher that the mechanic squirted the oil moments before, rather than that you really need new shocks. However, local mechanics have both less opportunity and less reason to try such stunts. First, they cannot keep selling you new shocks each week! Second, they know that if you catch them once at attempted fraud, your relationship will end, and you will also tell your friends to avoid them. Mid-desert service stations will never see you again, and thus have no such constraints on their behavior.

Consumers can protect themselves against fraud by learning more about the activity at hand. With auto repair, many people can learn to be effective mechanics on their own, and hence less likely to be subject to fraud. With the purchase of stereo equipment, we at least can listen to the quality of the sound. With these and many other activities, we also can return the product to the seller or the device to the repair person if it doesn't function correctly. You can always go back to your mechanic and say, "Do it again until you get it right!" Not only that, mechanics probably have incentives to try, if they value maintaining a lasting relationship with you.

With medical care, as with other areas in which "professionals" dominate the supply of the activity, things seem at least qualitatively different. First, the disparity of knowledge between the doctor and the patient is larger than that between the customer and the auto mechanic. A reasonably intelligent person can learn quite a bit about auto repair in a relatively short period of time. The frequency of do-it-yourself (DIY) books on this topic and the number of auto parts stores attest to the commonality of this practice. The Yellow Pages in Rochester, New York, for example, lists more than 200 auto parts stores. By contrast, only three establishments offer to sell surgical instruments, suggesting that DIY surgery seems unpopular relative to DIY auto repair.

Perhaps more important, it may prove difficult to trade in a "service" when it doesn't work properly. By its very nature, a "service" involves the participation of the patient's body. If a surgical mistake is made, trade-ins may be hard to come by. Obviously, many medical mistakes are self-correcting, and many others can be restored with further medical intervention, but it seems reasonable to state that, on average, mistakes are harder to correct with services than with goods, services having less recourse to trade-ins as an ultimate fallback strategy.

The ability of individual customers to learn about the activity they purchase from others places a constraint on the amount of fraud one might expect. Alas, there are so many things to learn about in this world that we cannot learn enough to protect ourselves on every possible front. Adam Smith pointed this out several hundred years ago, when he noted that "division of labor is limited by the extent of the market." In frontier communities, we would all operate as "Jacks (and Jills) of all trades"; in a larger society, we all specialize. Because we specialize, we must depend upon (and trust) others, leading to the possibility of fraud. Some of this fraud is not worth confronting. There is, in the words of one study, an "optimal amount of fraud" that we should learn to live with (Darby and Karni, 1973).

Fortunately, we are protected somewhat by our friends and neighbors who take the time to learn about auto repair (for example). They can help steer us away from clearly fraudulent mechanics toward those whom they trust. This process of acquiring information about the quality of mechanics (or doctors and dentists) proves important in the functioning of health markets, a topic to which we will return in Chapter 7.

Externalities

Another area importantly separating health care from many other (but not all) economic activities is the common presence of "externalities," both positive and negative. External benefits and costs arise when one person's actions create benefits for or impose costs on others, and when those benefits and costs are not privately accounted for in individuals' decisions. Many early successes in medicine dealt with communicable diseases, probably the purest form of an event with externalities. When people get sick with a communicable disease such as polio or the flu, they not only bear their own illness, they also increase the risk that their relatives, friends, and neighbors will contract the same illness. When they take steps to avoid such diseases, they confer a benefit not only on themselves, but on those around them. For example, the social benefit of getting a flu shot exceeds the private benefit. If people balance the costs of flu shots (including monetary costs, time, inconvenience, pain, and the risk of an adverse reaction) with their private benefits (the reduced risk of contracting the flu for a season), they will underinvest in flu shots from a societal perspective.

Many health care activities have little or no external benefit or cost, but surprisingly many other such activities do. Most of the major health care activities with significant externalities have become such a part of the background of our society that we seldom recognize their presence or consequences. Sewage control, mosquito abatement, quarantine rules for certain diseases, and massive inoculation programs for infectious diseases often pass unnoticed by the average person.

Other apparently private activities also create external costs. For example, every time a patient receives an antibiotic injection, the odds go up slightly that a drug-resistant strain of a bacterium will emerge, immune to the current antibiotic. In relatively closed communities such as nursing homes, this can become a serious problem (Phelps, 1989).

A number of other private actions affect other people's health and safety, but the health care system deals with them only at the end of the process. Most notable are individuals' decisions to drink and drive. Half of the vehicle fatalities in this country involve at least one driver who has consumed alcohol, and the number of "external" deaths caused by drunk drivers staggers the imagination. Every three years, for example, drunk drivers cause the deaths of more people on American roads than all deaths among U.S. soldiers in the entire Vietnam War. Although these issues typically are not considered as "health care economics," the death and injury associated with such events may be more important than most diseases (and their cures) in our society.

As with everything else discussed in this section, the issue of externalities is not confined to the health care sector. Such simple local activities as fire and police protection have at least some element of externality (or "public good") about them, and on a grander scale, national defense and the formation of alliances such as NATO create the same issues. Air and water pollution, obnoxious "boom boxes" at the beach, and cars with noisy mufflers provide other examples of externalities outside of the area of health. Thus, although externalities may be an important part of some medical activities, they are not unique to health care markets.

HOW MARKETS INTERRELATE IN MEDICAL CARE AND HEALTH INSURANCE

To gain a better understanding of health care economics, the next step should provide a framework upon which more detailed information can be assembled. This section provides that framework; it spells out the relationships between health care and health insurance, and establishes the major forces affecting supply and demand in each market. Later chapters focus on each of these subjects in greater detail; our purpose here is to set the stage, and to show more in outline form how these various factors relate to one another.

This analysis of health markets will be "static," assuming initially that the world stands still for a while. In this analysis, we seek to determine the sort of equilibrium toward which the health care markets would naturally move. Later, we consider dynamic issues, particularly those arising from development of new knowledge about medical care and health, and those arising from broad economic events (such as persistent economic growth). After we have this structure in hand, we will go back to the important elements in this world—supply and demand for insurance, supply and demand for medical care, and technical change—and study each in more detail.

Medical Care Markets with Fixed Technology

One fruitful way to analyze medical markets links together the supply and demand for health insurance with the supply and demand for medical care. In each separate market (as in any market), supply and demand interact to create the *observed quantity demanded* and the *observed price,* the product of which is actual spending in the market. Except for this direct interaction, the analysis of competitive markets assumes that supply and demand in a market are independent of one another. Put differently, consumers shouldn't care about the cost of the inputs for a good, just its output price. Similarly, producers (at least in a competitive market) don't need to know the incomes of consumers in order to decide how to price their products. In noncompetitive markets, different ways of analyzing behaviors of sellers and buyers are needed, as we shall see in later chapters.

Health care differs considerably from most other markets in the following way: The price consumers pay to buy the product is different from the price sellers receive. This happens because of health insurance, which *lowers the price* of medical care to the consumer at the time of purchase. Of course, the premium charged by the insurance company must eventually result in recovery of all of the costs of that insurance, including medical care purchased through the plan, but the net result of insurance still leads to a lower *relevant* price for decision making by the consumer. Chapter 4 discusses these ideas in detail, but for now, we need only to create a link between insurance and medical markets: We cannot talk meaningfully about medical markets or health insurance markets separately.

Figure 1.1 shows how these (and related) markets interact. Each box in the diagram characterizes either a supply or demand side of one of the relevant markets. Dotted "circles" show the phenomena we observe as these markets interact, such as prices and quantities consumed.

With this basic structure in mind, we now turn to a description of each component in these markets.

Figure 1.1 shows immediately why health care markets differ fundamentally from other areas of the economy. We cannot simply talk about "the supply and demand for medical care" (as we might with the study of other markets), but instead we must talk about two closely inter-related markets—those for medical care and for health insurance.

Health insurance (uniquely among insurance markets) directly affects the demand for medical care through the way it pays for health care. In other insurance markets, the insurance covers an asset that has a definable market

FIGURE I.I The interaction of medical, health insurance, and other markets.

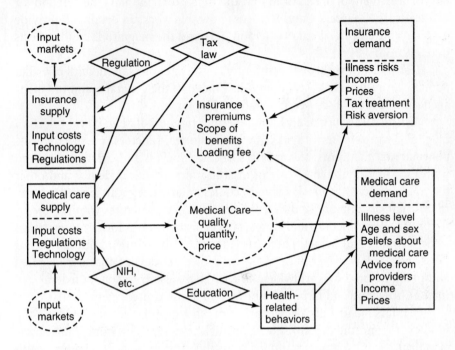

value (such as a home or an automobile), and if some harm or loss comes to that asset (fire, theft, collision, flooding, earthquake, etc.), then an appraiser can estimate the value of the loss and compensate the owner with a direct payment of cash, which the owner can use for any purpose whatsoever (repairing or replacing the damaged asset or any other use of the money).

With health insurance, no such objective valuation can occur because the "asset" is an ephemeral stock of health (more about this in the next chapter) for which no market exists and for which no objective valuation is possible. Because of that, health insurance instead insures the purchase of medical care, which (hopefully!) will recoup losses to one's health.[4] But this mechanism of

---

[4]The earliest health insurance in the New World—created by Carribean pirates—did indeed compensate people for health losses, all of which were precisely definable:

    loss of right arm = 600 pieces of eight
    loss of left arm = 500 pieces of eight (note the bias against left-handed people)
    loss of right leg = 500 pieces of eight
    loss of left leg = 400 pieces of eight
    loss of eye or finger = 100 pieces of eight
    loss of both legs or arms = 800 pieces of eight and a slave.

Source: Cordingly 1997.

protecting against financial risk (paying for health care) distorts the prices we pay for treatment of illness or injury, and hence directly alters the demand for medical care. Chapters 4 and 5 discuss how this works in detail and provide considerable empirical data to help understand the magnitude of the effects in operation.

Health insurance also directly enters into the choices of medical care that patients and their health care providers make in the general realm of "managed care," a topic discussed in detail in Chapter 11.

Medical care is not really a single service or good. Rather, it is a collection of goods and services provided by professionals (doctors, nurses, dentists, pharmacists, therapists of various sorts, technicians of various sorts, and more) through a dizzying array of organizations (medical, dental, and other therapists' practice groups; hospitals; clinics; pharmacies; nursing homes; and more) that operate under different organizational structures (not for profit, for profit, governmental) and almost always under various forms of regulation (federal, state, and local). These providers (and their organizations) use or prescribe various prescription drugs and medical devices that are invented and manufactured in worldwide markets. These also come under federal regulation (the Food and Drug Administration in the United States).

Chapters 6 and 7 discuss the primary type of professional provider ("the physician") and the organizations in which they typically work ("the physician firm"), and Chapters 8 and 9 discuss the most important separate health care organization ("the hospital") and some specific aspects of governance and decision making of these organizations in their most typical organizational structure (the not-for-profit firm).

Chapter 10 then discusses the market for insurance, focusing on the traditional economic model of why people purchase insurance ("risk-averse consumers"), and develops some important complications to this traditional model that arise because of the unique way that health insurance "covers" the risk of illness (by paying for medical care). Chapter 11 then discusses the evolution of the market for health insurance to consider "managed-care" mechanisms that help counteract some of the perverse incentives created by the basic structure of health insurance.

Subsequent chapters explore other aspects of health care markets that (visually) sit around the periphery of Figure 1.1, beginning with Chapter 12, discussing governmental provision of health insurance for various populations such as elderly people (Medicare), indigent individuals (Medicaid), children (Supplemental Children's Health Insurance Programs, or SCHIP), veterans, and others. We then turn to medical malpractice law (Chapter 13) and the issues involved in "externalities (Chapter 14). Chapter 15 emphasizes heavily the mechanisms by which new technologies enter U.S. health care markets, including regulatory structures and pricing as well as coverage decisions of public and private health insurers.

As we shall see later in Chapter 1, the health care economy has grown at prodigious rates over the last half-century in the United States (and around the world), and while we can "explain" much of the growth in medical spending through such traditional economic mechanisms as inflation (changes in the cost of living), population growth, and the systematic aging of the population, there remains an important component of the time trends in health care spending—approximately a 2.5-fold increase over the past half century—that most analysts attribute to technological change—the introduction of new ways of treating illness and injury. The role of technological change, and the best ways to control it, are in many ways the most interesting and complicated aspects of the study of health economics and the implementation of health care policy at a societal level.

Finally, Chapter 16 summarizes all earlier material in the textbook in a discussion of ways to think about "universal" health insurance in the United States. Most industrialized nations in the world have at least some form of universal health insurance for their citizens. The United States does not (at least as of the time this edition was sent to press), but the discussion of ways to think about those issues helps bring together every aspect of the economics of health care that have come in the first 15 chapters of the book. I hope you enjoy the excursion!

Dynamic Issues—Changes Through Time

In any economic system, changes in one part of the system trigger corresponding changes elsewhere, often with feedback to the original variables. Thus, although economic analysis often focuses on "long-run" equilibria, we might characterize the system we actually see and measure as a series of transitional short-run equilibria, always interacting and changing. Nevertheless, a series of important and persistent patterns appears in health care markets that bear discussion. These include (1) changes in the overall economy; (2) demographic changes, particularly the aging of our society; and (3) changes in medical knowledge, brought about mostly by biomedical research.

Economywide Income Growth Like almost all commodities and services, health care seems to be a "normal good," so that people's desires to use the good increase as their income increases. Studies of the effects of income on demand for care offer sometimes puzzling contradictions (see Chapters 5 and 16), but we should at least have in mind the overall change in per capita income in order to study the growth in health care spending.

Beginning after World War II (when modern health insurance began to flourish seriously), per capita income has increased with a steady if somewhat erratic pace. Overall price levels have also risen during this period

TABLE I.I PER CAPITA PERSONAL INCOME IN DOLLARS (IN 2000)

Year	Per Capita Income	Annual Growth Rate (Percent)
1950	$8,404	—
1960	9,735	1.5
1970	13,563	3.4
1980	16,940	2.2
1990	21,109	2.2
2000	25,472	1.9
2010^a	29,500	1.5

^{a}Figures are projections.
Source: Regional Economic Information System, Bureau of Economic Analysis.

(considerably!), so any meaningful comparison of per capita spending should adjust for inflation, to give "constant buying power." Table 1.1 shows the growth in per capita income over the years from 1950 to 2010 (the last year shown is a projection). With some obvious ups and downs in the growth rate, the U.S. economy has grown steadily since World War II, at an average annual rate of about 2 percent in real purchasing power. Although that might not sound like much, when compounded over 50 years, it makes real per capita buying power more than three times as large as it was a half century ago.

Demographics At the same time that our society has grown richer, it has grown older. After the famous postwar baby boom in the 1950s and 1960s, the population has settled in with a mere 6.7 percent under the age of 5. At the same time, the proportion of our population aged 65 or over has grown slowly but steadily from 8.1 percent in 1950 to 11.3 percent in 1980, reaching 13.2 percent in 2010. The important implication from this aging society stems directly from the underlying biological phenomenon of aging: As we get older, our health stock deteriorates faster, and we use more medical care. Table 1.2 shows these age-distribution patterns through time.

R&D and Technical Change

Still another important phenomenon in the dynamic health economy is technical change. As science and medicine progress, we learn how to do things we could not do previously. The most prominent examples in people's minds include spectacular surgical interventions involving artificial hearts, organ transplants, and the like, but the phenomenon of technical change pervades

TABLE 1.2 AGE DISTRIBUTION OF THE U.S. POPULATION

Year	Percentage over 65 Years Old	Percentage under 5 Years Old
1950	8.1	10.8
1960	9.2	11.3
1970	9.8	8.4
1980	11.3	7.2
1990	12.6	7.4
2000	12.4	6.8
2010[a]	13.2	6.7

[a]Figures are projections.
Source: Bureau of the 2007 Census, Population Projections Program.

every part of the health care system. Complex cancer therapies involving surgery, drugs, and radiation have increased tremendously. Genetic manipulation opens new realms of diagnosis and treatment. Complicated diagnostic devices such as the CT and MRI scanners depend on massive computing power, unobtainable even in the 1960s, and now nearly portable in size. Casts for broken arms can now be made lighter and waterproof. Even the humble Band-Aid differs significantly from its 1950s ancestor.

Much of this technical change has been fueled by biomedical research, supported by both public and private funds. The medical interventions deriving from this research have found ready financial support in a market with considerable (and growing) health insurance coverage.

Much of the private biomedical research has been funded by pharmaceutical companies, many in the United States, but many others elsewhere around the world. Almost all new drugs created (and tested) anywhere in the world find applications in most nations, so to refer to "U.S." private research, especially in pharmaceuticals, would provide a narrow and misleading picture. In addition, accurate and systematic data on research and development (R&D) spending in health care itself is almost impossible to obtain. Indeed, much of the research with health care implications, ranging from biology and chemistry to lasers and computers, begins in other sectors of the economy.

In government-funded biomedical research, however, the U.S. role in worldwide research is prominent and provides a reasonable portrayal of overall research activity. Table 1.3 shows the pattern of U.S. health research funded by various arms of the Department of Health and Human Services (formerly the Department of Health, Education and Welfare), primarily through the National Institutes of Health (NIH). The growth in research funding, particularly

TABLE 1.3 FEDERAL INVESTMENTS IN NEW KNOWLEDGE: THE NIH BUDGET THROUGH THE YEARS

Year	Total ($ Million)	Total (Year 2000 $ Million)	Annual Percentage Real Growth
1950	59	360	—
1960	81	431	1.8
1970	1,444	5,630	29.3 [!]
1980	3,573	6,823	1.9
1990	7,581	9,299	3.1
2000	17,800	17,800	6.7
2010^a	30,000	24,000	3.0

^{a}Figures are projections.
Source: www.nih.gov/about/budget.htm.

between 1955 and 1965, was spectacular by any standards, with a subsequent flattening out of real spending through time in the 1980s.[5]

Price and Spending Patterns These and other forces in the economy have led to a persistent growth in "real" medical spending in every year, at least since World War II. Indeed, this pattern of apparently ever-increasing spending growth has formed the basis of considerable private and public concern, provided the impetus for massive government regulation in health care, and created a large industry of "cost-conscious" health care plans in the United States over the past decade, all in an attempt to stem the flow of dollars before the "patient" bleeds to death financially. Our next goal here is to examine the temporal patterns of medical care prices and spending, and health insurance coverage and cost. These data form the background tapestry for the more detailed study of the health markets that follows.

Let's begin by examining the overall trends in health care spending. As before, all of these data occur in a world in which general inflation has taken place, and we really want to study a world "as if" no *general* inflation had occurred.

The Growth in Medical Prices Medical care prices are difficult to measure meaningfully, because the nature of the service changes. To understand this

---

[5]The NIH budget underwent a rapid doubling between 1998 and 2003, and then essentially flattened in nominal terms (creating reductions in spending power as inflation eroded the fixed budget). The $30 billion NIH budget forecast for 2010 in Table 1.3 includes a small projected increase for 2010 that may well not transpire. The budget proposal for fiscal year (FY) 2009 (the last available at this writing) asks for the same as the 2008 budget, $29.5 billion.

requires some understanding of how the Bureau of Labor Statistics (BLS) constructs the Consumer Price Index (CPI) and its component measures. For the overall CPI, they select a "basket" of goods that represents a typical pattern of purchases for urban consumers, including food, clothing, housing, transportation, medical care, entertainment, and other goods and services. Within each of these categories a specific set of commodities and services is chosen.

In medical care, the "medical CPI" has two main areas—medical care services (MCS) and medical care commodities (MCC). The former consists primarily of professional services (doctors, dentists, therapists, hospitals, nursing homes, and health insurance premiums), and the latter primarily prescription and nonprescription drugs and nonprescription medical equipment such as heating pads, wheelchairs, and condoms. In short, the BLS samples a large number of providers of the specific item in question (such as a physician office visit), carefully describes the item, and asks the provider how much it expects to receive (from patients and insurance) for one transaction. The BLS description of this process for a professional service (others are similar) follows. For professional services (such as a doctor visit), the BLS uses a standardized list (specific to each specialty) of procedures that the doctor might provide using standard medical references (the Current Procedural Terminology codes also used almost universally by insurance plans), and asks how much the provider expects to receive in total from the patient and insurance plans.

For hospital care, the "unit" is "the hospital visit"—either an inpatient stay or a single outpatient visit. The BLS actually obtains copies of individual hospital bills (sanitized of individual patient information) to generate the appropriate numbers, specifically the amount the hospital was paid for the visit from the patient and any relevant insurance coverage.

For prescription drugs, individual retail pharmacies (or Internet providers) are asked to provide the "last 20 drugs dispensed," and the BLS obtains prices of those 20 items (so long as the drugs are on a standard list it uses). Thus, the drug retailers' own prescription patterns (averaged over many retail outlets) provide a good random sample of the prescriptions actually filled in pharmacies across the country.

The CPI measures changes in this bundle of good and services, but even with the components in the bundle held constant, the CPI can misstate the "inflation" in some sense. The fly in the CPI ointment is technical change. As the quality of a good or service changes, its price will likely change as well, but if its "name" does not change, the CPI ignores the change in quality. This is important because generally people take increases in prices to be a "bad" outcome, diminishing people's buying power and hence their sense of well-being (utility). But if the price increased because of quality improvements, the price increase can actually signal an improvement in consumer well-being. Box 1.1 discusses this issue in more detail, and you will probably want to come back and reread this box after you have completed Chapter 4 (The Demand for Medical Care).

Several common examples will illuminate this problem. First, consider the most important element in the medical CPI, the "hospital room and board" charge, the basic fee charged for a semiprivate hospital room. Compared (say) with these in 1960, the services that come with that basic room have changed considerably through time: Standby emergency equipment pervades the hospital; the skill level of the nursing staff has increased; the bed's position is now controlled electronically by the patient, rather than manually by a nurse; the menu offers a variety and quality of food far surpassing the traditional fare in hospitals; the building is almost certainly air conditioned; and so on. All of these improvements appear as added costs in the CPI measure, but the added benefits tend to disappear behind the label of "semiprivate room and board fee."

BOX 1.1 QUALITY, PRICE, AND CONSUMER WELL-BEING

Does a price increase automatically signal that consumers are worse off? Many observers of the health care scene bemoan the increases in price (usually they look at "spending," not "price," but that's another matter) and decry the increases as a bad outcome for consumers. Can we use economic thinking to help illuminate this issue? Yes! (Did you expect an economics text to say no?)

First, let us look at the situation in which a price increase comes just because of an increase in the costs of production, with no change in quality. This is the situation presumed to take place when people make adjustments in the CPI because they make no adjustments for changes in quality. We'll use the idea of consumer surplus here, so if that concept is a bit rusty, *review the*

FIGURE A

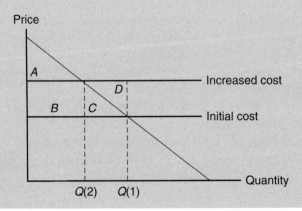

material in the Appendix to the book talking about consumer surplus. (Chapter 4 will review these concepts, too.)

In Figure A, consumers use $Q(1)$ at the initial cost, and the "extra" value they receive is the sum of areas A, B, and C. This is the "consumer surplus" associated with consuming $Q(1)$ at a price equal to the initial cost. If the costs go up (for any reason not associated with an increase in quality), then consumption falls to $Q(2)$, causing the loss of area C, and the higher price eats up area B in terms of consumer surplus, leaving only area A.

Two kinds of price index measurements exist, one called a Paasche index and the other a Laspeyres index. One (the Laspeyres) calculates the index at the original quantities consumed, and hence calculates a loss of areas $B + C + D$ (by failing to account for the reduced quantity in response to the higher price). The other (the Paasche) uses consumption at the new quantity, and thus calculates the loss as the area B (failing to account for the lost consumer surplus C). These two measures bracket the "true" loss, which is $B + C$. The standard CPI calculator is a Laspeyres index (except that the "shopping basket" used is updated periodically).

Now consider the case in which the cost goes up because the quality *goes up.* Because the quality is higher, the demand curve (willingness to pay) also goes up, and the consequences for consumer well-being depend on the relative shifts of price and quality. Figure B illustrates this situation, showing a case in which consumers are made better off by the increase in quality. [It is

FIGURE B

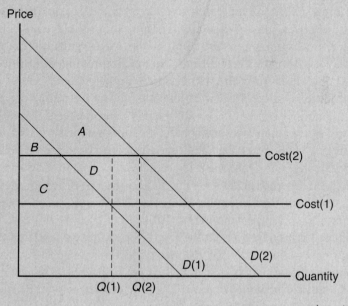

(continued)

BOX I.I QUALITY, PRICE, AND CONSUMER WELL-BEING (continued)

worth noting that if the quality increase is entirely market determined, then presumably consumers desired the higher quality and were willing to pay for it, so the suppliers responded. There could be other cases, for example, in which government regulation mandated the higher quality (and cost that comes with it), but consumers do not value the increase much. Then consumer well-being could fall, as in Figure A.]

In this situation, when price goes up, so does the quantity demanded [from Q(1) to Q(2)] because the demand curve's shift (due to the higher quality) is sufficiently great. With the initial quality, the consumer surplus is B + C. After the quality increase, the consumer surplus is A + B. (If these don't make any sense to you, it's time to review the section in the Appendix to the book that covers consumer surplus.) As drawn (and clearly these lines could be drawn to achieve a different outcome), consumer surplus increases with the increase in quality. Without recognizing the increase in quality, Monsieur Laspeyres would calculate the loss in consumer surplus as the rectangle consisting of C + D. Herr Paasche would have an even greater problem, because quantity increased as the price increased, and the Paasche index would presume that an increased price led to a decrease in quantity! The point is that without taking account of quality, one can make a serious mistake in assuming that price increases automatically lead to reductions in consumer surplus.

The same issues pervade almost every element in the CPI bundle of goods and services. Today's dental visit offers more highly trained dentists and staff; X-ray examinations are conducted at lower radiation levels, reducing side effects to patients; lighting is better, improving the ability of the hygienist to work carefully and with less pain to the patient.

In physicians' offices, nearly immediate laboratory results are available for many blood or urine tests, to complement the higher skill levels of the doctor and nurses there. Other diagnostic equipment abounds. In orthopedists' offices, a wide array of rehabilitation therapy equipment supplants the old hydrotherapy unit. Only one thing remains the same in the doctor's office between the 1970s and the 2000s—the magazines. The offices of most physicians in the country still contain *Time* and *Reader's Digest*. Some of these magazines may still show dates in the 1970s.

Figure 1.2 shows the overall time trends for the general CPI and the medical component of the CPI since 1960 with projections for 2010. You can see the general upward trend in prices during this past half century, but the two lines have different trajectories. The overall CPI has increased at a compound annual rate of 4.2 percent during this era (peaking at about 15 percent during the late 1970s). The medical care CPI has increased during the same period at a

FIGURE 1.2

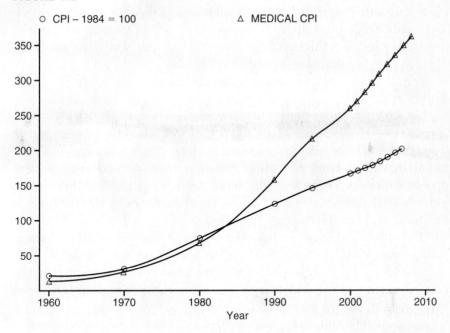

compound annual rate of 6.0 percent—a difference of 1.8 percent per year.[6] While that may not sound like much in any given year, it means that the relative price of medical care has increased by more than a factor of 2 in half a century.

Other potential problems pervade the medical CPI. The technical changes previously discussed mask an additional difficulty—one really wants to know the cost of treating an illness, not the cost of a particular activity (Scitovsky, 1967). Technological improvements, for example, shorten the length of stay for many hospitalizations, yet the CPI component shows only the rising per day cost, not the reduced length of stay. Shifting treatments out of the hospital, or treating diseases with drugs instead of surgery, provide additional ways in which technical change can lead the medical CPI to over-state the actual rates of increase.

---

[6]Except for a few years when price controls specifically affected health care (e.g., 1972–1973) and again in 1979–1980 (when the general CPI increased at 10–12 percent per year during the final years of the Carter administration), the annual changes in the medical care CPI compo-nent have hovered between 1 and 3 percent per year more than the general CPI, averaging (as noted before) about 2 percent per year. The general picture here is one in which medical care prices slowly but steadily increase at a faster rate than the overall CPI, but, more importantly, for a period of about half a century, with no changes in these trends in sight.

More recent studies of the cost of treating various illnesses demonstrate the same notion that Scitovsky found in 1967 about arm fractures: Technical change often appears to lower the costs of treating a particular disease or condition through time.[7] For example, the quality-adjusted cost of treating heart attacks appeared to fall by about 1 percent per year over the period 1983–1994, according to an index called "the Cost of Living" (Cutler et al., 1998).

Similarly, one finds that the costs of treating depression—a major cause of disability and income loss in the United States—have fallen greatly through time (Frank, Berndt, and Busch, 1999). Their work highlights the importance of studying the cost of the entire treatment: Some of the new drugs are more expensive than the older ones they replaced, but they require much less physician monitoring, hence, the overall costs of treatment fall as the (more expensive) new drugs come into use.

The global index of medical care prices masks important differences between component parts that make up "the health care sector." Table 1.4 shows the price index (1982–1984 = 100) for some important components (hospital care, physician services, dental services, and prescription drugs) in addition to the overall CPI and the medical CPI.

Between 1960 and 2010 (projected), overall prices increased by almost a factor of 8 and the medical CPI had increased by a factor of 17 (more than twice as much as the overall CPI). However, hospital prices in this period

TABLE 1.4 PRICE LEVELS THROUGH TIME (BASE 1982–1984 = 100)

Year	CPI	Medical Care	Hospital Room and Board	Physicians' Fees	Dentists' Fees	Prescription Drugs
1960	29.6	22.3	9.3	21.9	27.0	54.0
1965	31.5	25.2	12.3	25.1	30.3	47.8
1970	38.8	34.0	23.6	34.5	39.2	47.4
1975	53.8	47.5	38.3	48.1	53.2	51.2
1980	82.4	74.9	68.0	76.5	78.9	72.5
1985	107.6	113.5	115.4	113.3	114.2	120.1
1990	130.7	162.8	175.4	160.8	155.8	181.7
1995	153.5	223.8	253.0	208.2	205.3	238.1
2000	172.2	260.8	317.3	244.7	258.5	285.4
2005	196.8	323.2	439.9	287.5	324.0	349.0
2010[a]	225.0	400.0	600.0	340.0	400.0	425.0

[a]Figures are projections.
Source: Bureau of Labor Statistics, *Consumer Price Index*.

---

[7]For an excellent conference on this topic, see Triplett (1999).

increased by a whopping factor of 65.0, physician services by 15.5, dental services by about 15.0, and prescription drugs by about a factor of "only" 8.0—about at the general rate of inflation.

All of these "component part" indexes mask important changes in what is really being provided. For hospital care, the technology available within the hospital has dramatically improved within this half century, but perhaps equally as important (as we shall explore more in later chapters), the mix of patients within the hospital changed at least as much. With the advent of new drugs and outpatient (same-day) surgery, those patients who actually enter a hospital as "inpatients" are on average far sicker and require far more intensive treatment in 2010 than those in 1960.

The mix of patients within a physician's or dentist's office has probably not changed that dramatically (except for the general aging of the population), but the available technology has changed, as has the overall degree of specialization of providers.

Prescription drugs have also changed. (These drugs don't include those used with the hospital setting such as cancer therapy, but only those purchased by consumers and used outside the hospital setting.) A bottle of aspirin contains the same medication as it did in 1960 (a nonprescription item, of course), but many patients will have switched to alternative pain medications (ibuprofen, acetometaphin, naproxin, known by common brand names such as Advil, Tylenol, and Aleve) or prescription pain medications such as Celebrex (a new class of drugs). Thus, merely continuing to price "aspirin" would be misleading. The BLS sampling patterns ("the last 20 drugs prescribed from each pharmacy contacted") provide a natural way to rebalance such shifts in consumer demand. They will not, however, account for the appearance of new drugs that simply do things that were previously unavailable to consumers (including a wide array of drugs commonly advertised on television for such diseases as high cholesterol, erectile dysfunction, and peptic ulcers).

Medical Spending Patterns Medical spending is the product (literally) of quantities purchased and the average price per unit. The patterns of spending show better than any other measure the flow of real resources in our economy. Because dollars spent represent price × quantity, it is tempting to divide spending by price to get a measure of "quantity" consumed. In part, this exercise is meaningful, but in part, it is misleading. The difficulty arises, as discussed before, because of technical change. The price of hospital room and board has reflected some amount of technical change, but the "quantity" of care also changes in nature. In "hospital admissions," the scope of procedures has changed greatly through time. Some types of care no longer involve hospitalization (such as cataract removal), whereas other types of procedures occur now that simply did not exist in 1960, including organ transplants, attachment of artificial joints, and so on. Thus, even "quantity" of care has fuzzy meanings and boundaries when looking through time.

Despite these discrepancies, spending patterns can provide a useful backdrop for the study of health economics. Table 1.5 shows the personal consumption expenditures in the United States for the half century from 1960–2010.[8] In these "nominal" data, total spending increased by a factor of more than 100, with modest differences across categories, the most notable exception being for nursing homes, which increased by a factor of 200. This large increase is due almost entirely to the aging of the U.S. population, an issue discussed in more detail in relation to Table 1.8.[9]

Table 1.6 provides the same data, except that they are all adjusted to the 2005 general price level using the CPI. The most important difference between these two tables is the observation that the relative expenditure over the half century fell from 104 (in Table 1.5, for total spending) to 14 (in Table 1.6,

TABLE I.5 ANNUAL NOMINAL EXPENDITURES FOR MEDICAL SERVICES (BILLIONS OF DOLLARS)

Year	Total	Hospital	Physician	Drug	Other	Nursing Home
1960	23.3	9.2	5.4	2.7	5.3	0.8
1970	62.9	27.6	14.0	5.5	11.8	4.0
1980	215.0	101.0	47.1	12.0	36.2	19.0
1990	608.0	252.0	157.5	40.3	106.0	52.6
1995	864.0	341.0	220.5	60.9	168.0	74.1
2000	1,140.0	417.0	288.6	121.0	218.0	95.3
2005	1,661.0	612.0	421.2	201.0	306.0	122.0
2010[a]	2,435.0	900.0	615.0	330.0	430.0	160.0
Relative amount (2010/1960)	104.0	97.0	113.0	122.0	81.0	200.0

[a]Figures are projections.

---

[8]In all data that follow, the 2010 data are extrapolations from 2005 data (the last systematically available at the time of this writing). Typically, extrapolations use the annual growth rates for the previous five years, and are shown in generally "rounded" numbers to assist in remembering that these are extrapolations and not actual measurements of economic activity.

[9]As an exercise for the reader, it is instructive to calculate the shares of the total accounted for by each type of medical care, and observe how they change through time. For example, hospital care was 44 percent of the total in 1970, and fell to 37 percent in 2005, with prescription drugs and nursing homes accounting for much of the increase. The time path of prescription drug shares is particularly interesting, a topic for a later discussion on introduction of new technologies.

TABLE 1.6   ANNUAL EXPENSES IN CONSTANT 2005 DOLLARS (BILLIONS OF DOLLARS)

Year	Total	Hospital	Physician	Drug	Other	Nursing Home
1960	153	61	36	18	35	5.3
1970	316	139	70	28	59	20
1980	510	239	112	28	86	45
1990	908	376	235	60	158	79
1995	1,107	437	283	78	215	95
2000	1,293	473	327	137	247	108
2005	1,661	612	421	201	306	122
2010[a]	2,147	794	542	291	379	141
Relative amount (2010/1960)	14	13.1	13.1	16.4	9.7	26.8

[a]Figures are projections.

again for total spending). In other words, most of the increase in Table 1.5 is simply due to general inflation (changes in the CPI). Table 1.6 shows "real" spending in 2005 prices.

Table 1.7 makes a similar adjustment to account for population changes, putting all spending as if the population had been the same every year as it was in 2005. This accounts for almost half of the remaining increase: the ratio of 2010 to 1960 spending (again, focusing on the total amount) is now "only" 8.2. But an eightfold in "real, per capita" spending is still considerable.

Table 1.8 makes a further adjustment that rests on shakier footing: It adjusts for the change in relative prices between medical care and the overall CPI, acting as if the same relative prices existed in every year as in 2005. This use of the medical care component of the CPI brings the "grand ratio" comparison down to 2.8. As the previous discussion highlighted, this adjustment

TABLE 1.7   ANNUAL EXPENSE IN CONSTANT 2005 DOLLARS AND 2005 POPULATION ($ BILLIONS)

Year	Total	Hospital	Physician	Drug	Other	Nursing Home
1960	255	101	59.2	30	58	9
1970	461	202	103	40	87	29.3
1980	668	313	146	37	112	59
1990	1082	448	281	72	188	94
1995	1220	481	311	86	237	105
2000	1362	498	345	144	261	114
2005	1661	612	421	201	306	122
2010[a]	2091	773	528	283	369	137
Relative amount (2010/1960)	8.2	7.7	8.9	9.6	6.4	15.7

[a]Figures are projections.

TABLE 1.8 ANNUAL EXPENSES IN CONSTANT 2005 POPULATION AND CONTANT RELATIVE PRICES ($ BILLIONS)

Year	Total	Hospital	Physician	Drug	Other	Nursing Home
1960	672	265	156	78	153	23
1970	961	422	214	84	180	61
1980	1260	591	276	70	212	111
1990	1483	614	384	98	257	128
1995	1435	566	366	101	278	123
2000	1514	554	383	160	290	127
2005	1661	612	421	201	306	122
2010[a]	1884	696	476	255	333	124
Ratio 2010 to 1960	2.8	2.6	3.1	3.3	2.2	5.4

[a]Figures are projections.

is fraught with difficulty because of the change in the quality of component services and goods, and because even the "mix" of medical care has changed greatly through this intervening 50 years. So, take these adjusted data with a grain of salt. Taken at face value, however, this shows that "real, per capita" medical spending, even after adjusting for relative price changes, has still increased by almost a factor of 3 in the preceding half century.

Desirably, we would also adjust medical spending data by the age distribution of the population, merging data on the age distribution of the population over the past half century (or more) with average medical care use of each age group. To see how this might work, let's begin with ambulatory care visits (doctors' offices, outpatient clinics of hospitals, and emergency departments). Table 1.9 shows the pattern of use by age in 2005.

TABLE 1.9 SELECTED MEDICAL CARE USE BY AGE, PER PERSON, 2005

Age	Ambulatory Visits	Hospital Days	Ambulatory Prescriptions	Total Personal Spending ($2005)
Under 18	2.53	0.20	3.30	$2,650
18–44	2.24	0.33	4.70	3,370
45–54	3.44	0.47	8.40	5,210
55–64	4.58	0.71	12.40	7,787
65–74	6.47	1.40	18.40	10,778
75+	7.68	2.59	23.60	–
75–84				16,389
85+				25,691

Sources: CDC, *Health 2008,* Table 92 (ambulatory), Table 99 (hospital days), and Table 128 (prescription use). Total personal medical spending from personal communication, Sean Keehan, Center for Medicare Services, Office of the Actuary, National Health Statistics Group.

TABLE 1.10 AGE DISTRIBUTION OF THE U.S.
POPULATION—1960 AND 2005

Age	2005	1960
Under 18	26.2	37.5
18–44	36.9	32.4
45–54	10.0	11.7
55–64	10.2	8.9
65–74	6.3	6.3
75+	6.1	3.2

Source: CDC, Health 2007, Table 1.

Now couple these data with the age distribution of the U.S. population over the years, as shown in Table 1.10.

Between 1960 and 2005, the proportion of the population over 65 (the high-user group) increased from 9.2 percent to 12.4 percent (a 35 percent relative increase). Combining the data on the age distribution of the population in Table 1.10 and the age-specific spending patterns in Table 1.9, we can see that had the elderly population remained a constant proportion of the total population from 1960 to 2005, the annual ambulatory visits would average only 3.14 per person versus the actual average of 3.33 per person. Had the population not aged since 1960, ambulatory care use would be about 6 percent less.

We can make a similar calculation regarding the effect of aging on hospital utilization. As Table 1.9 shows, the elderly use much more hospital care than the non-elderly (1.4 days per persons between 65 and 74 years old, 2.59 days per person for those over age 75). The under-65 population uses about 20 percent of that amount. The actual overall hospital days per person in the U.S. in 2005 was 559 per 1,000 persons. Using the age-specific rates shown in Table 1.9 and the 1960 population distribution, we can calculate that the average would have been 468 days per 1,000 persons, or 84 percent of the actual 2005 rate of hospital use, had the population not aged at all. Thus hospital use would be 16 percent lower that it actually was in 2005 under that no-aging scenario.

Similarly, current estimates for drugs prescribed in ambulatory visits (based on a sample of doctors' offices and outpatient departments of hospitals) show that the average number of prescriptions per year rises steeply with age (Table 1.9), from 3.3 per child to 23.6 per person over age 75. Again, if we adjust the data as if the population had the same age mix as in 1960, the average would be only 6.79 per person per year. So, similar to hospital days, outpatient drug prescriptions would be about 12 percent lower in 2005 had the population not aged since 1960.

It would, of course, be desirable to be able to do the same sort of adjustments for other types of health care use, but the data do not exist to allow such time-trend comparisons within these other categories.

Data do exist, however, to make similar calculations for total medical spending by age group. The last column of Table 1.9 shows these patterns for total personal health care spending. If we calculate the weighted average using the 2005 population proportions and again using the 1960 proportions, we find that total medical spending has increased by one-eighth due to population aging.[10] Put differently, because health care is now about 16 percent of GDP, this means that about 2 percent of the GDP share is due to population aging—the GDP share would be about 14 percent with a constant age mix in the population, not 16 percent. And because the GDP share has grown from about 6 percent to 16 percent since Medicare was created in 1965 (a 10-point increase), more than one-fifth of that increase (2 percent of 10 percent) can be attributed to population aging.

If we apply this "aging population" adjustment to the bottom row of Table 1.8, we can account for still more of the overall increase in health care spending. The "ratios" in that bottom row would all be adjusted downward by one-eighth, so (for example) the 2.8 multiplier for total spending becomes about 2.5 with similar adjustments for all other columns in Table 1.8.

A final note here shows that as we look into the future, this issue becomes far more important: The "baby boom" of children born after World War II (late 1940s) are just now entering the over 65 population segment. Figure 1.3 shows population levels from 1950 to current times and projections through 2050. Census from 1900 through 2050. The proportion over 65 sits now at about 12.7 percent, but will rapidly accelerate (the "baby boom"), leveling off at about 21 percent by 2050. The proportion of in the 85+ age group—a population with very high average annual medical care costs—will increase from current levels of about 2 percent to about 5 percent by 2050. The effects of population aging portrayed here will greatly increase in the coming quarter of a century.

Even after all of these adjustments—CPI, relative prices, population size, and population mix (aging)—there remains about a 2.5-fold increase in medical spending over the past half century. What accounts for this? Most observers (present author included) would say "new technologies." Diagnosis and treatments for illnesses and injuries have changed dramatically over the past half century. In some sense, the cost of treating many illnesses and injuries has plummeted because they were previously not treatable (equivalent

[10]The average is $5,322 using the 2005 population mix, and $4,676 using the 1960 population mix. Since $4,676 is 88 percent of the 2005 spending of $5,322, we can see that the increase due to aging is about 12 percent, or about one-eighth of the total. Data through personal communication with Sean Keehan, Center for Medicare Services, 2008.

FIGURE 1.3 Actual and Projected Population Levels

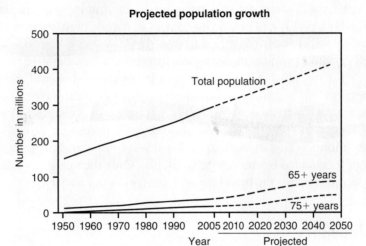

Sources: Centers for Disease Control and Prevention, National Center for Health Statistics, *Health, United States*, 2006, Figure 1. Data from the U.S. Census Bureau.

to having a prohibitively high price). Not only has the actual cost of treating some illnesses and injuries fallen (as the previous discussion about heart attacks and depression signaled), but also many new diagnostic techniques are now available that greatly add to health outcomes while adding new expenses.

The scope of these "new" technologies covers virtually every area of health care. Perhaps among the most dramatic in terms of effects on survival and lifestyle include treatments of heart disease, depression and schizophrenia, trauma care, and orthopedic repair (both through "minimally invasive" arthroscopic surgery and because of joint replacements for knees, hips, shoulders, and ankles). Angioplasty procedures (including stents to keep an artery open) and new medications—many quite expensive—reduce or eliminate the need for cardiac bypass surgery, lowering the cost and the adverse consequences of more invasive treatments.

Diagnosis has progressed perhaps even more rapidly in this era. Fifty years ago, the only diagnostic imaging technique available was plain X-ray films (first invented by Roentgen, who received a Nobel Prize in 1901 for his discovery of "X-rays" and their uses). Now we have sophisticated combinations of X-ray and computing in CT scanners, and nonradiation images using MRI that produce detailed "slices" and 3D reconstructions of the human body regularly. Ultrasound imaging can quickly and safely show both structure and things such as blood flow in human tissue. New Positron Emission Tomography (PET) scans can show metabolic function clearly, thus providing (for example) a precise way to determine whether a cancer has spread from its original organ.

A new wave of diagnostic and therapeutic technology is just emerging through the vastly increased understanding of the human genome, spurred greatly by both public and private investment to decode human genes. Genetic information will not only enhance diagnosis but will also alter treatment choices in many diseases. In addition, both gene therapy and "regenerative medicine" (the use of stem cells to form successful replacements of damaged tissue) will alter the treatment of uncountable numbers of diseases in the future.

These new treatments will add cost to our health care system. They will also add great health benefits. We should avoid becoming obsessed with "growth" numbers in data such as Tables 1.5–1.8 show, and focus as well on the benefits provided by the new technologies. Only then can we make intelligent decisions about the broad use of resources in our society.

AFTERTHOUGHT

In closing, we should emphasize that there is no "right" amount of spending on health care toward which we should aim. Optimally, we can evaluate spending on medical care in the same ways that we do other goods and services—namely, to ask how much our overall well-being increases or decreases as we change our use of resources in health care. The remainder of this book, and indeed much of the effort of health economics in general, provides ways to answer these questions. What forces have led to the spending patterns we now see? What benefits do we get from these activities? If we changed the patterns of resource use, how would our health and happiness change? The tools of economic analysis help us think about and sometimes answer these questions.

SUMMARY

Health care and health insurance markets are interrelated in complicated ways. Health insurance has the unique feature that it effectively alters the price in another market that consumers have to pay to buy the service (health care). No other consumer goods or services have this characteristic, making the study of health care both unique and complex.[11]

---

[11]Some financial markets have something similar—the "option" to buy or sell. For example, a standard "call" option gives the buyer of the option a right to purchase (say) 100 shares of IBM corporation stock at a specified price (say, $155) for a specific duration of time (say, until October 31). These options exist for many common stocks, and for certain commodities such as crude oil, hog bellies, gold bullion, and even foreign currencies. Health insurance differs considerably even from these options. Most "commercial" options are written for a price near the current price of the stock or commodity. By contrast, health insurance shifts prices by 75 to 80 percent or more.

Health markets also have interesting and complicated dynamic features. In addition to normal economic forces such as growth in income, health care markets change in response to the changing demographics of our society—older people use more medical care than younger people—and to changes in technology. The massive infusion of research funding by the federal government has surely created large changes in the capabilities and costs of our health care system. Understanding the patterns of spending through time will require an integration of all these factors.

RELATED CHAPTERS IN *HANDBOOK OF HEALTH ECONOMICS*

"Introduction: The State and Scope of Health Economics" by Anthony J. Culyer and Joseph P. Newhouse

Chapter 2, "An Overview of the Normative Economics of the Health Sector" by Jeremiah Hurley

Chapter 7, "The Human Capital Model" by Michael Grossman

PROBLEMS

1. Give at least four separate areas of medical care in which uncertainty creates an important, if not overriding, consideration in the economic analysis of related issues.
2. "Medical care is so special that normal economic forces don't apply." Comment.
3. Identify at least four things that will likely affect an individual's demand for *medical care*. Which will likely have the best ability to predict spending for a single individual? Which of groups of people (assuming that you do not know anything about individual health events)?
4. Identify at least four things that will likely affect an individual's demand for *health insurance*. Discuss how and why this list differs from the answer to question 3.
5. Which sectors of the medical care system (hospital, physician, drug, dental) have had the largest increases in relative prices between 1960 and the present time? (*Hint:* compare the bottom rows of Tables 1.7 and 1.8.)
6. The CPI for hospital care (as one example) measures the cost of a two-person "hospital room and board" charge as an important part of the CPI hospital index. Has the quality of that "hospital room" been constant for the last four or five decades? If not, what changes in quality have occurred? What does that tell us about the relevance and accuracy of the CPI for hospitals?

CHAPTER 2

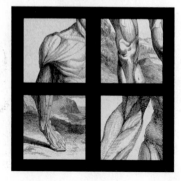

Utility and Health

Economists normally presume that individuals make decisions rationally with the ultimate goal of maximizing their lifetime utility, all subject to the "constraint" that one cannot purchase more than one's resources allow. The model gets very complicated in an intertemporal setting (when one makes lifetime investment decisions, can shift resources to later years by saving, and from later years to "now" by borrowing), and when uncertainty about the "horizon" is introduced (i.e., how long we'll live).

LEARNING GOALS

- Master the model of health as a durable good and asset that produces happiness ("utility").
- Learn how lifestyle choices affect health, including both direct effects on health and indirect effects on earnings.
- Discover how education affects health outcomes both directly and indirectly.

To think about this problem more clearly, it is useful to break the issue into component parts: How does health produce utility, and in turn, what affects health? What follows in this chapter discusses each of these issues in sequence. First we consider "health" as a durable good, even though it is not one we can buy and sell at the local mall or on eBay. Next, we consider things that affect health: your lifestyle choices and your medical care choices. Chapter 2 ends with the lifestyle choice issues, and Chapter 3 picks up by considering how medical care produces health.

HOW TO THINK ABOUT HEALTH AND HEALTH CARE (OR . . . HOW HEALTH ECONOMICS?)

Health as a Durable Good

To begin, think of the most fundamental of all building blocks of consumer demand theory, the "good" that increases a person's utility. Is anybody prepared to believe that having a dentist drill into a molar is a "good" in the traditional sense? Which of us really enjoys getting weekly allergy injections, or for that matter, once-in-a-lifetime yellow fever shots? These services—the actual events delivered and paid for in health care markets—can't meaningfully be thought of as "goods" in the traditional sense. They don't augment utility directly. They hurt. They cause anxiety. Sometimes they have bad side effects. These sound more like "bads" than "goods"!

We are better served by backing up a step, and asking what really does create more "utility" for an individual. The most helpful answer is also the most sensible: Health itself creates happiness. We can begin to think about a reservoir of "health" that people have, and ask how medical care fits into this picture. Michael Grossman has most prominently explored the idea of "health" as an economic good, and showed how a rational economic person would have a demand curve for medical services that "derived" from the underlying demand for health itself.[1]

The ideas flowing from the simple concept of a stock of health permeate modern health economics. Although we explore these ideas more fully in Chapters 3 and 4 on the demand for medical care, the basic idea deserves an early airing. You can think about health as a durable good, much like an automobile, a home, or a child's education. We all come into the world with some inherent "stock" of health, some more than others. A normal healthy baby has a relatively high stock of health. An infant born prematurely, with lung disease, the risk of brain damage, and possible blindness, has a very low initial stock of health. Almost every action we take for the rest of our lives affects this stock of health.

If we think of a bundle of other goods as X, and a stock of health (unobservable) as H, then we can say that a person's utility function is of the form

$$\text{Utility} = U(X, H)$$

---

[1]Highly recommended for the serious student, Michael Grossman's *The Demand for Health* (1972a) first explored the ideas of a stock of health and the derived demand for medical care. This work stems from a broader set of considerations of "household production" of economic goods, arising from the work of Gary Becker (1965) and Kevin Lancaster (1966). Grossman's most recent treatment of the issues appears in Grossman (2000), intended primarily for students at the graduate level.

FIGURE 2.1 (a) Increasing utility as a function of expanding goods. (b) Increasing utility as a function of expanding stock of health.

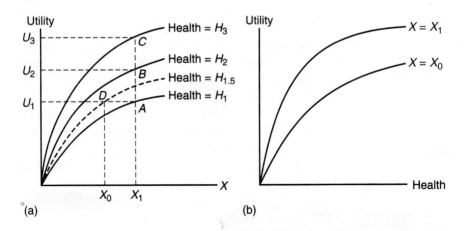

(a)

(b)

Technically, we should think of the flow of services produced by the stock of health that creates utility, just as the transportation services from a car produce utility. However, to keep the wording from becoming too clumsy, we can continue to say that the "stock of health" creates utility rather than the more technically accurate expression that "the flow of services from the stock of health creates a flow of utility."

In the usual fashion for "goods," we would say that "more is better," so that more health creates more utility. It also seems plausible that the pleasure of other goods and services, which we can designate as the ubiquitous X, might increase with health. It is more fun to go to the zoo when you do not have a headache, for example. Thus, as Figures 2.1a and 2.1b show, both X and H produce more utility as the consumption of each expands. Figure 2.1a contains a series of plots showing how utility grows with X, each having a different level of H associated with it (i.e., H is held constant at a specific value on each line in Figure 2.1a). Figure 2.1b shows how H increases utility for given X. We can combine these two figures into one, for example, by picking some specific value such as $X = X_1$, and finding the level of utility associated with various values of H (H_1, H_2, H_3, etc.), at the points labeled A, B, and C in Figure 2.1a.

These same points appear in Figure 2.2, on a map showing combinations of X and H that produce the same level of utility. For example, in Figure 2.2, the combinations of X and H at points A (X_1 and H_1) and D (X_0 and $H_{1.5}$) both create the level of happiness U_1. This being the case, the consumer would be wholly indifferent between having a bundle such as

FIGURE 2.2 The same level of utility produced by different combinations of X and H.

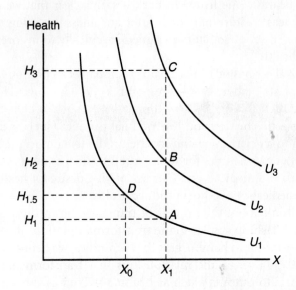

A or a bundle such as D. The point D has more H and less X than point A, but both create the same level of happiness. The same point D appears in Figure 2.1a, showing the same relationship to point A (with more H and less X). The only difference between the two is that Figure 2.2 identifies the consumption points in combinations that each create the same level of utility. We call curves such as the one labeled U_1 *indifference curves.* (Another name for them might be *isoutility curves,* stemming from the Greek *iso-,* meaning "the same.")

Maps such as these provide a particularly powerful way to describe many of the economic forces driving health care (and other) behavior, so we will use them frequently.[2] You see maps such as this commonly in everyday life, so they need not intimidate you.

---

[2]The appendix to this chapter develops some particular characteristics about indifference maps (and other ideas) in more detail, using mathematical concepts from the calculus. Those who wish to learn the concepts in this book at the more precise level allowed by formal mathematical structures can use the appendices. The main text, however, will remain free of such formalization, except in occasional footnotes.

THE PRODUCTION OF HEALTH

Where does health come from? In part, it seems clear that we can produce health, or at least restore part of it after an illness, by using what we call "medical care," a set of activities designed specifically to restore or augment the stock of health.

In the usual economic terms, an auto company can produce automobiles using steel, plastic, labor, tires, wires, and so on as inputs. The process of transforming medical care into health can be thought of as a standard production function. The demand for the final product (such as automobiles) leads in turn to a *derived demand* for the productive inputs (such as steel or auto workers), or sometimes for subassemblies (such as motors). The same is true for health and medical care: Our underlying desire for health itself leads us to desire medical care to help produce health.

We can think about the process of transforming medical care (*m*) into health (*H*) in a fashion similar to the transformation of meat, energy (heat), buns, and mustard into hamburgers. In economics, we define such a process as a *production function*, the relationships that transform inputs (such as medical care) into outputs (such as health). We can call this function anything we wish (Harry, Martha, or *g*), showing the functional relationship between various levels of *m* and *H*, "*g*" is more compact, making it a preferred name to Harry or Martha. Thus,

$$H = g(m)$$

We would normally presume that more *m* produces more *H*, that is, that *the marginal productivity of medical care is positive.* We would also presume, in common with other economic phenomena, that the *incremental effect* of *m* on *H diminishes as more m is used,* and after a while, may even become negative. This would occur if the negative side effects of a drug or treatment occurred so often that they swamped any good provided. (The Greeks provide another word for us here: *iatrogenesis,* combining the words for healer [*iatros*] and origin [*genesis*].)

Health outcomes also depend on the disease a person has, as does the productivity of medical care. For some diseases, modern medicine has highly effective therapies, and for others, not so effective. The initial (untreated) effects of different diseases on health are also obviously different. Thus, we really need to think of health as a function of both disease (*D*) and medical care (*m*), and the two interact. Thus,

$$H = g(m, D)$$

Figure 2.3 shows production functions for three different disease processes. Disease I does not make the individual terribly sick initially (without medical

FIGURE 2.3   Health production functions for three diseases.

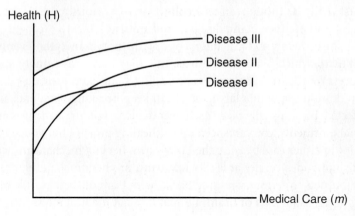

intervention), and medical care offers some help in healing, eventually reaching a near plateau. Allergies or asthma are useful examples. Disease II starts the individual out at worse health, but here doctors have more to offer, and they can return the person to a higher level of health finally, although it may take more medical care. A broken arm provides a useful example. Finally, Disease III does not start the person out very sick, but doctors have limited ability to help, in the sense that the level of health with no medical care is not much different from the level with a lot of care. Thus, the person's health will not vary much with m. A common cold provides a classic example, following the old maxim that it takes a week to get over a cold if you do not see a doctor, but seven days if you do. In cases such as these, the *productivity* of medical care is very small or zero over all ranges of use.

Several ideas deserve careful mention here. First, for almost every possible medical intervention, there reaches some point at which the *incremental productivity* ("marginal productivity") of medical care will fall very low, or possibly even become negative. However, the average productivity can be quite high. The production process for Disease II in Figure 2.3 represents a good case—on average, medical care had done a lot of good, but it is possible to expand the use of m to the point at which its marginal product also falls to zero—that is, the plot of health versus medical care flattens out. We should not confuse *average* and *marginal* effects. In later chapters, we will discuss the effects of changes *on the margin* in medical care in further detail, but it is important to remember that saying something has no marginal productivity does not mean that it is a worthless endeavor.

Second, it should be quite clear that the notation describing "medical care" as a homogeneous activity m is hugely simplistic. There are literally thousands of identifiable medical procedures, and similar numbers of identified diseases and injuries.[3] Thus, "the medical production function" must really be thought of as a collection of various medical interventions, each applying to specific diseases and injuries.

Third, many medical interventions do not change the eventual level of health to which a person returns, but they can considerably speed up the process of a "cure." The process of healing a cut hand provides an example. If you do nothing with a large cut, it can keep breaking open and may even get infected, but it usually heals itself eventually. If you use bandages and antibacterial ointments, you can speed up the healing process, but you get to the same point in either case because the body's own healing mechanisms work so well. This same idea carries at least some truth in phenomena ranging from intestinal upsets to seriously injured backs, with both of these people often returning to the same level of health no matter what medical interventions are used. The same holds for many important diseases for which there are no cures, but for which medical intervention can at best slow the process of decline to death. Prominent diseases in this category include (at this writing) acquired immunodeficiency syndrome (AIDS), Alzheimer's disease, and some forms of cancer.

Finally, we should always remember that medical care does not stand alone in affecting health. The production process contains much more than "medical care," including, most prominently, our own lifestyle. Also, the relationships between medical care and health may appear quite fuzzy, making it difficult to tell just how effective a medical intervention really is. This occurs because some people "get better" in ways unpredicted by doctors, and, sometimes, they get worse or die despite the very best medical treatment, or sometimes because of side effects of that treatment.

HEALTH THROUGH THE LIFECYCLE

Like any durable good, our stock of health wears out over time. We call this process *aging.* As the stock of health falls low enough, we lose our ability to function, and eventually die. Again, in economic terms, our stock of health

---

[3]The catalogs of diseases and procedures became more standardized as insurance became more important in health care. Insurers wanted ways to classify the procedures they pay for, and a number of competing systems emerged to provide that classification. The most commonly used system now is the Current Procedural Terminology system, now in Version 4 (called CPT4) and almost universally used in the health care system (American Medical Association, 1990). Similarly, as hospitals, doctors, and insurers sought common systems to classify illnesses, separate coding systems emerged. Most of these follow from the International Classification of Disease methods. The most recent version in common use is the International Classification of Diseases, Version 9, known more cryptically as ICD-9 (Department of Health and Human Services, 1980).

depreciates. "Normal aging" as measured in our society represents the average rate at which this depreciation takes place, but we should recognize that there is nothing biologically intrinsic about this process. Life expectancy has increased dramatically during this century, for example, implying that the depreciation rate on people's stock of health has slowed down through time. Public-health efforts (such as sanitation, and vaccination against communicable disease) and individual medical care all serve to slow down the rate of depreciation of health, or to restore health to (or near) its original level after all illness or injury. Thus, if we plotted a typical person's health stock through time, it would look something like Figure 2.4, with a steady increase during childhood, and then a gradual decline from "aging," all the while punctuated by random events of illness and injury that can cause precipitous declines in one's health. At some critical H_{min} the person dies. Medical care forms an important part of the process of restoring health after such events, unless H_{min} has been reached. For example, the appendicitis attack shown in Figure 2.4 would have continued in a rapid slide downward to death if the person's appendix ruptured and no medical care was obtained. Similarly, Table 2.1 shows aggregate mortality rates by age interval for U.S. citizens, dramatically portraying the decrease in the stock of health associated with aging.

Table 2.1 reveals something else that we will explore in more detail later—the consequences of "technical change" in health care. Even in the span of 20 years, medical progress has dramatically reduced the death rates in

FIGURE 2.4 Time path of health stock.

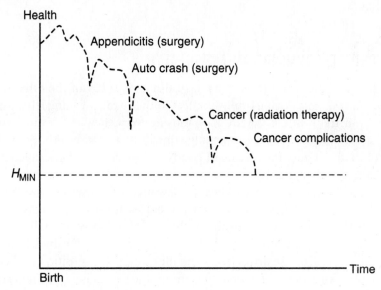

TABLE 2.1 OVERALL DEATH RATES BY AGE

	Aggregate Annual Death Rate per 100,000 Persons in Age Group		
Age (Years)	1985	1998	2005
1–4	52	35	29
5–14	26	20	16
15–24	102	82	81
25–44	167	161	92
45–64	875	680	670
65–74	2,848	2,495	2,137
75–84	6,399	5,703	5,260
Over 85	15,224	15,111	13,800

Source: U.S. Department of Health and Human Services, National Center for Health Statistics, *Death Rates for 72 Selected Causes, by 10-Year Age Groups* (1998, Table 250). Data for 2005 from CDC, *Health 2007*, Table 3.

some age categories, most notably for children, young adults, and the over 65 age groups. Much of this improvement is due to improved medical technology, but not all of it. For example, in the 15–24 age category, more than two-thirds of the improvement comes from reductions in vehicle-related fatalities, most of which arise from changes in drunk-driving laws and attitudes, and some of which comes from improved vehicle and highway safety. Nevertheless, the improvements in mortality rates in such a short period provide quite striking evidence on the consequences of improved medical care technology.

A MODEL OF CONSUMPTION AND HEALTH

In addition to the "random" events of health care, many of the other things we do and consume during our lives affect both the rate of aging (the slope of the smooth trend line in Figure 2.4) and the frequency and severity of the "spikes." Our own lifestyles can greatly contribute to our health. Behind the earlier broad portrait, the bundle of goods and services we have called X can take on many characteristics, some of which augment and others of which dramatically reduce our stock of health. New medical research shows increasingly that the old adage "you are what you eat" is at least partly correct. Perhaps a better notion comes from the Bible: "As ye sow, so shall ye reap." Prominent among such lifestyle choices are the decisions to smoke tobacco, consume alcohol, or use drugs (legal and illegal); the composition of diet; the nature of sexual activities; and the amount of exercise one undertakes.

Therein lies the rub: Many of the things we enjoy (goods in the composite bundle X) cause life itself to trickle away. Not only can X and H substitute for one another in producing utility (see the previous discussion on indifference curves), but also X affects H in a production sense as well. We should probably think about categories of X that have different effects on H. There are "good" types of X (X_G) that augment health. Moderate exercise provides a good example. There are clearly "bad" types of X (X_B) in terms of their effects on health, such as excessive alcohol consumption and high-cholesterol foods. Still other neutral goods, such as books or saxophone jazz concerts, will have no apparent effect on health, aside from possibly increasing or reducing tranquility for the person involved. Thus, we can expand the production function idea even further, to include these types of X, where the signs over each element of the production function indicate the direction of effect that these activities should have on the health stock:

$$ H = g(\overset{-}{X_B}, \overset{+}{X_G}, \overset{+}{m}) $$

We would be on very thin ice indeed to argue that people "shouldn't" consume "bad" items. Presumably, people's goals are to maximize utility as much as possible within their budget constraint, and X_B presumably increases utility. However, we should also understand the role of these choices in affecting health. In many ways, these behavioral choices dominate a person's health far more than the medical care system.

To see the importance of lifestyle events most clearly, we can turn to the most clear-cut of all measures of health, namely, whether people live or die. In particular, age-adjusted death rates, by cause of death, illuminate the role of lifestyle most clearly.

First consider the role of lifestyle in young adults. Table 2.2 provides the age-specific fatality rates for persons ages 15–24 in the United States in 2004. All of the really important single causes of death in this age group relate to "violence" in some way or another. The leading killer is "unintentional injuries" 80 percent of which are vehicle crashes. Homicide and suicide follow close behind. These four categories alone account for almost three-quarters of all deaths in this age bracket.[4] Most of these events lie outside the medical care system. Although doctors and hospitals (most probably emergency departments) can try to patch up the consequences of these events, it is clear that the role of medical care is quite small, relative to that of "life" itself.

---

[4]For young adult black males, the fatality rates from violence just stagger the imagination: In the 15–24 age category, the death rate is 176 per 100,000 (1997 data). The comparable rates for white males are 117, and (respectively) 37.4 for white females and 30.1 for black females. The death rate from homicide *alone* for black males age 15–24 exceeds the *all causes* death rate for comparably aged white males.

TABLE 2.2 FATALITIES BY CAUSE OF DEATH FOR PERSONS AGED 15–24, 2004

Cause of Death	Annual Deaths per 100,000 Persons	
Unintentional Injuries	36.7	
Homicide	12.1	
Suicide	10.3	
Subtotal: "Violent deaths"		59.1
Cancer	4.1	
Heart disease	2.5	
All other nonviolent causes	13.7	
Subtotal: All nonviolent causes		20.3
All causes		79.4
Percentage of all deaths due to violence	74.4%	

Source: U.S. CDC, *Health 2007,* Table 32.

In older adults, a different pattern emerges, but the story remains the same—"As ye sow. . . . " Here, the major causes of death shift to more familiar killers: heart disease, cancer, and stroke, all illnesses commonly associated with lifestyle choices. (Chronic obstructive lung disease is also heavily associated with tobacco consumption.) Table 2.3 shows death rates by cause of death for adults over age 65, and Tables 2.4 and 2.5 show the same data for

TABLE 2.3 CAUSES OF DEATH FOR PERSONS AGED 65 AND OVER, 2004

Cause of Death	Annual Deaths per 100,000 Persons
Heart disease	1,450
Cancer	1,049
Cerebrovascular disease (stroke)	355
Chronic obstructive lung disease	286
Alzheimer's disease	178
Diabetes mellitus	147
Influenza and pneumonia	143
Accidents	95
Kidney disease	95
Septicemia (systemic infection)	70
All other causes	904
All causes	4,772

Source: CDC, *Health 2007,* Table 32.

TABLE 2.4   CAUSES OF DEATH FOR PERSONS AGED 25–44, 2004

Cause of Death	Annual Deaths per 100,000 Persons
Vehicle crash and other accidents	35
Cancers	22
Heart disease	19
Suicide	14
Human immunodeficiency virus (HIV) infection	8
Liver disease and cirrhosis	4
Cerebrovascular events (strokes)	3
Diabetes mellitus	3
Pneumonia and influenza	1
All other causes	41
All causes	150

Source: CDC, Health 2007, Table 32.

TABLE 2.5   CAUSES OF DEATH FOR PERSONS AGED 45–64, 2004

Cause of Death	Annual Deaths per 100,000 Persons
Cancer	201
Heart disease	139
Accidents	36
Cerebrovascular events (strokes)	22
Diabetes mellitus	22
Chronic obstructive lung disease	21
Chronic liver diseases and cirrhosis	19
Suicide	15
Kidney diseases	8
Septicemia	8
All other causes	116
All causes	607

Source: CDC, Health 2007, Table 32.

persons at intermediate ages of 25–44 and 45–64. The leading causes of death in this intermediate group are blendings of those dominating the beginning and ending periods of adult life, as Tables 2.4 and 2.5 show although for the age groups in both tables, heart disease and cancers have become prominent killers.

The role of lifestyle choices in the causes of death for young adults seems clear. Yet, the same holds true for the major causes of death for the elderly: The risk of each of these events is strongly affected by lifestyle choices people make. Epidemiological data show systematically increased risks for most of these causes of death due to lifestyle choices. For heart attacks, to extend this point, consider the relative risks of a person with and without a particular lifestyle choice. Persons who smoke one or more packs of cigarettes daily have 2.5 times the risk of nonsmokers for fatal heart attacks. High blood pressure creates a 2.1-fold risk. Persons with elevated serum cholesterol have 2.4 times the heart attack risk of those with low serum cholesterol, and most doctors now believe that dietary intake can notably affect serum cholesterol. Finally, persons who lead a sedentary life have a 2.1 risk factor for heart attacks, compared with persons who exercise three times a week for at least 20 minutes.

A remarkable study appeared in 1993 that further illuminated the relationships between lifestyle and health outcomes. This study (McGinnis and Foege, 1993) calculated the deaths for various age groups associated with various identifiable sources, summing the effects of the "actual cause" across diseases (see Table 2.6). For example, they attribute to tobacco as the "actual cause" the "excess" deaths estimated to come from tobacco consumption from a wide variety of diseases, including lung cancer, other forms of cancer, heart disease, emphysema, strokes, low birth weight, and burns. They made similar imputations for other "actual causes."

The study was repeated a decade later with similar results (Mokdad et al., 2004). Their major results appear in Table 2.6. Strikingly, even with just a few "actual causes," they could account for half of all deaths occurring in the United States annually. Even more strikingly, almost all of the causes they

TABLE 2.6 ACTUAL CAUSES OF DEATH IN THE UNITED STATES IN 1990 AND 2000

Actual Cause	No. (%) in 1990[a]	No. (%) in 2000
Tobacco	400,000 (19)	435,000 (18.1)
Poor diet and physical inactivity	300,000 (14)	400,000 (16.6)
Alcohol consumption	100,000 (5)	85,000 (3.5)
Microbial agents	90,000 (4)	75,000 (3.1)
Toxic agents	60,000 (3)	55,000 (2.3)
Motor vehicle	25,000 (1)	43,000 (1.8)
Firearms	35,000 (2)	29,000 (1.2)
Sexual behavior	30,000 (1)	20,000 (0.8)
Illicit drug use	20,000 (<1)	17,000 (0.7)
Total	**1,060,000** (50)	**1,159,000** (48.2)

[a]Data are from McGinnis and Foege. The percentages are for all deaths.
Source: Mokdad AH, Marks JS, Stroup DF, Gerberding JL, *Actual Causes of Death in the United States, 2000,* JAMA 2004: 191: 1238–1245.

identified have much more to do with lifestyle choices than anything else. The top three causes—tobacco, diet/activity patterns, and alcohol—account for three-eighths of all deaths in this country, and of the nine major causes listed in Table 2.6, only "microbial agents" (infectious diseases) are arguably independent of lifestyle choices, and even some of these may actually be due to lifestyle because some will represent (for example) people who died of infections that arose because the person had AIDS, even though the death certificate listed the infection, rather than AIDS, as the cause of death. Finally, it is worth noting that of these actual causes of death, only "toxic agents" arise mostly from societal, rather than individual activities. In that case, exposure to chemicals and pollutants forms the major source of risk from toxic substances, and in many cases, these are mostly out of the control of single individuals. To summarize their results, one can accurately say that lifestyle choices dominate the health outcomes of the population of this country.

A More Detailed Look at Consumption and Health

"Whatsoever a man soweth, that shall he also reap."
Galatians 6:7

As outlined briefly in the discussion of the model of utility and health, we can observe a number of choices and activities that not only produce immediate pleasure ("utility") but also have known effects on health (and hence on medical care use). This section explores some of the economic aspects of the most important of these (as taken from Table 2.6): obesity, tobacco use, and alcohol use.

Obesity The most notable change in Table 2.6 between the 1990 and 2000 data is the rapid increase in deaths due to poor diet and physical inactivity. The United States (and other nations around the world) are experiencing an obesity epidemic of large proportions (pardon the expression). In the United States, the percent of adults who are overweight but not obese[5] has remained stable for decades at about 35 percent, but the fraction of adults who are obese has climbed from about 15 percent (40 years ago) to almost 40 percent currently (Figure 2.5). Almost certainly, when the next version of "the actual causes of death" is identified using 2010 data, obesity will have overtaken tobacco as the leading actual cause of death.

---

[5]Overweight is defined as a Body Mass Index (BMI) of 26 or more. Obese is defined as a BMI of 30 or more. For a person 6 feet tall, for example, a weight of 184 pounds creates a BMI of 25, and a weight of 221 pounds creates a BMI of 30. Take a moment to Google the terms "BMI calculator" on the Internet and calculate your own BMI.

FIGURE 2.5 Overweight and obesity trends in the United States, 1960–2004.

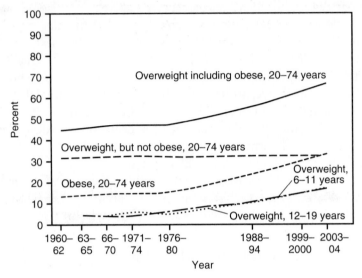

What underlying economic phenomena might cause this obesity epidemic? One "culprit" could well be technological change. First, as technology alters the general nature of the work we all do and increases the marginal productivity of workers, the number of calories expended in everyday work has fallen. Jobs have become more sedentary and less strenuous through time. In parallel, the increased value of time makes it "more expensive" to shed calories through dedicated exercise. At the same time, the cost of acquiring calories has fallen because of technological improvements in the agricultural sector and mass production marketing of food at all levels of production, including prepared meals. Lakdawalla and Philipson (2002) estimate that one-third of the increase in BMI in recent decades (see Figure 2.5) can be attributed to falling food prices and two-thirds due to decreased exertion in normal work activity.

The increased value of time also leads more people to shift to "fast-food" alternatives that are often calorie and fat laden. Americans spent about one-third of their food budget on restaurant meals in the 1970s, and now spend about one-half (Young and Nestle, 2002). This research also documents the increase in portion size for packaged food and restaurant meals. The authors identified 181 food items (packaged and chain restaurant meals) for which they could identify the specific time when larger portions were introduced. The trend began in the 1970s, and accelerated from 18 items (of their 181) in 1980–1984 to 65 items in the 1995–1999 period. Perhaps it is just a temporal coincidence, but these increases closely track the documented increases in obesity in U.S. adults (Figure 2.5).

Finally, Chou, Grossman, and Saffer (2002) analyzed obesity patterns in the United States, and found that the density of restaurants per capita is by far the strongest variable explaining these cross-sectional patterns. They further note that the number of fast-food restaurants per capita doubled in the 1970–1990 period, and the number of full-service restaurants rose by 35 percent in the same period.

Thus, economic thinking predicts the obesity epidemic to some extent. When something becomes cheaper (calories), we usually consume more, and when something becomes more expensive (expending calories), we usually use less of it. And when time becomes more valuable and more constrained (e.g., with more women in the workforce), consumers will naturally turn to prepared and "fast" foods. With that may have come at least part of the obesity epidemic we now observe.

Obesity is also linked to transportation choices (and hence to the relationship between where we live and where we work). If we live far from work, walking or bicycling to work becomes less of an option. Thus, in part, the urbanization of the modern world contributes to obesity through transportation issues. If it takes 20 minutes to walk to work, we'll drive or take mass transit.

Interestingly, even gasoline prices affect obesity in the United States. Courtemanche (2007) shows that higher gasoline prices cause weight loss, primarily because people begin to shift to mass transit from personal driving, which entails more walking to get from home and work to the mass transit stops. He estimates a considerable effect size: A $1 increase in gasoline prices would (by his work) reduce obesity-related fatalities by 16,000 per year and save $17 billion annually in health care costs.[6]

Obesity is strongly linked to mortality. Figures 2.6a and 2.6b show the relationship of overall mortality and BMI for men and women in the United States who participated in a prospective study (Calle et al., 1999). In these figures, the lowest-mortality group is defined as having a relative risk of 1.0 (on average), and everybody else has a relative risk of dying in a single year that is some multiple of that. The people with the lowest mortality had BMI values in the range of 22–25. The vertical white lines indicate relative risks of 2, 3, 4, and so on using a logarithmic in scale. The length of the horizontal bars in these charts show the statistical uncertainty around the average values. Thus, for example, a male with a BMI of 40 has

---

[6]Of course, because we consume about 400 million gallons of gasoline per day in the United States, paying an extra $1 per gallon would cost about another $145 billion annually, less by the amount that consumption fell due to the higher prices. Because gasoline prices did actually rise by more than $1 per gallon in the United States in 2008, an excellent "natural experiment" has taken place for future economists to study.

FIGURE 2.6 Relative risk of all-cause death for people who had never smoked and had no history of disease.

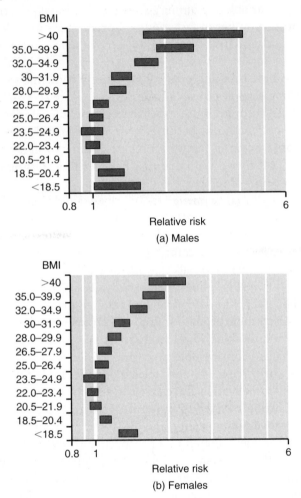

(a) Males

(b) Females

a relative risk of 2.58 (more than 2.5 times the risk of dying than a male in the lowest risk groups), with 95 percent confidence intervals—as shown in the horizontal bar—from 1.64 to 4.06. Heart disease was the most common cause of death from extra weight. For example, men with a BMI of 35+ have a threefold risk of dying from cardiovascular disease as the lowest risk group.

As one might expect, obesity has a strong effect on various forms of morbidity as well as mortality. Obesity has a strong association with numerous nonfatal diseases including diabetes, many types of cancer, heart disease, gall bladder disease, and others. In addition, orthopedic problems also increase with obesity. Coggon et al., (2001) estimated that a quarter of all knee surgeries in the United Kingdom could be eliminated if all of the population maintained ideal weights (BMI under 25). Obesity increases the burden on, and hence damage to hips, knees, ankles, and feet.

Tobacco and Health Tobacco consumption has long been known to degrade people's health. Despite that knowledge, many people continue to smoke cigarettes, cigars, pipes, and (in a new fad) hookahs or to chew tobacco or use snuff. Despite commonly held beliefs, most of these alternatives (including hookahs) are at least as dangerous as cigarettes. What does economics have to say about the use of tobacco?

First and most obviously, economics holds that the goal of life is to maximize utility, not longevity. Thus, obviously, if tobacco consumption increases people's utility, they might rationally and happily smoke or chew, even knowing the potential effects on their longevity. The famed Latin dictum, *"De gustibus non est disputandum"* ("there is no disputing of taste") suggests that one person's "tastes" are not the business of others. In an article bearing this Latin phrase as its title, two Nobel Laureates in economics (Stigler and Becker, 1977) show how a rational person might choose to become addicted to something such as tobacco, and also predict from basic economic principles that those who start down this path will increasingly end their addiction as they grow older.

Second, we can understand how consumers might be poorly informed about the risks of smoking (and other health-harming activities). If one does not understand the risks, consumption may take place in ways that would not exist if the consumer had complete information about the risks.[7]

One possible indicator of the role that information plays in the decision to smoke appears in smoking rates according to educational attainment: Throughout many decades, we can observe an inverse relationship between educational attainment and tobacco use. For example, in 2006, 20.3 percent of all U.S. adults smoked cigarettes. However, for those with less than a high school education, the rate was 28.8 percent; for those with a high school diploma, 26.5 percent; for those with some college attendance, 22.1 percent. Those with at least a bachelor's degree smoked at a rate of 8.2 percent.[8] Less than 3 percent of all U.S. physicians smoke tobacco. The big shift away from smoking occurs with college education.

---

[7]A later chapter assesses a similar problem by looking at the value of information about medical treatments in the section on Medical Practice Variations and demand curves. When you reach that point in the textbook, it would be a good time to circle back to this issue.

[8]Data on smoking rates by education from CDC, *Health 2007,* Table 64. Data on physician smoking from Nelson et al. (1994).

Even among "health workers," one can see an inverse relationship between education and smoking rates. In a survey using data from 1990–1991, Nelson et al., (1994) found that in the United States 3 percent of physicians (8+ years of posthigh school education) smoked, 18 percent of registered nurses (2–4 years of posthigh school education) smoked, and 27 percent of licensed practical nurses (typically one year of posthigh school education) smoked.

Alcohol and Health Alcohol consumption has very complicated effects on health. First, patterns and intensity of drinking have separate effects even if total consumption is held constant. Heavy drinking has worse health effects than light drinking, and binge drinking (very heavy drinking on sporadic occasions) has separate and distinct negative effects on health. Heavy drinking is known to increase the risks of liver cirrhosis, some cancers, and heart disease. Drinking and driving also increases the risk of vehicle crashes and fatalities.

The type of alcohol consumed appears to make a distinct difference as well. One recent study of Danish adults (Gronbaek et al., 2000) shows the all-cause, heart disease, and cancer mortality for people who primarily consume beer, distilled spirits, and wine.

Their data show that heavy drinking of beer and distilled spirits increases mortality from all causes and specifically for death from cancers, but with mixed results for coronary heart disease (CHD). The relative risk of cancer death for heavy drinkers of distilled spirits (more than 21 drinks per week) compared with non-drinkers is almost 2 (double the risk of cancer death).

Wine (as winemakers proudly advertise) appears to have beneficial health effects, reducing all-cause deaths by about 20 percent (even among heavy drinkers) and reducing heart disease by almost half for moderate drinkers of wine. New basic biomedical research not only confirms these effects but also has identified the underlying biological mechanisms.[9]

The relationship between education and alcohol use differs considerably from that observed for tobacco use and education. While increasing education lowers tobacco use, just the opposite seems to take place for alcohol use, as Figure 2.7 shows.

---

[9]It turns out that red wine is much better than white wine for protection against coronary artery disease, and especially red wines heavy in a particular compound known as *procyanadin*. For a good excursion into this literature, see Corder (2007). For those preferring to avoid alcohol consumption, other foods known to have a high content of procyanadin include chocolate (yes, it *is* good for you!), cranberry juice, pomegranates, and various apple species. It may well indeed be true that an apple a day keeps the doctor away!

FIGURE 2.7 Alcohol use in past month, adults 18+ years of age, by educational attainment.

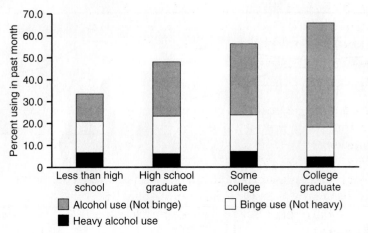

We can discern even more by linking the information from Figure 2.7 regarding alcohol consumption and mortality with information on the beverage of choice across people with different educational attainment. According to work from Klatsky, Armstrong, and Kipp (1990), wine drinkers tend to be more highly educated, distilled spirits drinkers less highly educated. Thus—for whatever reasons—more highly educated individuals opt more often for drinking patterns that are actually health increasing, and lower educated persons opt for more dangerous types of drinking. Thus, although on first appearance the relationships between education and alcohol and tobacco use appear to run in opposite directions, they actually show the same thing—higher education typically leads to lifestyle choices that improve health outcomes.

Alcohol use also has complicated effects on lifetime earnings. Without going into great detail, a review of this (very large) literature shows that moderate drinking may be associated with improvements in earnings (just as we see for the relationship between health and alcohol, especially wine). As with health effects, heavy drinking, particularly chronic alcoholism, lowers lifetime earnings, most notably (according to Mullahy and Sindelar, 1993) through reduced labor force participation, not wage effects. For a comprehensive summary of these and other issues relating to alcohol consumption, see Cook and Moore (1999).

Education and Health

Numerous analyses, many following the seminal work of Grossman (1972a, 1972b), have found positive associations between education and health outcomes. Furthermore, we can find not only links between education and the

FIGURE 2.8 Prevalence of overweight (BMI > 25) and obesity (BMI > 30) among U.S. adults.

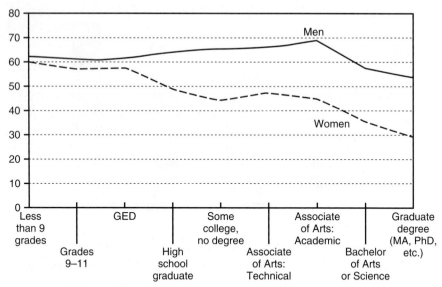

use of tobacco and alcohol that support the general notion that higher education increases health, but also the relationship in other health-affecting
behaviors. Just as we find with respect to tobacco, obesity declines with education, particularly among women (Figure 2.8). Similarly, the propensity to
undertake regular exercise rises with educational level (Stein et al., 1991).

Can we identify education as the *cause* of these health improvements? In
a provocative essay, Fuchs (1982) suggests that the underlying phenomenon
leading to both higher education and healthier lifestyle choices might be
fundamental differences in time preferences for different people. People with
a high "discount rate" (those who opt for immediate pleasure rather than
investing in the future), he argues, will not only opt against investment in
education, but will also engage in fewer health-producing behaviors. We have
no clear way to identify whether the underlying mechanism really is "time
preference" or not, nor do we really have any good understanding of how
time preferences are formed.

The issue becomes further confounded when we introduce the effect of
education on lifetime earnings. Education systematically increases people's
productivity and hence how much they earn over a lifetime. This additional
earning power provides the ability for people to live in healthier and safer
communities, and to buy things that improve health (vitamins, membership
in exercise clubs, and . . . yes . . . medical care). But it also gives people the
ability to purchase things that are less healthy (restaurant meals typically add
more calories to people's diets than home-cooked meals).

The problem becomes even more confusing when we consider the effects of health on earning power. For a given level of education, people who are healthier will be able to work more, will be more productive at work, and will typically get paid more as a result. And these effects accumulate through one's lifetime through "experience" factors. Thus, people with chronic diseases, particularly those with early onset, are likely to suffer a lifetime earnings loss in addition to their physical discomforts.

No matter how complicated we make the discussion, one thing remains evident: More education clearly improves health outcomes, and has many connections with healthier lifestyle choices that support the better health outcomes, including the use of tobacco and preferences for alcohol, proclivity to exercise regularly, and rates of obesity.

SUMMARY

This chapter begins by exploring a particular way of thinking about the relationship between health care and health itself, using the idea of a productive process. This formulation begins with the idea that utility is produced by health (H) and other goods (X). In turn, medical care systematically augments health. The relationships between health and other goods are more complicated than this simple model suggests, however. Some of the things we enjoy directly (part of the bundle of goods called X) enhance our health, and others reduce it. Exercise and proper dietary composition enhance health. Consumption of cigarettes, alcohol, and other drugs, as well as certain types of foods, reduce our health. Other lifestyle choices dominate health outcomes, particularly for younger persons, such as the combination of drinking and driving. The risks for most of the primary causes of death at any age are strongly affected by our own lifestyle choices.

This chapter explores the economics of several of these lifestyle issues in more detail, including economic issues related to smoking, obesity, and alcohol use. Each of these has distinct and important relationships to education. Tobacco use declines systematically with educational attainment. Obesity declines also with educational attainment, more so with women than men. Alcohol consumption is most complex because the type of drinking (heavy versus moderate, binge versus regular) affects health outcomes even for the same volume of drinking and because different beverage types (distilled spirits, beer, and wine) have different effects on health. As with the other health-related lifestyle choices, higher education appears to lead to less consumption of the most damaging types of alcohol (distilled spirits) and to more consumption of alcoholic beverages that actually improve health (wine, particularly some types of red wine). Much further analysis of the links between education and lifestyle choices is needed before we can fully understand these behaviors.

RELATED CHAPTER IN *HANDBOOK OF HEALTH ECONOMICS*

Chapter 3 "Medical Care Prices and Output" by Ernst R. Berndt, David M. Cutler, Richard G. Frank, Zvi Griliches, Joseph P. Newhouse, and Jack E. Triplett

PROBLEMS

1. What are the leading causes of death for young people? How much does the health care system have to do with their prevention?
2. What are the leading causes of death for older people? Which has more to do with their rates of occurrence—life style choices or medical care received throughout a person's lifetime?
3. Life expectancy in the United States has increased from about 55 years (at birth in 1900) to about 76 years (at birth in 2000). Yet, many studies suggest that most of the leading causes of death in modern America are due in important ways to our lifestyle choices. Can you reconcile these two points of view? To think about this, consider that the leading causes of death before World War II were infectious diseases that are now controlled well by antibiotics. You must also consider what time trends have occurred in lifestyle choices over this period. (Do people smoke more or less than before? Etc.)
4. If you were a powerful "Health Czar" in the United States and had the authority to change people's lifestyle, what would be your first priority (and why)? What mechanisms might you use to achieve these lifestyle changes (regulations, education, prohibition, etc.)? Do you think that these changes would improve the overall level of utility (in the economic conceptualization) compared to leaving them alone?
5. Discuss how general educational (rather than health-specific education) can affect health outcomes. In doing so, consider the links between education, income, income-related lifestyle choices, and health outcomes.
6. Taking into account the effects on people's physical activity (and hence health outcomes), do you think that the American population is better-off or worse-off with higher gasoline prices?

APPENDIX TO CHAPTER 2

A Formal Model of Utility Maximization

This appendix develops a formal model of a utility-maximizing individual who gains utility from both health (H) and other goods (X), and develops briefly the ideas of a production function for health.

Begin with a person who has a utility function of the form $U = U(X, H)$. If both X and H are normal goods, then the marginal utility of both X and H is positive. Using the notation of calculus, $U_X = \partial U/\partial X > 0$ and $U_H = \partial U/\partial H > 0$. An indifference curve (isoutility curve) as pictured in Figure 2.2 has slope $-U_X/U_H$. To see this, take the full derivative of the utility function, and then hold the *change in utility* equal to zero while allowing X and H to vary. This will show how X and H can vary while U does not—in others words, the set of combinations of X and H producing the same level of utility. The total change in utility is given by

$$dU = dX\, U_X + dH\, U_H$$

and if we hold $dU = 0$ while still allowing dX and dH to be nonzero, we can assess the trade-offs between the two that still keep total utility the same. Thus, set $dU = 0$ and solve for the ratio dX/dH, which gives the slope of the isoquant in Figure 2.2. Simple algebra gives

$$dX/dH = -U_H/U_X$$

This gives the usual economics notion of trade-off, called the "marginal rate of substitution" between X and H in producing utility.

We can model the production of health in a similar fashion. Begin with the simple production function $H = g(m)$. Then the marginal product of m is the derivative $dH/dm = g'(m)$, the slope of any of the various production functions shown in Figure 2.3.

Because we can convert m into H, we can embed that relationship in the utility function, so that

$$U = U(X, H) \rightarrow U[X, g(m)]$$

Using the chain rule, we can easily find the relationship between medical care and utility:

$$\partial U/\partial m = (\partial U/\partial H)(dH/dm) = U_H g'(m)$$

We will use these ideas more completely in Chapter 3, in which we expand on the transformation of medical care into health, and Chapter 4, in which we develop the demand for medical care more formally.

CHAPTER 3

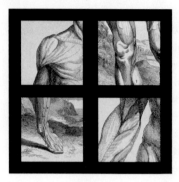

The Transformation of Medical Care to Health

We discussed in Chapter 2 the basic idea of a production function for health. Chapter 2 focused on ways lifestyle affects health. This chapter focuses on the way medical care affects health. First, we want to understand the relationships between the amount of health care used and resultant changes in health. Second, we can explore the predictability of outcomes in this process—the uncertainty associated with the production of health. A similar issue, related in many ways, is the uncertainty in the minds of doctors and other healers about the correct ways to use various health interventions. We will study this issue as well.

THE PRODUCTIVITY OF MEDICAL CARE

Marginal and Average Productivity

For every process ever studied, the productivity of inputs varies with the total amount of inputs used. A simple but revealing example involves the productivity of labor

LEARNING GOALS

- Understand the meaning of marginal productivity, the difference between average and marginal productivity, and the meaning of "extensive" and "intensive" margins.
- Review estimates of the productivity of medical care in producing health at an aggregate ("all medical care") level.
- Become familiar with examples in health care of the marginal productivity of specific medical interventions using cost-effectiveness measures, and understand how these vary along the extensive and intensive margins.
- Learn how cross-regional medical practice variations signal that providers (doctors) don't always agree about when to use various medical interventions.
- Learn about how, even within a single region, variations in practice style (and consequent medical resource use) occur.

in harvesting grapes. As a single worker begins to harvest a field, the worker must do every task alone and productivity (grapes harvested per worker per hour) is low. As a second worker is added, more than twice as many grapes are harvested. The *marginal product* with two workers is greater than that with one,[1] so the amount of product per worker increases.[2] This can occur, for example, because the two workers can specialize in various tasks (one picking, the other carrying grapes from the field) to which they are best suited. As more and more workers are added, the effects of specialization eventually begin to diminish, and finally the workers actually begin to get in each other's way.[3] Eventually, if you were to add enough workers to a vineyard of given size, they would begin to trample the grapes due to their crowding. When this happens, the marginal product of more workers is negative—total product would fall as the number of workers increased. Of course nobody would deliberately do this, unless the workers paid for the opportunity to work in the fields (rather than being paid for their work).

Productivity Changes on the Extensive Margin

Just as the productivity of workers can vary with the number of workers employed to accomplish any given task, the productivity of health care resources can also vary with the total amount used. Indeed, we can expect in general that the marginal productivity of health care resources will increase at low levels of use (such as might be found in a primitive or developing nation), and that the *marginal productivity* of health care resources will fall as more and more of such resources are used. With sufficiently large amounts of medical care used, the harm from iatrogenic illness could outweigh any gains, making the marginal product of health care resources negative.

One way to think about declining marginal productivity is to look at the populations for which a particular medical treatment might be used. For a particular example, consider the case of screening people for breast cancer. This disease primarily (but not exclusively) affects women, and the age profile of the disease

---

[1]The marginal product is technically the (partial) derivative of total output with respect to one input, holding all other inputs constant. For example, if the two inputs are labor (L) and acres of grapevines (A), and the output is pounds of grapes (G), the production function is $G = f(L, A)$ and the marginal product of labor is $\partial G/\partial L$, the rate at which G changes as L changes, holding A constant.

The language here carefully expresses an important point: It says "the marginal product of two workers" rather than the "the marginal product of the second worker." The extra productivity should not be connected with the actual second worker, but rather to the presence of two.

[2]The average product per worker is G/L.

[3]In this process, the marginal product, and, eventually, the average product will begin to fall.

suggests that the risks of breast cancer rise with a woman's age, at least for much of the life span. Epidemiological studies can characterize the risks that an "average" woman of a particular age will acquire breast cancer. Such studies might also sort out particular risk factors, such as dietary pattern, smoking habits, and so forth. Screening for breast cancer will have a *yield* of positive cases (say) per thousand examinations conducted that varies with both the population studied and the test's accuracy. The screening test (mammography, a very low-level radiation X-ray examination) might miss some actual cancer cases (false negative). The test's probability of detecting true cases—p—is called its *sensitivity*. The test might also inaccurately report breast cancer in somebody who does not have the disease, merely because something "looks like it" using mammography (false positive)—q. The yield of the test is composed of both true-positive and false-positive diagnoses. Suppose the fraction of true positives in the population being screened (as learned, for example, from epidemiology studies) is f. Then the yield rate of the test is $f \times p + (1 - f) \times q$. That is, p percent of the true positives and q percent of the true negatives will show positive on the test. Obviously, the higher the underlying probability of disease (f) in the population studied, the higher will be the yield of *true-positive cases* that can lead to cures of the disease.

Now think about the populations (age groups, for example) for whom mammography might be used. Intelligent use of the test will begin with those most susceptible to the disease, who turn out to be women over age 50. We could expand use of the test on the *extensive margin* by adding to (extending) the population base for whom the test was used—for example, to women between 40 and 50, and then to women between 30 and 40, and so on. The number of true cases detected per 1,000 tests would fall as we pushed the extensive margin as would the number of cures achieved.

We could even extend the population receiving this screening examination to the point at which its marginal product was negative. Even though the radiation used in mammography is very low, it creates a very slight risk that the X-rays themselves will induce breast cancer. If the population being screened has an extremely low underlying risk of breast cancer, it is possible that the *induced* (iatrogenic) cancers would actually occur more often than naturally occurring cancers would be found. This would quite likely be the case, for example, if women aged 20–30 received routine breast cancer screening with current mammography technology.[4]

---

[4]The issue of screening for breast cancer remains controversial, in terms not only of the populations who "should" be screened, but also of the best frequency of examinations. The U.S. Preventive Services Task Force currently recommends mammography every one to two years for women aged 40 and older. Chapter 5 provides an appendix that discusses the tools of medical decision theory more completely.

The same concepts apply to medical treatment as well as screening examinations. A common example might be the success of back surgery in eliminating the symptoms of low back pain, a common ailment of modern society. Studies show that 65–80 percent of Americans will have serious low back pain at some point in their lives, and at any time, over one in ten Americans has some low back pain, 10 million of whom have at least partial disability from the malady. Most do not receive surgical intervention (2 percent of American adults have had back surgery), and for those who do, the success rate reported varies considerably from location to location. One reason for this is the *case selection* methods various doctors use, another way of thinking about expanding the extensive margin of medical intervention. Some patients with low back pain are clear surgical candidates to almost any surgeon looking at them because of the mix of symptoms and diagnostic test results.[5] For these patients, surgery has a high likelihood of success. However, some surgeons are more "aggressive" and will operate without such clear signs and symptoms. In the economist's jargon, they are expanding the extensive margin of surgery. The yield of successful cases will surely fall, as the medical literature reports with great unanimity. Eventually, as with mammography, further expansion along the extensive margin (operating on every patient with mild symptoms, for example) would lead to more patients with bad backs as a result of surgical complications than were actually cured.[6]

Productivity Changes on the Intensive Margin

Another way to increase the use of medical care resources is the *intensive margin*. In this case, the population being treated is held constant, and the rate at which tests or procedures are used (the "intensity" of use) is varied. As with the case of variation in the extensive margin, variations in the intensive margin can produce first increasing, then decreasing, and finally negative marginal productivity of the medical resource.

The previous discussion of mammography provides an example of choices along the intensive margin. Should women receiving the test (say,

---

[5]The symptoms for this group include intractable pain that is not relieved by lying down, pain shooting down the leg (sciatica) if the patient's leg is raised up straight while the patient is lying supine, loss of sensation, and, particularly, loss of motor function in the leg or foot, and so on. CT or MRI imaging should also show a clear bulging disk at the point in the spine associated with the particular clinical symptoms.

[6]As is common in the study of the economics of medical care, a good deal of useful information resides in the medical literature, particularly in articles that appear occasionally in the medical journals summarizing the "state of the art" for doctors. In the case of low back pain, for example, useful summaries appear in Frymoyer (1988). These articles often provide good examples of such concepts as extensive and intensive margins in health care.

those aged 50–60) have the test every 10 years, 5 years, 2 years, 1 year, 6 months, monthly, or daily? Common sense tells us that daily is too often—breast cancer does not grow fast enough to show changes on a daily basis. Testing at 10-year intervals is probably too seldom as well—the tumor can begin, grow, and eventually prove fatal to the woman well within that time period. Testing more often than the 1- to 2-year recommended interval (e.g., monthly) would increase radiation exposure, false positives, and cost without commensurate benefits.

Evidence on Aggregate Productivity of Medical Care

How much health do we actually get from our current patterns of medical care use? The answer seems to be both "a lot" and "not very much" at the same time. We get "a lot" of gain on average, and considerable evidence supports this. It may also be true that we are not gaining very much on the margin, so that substantial changes in medical resource use might result in very little change in health outcomes. These ideas are not paradoxical, as the previous discussion on average and marginal productivity should suggest. Indeed, "smart" use of health care almost certainly would result in a level of health services at which the marginal product was declining (rather than rising or at the highest possible level of marginal productivity).

Aggregate Data Comparisons One type of evidence compares the health status of various nations and their use of medical care resources. These studies necessarily rely on the simplest measures of health outcomes, typically life expectancy, mortality rates, or (perhaps) age-specific mortality rates. One common indicator of health outcomes is the death rate for infants, although overall nutrition and broad public health measures (such as a sanitary water supply) have a significant effect on infant mortality rates, possibly more than that of personal medical care interventions.

One can also compare the life expectancy within regions of a single country, such as states, counties, or Standard Metropolitan Statistical Areas (SMSAs) in the United States and measure how variations in regional life expectancy vary with the use of medical care. These studies avoid some of the problems of cross-nation comparisons but introduce others.

Aggregate data studies of the relationships between mortality and health care (either multicountry or within country) invariably show that four things move in parallel: per capita income, per capita education, medical care use, and good health outcomes. All four are related to and affect each other. Higher per capita income directly creates better health through improved living conditions, including sanitary water supply, safer roads, and better nutrition. Higher per capita income also gives more buying power, which directly increases the amount of medical care used, also improving health outcomes. Higher income leads to the use of more education, which in turn leads to higher incomes in the future. Education is indeed a powerful engine for sustained economic growth. Better education also directly increases people's health, by making them more capable managers of their own lives and more adept at using those medical care resources available in the market.[7] Finally, better health also increases people's ability both to learn in school and to work productively, both of which eventually create more income.

The only exception to these findings occurs in some cross-state studies within the United States that find that for white males, the relationship between income and mortality is positive. One hypothesis to explain this is that the higher incomes of this group have led group members to purchase many things (such as fatty food and cigarettes) that reduce their life expectancy. However, in such data, complicated interactions of age, education, and migration patterns can obscure the true relationships, leaving us in a state of some ignorance about the true relationships between income and health. As the discussion in Chapter 2 suggests, it may well be that income has both positive and negative effects on health because (in our earlier notation), X_B (bad) "goods" decrease health, while X_G (good) "goods" (possibly including medical care) increase health. As income rises, one might first start purchasing X_G items, and then at still higher incomes, purchase more X_B items. At sufficiently high incomes, the "bads" might overwhelm the "goods" in their effect on mortality.

Unraveling the pure effects of medical care on health in this kind of setting has proven to be a difficult statistical problem because the data always show income, education, health care, and health outcomes moving relatively together through time (within a single country) or across countries (at a single time). One of the difficulties with such studies arises when trying to estimate how much medical care has actually been used. The most common approach takes reported medical spending (in the local currency) and converts that to some common currency (like dollars) using published exchange rates. However, because different countries have different ways (for example) of paying doctors, and different ways of counting the costs (for example) of hospital construction, *medical spending* may give only a fuzzy picture of the amount of *medical care* rendered.

Other studies make the same comparison (say) within a single country through time. These studies avoid the problems of finding the correct currency exchange rate, but they present a separate problem of converting

---

[7]Michael Grossman's studies of the demand for health emphasize the role of education in the process of producing health. See Grossman (1972a, 1972b).

spending in different times to the same "units" of measurement. Typically, the conversion of spending (say) from the 1950s to current years uses the medical component of the Consumer Price Index, just as the various versions of Tables 1.7 and 1.8 did in Chapter 1. These spending rates are then compared with longevity, age-specific mortality rates, or other measures of health outcomes through time. The general outcome of such studies is similar to the cross-national studies described previously. Income, education, health care spending, and health outcomes all seem to move together through time, and separating the effects of each has proven a difficult task.

In a recent analysis of U.S. time-series data, Hall and Jones (2007) used data from 1950 to 2000 (much as appear in Chapter 1 for medical spending) and combined these data with life expectancy at birth (which climbed steadily from about 66 years to 76 years over the same era), and estimated the production function for "health" as measured by life expectancy. Then, in a more complex analysis, they broke down life expectancy by age group, with 20 brackets ranging from 0–5 up to 96–100 years old. Hall and Jones have (over the years) life expectancies for each of these age groups ("conditional life expectancies"), which they then tie together with age-specific patterns of medical spending (much as in Table 1.9).[8]

One outcome from this analysis is an estimate of the "health elasticity of medical spending" by age group. This is a measure of the marginal productivity of medical care in producing increases in life expectancy—an important (but the only) benefit of increased medical care use. These results appear in Figure 3.1. In the figure, an elasticity of 0.3 (for example) says that a 10 percent increase in medical care spending will result in a 3 percent increase in health (in this case, increased life expectancy). The little "whiskers" show standard errors, which are (in every case) small relative to the actual estimates.[9]

These results provide one of the most powerful measures of the incremental productivity of health care in the U.S. economy to date. The age pattern is very interesting: The most productive ages for applying medical care are for young children. Then medical care becomes relatively unproductive (in extending life expectancy) for teenagers, and rises again with age until about age 50. The decline in the elasticity of health with respect to medical spending at teenage years should come as no surprise to anybody who looks at the main causes of death in these age groups (see Table 2.2); this age group

---

[8]The age-specific spending data appear only irregularly; Hall and Jones have them for 1963, 1970, 1977, 1987, 1996, and 2000. The authors used these data to distribute total national spending by age group, and interpolate between intervening years where no age-specific measures exist.

[9]For a more formal discussion of what this elasticity means, see the appendix to this chapter.

FIGURE 3.1   Elasticity of health with respect to medical spending, by age.

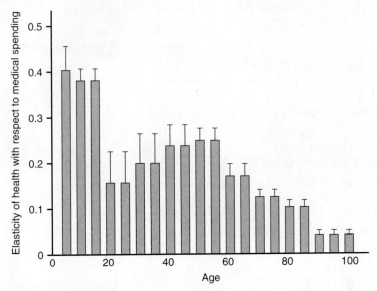

Source: Hall and Jones, 2007.
Note: "Whiskers" show standard errors of the estimates for each age group.

mostly dies from "violent" activities such as auto crashes and other accidents, homicide, and suicide. Medical care has little to do with many of these deaths.

After middle age (about 50), the health-spending elasticity falls steadily with age. Age not only reduces our stocks of health but also makes it more difficult for medical care to improve health, especially after age 80.

Finally, Hall and Jones (2007) estimated the marginal cost of saving a life and the marginal cost per life year saved for various age groups and time intervals. Table 3.1 shows that the marginal cost per life saved has increased at about 5 to 7 percent per year over this half century. The age patterns show essentially the same thing as Figure 3.1 does (as we should expect because a small elasticity of health with respect to medical spending is essentially the same thing as a high cost per year of life saved). For example, in 2000, the marginal cost per life year saved was very low for young children, leaped up for teenagers (because of the high rate of "violence" associated with observed deaths), and then falls until about middle age. After that, it rises steeply, becoming more than $.25 million per life year saved for persons over age 90.

These numbers reflect an average over all of the health care interventions provided to the population. As a later section in this chapter shows, we can find great variability in the cost per life year across not only different medical

TABLE 3.1 THE MARGINAL COST OF SAVING A LIFE AND ADDING ONE YEAR OF LIFE
(Thousands of Year 2000 Dollars)

Age	1950	1980	2000	Per Year of Life Saved 2000	Annual Growth Rates (percent per year) 1950–2000
0–4	10	160	590	8	7.8
10–14	270	2,320	9,830	150	7.2
20–24	1,170	3,840	8,520	153	4.0
30–34	500	2,120	4,910	107	4.6
40–44	160	740	1,890	52	4.9
50–54	70	330	1,050	38	5.4
60–64	50	280	880	47	5.9
70–74	40	280	790	66	6.2
80–84	40	340	750	123	6.1
90–94	50	420	820	373	5.6

Source: Hall and Jones, 2007.

interventions but also for the same intervention across different portions of the population (shifts along the extensive margin).

Randomized Controlled Trial Data

The cross-national and through-time data discussed in the section entitled "Aggregate Data Comparisons" all have the difficulty that many things "move together" in the data set, making it difficult to determine just what is responsible for the improved health that we see through time (within countries) and with higher income (across countries). An entirely different approach allows a completely different measure of the health-producing effects of medical care, using the results from a social science experiment using the standard techniques of the randomized controlled trial.

The study, begun in the early 1970s, was conducted by the RAND Corporation with funding from the federal government (Newhouse, 1974). The RAND Health Insurance Study (RAND HIS) had two major goals: to learn (1) the relationship between insurance coverage and health care use and (2) the resultant effects (if any) on actual health outcomes. The study was conducted in four cities and two rural sites, and encompassed more than 20,000 person-years of data. Some of the people were enrolled for three years and others for five years.[10] The enrollees were randomly assigned to several insurance plans, one of which provided full coverage for all health care used, and others of which required some copayment by the enrollees. As we will see in Chapter 5, the group with full-coverage insurance used substantially more health care than any of the enrollees who had insurance requiring some copayment. Thus, although the study did not experimentally vary the amount of health care received by enrollees,[11] it did experimentally vary the *price* of medical care. The resultant choices by individuals created the differences in medical use that were observed, and those in turn created the opportunity to study the effects of that added health spending on health outcomes.

The RAND HIS had three different types of measurement of health outcome for the enrollees. First, there was a series of questionnaires gathering data on the ability of individuals to participate in activities of daily living (ADL), their self-perceived health status, their mental well-being, and other self-reported (subjective) health measures. These data were collected at the beginning and at the end of the experiment from all adult enrollees and from parents for all children. There were also regularly collected data on sick-loss days (from work, from school, or from ability to work in the home). Finally, participants received a modified physical examination at the end of the experiment designed to measure conditions that the health care system *should* be able to affect, such as weight, blood pressure, vision, serum cholesterol level, hearing acuity, and the like. Some of the enrollees received the same measurements at the beginning of the experiment, allowing not only a comparison across plans (at the end of the study), but also a measure of how people's health had *changed* during the experiment.[12] Finally, all of the measurements were collected together statistically into a measure of "health-status age," a physiological measure that reports the apparent age of people's bodies.

The measure of health-status age has a common-sense feature: It should "age" by a year for each year the enrollees participated in the study, on average.[13] The HIS had a large enough sample size so that it should have been able to detect differences as small as 1 "year" of health-status age—that is, the difference in health levels associated with a year of normal aging, if such differences occurred in the different insurance plans.

---

[10]The different lengths of time in the study helped researchers determine whether the behavior at the beginning and the end of the experiment differed from that in the middle, a possibility given the design of the experiment. Chapter 5 provides a further discussion of this part of the HIS.

[11]To conduct such an experiment would probably be impossible in the United States because of ethical and legal restrictions on medical experiments.

[12]The physical examination at enrollment was given only to part of the enrollees to detect whether the information from the examination itself changed their use of the health care system.

[13]It did, on average, almost exactly.

For purposes of the health-status measurement, we need know at this point only that the low-coverage group used about two-thirds of the medical care used by the group with full coverage. Given that difference, we can ask, "What health differences occurred between these groups?"

The answer, although mixed, is generally "not much, if any." For adults, virtually every measure of health status was the same for the full-coverage group and the partial-coverage group except two: The low-income full-coverage group had better corrected vision than their counterparts in the partial-coverage group, and they had a very slightly reduced blood pressure (Brook et al., 1983). The corrected vision improvement was about 0.2 Snellen lines, equivalent to improving corrected vision from 20/22 to 20/20. On average, the blood pressure for the low-income fully insured enrollees was 3 mm of mercury lower than their partially insured counterparts. (Blood pressure is measured by the height of a column of mercury the pressure will support, usually reported at the peak and the trough of pressure as the heart goes through one cycle. A borderline high level of blood pressure will have a reading such as 145/90 for the two readings. Thus a 3-mm decline in blood pressure is about a 2 percent improvement.)

This improvement in blood pressure is more important than it might seem. For persons with relatively high health risks (e.g., from obesity, smoking, high blood pressure), the risk of dying was reduced by about 10 percent in the full-coverage group, but almost all of this improvement was due to the reduced blood pressure in that group. The RAND researchers conclude that targeted investment in health care activities known to produce lower blood pressure will produce a greater health yield than broad provision of free care. This conclusion underscores the importance of understanding the relationships between specific types of medical care use and specific gains in health.

The RAND HIS study has its own potential problems if we seek the definitive answer about the *marginal* effect of the medical care on health outcomes. The most obvious potential problems are (1) the short time horizon and (2) the potential lack of power to detect true effects (because the sample included only about 5,800 persons). We are unlikely ever to know fully the importance of the time-horizon problem; to do so would require a similar experiment to be conducted for (say) 10 or 20 years, and this seems very unlikely. The failure to detect differences in health habits (such as smoking, weight, and cholesterol levels) over the 3- to 5-year horizon of the experiment seems convincing evidence that full-coverage insurance (and the concomitant higher use of medical care) will not alter these important life-style choices, and altering them could have made large differences in the health outcomes of the enrolled populations. In terms of the statistical power, the study was able to calculate the chances that a true effect of the medical care wasn't detected; the estimates were precise enough that the study authors concluded they could "rule out the possibility of anything beyond a minimal effect" on various health measures.

An Important Caveat

Many of the outcomes assessed in the medical economics literature, particularly those looking at population-based data, rely on death rates (mortality) or life expectancy data (closely related) as the measure of health outcomes. When the major illness events in people's lives had risks of mortality (e.g., before dramatic improvement in the control of infectious diseases), this may have been appropriate, but it is clear now that relying on such measures alone can badly distort the value of medical resource use. Except for the small effect on suicide rates, for example, improvements in treatment of mental illnesses through new drug therapies (for illnesses ranging from depression to panic attacks, and even including some of the otherwise uncurable forms of schizophrenia) would never appear in mortality data. Similarly, knee and hip replacement surgeries allow elderly individuals to remain active in their homes for many years more than previously possible when these orthopedic problems limited the individuals' activities to within the home or even in a wheel chair or in bed. Medications that eliminate pain and nausea can provide important improvements in health outcomes, again not measured at all by mortality data.

Evidence on Productivity of Specific Treatments

A vast array of studies carried out by doctors and other health professionals shows that numerous specific interventions provide important health benefits. The strongest type of study is the randomized controlled trial, or more commonly, the RCT (see Box 3.1). The best of these studies provide important

BOX 3.1   RANDOMIZED CONTROLLED TRIALS

In a pure randomized controlled trial (RCT), patients agree to sign up for the "experiment" without knowing whether they will get the "new treatment" (here, dubbed *T*) or the customary therapy for the disease, known as the "control" (here, dubbed *C*). Patients are randomly assigned to receive either *T* or *C*, commonly (if possible) without either the patient or the treating doctors knowing which patient receives which. When both the patient and the doctor cannot "see" the treatment, this is known as a "double-blind" study. This is easiest with drugs, but harder with other treatments. In the "pure" design, research colleagues provide the drug or the control to the treating doctor in identical form. If the drug has no obvious manifestations such as creating a rash, then nobody except the statistical analyst on the project has any idea which patients received *T* and which received *C*. Sometimes it's impossible to keep the "secret" from the doctor, in which case one has a "single-blind" study, and sometimes even the patients know. (It's awfully difficult to run a

(continued)

BOX 3.1 RANDOMIZED CONTROLLED TRIALS (continued)

randomized trial on whether back surgery "works," for example, without having both the patient and the doctor know whether the patient had received an operation. On rare occasions in the past, patients have been deluded with a "sham operation" when they are put to sleep, an incision is made in the appropriate place in their bodies, and they are sewn up. These types of experiments are seldom conducted in this country.)

In a pure randomized trial, it's quite easy to measure how well the drug, device, or procedure "works": One looks at the outcomes for the treated group and compares them with those in the control group. The difference is the "treatment effect" and is the standard measure of treatment efficacy. For example, if 70 percent of the T group recover from their disease, but only 50 percent of the control group (i.e., those receiving existing therapy), we would commonly accept the idea that the treatment "works" if the sample size were sufficiently large. Studies such as these, incidentally, form the basis for some medical decision analysis "decision trees" as described in the appendix to Chapter 5 because they provide one type of estimate of the outcomes for people who do and do not receive treatment for a disease.

The beauty of the RCT is its simplicity: Because patients are randomly assigned to T or C, we have a strong presumption that "other factors" possibly affecting their recovery are also randomly distributed across the T and C groups. Thus, there is no need to measure other "covariates" or to worry about oddities of individual patients. If the sample is sufficiently large, the test is robust, and we can assert with strong confidence that "T is better than C" (or vice versa).

We should recognize that an RCT never "proves" that a drug or procedure works, in the sense that one can never "prove" anything with a statistical estimate. Take the previous example of 70 percent recovery versus 50 percent recovery. If the sample in the RCT included only 10 patients each in the T and C groups, then one could observe 7 "healed" patients in the T group by some chance, even if it worked no better than C. To see this for yourself, flip a coin 1,000 times and divide it into strings of 10 "outcomes." On average, about one out of every six of such groups will have seven or more heads. This means that an RCT with sample sizes of 10 patients each in T and C stands one chance in three of "finding" that T is better than C, even though they really have the same effect. (To see this, string out another set of 1,000 coins, divided into groups of 10, and call the first group T and the second group C. Now count the number of groups of 10 coins each in which T has more heads than C. This will happen about one-third of the time.) Elaborate statistical designs help to decide how large the samples should be in RCTs, but the problem persists with 100, 1,000, and even 1,000,000 patients in each "arm" of the trial. There's always a chance, albeit a very small one once the sample size grows to several hundred per arm, that the true effect is zero when the sample shows a benefit. This is why RCTs can never "prove" that a treatment works. More precise language would say that the RCT increases our confidence that it works, or we can even say that it works "with 99 percent confidence" (or whatever the appropriate statistical confidence turns out to be).

and highly reliable evidence on whether an intervention actually improves
health outcomes of patients, and (in more recent studies) at what additional
cost. Some of these studies provide important insights into the consequences
of extending treatments on either the intensive or extensive margins. Table 3.2
shows the incremental cost-effectiveness (CE) ratios (in year 2008 dollars) for a
series of interventions (i.e., the added cost for using the intervention divided by
the added life-years achieved in the target population). In each of the studies
shown, a strong RCT supports the estimate of incremental health benefits
(the marginal product), and in all cases, the studies allow comparison across
different target populations (moving along the extensive margin) or the rate

TABLE 3.2   ESTIMATED COST-EFFECTIVENESS OF COMMONLY USED MEDICAL INTERVENTIONS
(All Interventions Compared to "Usual Care" Unless Otherwise Noted)

Intervention	Cost/Life-Year (2008 Dollars)
Low-Dose Lovastatin for High Cholesterol	
Male heart attack survivors, aged 55–64, cholesterol level ≥250	3,237
Male heart attack survivors, aged 55–64, cholesterol level <250	3,440
Female nonsmokers, aged 35–44	3,035,160
Female hypertensive nonsmokers, aged 35–44	1,436,631
Exercise Electrocardiogram as Screening Test	
40-year-old males	186,561
40-year-old females	502,826
Hypertension Screening	
40-year-old males	41,279
40-year-old females	63,333
Breast Cancer Screening	
Annual breast examination, females aged 55–65	22,865
Annual breast examination and mammography, females aged 55–65	61,512
Physician Advice about Smoking Cessation	
1% quit rate, males aged 45–50	5,666
Pap Smear, Starting at the Age of 20, Continuing to 74	
Every 3 years, compared to not screening	36,017
Every 2 years, compared to every 3 years	711,671
Coronary Artery Bypass Graft	
Left main coronary artery disease	13,152
Single-vessel disease with moderate angina	132,131
Neonatal Intensive Care Units	
Infants 1,000–1,500 grams	16,391
Infants 500–999 grams	115,742

Source: Garber and Phelps (1997, and citations therein), converted to 2008 dollars using CPI.

of use of an intervention (moving along the intensive margin). An increasing CE ratio for any specific intervention (as the population changes) signals a declining marginal productivity (because the cost per treatment remains the same or similar in all cases shown here, no matter what the population treated).

For example, look at the use of low-dose lovastatin (a cholesterol-reducing drug) for various populations. For the highest risk population (older male heart attack survivors), the drug has an extremely high marginal product and, hence, a low CE ratio ($3,237 per life-year saved). Expanding the treatment to those with lower cholesterol slightly reduces the marginal productivity (expansion along the extensive margin). Expanding it again to female hypertensive nonsmokers hugely increases the CE ratio ($1.4 million per life-year saved) because the incremental benefit (marginal product) is so much smaller in this low-risk group, and expanding the treatment again to middle-aged nonsmoking females again doubles the CE ratio to $3 million per life-year saved.

Similar results appear in almost every intervention ever studied in RCTs. Exercise electrocardiogram screening for women is not as productive as for men (nearly $0.5 million per life-year for women versus about $0.2 million for men) because their underlying risk is lower. Treating low-weight infants in intensive care has a reasonably favorable CE ratio for infants in the 1,000–1,500 gram range (about 2–3 pounds), but when doctors expand the range of treatment to include infants under 1,000 grams, the incremental CE ratio rises rapidly to $116,000 per life-year saved because these newborns are so much sicker and harder to treat. Using coronary artery bypass grafts (CABG, usually pronounced "cabbage") for the sickest patients (those with the main artery supplying blood to the heart clogged up) has a very high productivity (and hence a CE ratio of only $13,000), but expanding that same surgical procedure to those with only mild symptoms (a single blood vessel other than the left main artery, producing chest pain upon exertion, known as angina pectoris, or more simply, "angina") increases the CE ratio by a factor of 10.

Some of these studies demonstrate how changes in the intensive margin (the rate or intensity of treatment of those treated) alters the marginal productivity of the intervention (and, hence, the CE ratios). For example, annual breast examination for women aged 55–65 saves life-years at a modest cost ($23,000 per life-year), but adding mammography (a more technologically intensive examination) increases the CE ratio to almost triple the level of breast examinations alone. Diagnostic tests for cervical cancer (the so-called Pap smear test) cost only $36,000 per life-year saved if conducted every 3 years, but increasing the rate to once every 2 years provides benefits only with vastly reduced marginal productivity, and the CE ratio rises to over $700,000 per life-year saved.

A new approach to understanding "the production of health" compares in great detail the procedures used (and costs thereof) to treat a specific medical condition and investigates how those costs—and the attendant health improvements—have changed over time. The increases over time in per-case spending can be matched with per-case changes in health outcomes, including survival or other aspects of health.

The first of these new approaches (Cutler and McClellan, 1998) measured the changes in costs and outcomes for treating heart attacks. Over the period 1984–1998, Cutler and McClellan found that costs had increased by $10,000 (in constant dollars) but that life expectancy of heart attack victims had increased by one year (on average). Thus, in this "across-time" comparison, the cost per life-year is $10,000. Most of the change in both health outcomes and cost comes from technological change.

Using a similar approach, Cutler and Meara (2000) looked at changes in low birth-weight infants over the period 1950–1990, an era marked by dramatic technological change in the way such infants were treated, the costs of such treatment, and survival. In constant dollars, they found an increased expenditure of $40,000 and an improvement in life expectancy of 12 years (on average). Thus, by this measure, technological change in newborn intensive care has a CE ratio of $3,300 per life-year.

These changes in costs and outcome are not quite the same as the sort of analysis reported in Table 3.2. Those studies (all RCTs using a fixed technology) give the CE ratio for a "snapshot in time." These "across-time" studies look at changes in the production function due to technological change, but one can still use the results to form the CE ratio for technological innovation. While there is no necessary reason to expect that such results will match those from the snapshot in time results, both of these estimates ($10,000 per life-year for treating heart attack victims and $3,000 per life-year for premature babies) are in the same ballpark as comparable technologies reported in Table 3.2.

More Finely Grained Outcome Measures

Much of the work just described looks at life expectancy as the "outcome," which means that medical interventions that improve the quality of life, but do not extend life expectancy, are somehow given short shrift in the analysis. A comparison of two international studies of treatment after heart attacks shows the importance of this issue.

The Canadian health care system rations the availability of many treatments extensively. Several studies have taken advantage of this "natural experiment" in treatment frequency and intensity to assess the marginal value of the extra treatments used on the U.S. side of the border. The key studies focused on invasive treatment for heart disease (coronary bypass surgery, angioplasty, etc.) and sought evidence on the efficacy of such interventions by looking at mortality due to heart attacks in the two populations. The results were rather disheartening (pun intended), even though the U.S. Medicare population received much more treatment. The U.S. population had about five to eight times as much invasive tests or surgery done within the first 30 days after the heart attack, a gap that narrowed slightly within 180 days after the heart attack, but persisted as a large difference in treatment rates. Yet the mortality rates, although showing a small improvement (21.4 percent versus 22.3 percent) a month after the heart attacks, did not differ when measured a year later. This seems to indicate that the *marginal productivity* of the extra treatments was quite small, at best extending life expectancy for less than a year for some of the patients.

However, this approach ignores potentially important improvements in health from the interventions. In an international study of patients hospitalized with heart attacks, Mark et al. (1994) showed the importance of measuring other dimensions of health outcomes. In their analysis, the Canadian patients stayed in the hospital (on average) a day longer during their initial heart attack event, but the U.S. patients were much more likely to receive "aggressive" diagnosis and treatment subsequently. The U.S. patients had a cardiac catheterization (a complex and potentially dangerous test of heart function involving inserting a catheter through an abdominal artery and into the heart) almost three times as often (72 percent versus 25 percent), and received some intervention to increase blood flow to the heart about three times as often as well. Two interventions were then available—"balloon angioplasty," which involves inserting a catheter into the coronary arteries and then pumping up a "balloon" on the end of it to compress the cholesterol-based plaques that clog up the arteries, and coronary artery bypass grafts (CABG), in which the clogged artery is actually bypassed with a graft.[14] The U.S. patients received the angioplasty intervention nearly three times as often (29 percent versus 11 percent) and had CABG surgery nearly five times as often (14 percent versus 3 percent). Overall, the U.S. patients had "revascularization" interventions at triple the rate of the Canadian patients. The outcomes showed the value of the extra treatment (the positive marginal productivity): The U.S. patients were less likely to have chest pain a year later (21 percent versus 34 percent of patients) and less likely to have shortness of breath (45 percent versus 29 percent). Measuring only mortality as the "health" outcome misses these important gains in health status.

---

[14]A third alternative has since emerged—metal "stents" that hold the artery open.

CONFUSION ABOUT THE PRODUCTION FUNCTION: A POLICY DILEMMA

The previous discussions blur somewhat an important problem in the discussion of "the productivity" of medical care: Doctors themselves seem to disagree about the right ways to use medical care, based upon a growing series of studies showing different patterns of use of various medical care services. Put another way, the medical profession within this country seems to have strong internal disagreements about the marginal productivity of various medical procedures. Not only that, similar variations in patterns of use for specific services emerge in medical care systems of other countries, ranging from Norway to Canada to Great Britain (where a unified National Health Service is responsible for providing health care). Much of the disagreement apparently centers on the appropriate *extensive margin*—that is, how many people should receive various treatments, given that they enter the health care system with a similar set of medical problems and conditions.

Medical Practice Variations on the Extensive Margin

The studies of medical practice variations have almost universally focused on the rate at which "standard" populations have received specific medical interventions. Almost universally, the studies have used hospital admission rates for various procedures as the basis for analysis, so the studies must define some geographic area, and then measure the rates at which a specific procedure has been used for that population. Most of these studies at least control for the age and gender composition of the populations. All of the good studies also carefully measure the rates of use for the populations in question, rather than the rates at which the activities are carried out in the region. (The two could differ considerably, for example, in a city with a large university hospital, and with a considerable referral practice for complicated procedures, or a rural area with no hospital or only a small hospital equipped for only routine surgery or medical treatment.)

The studies usually report the results in terms of a *coefficient of variation* (COV) in use rates across geographic regions. Box 3.2 describes the statistical basis of the COV measure. The COV is a useful measure here because it automatically scales each medical procedure the same way. Thus, a low or high COV has the same meaning no matter which medical activity is considered, and no matter which country the data come from. In its simplest terms, a low COV implies strong medical agreement about the way to use a specific medical procedure. A large COV implies considerable disagreement. Procedures for which large COVs repeatedly appear imply that the medical profession offers very different advice to its patients about when and how often to use those procedures. In economic language, large COVs in hospitalization rates imply substantial medical confusion or disagreement about the marginal productivity of various specific types of medical care. Because these studies look at the rates at which procedures are used in "similar" populations, the disagreement generally must arise on the extensive margin—how many people should receive the procedure.

The first of such studies (Glover, 1938) appeared within the British National Health Service. That study looked at the rate at which British schoolchildren had their tonsils removed in various regions of the country. The results appear startling in retrospect: A tenfold difference existed across regions in the rate of tonsillectomies for schoolchildren. This study sat unnoticed for three decades before a growing series of studies have expanded our knowledge of variations considerably: Kansas (Lewis, 1969), Maine (Wennberg and Gittelsohn, 1975), Iowa (Wennberg, 1990), Canada (Roos et al., 1986; McPherson et al., 1981), New England, Norway, and Wales (McPherson et al., 1982), Medicare patients in the United States (Chassin et al., 1986), and New York (Phelps and Parente, 1990) all provide grist for the mill. In each of these studies, substantial variation in the rate of hospitalization occurred for specific procedures in essentially "standard" populations. In every country or region studied, the medical community shows important disagreement about the appropriate rates of hospitalization for many surgical and medical interventions.

These studies produce a surprisingly uniform picture of medical practice variations: The procedures with relatively large variations in one region or country will likely have relatively large variation in another. The *absolute* variation will differ from study to study for a variety of reasons, but the patterns of *relative* variation show considerable stability.

BOX 3.2 STATISTICAL DISTRIBUTIONS

Suppose a risky world contains a fixed number of events that might happen. Rolling two dice, for example, gives 36 unique outcomes (1,1; 2,1; 1,2; 2,2; 3,2; 2,3; etc.) giving 11 possible total point counts (snake eyes through box cars). The total points on any roll of the dice occur with known probability (unless you are playing against somebody who has loaded the dice). The 11 possible outcomes occur with the following frequency:

Outcome	Number of Possible Combinations	Percentage of All Possible Outcomes
2	1	1/36 = 0.02777 ...
3	2	2/36 = 0.05555 ...
4	3	3/36 = 0.0833 ...
5	4	4/36 = 0.1111 ...
6	5	5/36 = 0.13888 ...
7	6	6/36 = 0.16666 ...
8	5	5/36 = 0.13888 ...
9	4	4/36 = 0.1111 ...
10	3	3/36 = 0.08333 ...
11	2	2/36 = 0.0555 ...
12	1	1/36 = 0.02777 ...

If we were to draw a frequency distribution of these outcomes, it would look like Figure A.

FIGURE A

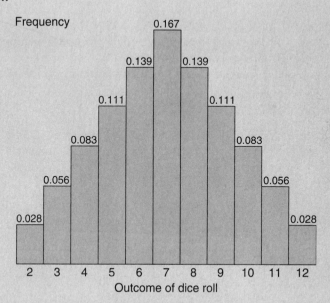

(continued)

BOX 3.2 STATISTICAL DISTRIBUTIONS (continued)

The average outcome is the sum of each numerical value, weighted by the proportion of times it occurs. If each possible outcome is described as x_i and p_i is the percentage of times outcome i occurs, the average for n possible outcomes is defined as

$$\mu = \sum_{i=1}^{n} p_i x_i$$

where μ (pronounced "myew," like the sound a cat makes) is the expected value of the random variable x. In the case of the dice, the expected value of the outcome is exactly 7.

The variance of the outcome is a measure of how spread out the distribution is. If many events are the same (e.g., if the dice were loaded and mostly came up as 7), then the distribution would be even more peaked than that shown above. If the dice were loaded to avoid 5, 6, and 7, the distribution would flatten out. The more peaked the distribution (more squeezed together), the less the variance. The less peaked, the flatter it is, and the more times things occur "in the tails" of the distribution. Such distributions have a high variance.

A common measure of variance is the expected value of the square of the difference between the outcome and its average, defined as

$$\sigma^2 = \sum_{i=1}^{n} p_i (x_i - \mu)^2$$

or sometimes just the square root of that, σ, known as the "standard deviation." (The Greek letter σ is pronounced "sigma.")

Finally, it can become useful to express the variability of a distribution in terms of a coefficient of variation, which is simply

$$COV = \sigma/\mu$$

If the variable is continuously distributed (as with the temperature of a body of water) rather than having a specific number of possible outcomes (as with the roll of two dice), then similar measures are defined, where $\phi(x)$ is the probability density function:

$$\mu = \int_{-\infty}^{\infty} \phi(x)\, dx$$

and

$$\sigma^2 = \int_{-\infty}^{\infty} \phi(x - \mu)^2\, dx$$

Figure B shows three distributions, each with an average value of $\mu = 10$, and variances of $\sigma^2 = 9$, 4, and 1, respectively. Thus, they have standard deviations of $\sigma = 3$, 2, and 1, and coefficients of variation of COV = 0.3, 0.2, and 0.1.

FIGURE B

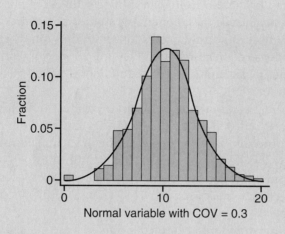

Normal variable with COV = 0.3

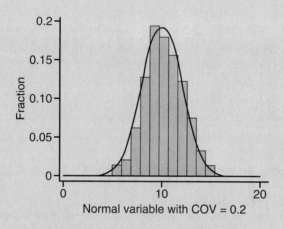

Normal variable with COV = 0.2

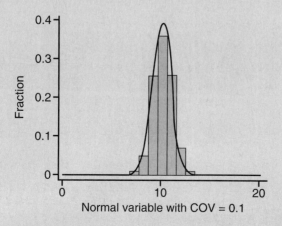

Normal variable with COV = 0.1

Table 3.3 shows the actual COVs for a variety of surgical procedures, either reported or calculated from data in nine different studies of medical practice variations. Among these commonly studied procedures, the greatest disagreement, almost uniformly, occurs for removal of tonsils and adenoids (T&A) and removal of hemorrhoids. The greatest agreement, in general, occurs for hernia repair and (except for the Kansas study) gallbladder and appendix removal.

The within-region variations in surgical rates (as in Table 3.3) do not necessarily correspond well with cross-nation agreement about the "proper" rates for these procedures, For example, although each region studied has a relatively small COV for hernia repair, the overall rates per 100,000 persons differ considerably across studies: 113 (England and Wales), 276 (New England), 186 (Norway), 235 (Canada), 309 (Kansas), 137 (West Midlands), 282 (United States).

The particular procedures identified in Table 3.3 are not necessarily those with large COVs; rather, they are the ones reported most commonly in studies. Larger COVs have appeared in several studies for some procedures. For example, in Medicare patients, Chassin et al. (1986) found high variation in such procedures as injection of hemorrhoids (COV = 0.79), hip reconstruction (COV = 0.69), removal of skin lesions (COV = 0.67), total knee replacement (0.47), and others. In a study of hospitalizations in New York State (Phelps and Parente, 1990), the largest COVs for hospitalization

TABLE 3.3 COEFFICIENTS OF VARIATION OF SURGICAL PROCEDURES IN VARIOUS STUDIES

	Prostate	Tonsil and Adenoid	Appendix	Hernia	Hemorrhoids	Gallbladder	Uterus
Kansas	—	0.29	0.52	0.22	0.40	0.32	—
Northeast United States	0.30	0.36	0.26	0.11	0.30	0.18	0.22
Norway	0.33	0.48	0.16	0.20	0.47	0.18	0.31
West Midlands	0.24	0.31	0.16	0.20	0.35	0.16	0.20
Maine	0.26	0.43	0.18	0.14	0.55	0.23	0.25
England and Wales	0.22	0.19	0.13	0.16	0.24	0.11	0.12
Canada	0.33	0.23	0.15	0.14	0.35	0.14	0.18
Four U.S. regions	0.15	0.17	0.11	0.15	0.13	0.14	0.17
New York counties	0.18	0.42	0.21	0.16	0.16	0.14	0.28

Sources: Lewis (1969) for Kansas; McPherson et al. (1981) for Canada, England, and Wales, and four U.S. regions; McPherson et al. (1982) for West Midlands, Norway, and Northeast United States; Wennberg and Gittelsohn (1975) for Maine; Phelps and Parente (1990) for New York counties.

occurred for within-hospital dental extractions (COV = 0.73) and false labor (COV = 0.75).

Several studies have also provided COVs for nonsurgical procedures, and these data show that the uncertainty about hospitalization is at least as great in these areas as for surgery. The first of such studies (Wennberg, McPherson, and Caper, 1984) found very high variations (COV > 0.4) in such areas as urinary tract infections, chest pain, bronchitis, middle-ear infections and upper-respiratory infections (both adults and children), and pediatric pneumonia. In a study of Medicare patient hospitalizations, Chassin et al., (1986) found moderate to large COVs for a number of nonsurgical conditions, including diagnostic activities such as skin biopsy (COV = 0.58) and coronary angiography (to detect clogging of arteries into the heart, COV = 0.32). In New York (Phelps and Parente, 1990), a large variation appeared for a substantial number of pediatric hospitalizations, even after controlling for the age mix of the populations, including pneumonia (COV = 0.56), middle-ear infections and upper-respiratory infections (COV = 0.57), bronchitis and asthma (COV = 0.35), and gastroenteritis (COV = 0.42). Large variations also occurred for adult admissions in categories such as concussion (COV = 0.41), chronic obstructive lung disease (COV = 0.43), medical back problems (0.31), adult gastroenteritis (0.26), and similar diseases. Psychiatric hospital admissions were also quite variable, including depression (COV = 0.48), acute adjustment reaction (COV = 0.52), and psychosis (COV = 0.28).

In another study, John Wennberg and colleagues (Wennberg et al., 1990) at Dartmouth Medical School reported on a comparison of the use of various medical procedures in two U.S. cities (Boston and New Haven), in both of which a large fraction of hospitalizations occurs in hospitals affiliated with medical schools (87 percent in Boston, 97 percent in New Haven). One important feature of this study is that it shows substantial variations in practice patterns even within the part of the medical community—academic medicine—that should be best informed about the efficacy of various medical interventions. The cities are quite similar in terms of age profiles, the level and distribution of income, and the proportion of persons who are nonwhite. By contrast with New Haven, Boston has 55 percent more hospital beds per capita, and each hospital bed had 22 percent more hospital employees, who were paid on average 5 percent more. On average, citizens of the Boston area spent 87 percent more on hospital care than those in New Haven.

The age-adjusted patterns of medical care use by citizens of the Boston area uniformly are higher than those of New Haven, with most of the variation occurring in (1) minor surgery cases and (2) medical diagnoses in which variations in admissions rates are high across the country. Small differences exist for major surgery and low-variation medical admissions, both in admission rates and lengths of stay.

Using a more finely tuned microscope, we can see diversity within this pattern of uniformity. Particularly within the major surgery category, a number of procedures appeared for which Boston had higher rates of use than New Haven, but an equal or larger number for which the use rate was larger in New Haven. For example, residents of New Haven received CABG at twice the rate of persons in Boston, but citizens of the Boston regions received treatment using carotid endarterectomy (a procedure to ream out clogged arteries) at over twice the rate of those in New Haven.

Wennberg (1990) has documented similarly large variations in the admission rates for numerous surgical procedures in the market areas of 16 major university hospitals and large community hospitals around the country, again, in medical centers with the greatest presumed medical knowledge of any part of the health care community. The variations in admission rates correspond closely to those found in other settings. Even medicine's elite systematically disagree about the proper use of many procedures. Table 3.4 shows Wennberg's findings for 30 surgical procedures. Notice the similarity of results for procedures that also appear in Table 3.3.

Table 3.4 also reveals a useful rule of thumb: In such studies, the ratio of highest to lowest rates of use will approximately correspond to 10 times the COV. For appendectomy, for example, the COV is 0.30, and the ratio of high to low is 2.86. This holds true for most procedures and studies in this literature, and provides a more intuitive way of comprehending the meaning of a COV.

PHYSICIAN-SPECIFIC VARIATIONS (MEDICAL PRACTICE STYLES)

All of the previous information about medical disagreement (variations) has relied on data comparing the use of medical interventions across different regions, looking at interventions (such as decisions to hospitalize, rates of surgery performed) one at a time. This requires a very different approach to studying differences in treatment choices than the cross-regional studies of single treatments.

A statistical dilemma underlies all studies of the phenomenon. To gain statistical reliability (and, hence, confidence that observed differences are "real" rather than just statistical artifacts), one must use a large number of treated patients, and one must have reasonable confidence that any differences in treatment rates are not due to differences in illness. In the cross-regional studies, this problem is solved by analyzing single diseases (or treatments). To gather together enough patients for statistical reliability, one must aggregate them by geographic region. This, in turn, requires that one "standardize" the

TABLE 3.4 COEFFICIENTS OF VARIATION IN 16 UNIVERSITY HOSPITALS OR LARGE COMMUNITY HOSPITAL MARKET AREAS

Procedure	Coefficient of Variation	Ratio High to Low
Colectomy (removal of colon)	0.12	1.47
Resection of small intestine	0.14	1.75
Inguinal hernia repair	0.15	2.01
Pneumonectomy (removal of part of lung)	0.21	2.72
Simple mastectomy (removal of breast)	0.27	2.71
Open-heart surgery	0.23	2.29
Extended or radical mastectomy	0.21	2.21
Hysterectomy (removal of uterus)	0.28	2.60
Cholecystectomy (gallbladder removal)	0.23	2.22
Embolectomy	0.36	4.10
Protectomy (rectal surgery)	0.27	3.01
Pacemaker insertion	0.28	2.63
Thyroidectomy	0.34	3.35
Appendectomy	0.30	2.86
Total hip replacement	0.35	2.99
Repair of retina	0.27	3.12
Prostatectomy (prostate surgery)	0.33	3.12
Coronary bypass surgery	0.33	3.62
Mastoidectomy	0.46	4.03
Aorto-iliac-femoral bypass	0.38	3.62
Diaphragmatic hernia	0.37	3.45
Stapes mobilization	0.48	4.28
Spinal fusion with or without disc removal	0.52	5.20
Peripheral artery bypass	0.36	4.36
Cardiac catheterization	0.44	4.48
Excision of intravertebral disc	0.43	5.09
Graft replacement of aortic aneurysm	0.40	6.26
Laparotomy	0.47	5.60
Total knee replacement	0.53	7.42
Carotid endarterectomy	0.83	19.39

Source: Wennberg (1990).

age and gender mix of populations in different regions because the rates of disease vary considerably by both age and gender. The traditional approach to accomplish this in the medical literature is the epidemiological method called "indirect standardization," which, in effect, computes the regional rates of treatment as if each region had the same age and gender composition. Previous statistical work has even provided ways to test whether observed regional variations arise from pure chance (Diehr et al., 1992).

However, if one wishes to study individual physicians' choices, other approaches must be used because no doctor treats enough patients with a single disease to make comparisons meaningful. Rather, one must add up patients across diseases within doctors' practices. This, in turn, requires the ability to control for case mix and severity of illness at the level of the individual patient, and until recently, the tools to do this have not been available. However, new methods are now available to "standardize" individual doctors' patient mix. With case mix and severity of illness standardized, one can estimate the medical costs used to treat the patients in each doctor's practice, and hence estimate each doctor's "style."

To do this, a research team used claims data from several hundred thousand patients in a Blue Cross and Blue Shield insurance plan that had no deductibles, and covered a wide array of inpatient and outpatient services (Phelps et al., 1994). The study focused on the treatment patterns of primary care doctors because in this insurance plan (called "Blue Choice") patients quite literally could not be treated without first seeing their primary care doctor. (The plan is an IPA-model HMO, as discussed more extensively in Chapter 11.) There were about 500 primary care doctors caring for these patients, representing nearly all of the primary care doctors in the Rochester, New York, region.

The research approach analyzed the medical care use of individual patients in the Blue Choice plan, using two new methods to calculate the severity of illness that each patient had during the year. In simple terms, after controlling for the illness of each patient, the unexplained portion was averaged over each patient in each doctor's practice, and those average "unexplained" amounts provide an estimate of each doctor's "style."[15]

Because of the way the Blue Choice plan worked, it made good sense to compare the total medical care costs incurred by each patient, and attribute all of those costs back to the primary care doctor. This is the right approach here because the patients could not get any treatment except when authorized by their primary care doctor, including direct patient visits, drugs, hospitalizations, and—importantly—referrals to specialists. Thus, the results

---

[15]For those readers with econometric training, the following provides a brief description of the actual approach. Individual annual medical care spending was regressed on a series of explanatory variables, including the case-mix and severity of illness measures, age, gender, and other available sociodemographic variables. These regressions accounted for an amazing 50–60 percent of the variation in annual medical spending at the individual level, far more than any previous studies on data such as these have ever been able to accomplish. The regressions also used "dummy" variables for each primary care physician, a so-called fixed effects regression model. The coefficients from those dummy variables formed the basis for the histogram shown in Figure 3.3.

described as follows relate to total medical care spending (as covered by the insurance plan, excluding only things such as long-term care), not just the treatment directly provided by the primary care doctors.

The results show that doctors do indeed have importantly differing styles, patterns of treatment intensity that are statistically reliable and consistent across years. Figure 3.2 shows a histogram that portrays the frequency of doctors' styles in a simple yet important way: It shows the frequency of doctors with practice styles that use relatively more or less medical care to treat their patients than the average in the community. Thus, a score of zero in this analysis means that the doctor's style is just at the average spending. A score of −0.1 means that the doctor's patients, on average, had 10 percent less medical care used for them than the overall average, and a score of 0.2 means (similarly) that those patients cost 20 percent more than average. As Figure 3.3 shows, there turned out to be a wide array of "styles" within this single medical community. The study could also calculate the standard deviation around the estimate of each doctor's "style," and hence could understand how much of the differences were likely due to chance and how much were systematic. For a number of the doctors with styles close to the average (scores near 0), the differences were not significantly different from the average (in a statistical sense of significance), but for most doctors with "styles" 10 percent or more away from the average, the differences are statistically significant.

The differences are also "important" in the sense that these doctors' style differences lead to considerably different medical spending to treat the same numbers of patients. (Remember, statistical techniques have created a comparison as if each doctor had the same mix of patients in age, gender, and illness

FIGURE 3.2 Distribution of primary care doctors' "practice styles" in Rochester, New York.

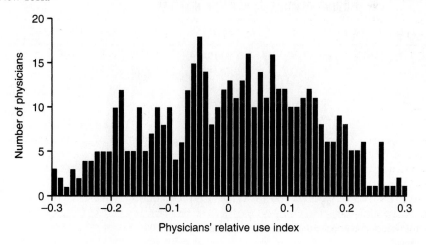

FIGURE 3.3 Distribution of doctors' "practice styles" for hospitalized Medicare patients in Oregon and Florida.

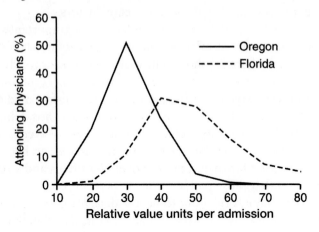

Source: Welch, Miller, and Welch (1994).

patterns.) On average, the lowest cost 10 percent of doctors used about half the medical care resources as the top 10 percent of the doctors. Table 3.5 shows the average medical spending for patients in this plan, arrayed by the relative costliness of the primary care doctors.

A similar study, focusing on hospitalized Medicare patients, demonstrated similar diversity in physicians' styles within regions, and strong differences in the average style across regions, thus (in a nice way) highlighting the importance both of physician-level variations within a single region and cross regional differences. In this study, Welch, Miller, and Welch (1994) used 1991

TABLE 3.5 DIFFERENCE FROM AVERAGE COST (BY DECILE OF PRACTICE COSTS) IN PRIMARY CARE PHYSICIAN PRACTICES IN ROCHESTER, NEW YORK

Decile	Number Doctors	Number Patients	Average Deviation ($)
1	49	10,224	−419
2	50	19,976	−205
3	49	15,688	−132
4	50	29,425	−83
5	49	24,133	−48
6	50	20,211	−12
7	50	25,597	46
8	49	20,716	115
9	50	17,658	223
10	49	7,263	594

Note: Average expense for this under-65 population was $879.00.

Medicare data, controlling for case mix, to "profile" 6,802 physicians from Florida and 1,101 from Oregon, selected from a larger group because they had at least 10 Medicare hospital admissions during the year. They measured the "resource units" billed by the physicians for their hospitalized Medicare patients, in each case using the national average resource units for that particular type of admission. They used the Resource Based Relative Value System adopted by Medicare in 1992 as the basis for assigning these "resource units" (see Chapter 12 for a discussion of this physician payment mechanism).

Figure 3.3 shows the authors' results, which provide further information on the degree of differences among physicians' practice styles within communities (although in this case the "communities" are entire states, not single metropolitan areas as in the work discussed previously from Rochester, New York) and across regions.

These data show extensive differences within both regions in doctors' behavior. In Oregon, the mean relative value unit (RVU) per hospital admission was about 30 (equivalent to the "work" of 30 routine office visits), with a range from 10 to 70. The mean RVU use in Florida was half again as large (46 RVU per admission). Recall that these data are all standardized by case mix, so that cannot account for the differences. In Florida, the range was even wider than found in Oregon. This study found the same patterns of behavior both across and within states when comparing physicians of the same specialty (e.g., comparing internists with internists, orthopedic surgeons with orthopedic surgeons).

EXTENSIVE AND INTENSIVE MARGIN DIFFERENCES: ARE THEY SIMILAR?

One might wonder whether regions (or doctors) that disagree about the extensive margin of care have related disagreements about the intensive margin of use. For example, if one knew that (say) Boston was very "aggressive" on the extensive margin (admissions to the hospital), would they more than likely be high or low on choices of the intensive margin (length of stay)? Unfortunately, few studies can make such a comparison. One study, looking at the use of ambulatory care by Medicare patients, concluded that the propensity to use care overall (per capita visits to physicians) was not related to the intensity of treatment rendered (Stano and Folland, 1988). This study uses a quite broad and general measure of medical care (visits), and thus may mask some important relationships. A study of Medicare patients (Chassin et al., 1986) looked at a specific surgical procedure and reached the same conclusion. The rate at which patients received coronary artery bypass grafts varied by a factor of 3 from the low-use to high-use regions studied, but the number of grafts made in each patient (the intensive margin) was unrelated to the overall use rate. Thus, from the (somewhat meager) evidence available, it appears that disagreements about the extensive and intensive margins of use may be quite different. Doctors who are "aggressive" or "conservative" on one margin may be the same or different on the other margin.

A study by Roos and colleagues in Manitoba used individual patient data from their provincewide claims system to address a similar question. They estimated the propensity of doctors to admit patients to the hospital, and also the average length of stay among those patients who were admitted. They found a slight but negative relationship between the two indexes for each doctor, suggesting that at least in this area, those who tend to admit more patients end up (on average) with less sickly patients. In other words, in their data, increases in the extensive margin (admissions) led to a slight decline in the average intensity (length of stay), as would be expected with appropriate "sorting" of patients into the hospital on the basis of illness severity (Roo et al., 1986).

The Policy Question: What Should We Do About Variations?

The apparently considerable disagreement over proper use of medical interventions disturbs many analysts of the health care system. The uncertainty demonstrated by these variations highlights an important question: How do medical interventions become accepted as standard medical practice, and what causes the medical community to change its beliefs about therapeutic efficacy? More particularly, what is the proper way to create and disseminate information about the efficacy of medical interventions—their marginal productivity?

These are complicated questions, deserving careful consideration. At this point, we can merely look ahead to subsequent points of this book: Information such as this is a "public good" and probably will not emerge spontaneously through private actions. Chapter 13 describes the role of the medical–legal system in affecting the quality of care in medicine. For now, we will stand on the observation already made: Most of what constitutes "modern medicine" has never been tested in a scientific fashion, and its marginal productivity in producing or augmenting health therefore remains an open question.

SUMMARY

Health can be produced by medical care, although the process is often uncertain and may not always proceed as intended. As with other productive processes, the production of health is almost certainly subject to diminishing returns to scale: The more medical care we use, the less incremental gain we get back in terms of improved health.

Available evidence shows both that the average effect of health care has been quite important in augmenting our health, and that the incremental effect of further health care might be quite small.

Further resources can be devoted to health care on both an extensive margin (more people treated) and an intensive margin (more treatment per person treated). Doctors seem to disagree considerably about the right amounts of health care to use on both of these margins of adjustment. On the extensive margin, numerous studies show substantial variations in the rate at which various medical interventions are employed. These variations *require* disagreement among doctors: They signal medical confusion. On the intensive margin, considerable disagreement exists as well about the proper length of stay (for example) for various hospitalizations. Doctors appear to have "signatures" characterizing their length-of-stay plans.

On balance, the differences of opinion about proper medical practice have considerable implications for resource use. Wennberg and his colleagues, for example, have estimated that if the 1988 practice patterns in Boston applied to the nation as a whole, we would spend 15 to 16 percent of our GNP on health care (rather than the then-current 11 percent). By contrast, if the practice patterns in New Haven applied to the country, we would spend about 8 percent of our GNP on health care. At present, we have little direct evidence on the differences in production of health arising from such diverse choices in the rate of use of medical interventions. The RAND HIS results suggest that the improvement in health from such radically different spending patterns may be small, at best. The econometric estimates by Hall and Jones (2007) are more encouraging, except for teenagers and the very elderly (see Figure 3.1).

RELATED CHAPTERS IN *HANDBOOK OF HEALTH ECONOMICS*

Chapter 4, "Advances in CE Analysis" by Alan M. Garber

Chapter 5, "Information Diffusion and Best Practice Adoption" by Charles E. Phelps

Chapter 32, "The Measurement of Health-Related Quality of Life" by Paul Dolan

PROBLEMS

1. "Most of the variability in average medical care use across regions is due to differences in insurance coverage." Comment.

2. Thinking about a diagnostic test such as breast cancer screening, describe what it means to increase use of the test (1) on the intensive margin and (2) on the extensive margin.

3. People living in Boston are hospitalized about 1.5 times as often as those living in New Haven, yet their health outcomes, based on age-specific mortality rates, appear to be identical. Does this mean that hospital care has no ability to improve health? (*Hint:* Think about the difference between average and marginal productivity. See also Question 5 that follows.)
4. "Variations in medical care use probably arise from the educational level of doctors, with less trained doctors using either too much or too little care and better trained specialists using about the right amount of care." Comment.
5. Most available studies of the effects of medical care on health outcomes use mortality as the measure of health. If there are other dimensions to health in addition to living versus dying that remain unmeasured (such as freedom from pain, mobility to move around freely, physical endurance to perform work) then how (if at all) might that alter our estimates of the marginal productivity of medical care? (*Hint:* Think about U.S. versus Canadian comparisons reported in this chapter.)
6. Cross-regional studies of medical practice variations and comparisons of individual physicians' "styles" show considerable differences between the rates of use of medical care across providers. Presuming (for the moment) that the populations being treated in these comparisons are equivalent (or sufficiently so to ignore the differences), would you say that these studies show (a) that some doctors treat too much; (b) some doctors don't treat enough; (c) both; (d) neither; or (e) we can't tell from data such as that? Explain your conclusion.
7. What evidence could you assemble to convince a skeptic that increased spending on medical care in recent decades has had a beneficial effect on people's health?

APPENDIX TO CHAPTER 3

Marginal, Average, and Total Productivity

This appendix summarizes the ideas of average and marginal productivity, stated in the most general of production functions—that is, where output varies with a single "composite" input, for example, producing "health" with a single composite input called "medical care." Thus, $H = f(M)$ describes the type of production function we are discussing. The central idea is that the input (M) yields different *incremental* returns of output, depending on how much of the input one uses. The production function shown here displays (initially) *increasing* marginal product, and then the more common *decreasing* marginal product. As we will see, it seldom makes sense to operate in a realm in which returns are increasing, so thinking about production functions with decreasing returns makes the most sense.

Figure 3A.1 shows the graph of output (H) plotted against M. The curve initially dishes up ("U shaped"), and then tips over to be "hill shaped." The point at which it tips over is called an "inflection point," labeled M_1 on the graph. Output H increases as M increases (corresponding to the idea that more M produces more H) until the point M_3, at which point H actually

FIGURE 3A.1

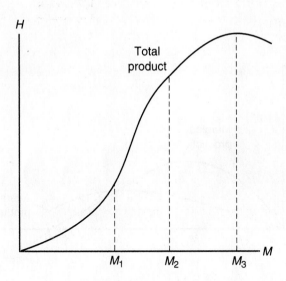

begins to decline as more M is used. In medical questions, this would be called "iatrogenic illness" because health would fall as medical care use increased.

The slope of the production function at any point along Figure 3A.1 is the marginal productivity of medical care—$\partial H/\partial M$. If one converts that slope to a measure of proportional change—$(\partial H/H)/(\partial M/M)$, where H and M are the values at the same point on the curve (e.g., at M_2), then that proportional change measure is the elasticity of health with respect to medical spending, the characterization of the health care production function estimated by Hall and Jones (2007) and appearing in Figure 3.1.

Figure 3A.2 shows the same production function, but it graphs on the vertical axis either the marginal productivity ($\partial H/\partial M$) or the average productivity (H/M), rather than the total output H (which appears in Figure 3A.1). The marginal product curve rises initially, until it tips over at output level M_1, the inflection point in Figure 3A.1, and begins to fall. Another point of interest occurs at M_2, the point at which the average product reaches its highest possible level in Figure 3A.2. (Note that this occurs in Figure 3A.1 at the point at which a ray from the origin to the curve is at its steepest.) It also must be true that, at that point, average and marginal product are equal.[16] This is why we

---

[16]The proof occurs as follows: Define average product = H/M, and find its maximum by taking the derivative and setting it equal to zero. The derivative of H/M is $(M\partial H/\partial M - H)/M^2$; setting that equal to zero gives $\partial H/\partial M = H/M$. However, because H/M = average output, this proves that when average output has reached its maximum, average and marginal product are equal to each other.

FIGURE 3A.2

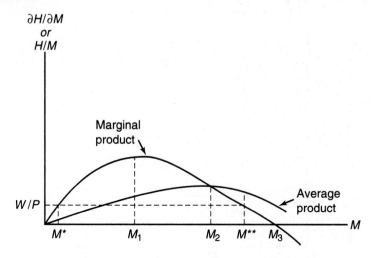

show the average product and marginal product curves intersecting in Figure 3A.2 at the input rate M_2.

If we say that another "unit" of H is worth P and that another unit of M costs W, then the optimal use of M is to expand its use until the value of the incremental product just equals the incremental cost of another unit of input—that is, $\partial H/\partial M = W$, or in a way that we can graph in Figure 3A.2, expand use of M until $\partial H/\partial M = W/P$. Now we can see why it makes sense always to operate in a realm of diminishing marginal product (that is, where marginal product is positive, but falling in Figure 3A.2). Look in Figure 3A.2: This "optimality" condition occurs at two points, indicated by M^* (at a very low rate of use of M) and M^{**}, at a larger rate of use, which mathematically must occur at an input rate exceeding M_2. If we "stopped" using M at the point M^*, we would "give up" a lot of output H that would cost less to produce, per unit, than its value P. Thus, it makes sense to expand use out to M^{**}, but not further, say to M_3, where the marginal product falls to zero.

Perhaps the key idea to remember from this in terms of the discussion of use of health care is that, in the realm of "sensible" use of medical care, *marginal product is less than average product.* That is to say, we'll get less than the average yield of health output when we use more medical care in the vicinity of the optimum. This is why we must continually think about marginal ("incremental") benefits rather than average benefits of medical care.

CHAPTER 4

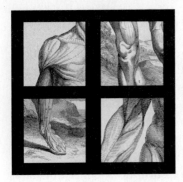

The Demand for Medical Care: Conceptual Framework

In this chapter we derive the consumer's demand curve for medical care from the utility function described previously and then analyze the effects of a health insurance policy on that demand curve and quantities demanded. Finally, we study the evidence showing how demand varies with systematic features such as income, age, gender, and location. We learn how much price and insurance coverage alter use of medical care. We see how time acts as a cost of care. Finally, we see how illness events—the level of sickness people actually experience—dominate individual choices of how much health care to buy in any given year. This, in turn, sets the

LEARNING GOALS

- Follow the logic for shifting from "demand for health" to "demand for medical care" with specific illnesses.

- Understand how to derive demand curves for medical care from indifference curves (and how these relate to the demand for health).

- Interpret demand curves as "value" measures.

- Learn how health insurance of various types alters the price of medical care and affects demand curves.

stage for analyzing the demand for health insurance in Chapter 10. The next few pages provide a fairly complete characterization of how the economic model goes from utility functions to demand curves. The remainder of the book relies intensively on the demand curve rather than the utility function, so those who are comfortable with the idea of a demand curve (or those who are willing to accept the idea on blind faith) might just skip directly to the discussion of demand curves themselves following the section on indifference curves. However, for those willing to invest the effort, the excursion through the terrain of utility theory that follows will add considerably to their final understanding of the meaning of demand curves and how various economic and health-related events alter those demand curves.

INDIFFERENCE CURVES FOR HEALTH AND OTHER GOODS

The economist's model of consumer demand begins with the utility function, as described in Chapter 2. This model makes the consumer's own judgment of something's value the only relevant judgment—*de gustibus non disputandum est.*[1] We assume that the consumer has a stable utility function, in the sense that it doesn't change from period to period or with new information, for example, about the value of medical care. We make this assumption because without it, we lose the ability to say much about consumer behavior. However, we need to remember that it is just an assumption.[2] Thus, our starting point is the utility function, Utility $= U(X, H)$.

We had developed in Chapter 2 the idea of an indifference curve, the set of all combinations of X and H that creates the same level of utility. As in standard consumer demand theory, the consumer tries to reach the highest indifference curve possible because utility is higher then. The budget constraint provides the limit to this process. The consumer must pay for X and for any medical care (m) used to produce H, and overall spending must be limited to the available budget. This presents the first "wrinkle" in applying standard economic theory to the demand for medical care. Somehow, we need to make the translation from health (H), which improves utility, to medical care (m), on which money is spent. The *production process* provides this translation, which we described in Chapter 2 as the relationship $H = g(m)$. As we saw in Chapter 3, this process is almost certainly subject to diminishing returns to scale, so the relevant question is how health changes as medical use changes. To provide a shorthand way to describe this, we will define $g'(m)$ as the *rate* at which health improves for a small change in m.[3] Thus, we can redraw the diagram in Figure 4.1a (which maps combinations of X and H) as Figure 4.1b,

---

[1]Literally, "There is no disputing of tastes."

[2]According to some schools of philosophy, the "realism" of assumptions matters. According to others, it doesn't matter, at least in one sense. Assumptions determine the structure of a *model* of human behavior. The *theory* corresponding to that model is that consumers act *as if* the model replicated human behavior. The *theory* can be refuted by finding human behavior that conflicts with the model, according to the philosophy of Karl Popper and others. Thus, the test of a theory is not its realism but the predictive value it has. Of course, if a model has assumed away critical parts of the problems, then it will fail the prediction test because it will not be able to predict behavior well. For a classic discussion of these issues in an economic setting, see Milton Friedman, *Essays in Positive Economics* (1966).

[3]In the notation of calculus, we need the marginal productivity, $\partial H/\partial m$. Since $H = g(m)$, we describe this throughout the book by using the notation g'(m), where g' $= \partial H/\partial m$ is the marginal productivity of m.

FIGURE 4.1 (a) Production possibilities curve. (b) Budget line for optimal consumption decision.

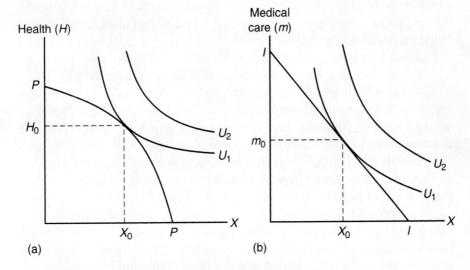

(a)   (b)

which maps combinations of X and m (not X and H). If $g'(m)$ were always constant for any amount of m chosen (i.e., if there were no diminishing returns to producing H), then these two panels would look the same, except that the units of measurement along the vertical axis would be in medical care units rather than health units. However, because the production of health exhibits decreasing returns to scale, the curves can also change shape.

Figure 4.1a also shows a *production possibilities curve,* labeled *PP.* This curve represents the feasible set of combinations of X and H the consumer can attain, given the available budget and the production function $H = g(m)$. It curves downward (it is concave) because of the diminishing marginal productivity of m in producing H. Figure 4.1b shows the same situation in a map with dimensions X and m (not X and H). Instead of a production possibilities curve, Figure 4.1b has a budget line II, showing the budget $I = p_x x + p_m m$ as a straight line (because individual consumers can treat market prices as fixed). It is as if the original Figure 4.1a were drawn on a rubber sheet and then stretched to create Figure 4.1b. The direction and extent of the stretching would depend on the production function for health, $H = g(m)$. In general, the map would have to be stretched in just such a way to straighten out the production possibilities curve *PP* into the straight budget line II.[4] The indifference curves would all get warped by the same stretching process. We

---

[4]Of course, one could begin with Figure 4.1b and then stretch it into Figure 4.1a, again using the production function (in the other direction) to describe the appropriate amount of stretching. To do this, Figure 4.1b would be stretched vertically at each point on the m-axis according to the *inverse* of the marginal productivity of m.

need know here only that the indifference curves comparing X and m have the same *general* shape as the indifference curves in Figure 4.1a, which most closely map the utility function directly.[5] As will become clearer in a moment, the translation from Figure 4.1a (showing X and H) to Figure 4.1b (showing X and m) has meaning only for a particular illness because the effect of medical care on health depends on the specific illness and its severity.

We will say that consumers act as if they wish to maximize utility $= U(X, H)$ within the constraints implied by their budgets, which they spend on X and m. If a consumer's income is I, then the budget constraint says that spending must not exceed income, or $I \geq p_x X + p_m m$. Because the consumer wants to reach as high a utility level as possible, the entire budget is always used, and $I = p_x X + p_m m$. This means that the consumer picks the point at which a single indifference curve is just tangent to the budget line II in Figure 4.1b. This point specifies that the best possible mix of X and m is (X_0, m_0). Because m_0 produces the level of health H_0, the companion point in Figure 4.1a is the point (X_0, H_0). This point is also tangent to the production possibilities curve PP at a single point. In either Figure 4.1a or 4.1b, the consumer has spent the entire budget in a way to maximize utility.

We can now show in Figure 4.2a and 4.2b the effects of the consumer's "getting sick." Begin in Figure 4.2a at the previously described optimum consumption, shown as point 1. An illness event immediately drops the level of health from H_0 to H_1. Call this health loss ℓ. At the same time, the set of achievable combinations of X and H shifts inward *for every level of X*. The shape of the new production possibilities curve $P'P'$ depends on the relationship between m and H for this disease. Its curvature reflects diminishing returns to using more medical care in general. The health loss ℓ acts the same here as a direct loss of income; it reduces the achievable opportunities to consume X and H. However, point 2 in Figure 4.2a is not the best achievable here. After the illness, the consumer can slide along the $P'P'$ curve to point 3, giving up some consumption of X to increase the level of health from H_1 to H_2. Point 3 is the best the consumer can do. The illness initially drops the level of utility from U_1 to U_2, and the purchase of medical care (at the sacrifice of some X) raises it back to U_3. (Note in Figure 4.2a that the subscripts on the utility curves refer to the sequence in which they are reached, not comparative levels of utility.)

---

[5] We had noted in Chapter 2 that some types of "goods" in the bundle of goods x in fact also lowered the level of health. The presence of such goods means formally that $H = g(m, x_B, x_G)$, and we need to define $g'(m)$ as the partial derivative of g, holding x_G and x_B constant, so $g'(m) = \partial H/\partial m$. In diagrams such as Figure 4.1a, the presence of some x_B just makes the PP curve lower or more concave (have more of a bend in it), but the general idea remains the same.

FIGURE 4.2 (a) When consumer "gets sick"—health. (b) When consumer "gets sick"—medical care. (c) When consumer "gets sick"—income loss.

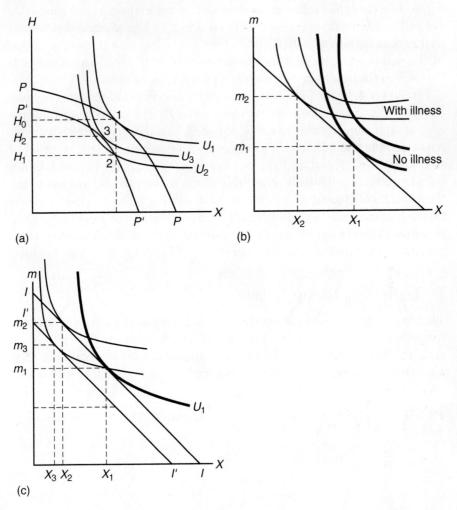

In Figure 4.2b, we can see the same situation in a map of X and m. Several important differences occur here. First, the indifference curves all shift when the consumer gets sick. In particular, they change slopes, so the marginal rate of substitution between X and m shifts. Although the *utility function* is stable, the *indifference map* with X and m as coordinates shifts with the illness level. In Figure 4.2b, the heavy curves show the preferences of the person before becoming sick, and the light indifference curves show the same person's preferences after the illness event. The decline in consumption from X_1 to X_2, coupled with the increase in use of medical care from m_1 to m_2, shows the effect of illness on patterns of spending in the market.

In addition, *if illness harms a person's ability to earn an income,* then the budget constraint in Figure 4.2b might also shift inward because of the illness. Figure 4.2c does this, with the same pattern of preferences as in Figure 4.2b, but with a decline in income as well from II to $I'I'$. The additional reduction in the consumption of both X and m reflects this loss of income. This is one of the reasons why income and health are positively correlated. Another is that more income allows the purchase of more medical care.

In Figure 4.2c, the pre-illness choice of X and m sits at the tangency of a heavy indifference curve with the budget line II. The utility level U_1 is the highest attainable for the income I_1. When illness strikes, indifference curves rotate and income falls to $I'I'$. The best post-illness choice is the tangency of the budget line $I'I'$ and the light indifference curve, at point (X_3, m_3). Illness has caused three potentially observable things to happen: Income has fallen, the amount of X has fallen, and the amount of m has increased. Even if illness does not cause income to decline (for example, the person might have good sick-loss insurance or sick leave), X will still fall and m will still increase, compared with the no-illness choices. The choice of (X_2, m_2) represents this case.

The Effects of an Increase in Income

We can use graphs such as Figure 4.3b to ask what the effects of income would be, holding everything else constant, on the consumption of medical care. This is the first step in deriving demand curves for medical care. As in any standard economic analysis, we portray this in Figure 4.3a with a shift

FIGURE 4.3 (a) The effects of income on health. (b) The effects of income on medical care.

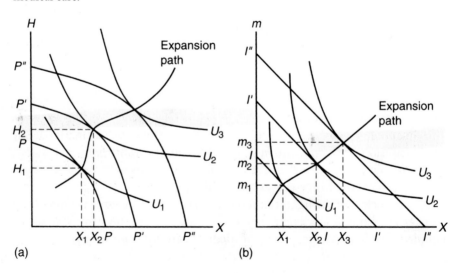

(a)   (b)

outward in the production possibilities (*PP*) line or in Figure 4.3b with a parallel outward shift in the budget line *II*. These panels show an "expansion
path" of how consumption of *X* and *H* or *m* would change with increasing
income, *holding everything else constant*.

It is important to remember this condition: In real-world data, people
with higher incomes often have better health insurance than those with lower
incomes, leading to more medical care use, as we will shortly see. They may
also get sick less often, leading to less medical care use. For some of them,
lifestyle choices at higher incomes (life in the fast lane) may cause health to
fall with higher incomes. On balance, a simple plot of medical care use versus
income would embed a complex set of phenomena affecting medical care use.
However, if we continue to hold everything else constant, as in Figure 4.3b, a
plot of the consumption of *H* versus income and *m* versus income taken from
Figure 4.3a and 4.3b would yield the Engel curves for *H* and *m* in Figure 4.4.[6]
The pattern of indifference curves in Figure 4.3 and the Engel curves in
Figure 4.4 are drawn to replicate (approximately) some empirical regularities
that we will study further—namely, that changes in individuals' incomes (if
all else is held constant) do not seem to alter greatly the amount of medical
care consumed.

In Figure 4.4, we see some (but not all) of the possible complications that
might enter a simple comparison of income versus health or the use of medical care. For example, in Figure 4.4a, a "sanitation" effect at low incomes

FIGURE 4.4   (a) Engel curve for *H*. (b) Engel curve for *m*.

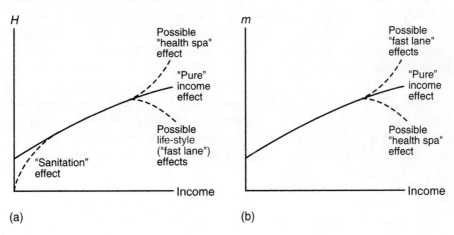

(a)   (b)

---

[6]Engel curves, a plot of income versus amount consumed, are named after the economist Ernst
Engel, to whom the development of the Engel curve is commonly attributed.

offers the possibility that health outcomes might rise very rapidly with initial improvements in income, as basic sanitary measures (e.g., water supply and vaccines) radically alter the conditions in which people live. This would be most pertinent, for example, in a poor rural village in a developing nation. In addition, we see a "life in the fast lane" effect, in which increasing consumption of X_B with higher income causes health to fall (Figure 4.4a) and medical expenses to increase even faster than the "pure" income effect would suggest (Figure 4.4b).

Figure 4.4 only hints at the many possible interactions of income and health. Some of them arise because changes in income alter the "external" production possibilities for health (e.g., public health measures). Others arise because of lifestyle choices and how they change with income. Other "external" and "internal" effects may work in the opposite direction. For example, increasing income (at the level of a society) may come only with an industrial process that generates more health hazards. Similarly, nothing says that higher income "lifestyle" effects have to be negative. Life in the fast lane might just as well be life in the health spa, so that higher income contributes more, not less, to the level of health, aside from the direct purchase of medical care.

FROM INDIFFERENCE CURVES TO DEMAND CURVES

The same sort of diagram can help us make an important shift, from indifference curves, showing how various combinations of H and X create utility, to demand curves, showing how the desired quantity of medical care (m) changes with its own price. Indifference curves, by their nature, are unobservable because we cannot measure utility. However, if consumers act according to the model portrayed by indifference curves, then we can infer something completely observable from this model, the standard demand curve, a plot of how much medical care people would consume at different prices. To do this, we use a standard technique. For a given level of illness (so the indifference curves are stable), we change the price of m (p_m), holding constant money income (I) and the price of other goods (p_x). In an indifference curve diagram such as the one shown in Figure 4.5a, *reducing p_m* means swinging the budget line outward, holding its intercept on the x-axis constant.[7] Increasing p_m would rotate the budget line in the other direction around the X-axis intercept.

---

[7]Here is an easy way to remember this: If the consumer spent everything on X, then the relevant part of the budget line would be where it intersected the X-axis because m would equal zero there. At that point, the price of m would be irrelevant, and the same amount of x would be consumed. By contrast, for the same money budget, if the consumer spent everything on m, purchasing power would be increased as p_m fell. Thus, more m could be purchased. In general, a change in p_m means a rotation of the budget line around the intercept on the X-axis of the indifference map.

FIGURE 4.5   (a) Lower price for m. (b) Demand curve for m. (c) Effect of income.

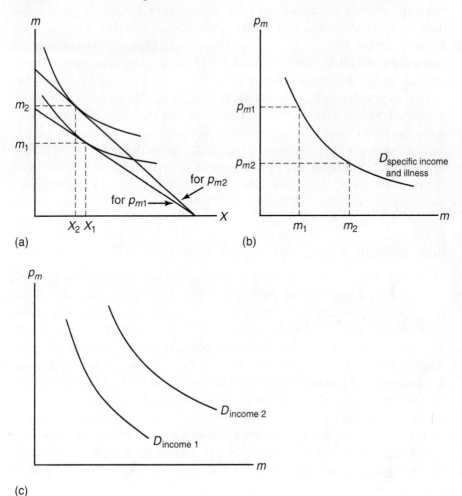

(a)

(b)

(c)

To trace out a demand curve, we simply vary p_m, holding everything else constant (in this case, income, p_x, and the illness level l), and see what amounts of m are chosen by the consumer. We begin with a particular value for p_m, for example, p_{m1}, which gives a particular value m_1 as the best choice. In the *demand curve* diagram, we can plot that combination of p_{m1} and m_1. Now decrease the price to p_{m2}, and find the matching amount consumed, m_2. Repeat the same process for every possible price to trace out the entire demand curve D shown in Figure 4.5b.

This demand curve is completely observable in the real world. Although it is derived from a fairly abstract utility theory, it offers an observable model of consumer behavior that (in concept) is refutable. Thus, the demand curve becomes one of the most important tools of the economist. If we had begun the entire process of tracing out the demand curve at some higher level of income, we would notice that at every price p_m we looked at, more m would be chosen at the higher income than at the lower income. As we trace out the demand curves for medical care, this would create a separate demand curve for each level of income a person might have. So long as health is a "normal" good (i.e., people want more of it as their income increases), demand curves associated with higher income will always lie to the northeast of demand curves associated with a lower income. Although it is common to portray such shifts as parallel, nothing requires this in general; the effects of income in shifting demand for medical care could differ considerably at different prices. Figure 4.5c shows how demand curves shift out as income rises, assuming that medical care is a "normal" good.

HOW DEMAND CURVES DEPEND ON ILLNESS EVENTS

The same theory of demand has the (commonsense) result built into it that people who are seriously sick will demand more medical care, other things being equal, than those who are less sick. The formal proof of this idea is somewhat messy, but the main idea appears in Figure 4.2. The bigger the illness event (larger ℓ), the more the health loss in Figure 4.2a and the flatter the indifference curves in Figure 4.2b become. As the slopes of the indifference curves change, the tangency (optimal consumption choice) must occur at a larger level of m, given a constant slope for the budget line.

In Figure 4.6, we can see a series of demand curves for various illness events. They represent a range from "normal health" (when the consumer would see a doctor perhaps only once a year), to a moderately serious automobile accident (emergency room visit, some X-rays, stitches, and a couple of

FIGURE 4.6 Demand curves for various illness events.

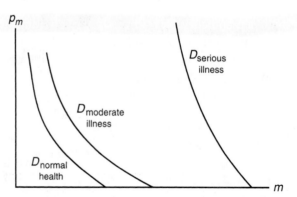

follow-up visits in the doctor's office), to a protracted bout with cancer (many diagnostic tests, surgery, therapy, etc.). Each of these demand curves also depends on the level of income. At a higher income, the demand curve associated with each event would sit somewhere to the right of those shown in Figure 4.6. Theory cannot tell us how much; empirical studies are needed to provide that information.

DEMAND CURVES FOR MANY MEDICAL SERVICES

The preceding discussion masks the idea that consumers have available not a single medical care service but a complex variety of such services. Again, although the formal theory is somewhat messier, the ideas to deal with such a world are in fact quite similar to those described here. The only adjustments we need to make are to recognize (1) that health can be affected by more than one type of medical care and (2) that various types of medical care can be either complements or substitutes. We discuss each of these ideas next.

Multiple Health Inputs

If multiple types of medical care affect health, then we need to write the production function for health as $H = g(m^1, m^2, \ldots, m^n)$, for the types of medical care available. Each type of medical care would then be demanded according to its marginal productivity, *given the amount of all other medical inputs* used. Each medical input would have its own demand curve, derived in the same way we have just seen for the single good m.

Complements or Substitutes?

One important question that appears when we consider more than one type of medical care is whether the various services are complements or substitutes. Complements are goods or services that are consumed together, and "help each other out" in producing health. Gasoline and tires are complements in the production of miles driven. Substitutes are just what they sound like: Using more of one allows use of less of the other in order to achieve the same result. Cars and airplanes are substitutes in the production of passenger transportation. Formally, we define medical care of various types as complements or substitutes based on behavior in response to price changes. If the amount of service m_i rises as the price p_j (the price of service m_j) rises, then the two goods are substitutes. If m_i falls as p_j rises, the two goods are complements. Because we expect m_j to fall as p_j rises (producing a downward-sloping demand curve), then saying that m_i and m_j are complements simply means that the use of both declines as p_j rises. In other words, their consumption patterns move together as the price of either one of them changes. Just the opposite happens if they are substitutes.

In health care, an important policy question was raised some time ago: Are hospital care and ambulatory care complements or substitutes? More generally, are preventive and acute medical care complements or substitutes? Among other things, the best design of health insurance packages depends on these relationships. If preventive and acute care are substitutes, then a "smart" health insurance program might encourage the use of preventive care, even though that care costs the insurer some money, because it would more than save that much with lower spending on acute medical care. (The same question arises with ambulatory care and hospital care.) The question first appeared in a provocative form: Was insurance that denied complete coverage for preventive/ambulatory care penny-wise but pound-foolish? Like other important features of the demand for medical care, theory alone cannot provide an answer. Empirical studies of the demand for care are needed to answer such a question. Chapter 5 summarizes the available evidence on these questions.

THE DEMAND CURVE FOR A SOCIETY: ADDING UP INDIVIDUAL DEMANDS

All of the discussion to date really centers on a single individual, but the transition from the individual to a larger group (society) is quite simple. The *aggregate* demand curve simply adds up *at each price* the quantities on each individual demand curve for every member of the society.[8] Figure 4.7 shows

FIGURE 4.7 Aggregate demand curve for a three-person society.

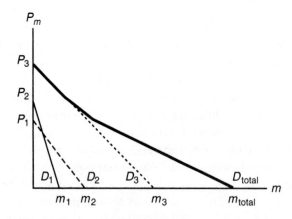

[8]This is called *horizontal aggregation* because of the economist's usual penchant for drawing demand curves with price on the vertical axis and quantity on the horizontal axis of a demand curve diagram. Adding things "horizontally" in such a diagram produces the correct picture.

such an aggregation for a three-person society, but it should be clear that the process can continue for as many members of society as are relevant. The demand curve called D_1 (the solid line) is for person 1, D_2 (the dashed line) is for person 2, and D_3 (the dotted line) is for person 3. The aggregate demand curve D_{total} adds up, at each possible price, the total quantities demanded. It coincides with D_3 at higher prices because only person 3 has any positive demand for m at prices higher than p_2. There is a kink in D_{total} at p_2, where person 1's demands begin to add in, and again at p_1, where person 2's demands begin to add in. At a price of $p = 0$, the total quantity demanded m_{total} would equal the sum of m_1, m_2, and m_3, the quantity-axis intercepts of each person in the society.

It is important to remember that the demand curves D_1 through D_3 all depend on the particular illness levels experienced by persons 1 through 3. Thus, because their demand curves would shift if their illnesses changed, so would society's demand curve D_{total}.

USE OF THE DEMAND CURVE TO MEASURE VALUE OF CARE
Marginal Value

The previous discussion shows how the quantity of medical care people demand is affected (for example) by price. Demand curves show this relationship, describing quantity as a function of price. They can also be "inverted" to describe the *incremental (marginal) value consumers attach to additional consumption of medical care* at any level of consumption observed. This is the *willingness to pay* interpretation of a demand curve. For this interpretation, one needs only to read the demand curve in the direction other than is normally done. Rather than say that the quantity demanded depends upon price (the interpretation given earlier), we can say equally well that the incremental value of consuming more m is equivalent to the consumer's willingness to pay for a bit more m. Just as the quantity demanded falls as the price increases (the first interpretation of the demand curve), we can also see that the marginal value to consumers (incremental willingness to pay) falls as the amount consumed rises. We call these curves *inverse demand curves* or *value curves*.

Inverse demand curves (willingness to pay) slope downward for two reasons: (1) the declining marginal productivity of medical care in producing health and (2) the decreasing marginal utility of H itself in producing utility. The first issue (diminishing marginal productivity of health care) would suffice to produce downward-sloping demand curves for an individual (see the discussion in Chapter 3 of the intensive margin) or for a society (see the discussion in Chapter 3 of the extensive margin). The second idea merely adds to the list of reasons why demand curves would slope downward. Empirically, we could separate out one concept from the other if we could accurately measure $g'(m)$ for each level of m consumed.

We can extend the same idea one step further by noting that the *total value to consumers of using a certain amount of medical care is the area under the demand curve.* It may be useful to think in specific terms, such as the demand for having one's teeth cleaned and inspected (Figure 4.8). Suppose the first dental visit each year created $100 in value to the consumer (better looking teeth, reduced concern about cavities, etc.). If the visit cost $30, the consumer would get $70 in *consumer surplus* out of that visit. A second visit per year (i.e., at 6-month intervals) might create a further $75 in value, again costing $30 and $45 in consumer surplus. A third visit per year (every 4 months) might create a marginal value of $35 and a consumer surplus of only $5. A fourth visit per year would create only $20 in marginal value and would cost $30. No intelligent consumer would do this because it would cost more than it was worth for the fourth visit each year. We should observe three visits by such a consumer each year, unless some illness event (cavities or a broken tooth) caused other visits.

Two ideas appear in this discussion. First, demand curves can tell us how to predict quantities consumed. Intelligent decision making will continue to expand the amount consumed until the marginal value received just equals the marginal cost of the service. (In the case of the dental visits, we don't quite achieve "equality" because we described the incremental value of dental visits as a lumpy step function, dropping from $100 to $75 to $35 to $20 visits, and the cost was described as $30.)

FIGURE 4.8   Consumer surplus for dental visits.

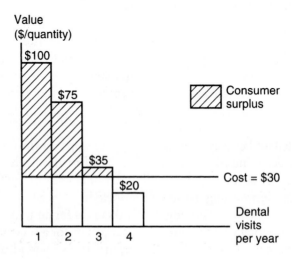

TABLE 4.1   CONSUMER SURPLUS FOR DENTAL VISITS
(Fictitious Data)

Quantity Consumed per Year	Incremental Value of Care ($)	Net Value of This Visit with $30 Cost ($)	Total Net Value (Consumer Surplus) ($)
1	100	70	70
2	75	45	115
3	35	5	120
4	20	−10	110

The second concept is that of *total consumer surplus* to the consumer from having a specific number of dental visits each year. As noted, intelligent planning would stop after the third visit each year. Total consumer surplus sums up all of the extra value to consumers (beyond the costs paid) for each unit of care consumed. Figure 4.8 shows how this would look for the dental visits described here, and Table 4.1 shows the same data numerically. It is easy to prove that consumer surplus is maximized by a simple rule: Expand the use of the service until the marginal benefit has just fallen to match the marginal cost. In this case, at the third visit per year, the marginal benefit has fallen to $35, the marginal cost is $30 per visit, and stopping at that rate of visits maximizes consumer surplus, as the last column of Table 4.1 shows.

Of course, the type of "incremental value" data shown in Figure 4.8 and Table 4.1 is just a lumpy version of a demand curve. One could easily draw a smooth line through the midpoints of the tops of each of the bars in Figure 4.8 and call it a demand curve; adding up such curves across many individuals would smooth things out even more.

HOW INSURANCE AFFECTS A DEMAND CURVE FOR MEDICAL CARE

We now come to one of the key ideas in all of health economics: Health insurance is usually structured in such a way that it reduces the price consumers pay at the time they purchase medical care. *Health insurance lowers effective prices.* If medical care obeys the normal laws of economics, providing people with a health insurance policy should increase their use of medical care. (The major function of insurance is to reduce financial risk. The mechanism of doing that—lowering the price of medical care—produces a side effect of increased medical care use. Chapter 10 discusses the demand for health insurance in detail.) Health insurance can be structured in numerous ways, but several standard features appear in many policies, and understanding how they work and how they affect demand for medical care provides important insight into many health policy issues. The typical features are (1) copayments, (2) deductibles, and (3) upper limits on coverage. Following is a discussion of each.

Copayments

A copayment is simply a sharing arrangement between the consumer and the insurance company, specified in the insurance contract. When the consumer spends money on medical care, the insurance company pays some of it and the consumer the remainder (the copayment). Copayments come in three traditional forms, a proportional *coinsurance rate* and a flat *indemnity payment* by the insurance company, or a fixed dollar consumer-copay. The last of these is easy to analyze because the copay *is* the price, and the quantity consumed is simply the relevant quantity on the demand curve. The other arrangements require more analysis to understand.

Coinsurance Rate In a *coinsurance* arrangement, the consumer pays some fraction of a medical bill (such as 20 percent or 25 percent, sometimes 50 percent in dental insurance), and the insurance company pays the remainder. If we call the consumer's copayment share C, then the insurance company pays a share $(1 - C)$. Using the methods of demand theory previously developed, we can now see precisely how coinsurance-based insurance plans alter consumer choices for medical care.

Figure 4.9 shows a consumer's demand curve for a particular illness, *without any insurance*. Suppose the price of care is p_{m1}. If the consumer has

FIGURE 4.9 Consumer's demand curve with a particular illness.

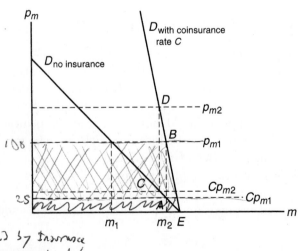

{handwritten:} $C(m, -P_m, : P_{m})$ by Insurance
{handwritten:} $C(pm, - m : $ Out by patient/consumer

an insurance plan that pays $(1 - C)$ percent of all medical bills, then the effective price of medical care has fallen to Cp_{m1} when the consumer seeks medical care. To construct the consumer's demand curve with this insurance policy in place, find the quantity demanded at Cp_{m1} (point A in Figure 4.9). This is the quantity demanded at p_{m1} with the copayment insurance policy in place. Thus, on the insured person's demand curve, we can place the point B at the same quantity of point A, but at the price p_{m1}. Now do the same thing at some higher price p_{m2}, producing the point C on the original demand curve and the point D on the insured demand curve. The points B and D begin to trace out the insured demand curve. Another point (which is easy to find) is where the original demand curve shows $p_m = 0$. When p_m equals 0, Cp_m also equals zero, so the quantities consumed are the same at a zero market price with or without insurance (point E). Thus, at least as a first approximation, we know that a coinsurance-type plan must go through the same quantity-axis intercept as the uninsured demand curve.

The effect on quantities consumed comes by comparing quantities demanded on these two demand curves (insured versus uninsured) at a specific market price such as p_{m1}. In Figure 4.9, the uninsured person will consume m_1 at market price p_{m1}. The same person, with the coinsurance policy in place, will consume m_2 at a market price p_{m1}.

More generally, we can expect that the effect of a coinsurance plan will always be found by *rotating* the insured demand curve clockwise around the quantity-axis intercept of the uninsured demand curve. The smaller the coinsurance-rate C, the larger the rotation. At the extreme ($C = 0$, or full coverage by the insurer), the demand curve is a vertical line (slope equal to infinity). If quantity were on the vertical axis and price on the horizontal axis, the slope would become zero because the graph would show a flat line. In this case, no matter what the market price, the consumer will always consume the same amount because the insurance plan pays all costs when $C = 0$. In a straight-line demand curve, the slope of the demand curve is related to the "uninsured" demand curve in the following simple way: For a coinsurance rate of C, where the slope dp/dm of the uninsured demand curve is β, the insured demand curve has a slope of β divided by C. Thus, for example, if C equals 0.2, then the slope would become five times as great. (Graphed the other way around, the slope dm/dp would become C times its original slope.)

The insurance policy also makes the demand curve less elastic in general (when evaluated at the same price). The elasticity of a demand curve describes the percentage change in quantity arising from a 1 percent change in price. (See Box 4.1 for a summary discussion of the concept of demand elasticities.) When $C = 0$, the elasticity is zero, which is another way of saying that the consumer ignores price in making decisions about purchasing medical care. In the case of linear demand curves, there is no simple relationship between the uninsured and insured elasticities, except to say that, at the same market price, insured-demand curve elasticities fall steadily toward zero as C falls toward zero.[9]

The appendix to this chapter proves that the elasticity with respect to coinsurance equals the elasticity with respect to price—no surprise because coinsurance acts to change price, and the net price *is* C times the market price. Thus, for example, if demand falls 5 percent for a 10 percent increase in price, say from $p_m = \$20$ to $p_m = \$22$ ($\eta = -0.5$), then demand will also fall 5 percent for a 10 percent increase in the coinsurance rate, such as from $C = 0.4$ to $C = 0.44$. If the price elasticity is -0.1, then the elasticity of quantity demanded with respect to the coinsurance rate is also -0.1.

We must remember that demand curves such as those derived in Figure 4.9 (and similarly for Figure 4.10) show two important aspects of *behavior*, but they should not be treated as *marginal value* curves in the sense described in a preceding section. They describe both changes in quantities consumed and also the changes in price responsiveness created by the insurance, but

FIGURE 4.10 The effect of an indemnity plan on consumer demand.

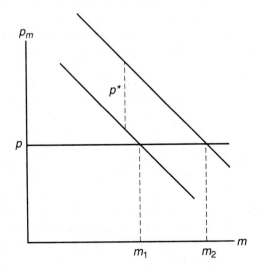

[9]For linear demand curves, the relationship is rather odd looking: Evaluated at the same price, the elasticity on the insured demand curve (η_c) is related to the elasticity on the uninsured demand curve (η) by the formula $\eta_c = C\eta/[1 - (1 - C)\eta]$. For small values of η, this means that η_c is approximately equal to $C\eta$. For example, if the uninsured elasticity is -0.2 and the coinsurance rate is 0.25, then the exact calculation for the insured elasticity is -0.043, and the approximation is -0.05 (about a 15 percent error). The approximation works even better for larger values of C. For the same initial value of η and $C = 0.5$, the approximation is -0.1 and the exact value is $-0.90909\ldots$ (about a 9 percent error).

BOX 4.1   ELASTICITIES OF DEMAND CURVES

A demand curve shows the relationship between quantities demanded by consumers and the price, holding constant all other relevant economic variables. The *slope* of the demand curve tells the rate of change in quantity (q) as the price (p) changes. Suppose we have two observations on a demand curve, (q_1, p_1) and (q_2, p_2), where something has caused the price to change and we can observe the change in quantity demanded. Define the change in q as $\Delta q = q_2 - q_1$ and the change in p as $\Delta p = p_2 - p_1$. The rate of change in q as p changes is then $\Delta q/\Delta p$. [If we allow the change to become very small, using calculus techniques, we would define the rate of change at any point as dq/dp, the first derivative of the demand curve $q = f(p)$.]

The *elasticity* of a demand curve is another measure of the rate at which quantity changes as price changes. The advantage of elasticities is that they are scale free, so you don't need to know how quantity and price were measured to understand the information. For example, quantity could be measured in doctor visits per 100 persons per year or doctor visits per 1,000 persons per month. Changes in that measure as the price changed—the *slope* of the demand curve—would depend on how quantity was measured. To "descale" slope measures, we simply put everything in proportional terms. That is, instead of asking how quantity changes with price ($\Delta q/\Delta p$), we ask what the *percentage* change in quantity (% Δq) is in response to a percentage change in price (% Δp). That's all an elasticity is—a ratio of % Δq to % Δp.

Economists commonly use the Greek letter η (eta) to describe a demand elasticity; we follow that convention here. When we can meaningfully treat the data as having come from a demand curve of the form $q = f(p)$, with a slope $\Delta q/\Delta p$, the elasticity is defined as $\eta = (\Delta q/q)/(\Delta p/p) = \%\ \Delta q/\%\ \Delta p$. Each variable (quantity and price) is "normalized" to its own value, which makes the elasticity scale free. (It has the dimension of a pure number, whereas a slope has the dimension of quantity/price.) Notice that the elasticity commonly will change as you move along a demand curve, so a carefully defined elasticity will also report the range of data (quantity, or price, or both) to which it pertains.

The distinction between slopes and elasticities is important because the language economists use has particular meaning in each case. Begin with a simple straight line demand curve such as shown in Figure A. This curve has a *constant* slope because it's a straight line. In this case, the slope is -1 because the price falls by 1 unit for each 1 unit the quantity increases. The elasticity changes as you move along this curve. At a quantity of 5 units of care, the relevant price is 15 and the elasticity is $(\Delta m/\Delta p)(p/m) = -1/(15/5) = -3$. At a quantity of 10 units, the price and quantity are both 10 and the elasticity is -1. At a quantity of 15 units, the price on the demand curve is 5 and the elasticity is $-1/(5/15) = -1/3$. This generally holds for straight-line demand curves; the elasticity increases as you slide up the demand curve.

(continued)

BOX 4.1 ELASTICITIES OF DEMAND CURVES (continued)

FIGURE A

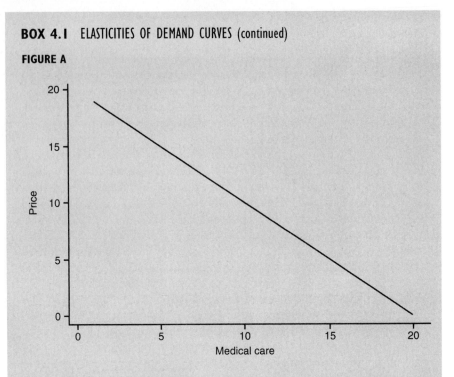

Figure B shows a different type of demand curve, one that's really "curved," and in this case in a particular way. The elasticity is constant all along the demand curve at $\eta = -1$. Here, the *slope* changes constantly, but the elasticity stays the same as you slide along the demand curve.

Figure C demonstrates a separate issue: how elasticities change for demand curves of similar "slope" but where one illness is more severe (and, hence, quantities demanded at any price are larger) than for the other. In this case, demand for the serious illness is always 30 units more than in the case of the mild illness. At the price of 10 (where quantity is also 10 in the mild-illness demand curve), the elasticity is -1. On the demand curve for the serious illness, the slope is the same (-1), but at the same price, the quantity is 40, not 10. This makes the demand elasticity at that price equal to -0.25 a quarter as large. Although the demand is changing at the same rate (reflected by the slope $\Delta m/\Delta p$), the *proportional change* in demand is smaller in the second case because the quantity demanded is larger.

Figure D shows a similar phenomenon with constant-elasticity demand curves (both with elasticities of -1). The serious illness has quantities demanded at every price that are exactly five times the amount demanded for the mild illness. At any price, the quantity is one-fifth as large in the mild-illness case, and the slope (remember, the relevant slope is $\Delta m/\Delta p$) is five times as large. Thus, both demand curves have the same elasticity everywhere.

FIGURE B

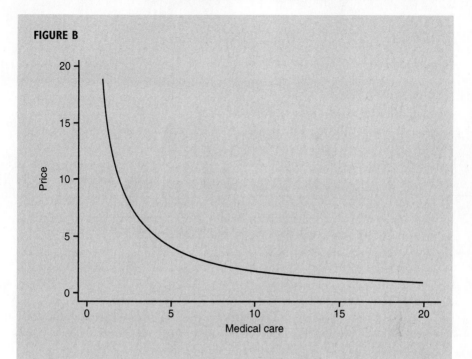

FIGURE C

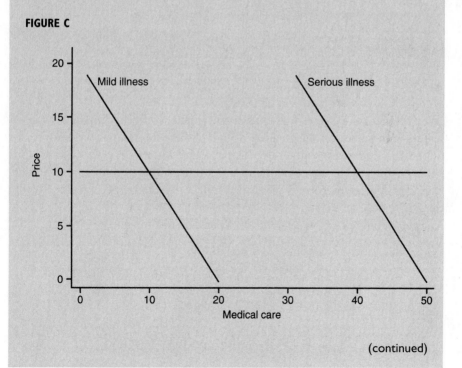

(continued)

BOX 4.1 ELASTICITIES OF DEMAND CURVES (continued)

FIGURE D

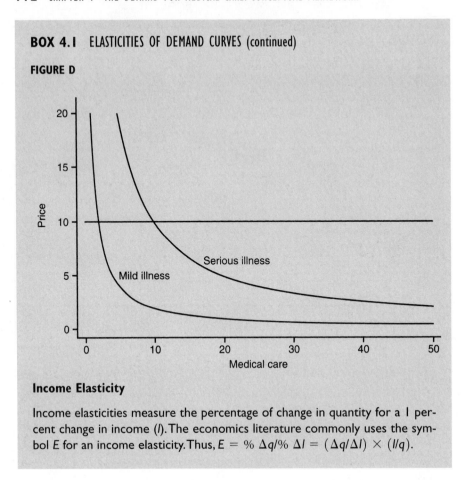

Income Elasticity

Income elasticities measure the percentage of change in quantity for a 1 percent change in income (I). The economics literature commonly uses the symbol E for an income elasticity. Thus, $E = \%\ \Delta q / \%\ \Delta I = (\Delta q / \Delta I) \times (I/q)$.

since the insurance does not change the intrinsic effect of medical care on health, and, hence, on the creation of utility, these demand curves should not be used to determine value to the consumer. *Consumer surplus* calculations should always be made using the original uninsured demand curves, understanding that the quantities consumed reflect the altered price created by the insurance policy.

One final technical addendum bears mentioning here. The demand curves just described must also be shifted inward to account for the income effects of the insurance premium. Suppose the premium costs $R per year. Paying for the insurance policy at the beginning of the year reduces the consumer's income by $R for the year. Thus, demand curves for every good, including medical care services, must be shifted inward to account for the reduced income. (See the previous discussion about income effects.) Put differently, the demand curves must all be calculated for an income of $I - R$, instead of an income I, once the consumer has committed to buy the insurance policy.[10] Of course, if the effects of income on medical care use are small, such an adjustment would be small, and perhaps best ignored empirically.

Indemnity Insurance The second form of copayment, a flat *indemnity* payment, is less common than coinsurancelike plans. Quite simply, an indemnity plan pays the consumer a flat amount for each medical service consumed, with the amount preestablished in the insurance contract. Some hospital insurance policies do this, for example, by paying to the insured person some specific amount, such as $500 per day in the hospital. Their effect on demand for care is easy to describe using our standard models. Suppose the insurance plan specifies that p^* will be paid each time the consumer uses a particular medical service. Then the consumer's demand curve just shifts upward by p^* for every possible quantity consumed. Figure 4.10 shows this arrangement. The quantity consumed with no insurance is m_1; with the indemnity plan paying p^* per unit, the quantity consumed is m_2.

Deductibles

Deductibles are a common feature of many insurance plans, both in health insurance and elsewhere. A deductible is some fixed amount—for example, $150—that the consumer must pay toward medical bills each year before any insurance payments are made. The deductible can be any size (ranging from $25 or $50 in some plans to more than $1,000 in others). The idea is to not bother insuring "small" losses and to save insurance costs in return.

The effect of a deductible on the demand curve is quite complicated, and depends on the degree of illness severity (i.e., how far out the demand curve is shifted by the illness) in relationship to the size of the deductible. Figure 4.11 shows the effect of a deductible on the apparent price of care, dropping the price to 20 percent of its normal level after a deductible of size $\mathbf{D}$ has been met, where $\mathbf{D} = pm^*$ (where m^* is the quantity such that buying just that amount of medical care at a price of p leads to an expenditure of amount $\mathbf{D}$).[11] The 20 percent is arbitrary, but is a common feature of many "major

---

[10]Chapter 10 describes modifications to this picture when the insurance is provided through an employment-related work group, and how such insurance premiums (such as R) are formed.

[11]Of course, if the price were higher, the amount of medical care needed to exceed the deductible would fall. The mathematically astute reader can draw a rectangular hyperbole of the form $\mathbf{D} = p \times m$ that will show the combinations of p and m that create just enough expenditure to satisfy the deductible. Once p is known, then a given m (such as m^* in the figure) satisfies the deductible.

FIGURE 4.11 The effect of a deductible on consumer demand.

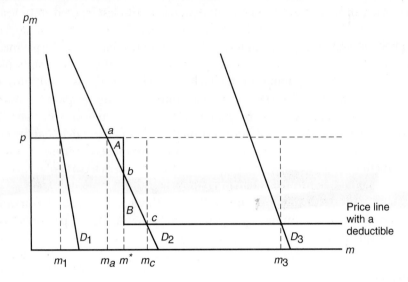

medical" insurance policies. It could be any coinsurance rate after the deductible is met, including $C = 0$. As we shall learn in Chapter 12, Medicare's "Part B" insurance for physician services for the elderly has a 20 percent copayment once a deductible of a given size has been reached, $135 in the case of Medicare in 2008 (and indexed annually).

Consider first the demand curve for a mild illness, D_1, that cuts the kinked price line to the left of the kink. For an illness of this size, the deductible has no effect. The quantity demanded is m_1, just as if the consumer had no insurance policy. Next consider the demand curve D_3 for a very serious illness, cutting the new price line considerably to the right of the kink. Here the situation is just as if the consumer had an insurance policy paying 80 percent of the care, just as in Figure 4.9. The consumer will purchase the amount m_3, where the demand curve D_3 crosses the new price line (at 20 percent of the market price). In both of these cases, the quantity demanded is chosen by finding the intersection of the demand curve with the price schedule.

But demand curve D_2 in Figure 4.11 is tricky! It cuts the price schedule at three places, labeled a, b, and c. Which reflects the amount that the consumer will rationally demand? The answer depends on the sizes of the triangles A and B, representing areas of consumer surplus. (Review the discussion around Figure 4.8.) Suppose the consumer stopped at point m_a, and received the commensurate amount of consumer surplus between the price line P and the demand curve D_2 out to the point m_a. Now think about expanding consumption out to quantity m_b, consuming exactly m^* of medical care. (Remember, m^* is the amount that just leads to an expenditure of **D** at the

price p.) The consumer would automatically lose the area of consumer surplus of triangle A by making such a move, so it would always be irrational.
What if the consumer were to continue increasing the amount of medical
care until point c, where the demand curve intersects $0.2P$ and the quantity
consumed is m_c? The consumer would then gain back a consumer surplus
triangle of size B. Whether it was intelligent to consume m_c or m_a would
depend on the relative sizes of triangles A and B. If $B > A$, then m_c creates
more well-being than m_a (and vice versa). So, the consumer will consume
either at m_a or m_c, but never at m^*.[12] Figure 4.11 is drawn such that the area
of triangle B exceeds that of triangle A, so the consumer's best choice here is
to consume m_c, essentially ignoring the presence of the deductible.[13]

Alas, life is not quite so simple if one wants really to understand the
effects of an insurance policy with an annual deductible because the
deductible accumulates over more than one illness episode. A simple example
explains the problem more fully. Suppose the consumer has an insurance
policy with an annual deductible of $200, beginning January 1. On February
15, the consumer becomes ill after a lovely Valentine's Day dinner with a date,
perhaps from food poisoning. A trip to the doctor and some laboratory tests
($75) relieve the anxiety about the problem, which gets better. For that ill-
ness, the consumer receives no insurance payment. However, for any future
illnesses during the year, the consumer has an insurance plan with only $125
remaining on the deductible. Thus, the visit to the doctor produced not only
the direct benefit of treatment but also the added benefit of "trading in" the
$200 deductible insurance plan for a $125 deductible plan. The economic
value of that bonus (the "improved" insurance plan) acts as an offset to the
$75 cost of the doctor visit. In a complicated fashion, the "apparent price"
facing the patient falls as total spending gets nearer to the deductible amount,
but the rate at which this happens varies with the time of year. (It doesn't do
much good to spend your way past a deductible on December 28 if a new
deductible starts up again on January 1.)

However, the clear effect of a deductible remains: Demand for care
should resemble demand from an uninsured consumer for small illness
events and be similar to demand from an insured consumer for large illness
events. The overall effect on demand remains an empirical issue, which we

---

[12]There is, of course, one situation in which consuming m^* would be rational—when the illness level was such that the demand curve just touched the kink in the price line at m^* as the single point of intersection between the price line and the demand curve for that particular illness.

[13]Even this is not technically correct, but it is "nearly so." The expenditure represented by the
deductible **D** reduces income available for all other goods and services, so all demand curves,
including those for medical care, shift inward slightly because of this small income effect. But
the effect is so small as to be trivial in the real world, and can safely be ignored.

discuss in the next chapter in more detail. For a more complete discussion of this problem, see Keeler, Newhouse, and Phelps (1977).

Maximum Payment Limits

Some insurance plans also have a cap on the amount the insurance company will pay. Early hospital plans put this cap at 30 hospital days, after which the consumer was uninsured. Many "major medical" insurance plans also put a cap on total spending, such as $100,000 per year and $300,000 for a lifetime.

The effects of a cap on insurance are the reverse of a deductible—they make really serious medical events "uninsured." Because of this, one might think that this would be a very unpopular insurance plan, but they were quite common in the past. (See Chapter 10 for discussion.) Many private insurance plans now have a "stop-loss" feature that places an upper limit on out-of-pocket spending by the consumer, even if there are copayments for some care.

Mixed-Bag Insurance

Many insurance plans pay some constant percent of all medical bills above a deductible (such as $150 per year). "Major medical" insurance plans commonly have this feature. Some insurance plans pay with some combination of indemnity and coinsurance. An important example of this is Medicare Part B, which pays for physician services for Medicare enrollees. That plan pays 80 percent of a physician's bills (above an indexed annual deductible), but *only if the physician's fee is no higher than a predetermined amount,* such as $40 per visit. (The amount varies by region and type of service provided.) If this occurs, Medicare Part B pays 80 percent of the maximum fee. In the example, it would pay 80 percent of $40 ($32). Thus, Medicare Part B combines a 20 percent coinsurance plan and an indemnity plan.

TIME COSTS AND TRAVEL COSTS

We should also recognize the role of time as a "cost" of acquiring medical care. As with any service, medical care requires the presence of the patient. (Why do you think we're called "patients" while we're waiting for the doctor?) Travel to and from the doctor also creates costs, both in time and the direct travel costs.

The appropriate "value" of time to use in calculating the "time cost" of medical care can become quite complicated. For a working person on an hourly wage rate with no sick leave available, the cost of going to the doctor during the workday is obviously equal to the wage rate. If the person earns

$20 an hour and it takes 2 hours to see the doctor, he or she has lost $40 in wages, and the "time cost" of the doctor visit is $40. If that person has a generous sick-leave policy at work, the time cost may be much smaller, if not zero. For persons not working directly in the labor market (such as a homemaker), there is still a related time cost—the value of that person's time in the household. Because most persons working in a household setting have the opportunity to work in the labor market, we can infer that their time is more valuable to them in the home than their best market opportunity because they have chosen the home, rather than the labor market, as their place of work. Thus, their time is worth *at least* as much as their market opportunity wage, and medical care visits have a time cost proportional to that amount. Of course, persons working in the household setting don't have anything resembling the sick leave that an employed person might have, so they bear the brunt of any time costs incurred.

Time costs act just as money costs do in affecting demand for medical care. If time costs rise (either because the actual time spent rises or the value of time rises), then demand for medical care falls. Sick leave from places of employment plays the same role for time costs as health insurance does for money costs. The better the sick leave policy (the better the insurance), the more medical care use we should expect.

As with other aspects of the demand for medical care, we must turn to empirical studies to determine the importance of time costs in affecting demand for care.

Waiting (Delay to Appointment)

A separate type of "waiting" occurs often in health care systems (including market-based systems such as the United States and government-operated systems such as the British National Health Service)—delays to appointment. In concept, delays to appointment differ from pure "waiting time" (say, in a doctor's office) because the patient's time is available for other activities during the delay, at least in some cases.

However, systematic delays can serve to reduce demand for medical care. The mechanism in play here does not rely so much on the opportunity cost of time (which is the issue in actual waiting times) but rather on the fact that the value of the medical intervention may change through time. In some cases, illnesses heal spontaneously, so treatment becomes moot. Treatment for common colds, for example, almost always falls into this situation. The common aphorism says that it takes a week to get over a cold if you see a doctor, and seven days if you don't. So if you can't get an appointment to see a doctor for at least a week, the delay to appointment serves to reduce your demand for physician services.

At the extreme form (and this matters with more than trivial frequency in such settings as the British and Canadian health systems), the delays for treatment are so long that the patient dies of the illness before treatment is rendered. Recognizing this, some patients in these health care systems "opt out of the queue" by purchasing health care elsewhere. In many cities along the common border between the United States and Canada, for example, a good number of patients seeking hospital-based treatment come from Canadian cities across the border, with the patients choosing to pay out of pocket for the private care in the United States rather than waiting for (insured) treatment within their own health care system.

For a more extensive discussion of queues and waiting delays, see Cullis, Jones, and Propper (2000).

THE ROLE OF QUALITY IN THE DEMAND FOR CARE

Quality of care has (at least) two important facets. First, medical care "quality" assesses how well the medical care produces outcomes of improved health. Thus, *quality of care* has to do with whether the medical intervention was appropriately selected and properly carried out. In an office visit to a doctor, for example, consumers may judge this quality by assessing the training of the doctor (good medical school? board certified? relevant subspecialty training?) or the time the doctor spends with the patient.

Consumers also place value on the amenities associated with medical care because they must participate in each step along the way. In a doctor's office, this may mean that the office is neat and orderly, the magazine supply is refreshed more than occasionally, and the air conditioning works in the summer. In a hospital, the quality and diversity of the food, the quality of the TV reception, and the friendliness of the staff—in short, the "hotel" aspects of the hospital—are important aspects of this type of quality. Consumers should value both types of quality, although they may be able to judge the latter much better than the former. (We will return to the question of how consumers can infer the technical quality of care when we discuss licensure of physicians and other healers in Chapter 15.)

Thus, when we say that a consumer has a willingness to pay $X for an office visit to a doctor, we must be certain to specify the quality of care. Perhaps the most useful idea (which resurfaces later in our studies of hospital behavior more directly) is that we can actually construct an entire *family* of demand curves for medical care, each "member" of the family representing a different quality. If we think of these as willingness-to-pay curves, the idea becomes quite clear. At each quantity consumed, the rational consumer's willingness to pay will increase with quality. Thus, if we "index" demand curves on the basis of quality, the family of demand curves has a very clear structure: The higher up the demand curves sit (the higher willingness to pay), the higher the quality. Figure 4.12 shows a set of three demand curves for medical care (m), at three levels of quality, so that Quality 3 > Quality 2 > Quality 1, and so on.

We could define *quality* tautologically as those features of medical care (aside from quantity) that lead consumers to pay more.[14] Fortunately, we can avoid this approach, at least partly, in medical care by noting that quality can denote, in part at least, the efficiency with which medical inputs produce health. Thus, for example, if more highly trained providers such as medical specialists produce health with greater precision or certainty than do lower trained providers, we can truly say that the more highly trained providers have higher quality. Of course, some aspects of quality remain subjective, such as the bedside manner of a provider, but quality does have real and measurable meaning in health care, and we should expect that an informed consumer would be willing to pay more for higher quality care.

Quality can be measured directly in ways that have importance to consumers, and (as we might expect) consumers react to such information when it becomes available. A good example has occurred in New York State, where the Department of Health (NYSDOH) began publishing (in the 1990s) mortality rates for doctors and hospitals doing open heart surgery (a *very* relevant

FIGURE 4.12   Quality and demand curves.

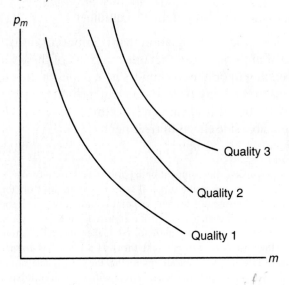

---

[14]The old real estate joke reflects on this: "If a 'house with a view' and a 'house with no view,' otherwise the same, sell for the same price, then the 'house with a view' has no view."

indicator of quality of care if you are thinking about having the surgery!). The NYSDOH reports carefully adjust for information known about the patients' underlying severity of illness, so they report "adjusted" mortality measures that (to their best ability) give prospective patients exactly the information they want: "What are the survival odds for a patient like me?"

Doctors and hospitals initially complained when the study was first released that the "best" hospitals appeared to have the worst outcomes because of the selection of the "best" hospitals by patients who are the sickest and have the most complicated illnesses. However, once the risk adjustments were completed, some important differences persisted across hospitals and doctors. Perhaps most importantly for our purposes, the NYSDOH publishes (and widely publicizes) these measures annually. How do patients respond?

In an analysis of these data, two important results emerged. First, patients did indeed shift their treatment choices away from the poorer and toward the better doctors and hospitals (as measured by survival rates) (Mukamel and Mushlin, 1998). Indeed, a 1 percentage point improvement in mortality rates led to a 7 percent increase in market share. Furthermore, the market responded by having higher prices for the better outcomes, with prices increasing on average by $250 for each percentage point improvement in mortality.[15] Second, and quite remarkably, the overall state mortality data improved considerably as doctors and hospitals all worked to improve their outcomes in the harsh glare of public information about mortality outcomes.

Patients' Beliefs and the (Un)Informed Consumer

Figure 4.12 has another interpretation that is important in later discussions about the role of physicians. It is that one can think of these various demand curves as depending upon the consumer's *perceptions* of the quality, productivity, or general desirability of medical care, including both general beliefs about the efficacy of medical care and treatment-specific beliefs about the benefits and possible side effects of treatment.

---

[15]This result implies considerable competition by price. The typical cardiac surgery patient is elderly, and has (if not harmed by the surgery) an expected life span of (for discussion purposes) 10 years. Thus a decrease of 1 percentage point in mortality creates about 0.1 "expected life-years." (The idea doesn't change much if life expectancy is 5 or 15 years.) This implies a cost per life-year to the patient (paying more for the higher quality) of about $2,500 per life-year, a remarkably low cost. (Compare this with the costs per life-year for many medical interventions as shown in Table 3.1!) This result implies that the price is determined mostly by costs of supplying the services, and does not reflect any significant markup that monopoly power would permit. At the extreme of things, a pure discriminating monopolist could extract all of the extra value of the lower mortality risk with higher prices, but that clearly has not happened in the New York cardiac surgery markets.

Some patients come from families and backgrounds that hold distinctive views about the general efficacy of medical care. Those who strongly believe that medical care is highly efficacious tend to have a higher willingness to pay (marked by curves such as those labeled "Quality 2" and "Quality 3" in Figure 4.12). In contrast, those who distrust medical treatment in general have a lower willingness to pay (marked by a curve such as the lowest one in Figure 4.12). Some religious beliefs, such as those held by Christian Scientists, alter general patterns of medical care use, while others, such as treatment-specific beliefs held by members of the Jehovah's Witness faith, strongly affect demand for care. (The beliefs of Jehovah's Witnesses forbid the use of blood transfusions.)

One can also consider patients' beliefs about specific therapies. Think for a moment, for example, about a dentist's characterization of a root canal procedure. If the procedure is described as nearly painless and promises continued functional use of and desirable aesthetic appearance of a tooth that will otherwise become discolored and eventually die (and have to be removed), then a root canal will seem more desirable (higher willingness to pay). Alternatively, if the dentist describes the outcome more cautiously ("we can probably save the tooth") and emphasizes the possible unpleasantries of the procedure ("it's quite uncomfortable for many people"), then the demand will be lower.

A key point here is that, particularly for specific treatments, patients will likely get much (if not all) of the relevant information they have from the provider who will perform the treatment (if the patient agrees to receive it). In any such case, when the "advisor" also provides the treatment, an economic incentive arises for the provider to deceive the patient, increasing the patient's demand and hence willingness to pay for treatment. This problem, known as "induced demand" in the medical economics literature, is discussed more fully in Chapter 7.

REVISITED: THE PRICE INDEX FOR HEALTH CARE

Chapter 1 shows the path of medical care prices through time, but notes that a major problem persists with the changes in quality that have occurred through the last half century. *Now is a good time to reread Box 1.1, showing how changes in quality of care (and hence in willingness to pay) can affect one's interpretation of the welfare effects of a price increase on consumer surplus.* Quality matters, and the failure to take quality improvements into consideration can badly distort one's understanding of how consumers have been made better or worse off by changes in health care.

A few recent studies on the costs of treating particular illnesses suggest that, in fact, when quality adjustments are taken into account, the costs of health care are falling, not rising through time. This conclusion emerged both from analysis of treatment of heart disease (Cutler et al., 1998) and treatment of depression (Frank, Berndt, and Busch, 1999): Costs of treating these illnesses have actually fallen through time, in striking contrast to the portrait of ever-rising medical prices shown in Chapter 1.

An early analyst of health care economics (Reuben Kessel, University of Chicago's Graduate School of Business in the 1960s and 1970s) put the issue very clearly. Updating his remarks to the current era, he often asked: "Would you rather have 1950s medicine at 1950s prices or 2000 medicine at 2000 prices?" The usual answer to his question was "I'd rather have current medical care at current prices," which implies that consumers are better off, despite the "inflation" that has occurred in health care. Most readers of this textbook probably cannot envision what health care in the 1950s, let alone the 1970s or perhaps even the early 1990s, was like, but a quick review of most of the major health care activities in the early twenty-first century would reveal that few of these were available even as recently as 1975, including (among others) CT and MRI diagnostic scanning devices, organ transplants, medications to control hypertension and cholesterol, most current cancer therapies, open heart surgery and angioplasty to open clogged coronary arteries, hip and knee replacements, and laser correction of vision to avoid use of eyeglasses. The newly evolving molecular and gene therapies will likely make even these interventions seem crude by comparison, although they will surely add to the total health care spending bill.

SUMMARY

The demand for medical care derives from the more fundamental demand for health itself, which produces utility. As long as medical care helps to augment health (for example, by restoring the health of a sick person), rational decision making will create systematic demand curves for medical care by individuals. These demand curves slope downward, so that less care is demanded at higher prices, other things held equal. More serious illnesses shift the demand curves for medical care outward, so that (other things held equal) more medical care is demanded by people who are sick than by those who are well. Income (among other things) also causes the demand curves for medical care to shift outward, so that (at constant prices) people with more income buy more medical care. This relationship can be confounded seriously (perhaps *incredibly* would be a better word) by such things as the patterns of consumption (X_G, X_B, etc.), loss of income with illness, and other factors. At the societal rather than individual level, the relationship is further confused by such things as pollution and industrial accidents, "byproducts" of industrialization that can create more income, but which can also cause poor health.

Insurance coverage generally acts in some way to reduce the price of medical care, although the explicit mechanisms are diverse. Standard economic models are useful in analyzing the effects of insurance on quantities of medical care demanded.

RELATED CHAPTERS IN *HANDBOOK OF HEALTH ECONOMICS*

Chapter 7, "The Human Capital Model" by Michael Grossman
Chapter 10, "Insurance Reimbursement" by Mark V. Pauly

PROBLEMS

1. For a specific consumer and for a specific illness, draw the demand curve for medical care without insurance. Then carefully draw the demand curve for the same person and illness when the person has an insurance policy that pays (1) for 50 percent of all medical costs and (2) for 100 percent.

2. Describe the effect on demand curves for office visits to a physician when an insurance policy pays a flat amount, for example, $25, per doctor visit.

3. For a single consumer, show the demand curves for three illnesses, ℓ_1, ℓ_2, and ℓ_3, where the degree of illness increases as the subscript increases from 1 to 3. Need the demand curves be parallel? Could they ever possibly cross?

4. For a single illness (such as a sore throat and cough), show the demand curves for three different consumers with different preferences about medical care and other goods. Need the demand curves be parallel? Could they ever cross? Now aggregate those three demand curves into a demand curve for them together. If these three people constitute the entire population in a market area, then this demand curve is the "market" demand curve. Think about what would happen when you aggregated the demand curves of thousands of individuals.

5. Demands for medical care are specific to each illness, and each illness can create demand for more than one type of medical care (e.g., hospitals, doctors, drugs). Should we think about demand curves that are specific to the illness (e.g., sore throat) or the medical intervention (e.g., office visit, antibiotic injection)? Explain your conclusion.

6. When the quality of a medical service rises, what happens to the demand curve for that service? What if quality increases in ways that are unobservable to the consumer, such as a reduction in the probability of adverse side effects?

7. Describe the concept of consumer surplus in terms that can be understood by a person untrained in economics.

8. Suppose that there's only one type of medical care (office visits) and that each visit costs $20. Consider now an insurance policy with a $100 deductible that pays for 80 percent of the consumer's medical costs after that. The price schedule confronting that consumer has a step in it at a quantity (five visits) such that total spending (price $\times$ quantity) equals the amount of the deductible ($100).

Draw such a price schedule. Now draw a consumer's demand curve that intersects the price schedule at two visits (on the top step), at five visits (somewhere in the vertical portion of the price schedule), and at seven visits (on the lower step). Question: What is the optimal quantity for this patient to consume, two visits, five visits, or seven visits? Why?

9. What would happen to demand curves for medical care if consumer income increased? (Don't forget the effects of income on consumption of health-affecting commodities such as running shoes, cigarettes, fatty foods, automobile air bags, etc.)

10. Suppose a demand curve has the form $q = 100 - 10p$. What is the quantity consumed at $p = 5$? What is the elasticity of demand at $p = 5$?

APPENDIX TO CHAPTER 4

Demand Curves and Demand Elasticities

The price consumers pay for medical care with a simple insurance policy is $C \times p_m$, where C is the coinsurance rate and p_m is the market price. The insurance policy costs $\$R$ per year. Thus the budget constraint for the consumer with insurance, at the time medical care will be purchased, is $I - R = p_x x + C p_m m$. We have seen in the text how this can lead to a demand curve for the consumer of the form

$$m = f(\text{income, price, illness level})$$

Suppose we take a linear approximation to such a curve, so

$$m_{ni} = \alpha_0 + \alpha_1(\text{income}) + \alpha_2(\text{price}) + \alpha_3(\text{illness level})$$

The derivative of m with respect to price is α_2, and the price elasticity of the demand curve is $\alpha_2 \times (\text{price}/m_{ni})$ where m_{ni} means the amount of m purchased with no insurance (ni), and, of course, this depends on income, price, and so on. If the consumer obtains an insurance policy with coinsurance C, then everywhere that "price" appears in the demand curve is replaced by $C p_m$ and income is replaced by $I - R$. Thus, the demand curve with insurance (m_{wi}) is

$$m_{wi} = \alpha_0 + \alpha_1(I - R) + \alpha_2(C \times \text{price}) + \alpha_3(\text{illness level})$$

The derivative of m_{wi} with respect to price is $\alpha_2 C$, and the elasticity is $\alpha_2 C \times \text{price} \div m_{wi}$, where $m_{wi} > m_{ni}$.

Similarly, the derivative of m_{wi} with respect to C is $\alpha_2 \times \text{price}$, and the elasticity is $\alpha_2(\text{price}) \times C \div m_{wi}$, the same as the derivative with respect to m_{wi} with respect to price. Thus the elasticities with respect to price and coinsurance are equal.

Of course, as the text points out, when more than one type of medical care is available, the demand for one type of care may depend on the prices (and insurance coverage) of other types of care. Suppose that two types of medical care (such as ambulatory and inpatient) could treat the same patient's illness. Then we would have two demand curves, shortening *price* to P and using subscripts of A for *ambulatory* and I for *inpatient*:

$$m_I = \alpha_0 + \alpha_1(I - R) + \alpha_2(C_I \times P_I) + \alpha_3(C_A \times P_A) + \alpha_4(\text{illness level})$$

and

$$m_A = \beta_0 + \beta_1(I - R) + \beta_2(C_I \times P_I) + \beta_3(C_A \times P_A) + \beta_4(\text{illness level})$$

Demand for each type of care depends on its own price and the "cross price" of the other type of care. As discussed in the text, if the goods are substitutes, then α_3 and β_2 would have positive signs; they would have negative signs if the goods were complements. This idea obviously generalizes to the case of multiple types of medical care.

Notice that each type of care can have its own coinsurance rate. Hospital and ambulatory care commonly do have differing coinsurance rates, as do dental care and other specific types of care. The benefits package of an insurance plan determines the coinsurance rates for a given plan.

Proof that aggregate demand curve elasticity is the quantity-weighted average of individual elasticities:

Define $M = \sum_{i=1}^{n} m_i$ as the aggregate spending for a society composed of n individuals, each with demand equal to m_i, rate of change in demand $dm_i/dp = \beta_i$ and demand elasticity η_i. The change in M with respect to p is

$$\frac{dM}{dp} = \sum_{i=1}^{n} \beta_i = \sum \eta_i \times (m_i/p)$$

so

$$\eta = \frac{dM/M}{dp/p} = \sum_{i=1}^{n} \eta_i \times (m_i/M) = \sum_{i=1}^{n} s_i \eta_i$$

where $s_i = m_i/M$ is the ith person's share of the total quantity M. Thus, aggregate demand elasticities are a quantity-weighted mixture of individual demand elasticities.

CHAPTER 5

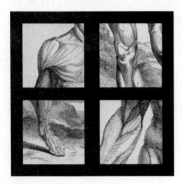

Empirical Studies of Medical Care Demand and Applications

The previous chapter developed a conceptual model of the demand for medical care, showing how we can move from the basic model of utility for health (unobservable) to an observable demand curve. The key relationships that we expect to find include the following predictions about quantities of medical care demanded, in each case with all other relevant factors held constant. Quantity demanded should increase

As price falls

With illness severity

With the generosity of insurance coverage (either with lower copayment or lower deductibles)

As the cost of time decreases

As the time used to obtain care decreases

With age, for adults

LEARNING GOALS

- Understand the distinction between a *model* (as in Chapter 4) and *evidence* (as in this chapter.)

- Gain at least a general understanding of the magnitude of demand elasticities for medical care of various types.

- Understand how specific variables (age, illness, income, and lifestyle) affect demand for medical care.

- See how cross-price elasticities (e.g, drugs and acute medical care) can matter.

- Apply consumer demand models and evidence to measure the economic importance of medical practice variations.

We also know that income increases demand in the aggregate for all goods and services. Although there is no specific prediction for any good or service (including any specific type of medical care), higher income may well increase demand for care. Finally, when the prices of two services (such as hospital care and office visits) move separately or are insured differently, how the use of one service changes as the price or insurance coverage of the other changes depends upon whether they are complements or substitutes. With this information in hand, we can now turn to studies of how people actually have used medical care and how these various factors actually affect demand.

STUDIES OF DEMAND CURVES

A number of economists have estimated demand curves for various types of medical care in various settings using various types of data available in the literature or (occasionally) collected for the purpose. These provide an unsettlingly wide range of information. The estimated price elasticity of demand found in these studies varies by an order of magnitude or more from the largest to the smallest. For example, this past literature finds estimates of the price elasticity for hospital days ranging from −0.67 (Feldstein, 1971) to −0.47 (Davis and Russell, 1972) to 0 for some illnesses (Rosenthal, 1970). For physician care, estimates range from −0.14 (Phelps and Newhouse, 1972; Scitovsky and Snyder, 1972) to −1 (for hospital outpatient visits, Davis and Russell, 1972). One study reported an overall elasticity of demand for medical care as large as −1.5 (Rosett and Huang, 1973). Many of these studies had complicated statistical problems embedded in them that made their results difficult to interpret (Newhouse, Phelps, and Marquis, 1980), and the wide diversity of estimates made it difficult to know what to make of any of them individually. Perhaps the only agreement in the literature by the mid-1970s was that "price mattered."

In part because of the difficulties found in previous studies, in the mid-1970s the federal government launched a randomized, controlled trial of health insurance to learn more about how insurance affects demand for care. Conducted by the RAND Corporation, it was called the Health Insurance Study (HIS). For many purposes, we can treat these results as the best available because the statistical difficulties surrounding previous studies are essentially eliminated in the RAND HIS analysis and the sample sizes far exceed those available in most studies. Thus, although other estimates exist, we focus here on the RAND HIS results for most types of medical care.

The RAND Health Insurance Study (HIS)

The RAND HIS was one of several large social science experiments conducted under federal government auspices in the 1970s. This study basically followed standard "laboratory" experimental design methods, modified only as necessary for ethical and administrative purposes. A total of 5,809 enrollees was chosen from four cities (Dayton, Ohio; Seattle, Washington;

Charleston, South Carolina; and Fitchburg, Massachusetts) and two rural sites (one in South Carolina, the other in Massachusetts). Enrollees were asked to participate for either 3 or 5 years[1] and to give up the use of any insurance plan they might be holding, using only the randomly assigned insurance of the HIS for that period. The total number of person-years available for analysis was 20,190. The eligible population consisted of persons less than the age of 65 who were not institutionalized.[2] At enrollment, the persons were told which of the following insurance plan they would use: (1) full coverage $(C = 0)$ for all services, (2) 25 percent copayment $(C = 0.25)$ for all services, (3) 50 percent copayment $(C = 0.50)$ for all services, (4) 50 percent copayment for dental and mental services $(C = 0.25$ for other care, $C = 0.50$ for dental and mental services), (5) an individual deductible *for ambulatory care only* of $150 per person in the family ($450 total per family),[3] and (6) essentially no coverage until a catastrophic cap had been reached (5, 10, or 15 percent of family income, subject to an overall maximum of $1,000). This latter plan actually had a 5 percent payment rate $(C = 0.95)$ in order to provide an incentive for families to file claims, from which medical use information was derived. Separately, some persons were enrolled in a health maintenance organization (HMO) in Seattle, the results of which are discussed in Chapter 11.

In every plan, the enrollees had a cap on their financial risk, just as for the "catastrophic coverage" plan, so that no family ever had to spend more than 5, 10, or 15 percent of their income (up to a maximum of $1,000) on medical care out of pocket. (If 15 percent seems large, recall that well more than 10 percent of the GNP is spent on medical care.) If the family's medical spending exceeded that limit, they received full coverage $(C = 0)$ for all remaining expenses for the year. Of course, a family on the $C = 0.25$ plan was much less likely to reach such a cap than a family with the $C = 0.95$ plan.

-----

[1] The different time horizons provided the opportunity to learn whether the relatively short time horizon of the study affected results. In general, it did not, with the exception of dental care use, which was abnormally high in the study's first year for persons on the plans with most complete coverage.

[2] The population that was older than 65 was excluded because government rulings prohibited Medicare participants from waiving their right to Medicare coverage. Because all enrollees had to stop using their previous insurance to participate, this ruling eliminated the possibility of studying this older age group.

The study also eliminated persons from the very highest part of the income distribution, mostly for political appearances; the study was initially funded by the Office of Economic Opportunity, the administration's program for combatting poverty.

[3] This plan was designed to test whether inpatient and outpatient care are complements or substitutes.

The cap was put in place to provide people with an incentive to enroll and was coupled with a "participation incentive" payment equal to the maximum risk the family faced. For example, if a family had an income of $15,000 and had a 5-percent-of-income catastrophic cap, they had a maximum risk of $750 and would receive $750 just for participating in the experiment. This feature of the experiment had positive ethical properties (nobody was made worse off financially for participating) and good experimental design properties (it successfully eliminated almost all enrollment refusals and attrition during the experiment), but it obviously complicated the analysis somewhat, compared with plans that might have been used. However, subsequent analysis based on episodes of illness (Keeler, Buchanan, Rolph, et al., 1988) rather than on simple plan comparisons allows one to project the results from the HIS for other complicated insurance plans, some with designs quite different from the small set used in the study.

The primary results from the HIS compared means across the plans, the simplest approach, and one allowed by the randomized-trial design. The use of regression analysis to control for other factors increased the precision of the estimates and shows the effects of other variables (such as age and income) that are explored shortly. Table 5.1 shows the basic results for outpatient care and total medical spending. Table 5.2 converts these data into arc-elasticities. (See Box 5.1 on arc-elasticities.)

Using episode-of-illness analysis, Keeler et al. (1988), broke down the price response into two components: the number of episodes and the spending per episode. Table 5.3 shows the resultant arc-elasticities broken down more finely by type of care received. In general, the price responsiveness of medical services was still fairly small, but it is larger than the simple comparison of plan means shows.[4] The patterns of demand elasticities correspond to intuition about "medical necessity." Demand for hospital care was least price responsive (particularly at higher coinsurance rates), "well care" (preventive checkups, etc.) was most price responsive, and acute and chronic outpatient care fall in between.[5] For all medical services, the price elasticity was estimated to be -0.17 in the range of nearly complete coverage ($C = 0$ to $C = 0.25$), and -0.22 for higher coinsurance rates. The largest price response found was -0.43 for "well care" in the higher coinsurance range. As a summary measure, we can now say with considerable confidence that

---

[4]We should expect this to occur because of the catastrophic cap built into the HIS plans. For serious illness events (large medical spending), all of the plans provided full coverage. Thus, there was not as much "difference" between the plans as there would be without the catastrophic cap, and differences in medical use across plans will be somewhat compressed.

[5]The categorization of *acute, chronic,* and *well care* comes from a check-off box on the insurance form, filled out by the physician.

TABLE 5.1 SAMPLE MEANS FOR ANNUAL USE OF MEDICAL SERVICES PER CAPITA

Plan	Face-to-Face Visits	Outpatient Expenses (1984 Dollars)	Admissions	Inpatient Dollars (1984 Dollars)	Probability Any Medical (%)	Probability Any Inpatient (%)	Total Expenses (1984 Dollars)	Adjusted Total Expenses (1984 Dollars)
Free	4.55	340	0.128	409	86.8	10.3	749	750
	(0.168)	(10.9)	(0.0070)	(32.0)	(0.817)	(0.45)	(39)	(39)
25%	3.33	260	0.105	373	78.8	8.4	634	617
	(0.190)	(14.70)	(0.0090)	(43.1)	(1.38)	(0.61)	(53)	(49)
50%	3.03	224	0.092	450	77.2	7.2	674	573
	(0.221)	(16.8)	(0.0116)	(139)	(2.26)	(0.77)	(144)	(100)
95%	2.73	203	0.099	315	67.7	7.9	518	540
	(0.177)	(12.0)	(0.0078)	(36.7)	(1.76)	(0.55)	(44.8)	(47)
Individual deductible	3.02	235	0.115	373	72.3	9.6	608	630
	(0.171)	(11.9)	(0.0076)	(41.5)	(1.54)	(0.55)	(46)	(56)
Chi-squared (4)	68.8	85.3	11.7	4.1	144.7	19.5	15.9	17.0
P value for chi-squared (4)	<0.0001	<0.0001	0.02	n.s.	<0.0001	0.0006	0.003	0.002

Note: All standard errors (shown in parentheses) are corrected for intertemporal and intrafamily correlations. Dollars are expressed in June 1984 dollars. Visits are face-to-face contacts with M.D., DO, or other health providers; excludes visits for only radiology, anesthesiology, or pathology services. Visits and expenses exclude dental care and outpatient psychotherapy. n.s. = not significant.
Source: Manning, Newhouse, Duan, et al. (1987).

TABLE 5.2 ARC-ELASTICITIES FOR DEMAND

Range of Nominal Coinsurance Variation (%)	Range of Average Coinsurance Variation (%)	All Care	Outpatient Care
0–25	0–16	0.10	0.13
25–95	16–31	0.14	0.21

Source: Manning, Newhouse, Duan, et al. (1987).

TABLE 5.3 ARC-ELASTICITIES BY TYPE OF CARE

Coinsurance Range %	Outpatient			Total Outpatient	Hospital	Total Medical	Dental
	Acute	Chronic	Well				
0–25	0.16	0.20	0.14	0.17	0.17	0.17	0.12
	(0.02)	(0.04)	(0.02)	(0.02)	(0.04)	(0.02)	(0.03)
25–95	0.32	0.23	0.43	0.31	0.14	0.22	0.39
	(0.05)	(0.07)	(0.05)	(0.04)	(0.10)	(0.06)	(0.06)

Note: Standard errors are given in parentheses. For their method of computations, see Keeler, Buchanan, Rolph, et al. (1988).
Source: Keeler, Buchanan, Rolph, et al. (1988).

although medical care use does respond to price, the rate of response is fairly small compared with some other goods and services, with elasticities generally in the range of −0.1 to −0.3 for most medical services.

The study by Keeler, Buchanan, Rolph, et al. estimated the expenses for persons with a number of plans, including "no insurance," although this plan did not actually exist in the HIS. Converting their results (see Table 5.6) to 2000 spending levels using the medical CPI (see Box 1.1 and Table 1.4), the uninsured under 65 person is predicted to spend $1,330 per year and the fully insured person, $2,315. Thus, their models indicate that a person with full coverage will spend about 75 percent more per year on medical services than a completely uninsured person. This same phenomenon occurs in very diverse settings.

These results stand in sharp contrast to much of the previous nonexperimental literature, as might well be expected, because (with a few exceptions) the previous literature confronted serious statistical problems. The few older studies that relied on "natural experiments" prove in retrospect to be remarkably close to the "gold standard" of the HIS,[6] while those relying on aggregated

---

[6]Most notable were the data collected by Anne Scitovsky and Nelda Snyder from a natural experiment using Stanford University employees (Scitovsky and Snyder, 1972). In a multiple regression analysis of those data (Phelps and Newhouse, 1972), the estimated elasticity for outpatient care in the range of $C = 0$ to $C = 0.25$ was −0.14, remarkably close to the estimate of −0.17 in the HIS. The Scitovsky and Snyder data did not feature a catastrophic cap on spending.

BOX 5.1 ARC-ELASTICITIES

This chapter discusses a form of elasticity—arc-elasticity—that is different from the one that was mentioned in Chapter 4. GO BACK TO BOX 4.1 TO MAKE ABSOLUTELY CERTAIN THAT YOU UNDERSTAND THE BASIC IDEAS OF SLOPES AND ELASTICITIES.

Done? OK, you can read ahead. You still don't have the ideas firmly in place? GO BACK AND READ BOX 4.1 AGAIN! Now we can talk about arc-elasticities:

In some data, only two points on the demand curve are available, in which case we usually compute an arc-elasticity. This measure computes the change in quantity and price relative to the average of the two observed values. Thus,

$$\bar{\eta} = \frac{\%\Delta Q}{\%\Delta P} = \frac{\Delta Q / \bar{Q}}{\Delta P / \bar{P}} = \frac{(Q_2 - Q_1)/[(Q_2 + Q_1)/2]}{(P_2 - P_1)/[(P_2 + P_1)/2]}$$

Because the 2s cancel out, the formula is commonly written as

$$\bar{\eta} = \frac{(Q_2 - Q_1)/(Q_2 + Q_1)}{(P_2 - P_1)/(P_2 + P_1)} = \frac{(Q_2 - Q_1) \times (P_1 + P_2)}{(P_2 - P_1) \times (Q_1 + Q_2)}$$

This provides a way to estimate an elasticity when only two data points exist, a situation that occurs with surprising frequency in real-world data-gathering efforts.

data now seem in retrospect to be far off the target, some by as much as an order of magnitude.

Are Hospital and Outpatient Care Substitutes or Complements?

The HIS was designed to show whether hospital and ambulatory care are complements to one another (as tires and gasoline are) or substitutes (as automobiles and airplanes are). The $150 individual deductible provides just this test because the deductible applied only to ambulatory care. Enrollees on this plan had full coverage for all hospital care. Thus, any differences in hospital use between that group and the overall full coverage plan ($C = 0$ for all care) can answer this important question. Table 5.4 shows hospital admissions and spending by plan. The groups with a $150 individual deductible for ambulatory care had only 10 percent fewer hospital admissions and 9 percent less total cost of hospital care than the full coverage group. Although the statistical precision is not terribly strong, these results indicate that the two services are complements, not substitutes. That is, as the insurance generosity for ambulatory care fell, both ambulatory and hospital use fell.

TABLE 5.4   HOSPITAL USE IN THE HIS

Plan	Admissions per Year	Inpatient Cost (1984 Dollars)
$C = 0$	0.128	409
$C = 0.25$	0.105	373
$C = 0.5$	0.092	450
$C = 0.95$	0.099	315
Individual deductible $150	0.115	373

Source: Manning, et al. (1987).

Dental Care

The HIS data also show demand elasticities for other services, including dental care, mental health care, and emergency room care. For dental care, previous studies provided sparse information on price responsiveness, all with potential methodological problems (Phelps and Newhouse, 1974). If anything, these data suggest that demand for dental care would be more price responsive than for other medical services. The HIS results confirm this, at least partly, as Table 5.5 reveals. For higher levels of coinsurance ($C > 0.25$), the arc-elasticity of dental care demand is -0.39, larger than all other medical care except well care. However, in the $C = 0$ to $C = 0.25$ range, dental demand had an estimated elasticity of -0.12, lower than most other medical services, including hospital care. Dental care was one area in which behavior differed between early experimental years and later years. Intuitively, people can "store up" dental visits easier than other types of care. Those patients who went from relatively poor dental insurance onto a generous HIS plan ($C = 0$

TABLE 5.5   ANNUAL SPENDING RELATIVE TO $C = 0.95$ PLAN
($C = 0.95$ Plan $= \$100$)

Insurance Plan (Nondental/Dental)	Year 1		Year 2	
	Nondental ($)	Dental ($)	Nondental ($)	Dental ($)
Free/free	200	252	177	152
25%/25%	145	158	128	109
25%/50%	144	181	122	98
50%	111	118	105	112
95%	100	100	100	100
$150 per person deductible	143	163	124	94

Source: Manning et al. (1985).

or $C = 0.25$) would have a "bargain basement" price for dental care during the experiment. We should expect them to take advantage of that by correcting any backlog of dental problems. Table 5.5 shows that this is exactly what happened. In Year 1, the difference in spending for any of the better insurance plans versus the 95 percent coinsurance plan was greater for dental care than for other medical care, and the differences become more pronounced the better the insurance coverage. Yet in Year 2, the differential spending in the better insurance plans was almost always less for dental care than for other medical care. Once the "backlog" of dental problems is dealt with (in Year 1), people with good insurance seem not to purchase much more dental care than those with poorer insurance, with the notable exception of the full coverage ($C = 0$) plan. These results suggest the importance of some coinsurance to control spending within dental plans, even if relatively modest in size.

Other Specialized Services

The RAND HIS also allows the study of numerous other "specialized" services in addition to dental care. These services were particularly difficult to study using nonexperimental data before the HIS was carried out because there was so little private insurance coverage for some of these services. Of particular interest are the estimated price responses in demand for prescription drugs and in demand for mental health services, two important services for which insurance coverage is often "optional" in private insurance plans.

In the case of prescription drugs, demand appears to be somewhat more price responsive than for other medical services. Fully insured persons on the RAND HIS used 76 percent more drugs (measured by annual expenditures) than those with the 95 percent coinsurance plan. About half of that shift occurred with the move from free care to a 25 percent coinsurance plan, and the remainder is attributable to the shift from 25 percent coverage to little or no insurance (the 95 percent coverage plan). (For details, see Liebowitz, Manning, and Newhouse, 1985.)

In the case of mental health services, there is reason to expect a larger price responsiveness in advance because there are (at least by "common-sense" definitions) more nonmedical substitutes for mental health treatment than there are, for example, for brain surgery. In the case of mental health treatment, the services of psychologists, counselors, the clergy, and even bartenders (at least by anecdote) serve as possible substitutes for medical treatment by psychiatrists. Thus, insuring one type of care but not another has the potential for tipping the balance among those substitutes heavily.

A simple comparison of the mental health care utilization of those on various health insurance plans leads one to the conclusion that its use is about as sensitive to price as other types of ambulatory medical care (Manning, Wells, and Benjamin, 1984). However, critiques of this work by Ellis and McGuire (1984) suggested that a particular feature of the RAND experiment might have distorted the results. Because mental health care users are relatively large users of all health services, they are more likely to exceed the spending cap in the experimental treatments (see preceding discussion) and, hence, to have full coverage for much of their mental health care. In a reanalysis of the data looking at episodes of illness rather than annual spending (and hence allowing study of behavior before and after a spending cap might be exceeded), Keeler et al. (1986) found a larger behavioral response: Those with full coverage, according to the new estimates, used about four times the care of those without insurance. Interestingly (and somewhat uniquely among medical services), the effect of changing coinsurance in the higher ranges (50 percent to 100 percent coinsurance) was quite large. In other health services discussed here, we can recall that most of the "action" with coinsurance happens when the plan shifts from full coverage to 25 percent coinsurance, with relatively little additional reduction in demand occurring as the coinsurance rate increases from 25 percent to higher levels. For mental health care, however, this does not hold true. Although the effect of shifting from full coverage to 25 percent coinsurance was about the same as for other medical services, the effect of shifting from a 50 percent to a 95 percent coinsurance was about twice as large as for other medical services.

Effects of a Deductible

The HIS results allow a simulation of the spending patterns under insurance policies that were not actually tested, such as a plan with 25 percent coinsurance and a $100 deductible or a $500 deductible. All of the dollar figures in this discussion refer to 1984. As briefly described earlier, the expected effects of such a plan are complicated, with the one obvious quality that higher deductibles should lead to lower total costs for care because higher deductibles make the price of medical care higher for more types of illness events. Table 5.6 shows the simulation results from the RAND analysis (Keeler, Buchanan, Rolph, et al., 1988), relying on the estimated responses from the actual experimental plans and mathematically interpolating and extrapolating as needed. The results seem quite striking. The initial effect of a small deductible ($50) is considerable, and then little happens to demand until the deductible exceeds $500, particularly for hospital care.

We can compute the elasticity of demand in response to changing a deductible, just as we can for a coinsurance rate, a price, or income. The data in Table 5.6, for example, show that the elasticity of total expenses with

TABLE 5.6 PREDICTED TOTAL MEDICAL CARE COSTS FOR INSURANCE PLANS WITH DEDUCTIBLES

Deductible ($)	Annual Spending by Type of Medical Treatment ($)				
	Hospital	Acute	Well	Chronic	Total
0 (free care)	400	226	68	148	842
50	387	166	47	112	713
100	384	152	43	104	682
200	379	136	37	92	644
500	376	121	33	83	613
1,000	291	114	32	78	515
2,000	283	111	31	76	501
No insurance	280	109	30	73	492

Note: All data are 1984 dollars.
Source: Keeler et al. (1988).

respect to the deductible is -0.07, and for hospital expense, -0.04.[7] Hospital care does not respond very much until the deductible exceeds $500. Acute care use falls off rapidly with the first small deductible and then smoothly (and slower) thereafter. Total ambulatory care use is near the level of an uninsured person by the time the deductible has reached $500. Interpolating between results in Table 5.6, a deductible of approximately $150 moves a person halfway between the total medical use of a fully insured person and a person with no insurance.

To preview the results in Chapter 10 on demand for insurance, we can simply note here that the cost-saving effects of a moderate-deductible plan are similar to those of coinsurance plans that confront the consumer with a somewhat larger financial risk. Thus, based on these experimental results, the "best" types of insurance plans may include deductibles of moderate size.

Income Effects

The HIS results allow estimates of the effects of income on demand for care, including an interaction of income and insurance plan generosity. Both commonsense and the full use of economic theory suggest that pure income effects should be small, if not zero, with full-coverage insurance.[8] The HIS

---

[7] These estimates come from regressions with the logarithm of total expense (or hospital expense) regressed on the logarithm of the deductible.

[8] Even with full coverage for medical care, there might be a positive income effect on demand. This can occur because better health can raise the value (marginal utility) of other goods (x), and greater income allows the purchase of more x. For example, because bicycling and golf are more enjoyable when you're healthy, higher income people might seek more medical care so they can enjoy their sporting activities more.

data in general show small positive effects of income on medical care use, with the exception of hospital admissions. Comparisons of use rates by the lowest, middle, and upper third of the income distribution shows a slight U-shaped pattern of care for most services, with low- and high-income families using the most care, and middle-income families using the least. In part, this reflects the effects of illness on family income. In particular, persons with higher income enter the hospital less frequently than those with lower income. Using data from the RAND study, the calculated income elasticities for the number of episodes of illness appear in Table 5.7. A quick summary number suggests that the income elasticity of demand is 0.2 or less for medical care.

When considering the effects of income on demand, we must be careful to recognize that cross-sectional studies such as the RAND HIS hold constant the available medical technology (broadly defined, including equipment, medicines, surgical techniques). As income increases, so does the demand for new approaches to healing. Furthermore, technical change that emerges alters the patterns and amounts of medical care demanded. Indeed, much of the growth in health care spending in the years since World War II has surely come from technical change.

One way to understand how important technical change is in the long run is to see how different are the estimates of income elasticities taken from time series data, which incorporate the effects of technical change, rather than taking technology as fixed (as a cross-sectional study does). Several studies have done this, and the estimated income elasticities of demand are generally much higher than those found in the HIS. Another way to derive such an estimate is to compare the incomes and medical care use across different countries. A number of studies, discussed in detail in Chapter 16, have found an income elasticity of demand for health care of more than 1.0.

TABLE 5.7 INCOME ELASTICITIES FOR EPISODES

Type of Care	Income Elasticity for Number of Episodes of Illness
Acute	0.22
Chronic	0.23
Well care	0.12
Dental	0.15
Hospital	n.s.[a]

[a] Not significant.

Source: Calculated from Keeler et al. (1988), Table 3.6 (for average numbers of episodes) and Table E. I (for coefficients of income in regression equation). Estimated equation used SQRT (visits + 0.375) as the dependent variable and log (Income) as the explanatory variable. Elasticity is calculated as β SQRT (visits + 0.375)/visits, where β is the coefficient in the estimated regression.

EFFECTS OF AGE AND GENDER ON DEMAND

As the discussion of aging in Chapter 2 suggests, as people "wear out" faster (get older), they should logically demand more medical care. Almost any population will show this phenomenon: Utilization of almost all health services rises with age.[9] Table 5.8 shows the patterns of medical care use by age and gender for three types of medical care. In each case, increasing age leads to significantly more health care use. The ratio of use by the oldest segment (75+) to that of children is about 3:1 for out-of-hospital use (ambulatory care and prescription drugs in the ambulatory setting), and more than 10:1 for hospitalization. For hospitalization (presumably the most severe illnesses and injuries), even in the above-65 population, hospital use doubles for those over 75 compared with those 65 to 74. Would the data exist, they would surely show another large increase in a population of age 85+.

The effects of gender on utilization are more complex to follow. First, the obvious effects of childbearing appear in the 19–44 population measures. Of the 434 hospital discharges per 1,000 persons for females, 180 of those are for delivering children. The remaining amount (254 per 1,000) are similar to the same-aged male population, but still slightly higher. In all subsequent age groups, females have slightly lower hospitalization rates than males.

Patterns of ambulatory care use (physician office visits, clinic visits and emergency room visits) show a reverse effect: In every adult age bracket, females use more ambulatory care than males, markedly so again in the childbearing years, but continuing into older age brackets as well. The same

TABLE 5.8   AGE AND GENDER EFFECTS ON DEMAND

	Hospital Discharges per 1,000 persons/year		Ambulatory Visits per Person/Year		Prescription Drug Use in Past Month (percent)	
Age	Male	Female	Male	Female	Male	Female
Under 18	201	183	2.65	2.40	26.2	22.0
19–44	228	434	1.58	2.90	27.1	44.6
45–64	577	566	2.78	4.08	55.6	72.0
65–74	1,450	1,355	6.19	6.71	80.1	88.1
75+	2,745	2,501	7.41	7.85		

Sources: Health, United States, 2007, Hospital Discharges from Table 100, Ambulatory Visits from Table 92, Prescription Drug Use in Past Month from Table 96.

---

[9] A few counterexamples will exist, of course, such as acne medication.

pattern appears (not surprisingly) in the estimated rates at which people have used a prescription drug in the past month.[10]

The differences between ambulatory care use and hospitalization rates are probably partly biological and partly cultural. The effects of maternity-related health care use are obvious in these data. In addition, the lower hospitalization rates for adult females past the childbearing age are just another facet of the longer life expectancy for women than men. At any chronological age (e.g., age 62), women are biologically "younger" than men on average. Thus, in any specific age group, we should expect less medical care use. However, the higher rates of ambulatory care use show a different pattern: Women in all adult age groups use more care than men of the same age. This may be due to common patterns of medical care use; many women have both a "primary care doctor" (e.g., an internist) and a gynecologist, and indeed, many heath care plans that use a "gatekeeper" model (as Chapter 11 will discuss in more detail) allow women both a primary care "gatekeeper" and a gynecologist "gatekeeper."

THE EFFECTS OF ILLNESS ON DEMAND

Commonsense, theory (see Chapter 4), and much empirical observation indicate that medical care use rises directly with illness. The relationship between age and medical spending just discussed provides one way of looking at this effect because older people get sick more often than younger people. Other studies have shown precisely the same effect using direct measures of patients' illnesses and relating those illnesses to their use of medical care. Perhaps the most carefully conducted of these studes uses doctor's assessments of the seriousness of many illnesses (experts' ranking of disease severity for hundreds of specific diseases) and then links people's use of medical care to the severity of their illnesses. One study using this approach (Handy et al., 1994) found that disease severity measures such as this could explain up to 60 percent of the variance in annual medical spending in an employed population. Although this should come as no surprise to even the most casual observer of health care use, it is nice to see that carefully constructed measures of illness severity do indeed have high predictive power regarding medical care use.

LIFESTYLE AND ITS EFFECTS ON DEMAND

The link between illness and medical care use is both obvious and (as just noted) well established empirically. This raises a second-order question (from Chapter 2), namely the effects of lifestyle choices on illness (and hence

---

[10]This measure is limited to drugs prescribed in ambulatory settings, so it omits drugs prescribed and used within an inpatient hospital stay.

on demand for care). Estimating these "lifestyle" effects happens to be a common territory for analysis by epidemiologists (those who study patterns of illness).

We can think about this issue most readily by focusing on the discrete question of "who uses medical care?" The probability that a single person will use medical care depends on a number of things (including health insurance coverage, as discussed earlier) and illness. We can focus on the illness aspects of the problem. Some people who are sick use care, and some don't (depending on their attitudes about seeing doctors, etc.), but we can capture the relationship as $P(\text{use care} \mid \text{illness})$, to be read as probability of "using medical care" *given* (or conditional upon) an illness. Then the overall probability of using care becomes $P(\text{use care}) = P(\text{use care} \mid \text{illness}) \times P(\text{illness})$.

Epidemiologists focus further on why illness occurs; that is, they study determinants of $P(\text{illness})$. Consider any "lifestyle" event (cigarette smoking, obesity, promiscuous sexual activity, for example), and, for simplicity, let us just call this event X. Then $P(\text{illness})$ becomes $P(\text{illness} \mid X) \times P(X)$. Now $P(X)$ simply describes how likely a person in the population is to "do" X. The effects of lifestyle choice X on medical care then directly hinge on their effects on illness rates $[P(\text{illness} \mid X)]$.

We can understand the role of lifestyle on medical care demand by looking carefully at the role of lifestyle on illness because we know that medical care demand follows illness patterns closely. Box 5.2 provides a further exploration of the common approach to this question taken by epidemiologists. This provides yet another example of how the study of health economics can borrow from other disciplines. In this case, there is a close and fruitful link between epidemiology and health economics that bears extensive exploration by the serious student of medical demand.

BOX 5.2 EPIDEMIOLOGISTS' APPROACHES TO MEASURING RELATIVE RISK

The most common way to estimate the effect of lifestyle choices on illness is to estimate the relative risk of illness for persons who "do" and "don't do" some particular activity, which we can generically call X. There is an efficient and an inefficient way to study this. The inefficient way is to identify a lot of people who "do" X and then to find out how many of them have the related illness (and similarly for those who "don't do" X). Then the relative risk becomes $P(\text{illness} \mid X)/P(\text{illness} \mid \sim X)$. These are conditional probabilities and should be read (for example) as $P(\text{illness} \mid X)$ meaning "probability that illness is observed, given that X is observed." Also, you should read $\sim X$ as "not X," meaning that "X has not occurred." Epidemiologists could measure the relative risk directly, but, as noted, one must study a lot of people to get a good answer, particularly if $P(X)$ is small in general (even among people who "do" X).

The alternative relies on the magic of Bayes Theorem. In general, we can write $P(\text{illness} \mid X) = P(X \mid \text{illness}) \times P(\text{illness})/P(X)$. (This is the basic formulation of Reverend Bayes' important theorem in probability theory.) Using this approach, we can write down the relative risk for illness for those who "do" and "don't do" X as follows:

$$RR = [P(X \mid \text{illness})/P(\sim X \mid \text{illness})]/[P(X)/P(\sim X)]$$

As complicated as this looks, it comes down to a simple notion: Measure the relative frequency of the behavior X in the population with the illness, and compare that with the relative frequency of the behavior X in a comparable population without that illness. To start out, one simply needs to find a population of people who actually have the relevant disease (easy to track down in hospitals, doctors' offices, clinics, etc.) and then to ask them about their choices relative to behavior X. Then, to complete the puzzle, epidemiologists must also measure the frequency of behavior X in a control population, that is, a group of people matched in as many ways as possible to the case patients, except that they don't have the illness in question. (This matching tries to hold constant other factors that might affect the risk of illness, such as age, income, and race.)

The relative risk of illness (using the Bayes Theorem "trick") can be estimated directly by comparing the relative frequency of X among the sick case population $[P(X \mid \text{illness})/P(\sim X \mid \text{illness})]$ with its relative frequency among the control population $[P(X \mid \sim\text{illness})/P(\sim X \mid \sim \text{illness})]$.

As a numerical example of this process, consider the following data. Researchers wanted to determine the effect of secondhand smoke in households on the frequency of lung cancer. They studied people who had never smoked more than 100 cigarettes themselves in their entire lifetime. They measured exposure to secondhand smoke in "smoker-years," the number of years they were exposed to each smoker within their household. For example, during childhood and adolescence, a child could receive anything between 0 smoker-years exposure (neither parent smoked) to 40 smoker-years (both parents smoked for all 20 years of childhood and adolescence). In 191 pairs of matched cases (those with lung cancer) and those without lung cancer (controls), the following was found:

Exposure	Cases	Controls
Less than 25 smoker-years	139	162
25 or more smoker-years	52	29

(continued)

BOX 5.2 EPIDEMIOLOGISTS' APPROACHES TO MEASURING RELATIVE RISK (continued)

From these data,

$$P(X \mid \text{illness}) = 52/191 = 0.272$$
$$P(\sim X \mid \text{illness}) = 139/191 = 0.728$$
$$P(X \mid \sim \text{illness}) = 29/191 = 0.152$$
$$P(\sim X \mid \sim \text{illness}) = 162/191 = 0.848$$

The relative occurrence of X among the ill population is 0.272/0.728 = 0.373. The relative occurrence among the not-ill population is 0.152/0.848 = 0.179. The relative risk of lung cancer among those with behavior X (25 or more smoker-years of exposure) is 0.373/0.179 = 2.08. Thus, the risks of getting lung cancer among nonsmokers is twice as high among those people who grew up in a household with large exposure to other people's smoking (measured by 25 or more smoker-years exposure) as among those with little or no exposure to secondhand smoke. This study also estimated the relative risks from exposure during adulthood and during the entire lifetime of the cases and controls. This example uses the childhood exposure only to illustrate the general idea of calculation of relative risks. The interested reader can find more details in Janerich et al. (1990).

THE DEMAND FOR "ILLNESS"

Nobody, of course, unless afflicted by unusual mental disorders, would really "demand" illness in the economic sense because we typically understand illness as a "bad" that reduces utility. However, as we saw in Chapters 2 and 3 and in the previous section on relative risk calculations, the production of health involves both medical care and lifestyle choices, and the reverse side of the "production of health" coin is the production of illness (or the destruction of health, take your choice). Does economics have anything to say about "the demand for illness"?

Perhaps not surprisingly to those studying the economics of health care, the answer is an affirmative "yes!" Economic analysis can indeed help us understand why people consume "things" that afflict their health. The key issues fall into three categories: (1) joint production of pleasure and illness, (2) addiction, and (3) the degree to which the consumer understands the risks of illness. Let's take each of these in turn.

① Joint Production of Pleasure and Illness

By common economic analysis, the goal of a rational human being is to maximize utility, subject, of course, to the spending constraint provided by that person's income. The model also generalizes over a multiperiod ("lifetime") model in which people not only choose between various consumption choices "today" but also can do things "today" that affect health outcomes in the future ("tomorrow").

We can readily understand, given this framework, why a rational person and fully informed person might deliberately consume alcohol, tobacco, or other dangerous substances. Similarly, a person might deliberately engage in risky activities such as race car driving, bungee jumping off of a bridge over the Black Canyon of the Gunnison River in Colorado, or engage in unprotected sex with others. Why? Because it's fun! It creates utility. Certainly not for everybody, but if one's preferences tilt in those directions, economic analysis says that it can be rational behavior, even if the activity creates a risk of illness, injury, or even death.

We have already seen (Chapter 2) how education is linked to these choices: Higher education typically leads to persons engaging in fewer "risky" behaviors. One explanation (see the following discussion) is that higher education (by increasing the overall value of one's "human capital" makes it less desirable to engage in activities that put the human capital investment at risk.

② Addiction

Psychologists classify many risky activities as addictions, most notably the use of illicit drugs such as cocaine and heroin and their derivatives, methamphetamines and other "designer drugs," tobacco, and alcohol, as well as gambling. Can economic analysis help understand addiction? Again, the answer seems to be "yes." In a highly influential paper, Becker, Grossman, and Murphy (1991) analyzed the demand for addictive substances using a model of "rational addiction." In this model, people choose to become addicted to gain the pleasure of consumption, but their behavior changes through time in predictable ways that imply a deliberate ("rational") choice to become addicted (and often to quit later). A key feature of the model says that past consumption increases the marginal utility of current consumption.[11] In this

---

[11]The same sort of model applies to consumption of other things such as classical music concerts or other things that we usually call "acquired tastes." It might be useful for readers to discuss with their friends why tobacco and cocaine are considered "addictions" but classical music or stinky cheeses are considered "acquired tastes." *Hint:* There is no "right" answer!

model, higher prices in the past (hence, reducing previous consumption) should cause lower demand in the current period (with parallel but reversed effects for lower prices in the past). Thus, the model predicts that past, present, and future consumption are all "complementary goods" (and should have negative cross-price elasticities). One strong implication of the "rational addiction" model is that long-run elasticities of demand should exceed short-run elasticities. Studies of demand for addictive substances repeatedly show this phenomenon:

- *Tobacco:* The short-run elasticity of demand for tobacco is about −0.4. The long-run elasticity is about −0.7 (Grossman and Chaloupka, 1998).
- *Gambling at the racetrack:* "Demand" is measured by betting volume (dollars) per person attending the racetrack, and price is the "takeout" from the track (the proportion of dollars wagered that the track keeps instead of returning to bettors). The short-run demand elasticity is −0.3. The long run elasticity is −0.7 (Mobellia, 1991).
- *Heavy drinking:* A change in the excise tax that various states levy on alcohol has two effects. The short-run effect appears in immediate changes in consumption. The long-run effect appears in changes in deaths from liver cirrhosis. Changes in excise taxes on alcohol have a larger proportional effect on liver cirrhosis deaths than on immediate consumption (Cook and Tauchen, 1982).
- *Cocaine:* Even the use of a highly addictive drug such as cocaine responds to price. Grossman and Chaloupka (1998) find the elasticity of demand in response to a temporary price increase to be −0.3, the short-run response to a permanent price increase to be −0.7, and the long-run price response to be −1.4. Quintessentially, past use is a strong predictor of current use.[12]

Incomplete Information

Information can affect demand. If people do not understand the risks of illness or injury arising from some consumption or behavioral choice, their demand will shift away from what a "fully informed" consumer would choose to do. This could appear in several disguises. First, the person might not know the information, in which case providing it could alter behavior. Second, the person might know but ignore it. This behavior is termed "myopic

---

[12]As an aside for econometrics junkies reading this book, the rational addiction model also says that past consumption should enter models of demand for the "good" as an explanatory variable, and if omitted, the estimates of the true price elasticity of demand will be biased toward zero. Many empirical studies using the "rational addiction" approach find that omitting measures of previous demand have precisely this effect.

addiction" as distinct from "rational addiction." Third, the adverse consequences might occur in the distant future and (with a sufficiently high discount rate) essentially be ignored in current consumption choices.

A classic example of the provision of information occurred when the U.S. Surgeon General published a report in 1965 detailing the many adverse consequences of tobacco consumption. In response, after decades of steady increases in smoking rates, annual demand in the United States for cigarettes began to fall, and by 2005, smoking participation rates (the percentage of the U.S. population who smoke cigarettes) had halved from more than 40 percent in 1965 to 20 percent by 2005.

THE DEMAND FOR QUALITY: CHOICE OF PROVIDER SPECIALIZATION

One common indicator of quality is the amount of training a doctor has received. Doctors with added specialty training beyond medical school can take privately administered examinations offered by various medical specialty boards of examiners, usually only after completing 3 to 6 (or more) years of specialty training in an approved hospital residency program. This specialty training allows a doctor to use the description "Board Certified" (or "Board Eligible" if the training but not the examinations has been completed successfully). If the extra training raises doctors' quality, then people should be willing to pay more for visiting a doctor with that training than for a less trained physician.

In the RAND HIS, some weak evidence of this pattern of preferences appeared. First, the average price of a routine office visit paid by patients in that study was about 10 to 20 percent higher for a specialist in internal medicine (an internist) than for a general practitioner, who had not received any particular specialty training. This provides one estimate of the aggregate willingness to pay for higher quality, although it is a weak comparison. (For example, it doesn't indicate anything about how much time the doctor spends with each patient.)

Another more direct test emerged from the RAND HIS study. People with more generous insurance coverage should choose doctors with specialty training more than those persons with high deductibles or coinsurance if higher quality (as indicated by board certification) is recognized as desirable. The second piece of evidence showed, however, that among all patients in the study, the choice of provider specialization was not significantly related to the insurance plans (Marquis, 1985).

This finding alone should not create great surprise. Remember that the HIS randomly assigned people to the experimental insurance plans, so the types of doctors they were using before the study began would be randomly mixed across plans. Because the study would carry on only for 3 years for most participants (and 5 years for others), they may have been quite reluctant to break up an existing arrangement with their current providers. However, some patients changed doctors during the study. They form a more interesting group to study the effects of insurance on demand for quality.

Among those HIS enrollees who changed doctors during the study, the effects of insurance generosity on provider choice were still weak, at best. Statistically significant effects appeared; only among children in the study those with full-coverage insurance were 10 to 20 percent more likely to have a specialist (usually a pediatrician) as the new provider than were persons in the other insurance plans (Marquis, 1985).

On net, we know little empirically about the role of insurance in demand for quality. All of our intuition tells us that those with better insurance would more likely seek higher quality providers, both for quality of medical treatment and for amenities. Unfortunately, direct studies of this question are more difficult to find.

OTHER STUDIES OF DEMAND FOR MEDICAL CARE

A wide unstudied frontier still remains to explore more about the demand for various types of medical care and the demands in various settings. Demand varies with the income and education of the population, the quality of care, and the institutional settings in which care is delivered. Thus, it is useful to know how to find data that produce useful information on consumer demand. The following section provides some examples.

Natural Experiments I: The Demand for Physician Care

Sometimes, the real world conducts a "natural experiment" that allows careful study of the demand for medical care. Perhaps the classic of such studies resulted from the work of Scitovsky and Snyder (1972) at the Palo Alto Medical Clinic. Anne Scitovsky learned that Stanford University had changed its employees' insurance coverage because the insurance was costing more than the university wished to pay. The university had the choice of either making the employees pay more for the insurance or changing the insurance plan's structure to make it less costly. Fortunately (from a natural experimentalist's point of view), they chose the latter. Under the new insurance plan, the coinsurance for doctor office visits was raised from $C = 0$ (full coverage) to $C = 0.25$ (25 percent copayment). Scitovsky and Snyder studied the medical care use (using insurance claims data) for the year before the change (1966) and the year after the change (1968). *If nothing else had changed in the picture,* any differences in use of medical care should be due to the increase in copayment.

The results (reported in detail by Scitovsky and Snyder, 1972, and Phelps and Newhouse, 1972, in a different type of statistical analysis) closely match those found over a decade later in the RAND HIS. The average number of doctor office visits fell by a quarter, and the use of diagnostic tests fell by 10 to 20 percent (depending on the type of test). The change was about the same for "preventive" annual physical examinations as for other types of care.

The potential weakness of any such "natural experiment" is that something else might have changed during the period in question, complicating the analysis. For example, if in 1966 an unusually large flu epidemic had been experienced, then doctor visits in 1966 would have been abnormally high, and (had it been a "normal" year) the apparent effect of the coinsurance in reducing demand would have been even greater. Of course, the reverse is also true: If 1968 had had an unusually large epidemic of flu, then we might have seen no effect at all and incorrectly concluded that price didn't matter. In the Scitovsky and Snyder data, no such unusual events seemed obvious upon study of overall health care use in the region, but it always represents something to be alert for in studying natural experiments. In this case, a repeated analysis 5 years later by the same two researchers found that the effects persisted almost unchanged, lending further strength to the validity of their earlier work (Scitovsky and McCall, 1977).

An Important Cross-Elasticity of Demand

Most demand-curve information looks at how the "own price" affects demand (i.e., the price of the good or service being studied). Thus, demand curves show (for example) P_x on one axis and X on the other (price and quantity). We summarize the nature of such demand curves with the slope (dX/dP_x) or the same information in relative-change form (the elasticity, usually denoted simply as η). Sometimes, however, a "cross-price" elasticity has great interest: How does the demand for X change as the price of Y changes? If the cross-price elasticity of X with respect to P_y is negative, then X and Y are said to be complements (consumed "in synch") so that when either P_x or P_y rises, demand for X falls. If the cross-price elasticity is positive, then X and Y are said to be substitutes.

In the world of health care, several interesting questions relating to cross-price elasticities arise. Most particularly, what happens to utilization of hospital and ambulatory care if (say) the price of preventive care or prescription drugs falls? An earlier section described results from the RAND HIS regarding ambulatory care and hospital care. More recent data show a very interesting and potentially useful cross-price result regarding prescription drugs.

Gaynor, Li, and Vogt (2006) studied the effects of changes in prescription drug coverage in a series of employer-based plans. As these health plans change prescription drug copayment levels, one can also track subsequent changes in total prescription drug expenditures. The authors of this study found an own-price elasticity of −0.6 in the short run and −0.8 in the long run. Presumably the long-run adjustment allowed time (for example) for people to switch to generic drugs instead of higher cost brand name drugs.

Each $1 increase in the prescription drug copayment saved the insurance plans about $24 in the first year's drug costs and another $9 in annual drug costs subsequently (the long-run effect), for a total "savings" of $33 per patient per year.

This is not the complete story, however. Patients also substituted physician ambulatory care visits for drug treatment to some extent—the "cross-price" effect. In the first year, spending on ambulatory care rose by a bit more than $6 per year in the first year and rose to a total of almost $16 per year in the second year, so increased use of physician services wiped out about half the savings in prescription drugs. These results show that prescription drug use and physician services are substitutes; Gaynor, Li, and Vogt estimate the cross-price elasticities at +0.1 in the short run and +0.2 in the long run. They found no effect at all on use of inpatient hospital services.

Time Series Information: The Demand for Drugs

We have another source of information available that can sometimes shed light on the nature of demand for medical care—the behavior of aggregate data over time. One example of this occurred in the British National Health Service (BNHS). Over the span of 15 years, the BNHS changed the price it charged patients for prescription drugs on a number of occasions, primarily as budget or cost-control choices. The price varied from 0 to 2.5 shillings per prescription.[13] The payments by patients in the BNHS represented anywhere from 0 to 23 percent of the total cost of the drugs used ($C = 0$ to $C = 0.23$). Using the techniques of multiple regression analysis, Phelps and Newhouse (1974) estimated the effect of the out-of-pocket payments on total drug use within the BNHS. On average, total drug use was 15 percent higher at full coverage ($C = 0$) than with a 25 percent coinsurance ($C = 0.25$).

These results closely match those of Mississippi Medicaid behavior (Smith and Garner, 1974) and a Windsor, Ontario, prescription drug plan's outcomes (Greenlich and Darsky, 1968).

---

[13]A shilling is the British currency equivalent to the American nickel (i.e., one-twentieth of a pound). At that time, a pound converted to about $2.40, so a shilling was about $0.12. A 2-shilling fee for a prescription would be roughly equivalent to a $0.25 fee at the same time (in the 1950s and 1960s), or about $1.50 currently.

Natural Experiments II: The Role of Time in Demand for Care

One natural experiment demonstrates the importance of time costs in the demand for medical care. In this case, the student health service at a major university was changed from one location (5–10 minutes average travel time for students) to another (20 minutes average travel time). The study reported the number of student visits (Simon and Smith, 1973). Again using the technique of multiple regression analysis, Phelps and Newhouse (1974) estimated the systematic effect of the change in location of the health service. Visits fell by one-third from previous levels, despite the apparently improved surroundings and (if anything) less crowded atmosphere. The arc-elasticity of student health service visits with respect to time would be about −0.25 to −0.50, depending on whether the initial travel time is better characterized as 5 minutes or 10 minutes.

The Interaction of Severity of Illness with Demand Elasticities

Several recent studies have added to the body of knowledge about demand for specific medical services, focusing particularly on how demand elasticities change with illness severity. For example, Magid et al. (1997) studied the effect of copayments on decisions to seek medical care following a heart attack. For this most severe of medical events, they compared the behavior for groups that had no copayments in their health insurance versus those that had copayments of $25 to $100 in a period from 1989 to 1994 (using records for ambulance and hospital care in Seattle, Washington). They found (adjusting for observable differences in patients) that the time to arrival at medical care after onset of symptoms was virtually identical for those with and without the copayments. Although it would be surprising to find otherwise, this study confirms what many would suspect—for really major illness events, "moderate" copayments have no effect on patients' decisions.

In a separate study using national health care survey data, Wedig (1988) studied how differences in reported health status affected demand elasticities. He found that those in fair or poor health showed demand elasticities of about half the magnitude of persons in good or excellent health. This suggests (as intuition has led many to conclude) that sicker people pay less attention to price—that is, they respond less to price than healthier persons.

More on the Role of Time in the Demand for Care

Travel Time in Palo Alto
In the studies using Scitovsky and Snyder's data, it is also possible to see systematic effects of travel time on use of medical care because they coded the patients' home location and calculated the travel distance to Palo Alto, where the patients had to go to receive care.

The effects of travel distance on physician visits and expense look precisely the way we would expect in theory: Those who live further away used less care because the time and travel costs were higher. Particularly for families who lived more than 20 miles away, the effect was considerable: They had 30 percent fewer doctor visits than those who lived very close to the clinic.

Some of this could be the effect of the patients' just seeing a different doctor rather than going to the Palo Alto Clinic for care, but the insurance plan paid only for care at the clinic. Thus, if these families did decide to go elsewhere, they would have had to pay full price (about $15 per visit at the time), rather than a quarter of that at the Palo Alto Clinic.

An Interaction of Time Costs and Quality of Care

We first saw how time can act as a price, so that demand for medical services decreases when the time costs increase. One carefully conducted study looked at the interaction of time costs and provider choice. In this study (Coffey, 1983), the data provided a good measure of the opportunity cost of time to women (i.e., the value of their time in their best alternative use, whether at work in the job market or in other settings). Coffey studied the use of female medical services (e.g., gynecologists) and the role of time. She found not only that overall use of such services did not vary much with time cost—a 10 percent increase in time cost led to only a 1 percent decrease in overall use—but also that the choice of provider type was much more sensitive to time costs. In particular, a 10 percent increase in the time costs associated with seeing a public provider (hospital clinic, etc.) led to a 5 percent decrease in use. Apparently, as the waiting time in public clinics increases, some patients become willing to pay a higher price to receive faster service in private settings.

APPLICATIONS AND EXTENSIONS OF DEMAND THEORY

The methods of demand theory allow us to expand our understanding of other events and studies in the health care area. In one important application for the tools of demand analysis, we return to the problem of variations in medical practice.

Son of Variations: Welfare Losses and Medical Practice Variations

Using the tools of demand theory, we can extend further the analysis of variations in medical practice patterns that was discussed in Chapter 3. With the ability to calculate the incremental value of medical interventions using the consumer demand model, we can calculate the dollar value of the costs of variations, or at least a lower bound to such costs.

FIGURE 5.1   Welfare loss from wrong use of medical practices.

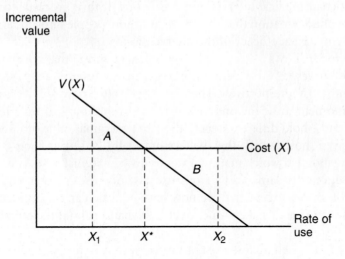

Figure 5.1 shows the basic construction of the problem. Suppose that two otherwise "identical" regions exist with different rates of use of a particular medical intervention (X) and that the *average* rate between the two regions is correct—that is, where the marginal cost (C) and the marginal value (the demand curve) are equal. (We will see the effect of a systematic error; for now, we assume the average is correct.) Each region (by construction) has the same demand curve for X. Only mistakes in judgment lead to the differences in use rates. Region 1 uses the procedure at rate X_1, and Region 2 uses it at rate X_2. In Region 1, too little of X is used, and consumers suffer a welfare loss because they would be willing to pay more for X (at the use rate X_1) than it costs to produce. The exact loss they suffer is the area under the demand curve but above the cost curve, between X_1 and X^*. In other words, they lose their consumer surplus on the consumption between X_1 and X^*, which is identified as triangle A in the figure. Similarly, consumers in Region 2 lose their consumer surplus on the excess consumption between X^* and X_2, identified as triangle B in the figure. Their welfare loss occurs because they spend more on each unit of care above X^* than it is worth to them.

The discussion of Figure 5.1 does not state what might cause people to use the wrong amount of care but rather describes how to calculate the welfare loss once we observe a region using the wrong amount. One way to find people consuming the wrong amount is simply to look for those who make a mistake, which they would do, for example, by selecting an amount of care for which the marginal value does not equal the marginal cost. Sometimes taxes, subsidies, or supply restrictions lead to that type of behavior. An alternative approach that we can explore hinges on the role of information. This approach asks what would happen if people's information about the efficacy of a particular medical intervention was wrong. It then proceeds to measure the value of information that would correct those people's misunderstanding about the marginal efficacy of the intervention.

Figure 5.2 shows a society with two cities (1 and 2) that have incremental value curves (inverse demand curves) for intervention X described as $V_1(X)$ and $V_2(X)$, respectively. Their "average" value curve $V^*(X)$ is assumed for the moment to be the one to which they would move if fully informed. Cities 1 and 2 hold different beliefs about the marginal value of intervention X, but given those beliefs, they behave optimally, by setting their consumption at the point at which marginal value equals marginal cost. As we can see, this produces the same sort of overuse or underuse of intervention X as Figure 5.1 shows, except that we now have a particular reason identified as the cause of those mistakes—incorrect information about the efficacy of the intervention.

How much welfare loss exists from variations in practice patterns? First consider City 1 [with value curve $V_1(X)$]. The triangle A has a dollar value equal to its area (because the vertical axis has dimension $/X$ and the horizontal axis has dimension X, their product has dimension $). The area of a triangle is the product of one-half of its base times its height. In this case, the base has length $(X^* - X_1)$. We can infer the height if we know how demand responds to price, or (the inverse question) how marginal value changes as the rate of use changes. In more precise terms, we want to know $dP(X)/dX$, where $P(X)$ is the marginal value at consumption rate X. If we have estimates of demand curves (where quantity varies as a function of price), we have

FIGURE 5.2 Incorrect information carries welfare losses.

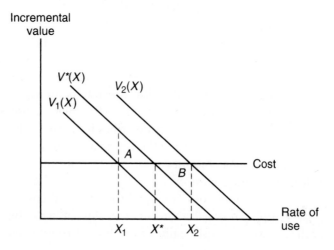

estimates of dX/dP, the rate at which consumption changes as price changes. In this case, we want just the inverse of that. The height of the triangle A is just $(dP/dX) \times (X^* - X_1)$. Thus, the area of triangle A is

$$0.5(dP/dX)(X^* - X_1)^2$$

Triangle B has a similar area, except that it uses $(X^* - X_2)^2$.

Now if we consider N regions similar to the two we have discussed, each with use rates X_i, then we could characterize the average use rate for all such regions and the variance around that average. The variance is the expected value of $(X_i - X^*)^2$, adding up each observed value of X_i weighted by the likelihood that it occurs. Thus, it is easy to show (again, if the average use rate is correct) that the expected welfare loss for a large number of regions associated with varying rates of use of intervention X is

$$\text{Welfare loss} = \frac{dP}{dX} \times \text{variance}(X) \times N$$

where variance(X) is the observed variance in use rates. A little algebraic manipulation converts this into a simpler formula:

$$\text{Welfare loss} = 0.5 \times \text{price} \times X^* \times N \times \frac{\text{variance}(X)}{(X^*)^2 \eta}$$

where η is the demand elasticity for intervention X (more precisely, the elasticity of a fully informed demand curve), and X^* is the average consumption. The *square* of the coefficient of variation (COV^2) described in Chapter 3 is equal to variance$(X)/(X^*)^2$. Thus, the information on coefficients of variation in Chapter 3 is an important but incomplete part of the welfare loss measure. The final welfare loss measure is

$$\text{Welfare loss} = (0.5 \times \text{total spending} \times \text{COV}^2)/\eta$$

This formula defines a direct measure of the likely importance of information about procedure X. Good information could move all consumers to the informed demand curve, away from their current uninformed demand curves. We can think of this measure as having three components: (1) Sutton's Law,[14] (2) the Wennberg/Roos Corollary,[15] and (3) the Economist's Addendum. Sutton's Law is simple: Money is important. The terms price

---

[14]Willie Sutton, a famous bank robber, was asked after he was arrested why he robbed all those banks. His response was "because that's where the money is."

[15]This term receives its name from the two most prominent researchers in the variations literature, John E. Wennberg, M.D., MPH, and Noralou Roos, Ph.D.

× quantity (total spending) reflect this idea. The Wennberg/Roos Corollary to Sutton's Law is also simple: Confusion magnifies the importance of money. The Economist's Addendum simply says the following: For a given amount of variation, the welfare loss is greater if the incremental value changes rapidly as consumption changes. In other words, the demand curve is "inelastic," which (in its usual form) indicates that the quantity demanded is fairly insensitive to the price charged.

The welfare losses from variations in practice patterns have been calculated using New York State data (Phelps and Parente, 1990). The largest single welfare loss arose from hospital admissions for coronary artery bypass surgery, with an annual welfare loss of $4 per person. Hospitalizations for psychosis created an annual welfare loss exceeding $3 per person. Other nonsurgical hospitalizations with high welfare loss included adult gastroenteritis ($1.60), tests of heart function ($2.60 per person), congestive heart failure ($2.30), adult pneumonia ($1.35), and nonsurgical patients with back problems ($1.15).

These losses may seem small on a per capita basis, but collectively they add up to very large losses. For example, for the United States with a population in 1990 of about 275 million people, the annual welfare loss from just the variations in use of coronary bypass surgery was $0.75 billion. However, because the knowledge needed to reduce variations would be valuable for many years, the value of that knowledge far exceeds $0.75 billion. For example, if the knowledge persisted for 20 years before it became outmoded (at a 3 percent real discount rate), the present value of the knowledge would exceed 15 times the annual welfare loss, or about $6.5 billion. Thus, given the variations in use of coronary bypass surgery, even a study costing several billion dollars would have a positive expected payout. Fortunately, the cost of careful studies to assess the outcomes of medical and surgical interventions is only several million dollars, at most. Thus, the case for careful studies of medical practices is overwhelming. The expected returns are probably hundreds if not thousands of times more than the costs of such studies.

All of the preceding analysis depends upon the assumption that the average rate of use is somehow correct. Of course, this is unlikely to be true, given the uncertainty about correct use. A systematic bias may have descended on medical choices. If so, then it is easy to show that the welfare loss measures indicated above are too low. The correct measure is the sum of the component described earlier (involving the coefficient of variation) plus the term

$$\text{Welfare loss from bias} = 0.5 \times \text{spending} \times (\%\text{bias})^2/\eta$$

where (%bias) is the bias as a percent of correct use (Phelps and Parente, 1990). To see the importance this could make in welfare loss, consider a procedure such as back surgery (laminectomy). The welfare loss from variations in back surgery calculated by Phelps and Parente was $1.10 per capita per year, or $0.25 billion for the total country. Annually, about 190,000 such operations are performed, at an average cost of about $5,000, so total spending is about $0.94 billion, or about $3.90 per capita. Using the demand elasticity for all hospitalizations in the RAND HIS, we can set $\eta = 0.15$ in absolute value. If the use rate is, for example, 10 percent too high (or too low), the loss from *biased* use rates (in addition to the loss from variability) is another $0.26 per year ($62 million total). The loss from bias rises with the square of the percent bias. For example, if the bias is 20 percent of the current rate, the bias-related loss is four times that arising from a 10 percent bias rate, or about $250 million per year. Again, the value of learning about such a bias is the discounted present value of all future years when the knowledge remains useful (i.e., until a new treatment for the illness emerges), and thus could be 15 to 20 times larger than the annual rate, or about another $4 billion.

Of course, we cannot learn the "proper" use rate (that at which a fully informed demand curve would indicate) by looking at variations. We can only infer that where variations exist, the likelihood that confusion exists is much greater and, therefore, that a complete study of the procedure will produce considerable value. If such studies detect systematic bias in the use of a procedure, even more value can emerge from such studies than from those just revealing and correcting the causes of inappropriate variations.

DECISION THEORY: DERIVING THE "RIGHT" DEMAND CURVE FOR MEDICAL CARE

The widespread findings of variations in the use of medical care indicate that many, perhaps most, doctors do not correctly use the medical interventions at their disposal. If they cannot advise their patients correctly, it may be illogical to expect patients to act as informed consumers. In part, the reason for the highly variable patterns of use may be that doctors are not taught well how to make decisions. Clinical decision making is an acquired art for most doctors, learned by example during their clinical years of medical school and in their residency training.

Fortunately, formal methods that could help doctors sort out the highly complicated problems of making medical decisions exist. Through the application of formal decision theory to medical problems, doctors are learning better how to advise patients about the use of medical interventions. In the terms of economic demand theory, medical decision theory spells out the best possible ways of using medical care to produce health, possibly even to show the best ways of producing utility. Properly done, medical decision analysis helps find the "best" demand curve for medical care. To put it slightly differently, formal medical decision analysis derives what the demand curve for medical care "should be" for a consumer trying to maximize a utility function that includes both health and other goods—$U(x,H)$—in a consistent and organized manner.

The appendix to this chapter provides an example of how medical decision theory works, studying the problem of using a diagnostic study for a patient to help diagnose whether a disease is present. This example shows the interested student how medical decision theory and medical demand theory are intimately related.

COST-EFFECTIVENESS RATIOS AND DEMAND CURVES

A common approach in the study of medical care, often built into a decision analysis regarding "proper" use of a medical intervention, is an assessment of the cost-effectiveness (CE) ratio of a medical intervention. More properly, we should use the phrase *marginal cost-effectiveness ratios,* because this research, when properly carried out, studies the incremental (or "marginal") consequences of "doing more" compared with "doing less" medical intervention. For example, one can study the marginal cost effectiveness of various interventions (as shown in Table 3.1) for various expansions of medical care use. Do we have any basis for believing that CE ratios can guide our thinking about when (or when not) to use medical interventions, based on the same principles that lead us to create demand curves for medical services from the original utility function $U(X, H)$?

Recent studies have shown that CE ratios can, in fact, be used legitimately to guide the use of medical interventions and, indeed, point the way to finding the "proper" CE cutoff value (values of CE ratios above which the intervention is deemed undesirable). Using the basic principles of utility maximization, Garber and Phelps (1997) and Lee (2008) show that one can indeed maximize expected utility in a lifetime consumption model by using interventions with CE ratios at least as favorable as a specific CE cutoff value. In addition, this study shows that one can use information from other (nonmedical) decisions to help determine that optimal cutoff and that it appears to be on the order of twice a person's annual income (as a general approximation). This approach says, for example, that a person with an annual income of $40,000 would be made best off by selecting interventions with CE ratios of about $80,000 per quality-adjusted life-year or lower and by choosing not to use medical interventions with poorer CE ratios than that. The logic behind the twice-annual-income rule is not easy to describe, and it is only a rule of thumb, but the point of the analysis is to show that the same principles of utility maximization used in finding demand curves (and interpreting them) can also be used to guide decisions about using medical care in an entirely different way—using CE ratios as the determinant of when to use medical care and for whom.

WHY VARIATIONS IN MEDICAL PRACTICE?

The availability of formal decision theory heightens the puzzlement about the significant variations in medical practice use from region to region. Do doctors disagree about the values to patients (or do patients have different values in different regions of the country)? This hardly seems plausible, at least not enough to account for the large variations in practice patterns. Do doctors disagree about the probabilities of illness? One way to answer that question is to use information on the patterns of using diagnostic tests and then the subsequent treatment. In the study of Medicare patients, Chassin et al. (1986) found that in regions in which the use of tests was high, so was the use of the parallel treatment. This may just put the question back one step further: Why do doctors use diagnostic tests differently? Doctors may also hold different beliefs about important aspects of the treatment's safety and efficacy. Doctors in a specific community may have shared experiences and beliefs that begin to form a local medical "culture," identifiably different in various regions. It seems important to learn what forms doctors' and patients' beliefs about therapeutic safety and efficacy, their beliefs about the probability of disease, and their use of diagnostic tests. As we learn more about these issues, we can better define the correct therapeutic strategies for patients and thus give patients a better informed judgment about medical interventions. As the welfare analysis of variations in medical practice shows, the gains from this type of study can be very large indeed.

Using the "decision tree" approach helps illuminate sources of mistakes that doctors can make in reaching a diagnosis for their patients. Four specific elements affect the simple decision to treat or not to treat: (1) beliefs in the efficacy of the treatment (how well does the therapy work?); (2) what the probability is of disease [earlier, discussed as P(illness)] in the patient; (3) costs of treatment; and (4) misunderstanding of patients' preferences for various health outcomes. When diagnostic tests enter the decision, additional sources of possible error arise from mistakes in understanding the accuracy of the tests (the rate of false-positive and false-negative diagnoses). A careful look at what is known about each of these issues suggests that, if anything, doctors' errors in each of these component parts of a decision-making process will lead to overtreatment of patients rather than undertreatment. That is, doctors tend to overstate probabilities of illness, treatment efficacy, patients' preferences for "cures," and the accuracy of diagnostic tests. They also tend to ignore actual costs of treatment more often than not because of the pervasive effects of health insurance (which takes cost out of the picture to a great extent). For a more complete discussion, see Phelps (1997).

SUMMARY

Empirical studies of demand for medical care have confirmed the role of price in people's choices of medical care of all types. Because insurance alters the net price of care to people, most of these studies have used people's responses to different insurance coverage as a proxy for different prices, because economic theory tells us that elasticities with respect to either price or coinsurance are equivalent. Early studies of demand elasticities found a wide range of elasticities, ranging from 0 (for some types of hospital care) to -1.5 or larger (for aggregate medical spending). This range of uncertainty, coupled with a strong desire by the federal government to know demand responsiveness with more certainty, led to the funding of a major randomized controlled trial, the RAND Health Insurance Study.

The RAND HIS offers the cleanest and most precise estimates of the effects of price on demand for medical care. These estimates confirm that price does matter, but probably not as much as earlier studies showed. Demand for hospital care is the least price sensitive, and ambulatory care (acute, chronic, and well care) and dental care are more price responsive. Nevertheless, it is certain that demand is price inelastic (i.e., $|\eta| < 1.0$) for all these services. A wide variety of quasi-experimental evidence augments the data from the RAND study, adding to our knowledge of how demand responds to price, income, time and travel costs, illness, and other determinants of demand.

We can also apply demand theory to understand further the importance of medical practice variations, described previously in Chapter 3. By adopting a model of misinformation about the marginal efficacy of medical interventions as the underlying cause of variations, we can estimate the welfare losses associated with variations. If the underlying model of misinformation is correct, these estimates strongly support the value of conducting studies (and disseminating the results widely) about the correct approaches to using various medical interventions because the value of such studies would greatly exceed their cost, even for very infrequent and relatively low-variation interventions. For common, expensive, and high-variation procedures, the yields from improving information vastly exceed the apparent costs of such studies.

RELATED CHAPTERS IN *HANDBOOK OF HEALTH ECONOMICS*

Chapter 8, "Moral Hazard and Consumer Incentives in Health Care" by Peter Zweifel and Willard G. Manning

Chapter 23, "Waiting Lists and Medical Treatment" by John G. Cullis, Phillip R. Jones, and Carol Propper

Chapter 24, "Economics of Dental Services" by Harri Sintonen and Ismo Linosmaa

PROBLEMS

1. "The RAND Health Insurance Study gave every subject a fixed amount of money that covered the maximum possible expenditure that each subject might have. Because of this, all participants could act as if they had full coverage, and the experiment was invalid." Assuming the validity of the first sentence, comment on the inference drawn in the second sentence.

2. Previous studies of demand for insurance had elasticities of demand in the neighborhood of -0.7 to -1, and sometimes -2. Compared with the results from the RAND experiment, which demand curves would lead to larger welfare losses associated with an insurance plan providing, for example, a coinsurance rate of $C = 0.2$?

3. For a person who previously had no insurance and received an insurance plan paying for 80 percent of all types of medical care, what increase in use would you expect for hospital care, dental care, and physician services, on average?

4. In the RAND study, two plans had full coverage for spending within the hospital, but one had a $150 deductible for ambulatory care. The plan with the ambulatory care deductible had a lower probability of hospital admission (0.115) per year than did the plan with full coverage for everything (0.128), even though both plans covered hospital care fully. (See Table 5.4.) What does this tell you about the use of hospital and ambulatory care? Are they substitutes or complements? Explain how this happens in plain English, without resorting to fancy economic jargon.

5. Looking at Figure 5.2, explain why triangles A and B represent welfare losses, given the presumption that the demand curves V_1 and V_2 differ from each other because of differences in beliefs about the productivity of medical care between doctor–patient combinations in Cities 1 and 2.

6. Describe one or more studies that would demonstrate how time acts just as price does in its effects on medical care use, for example, how increased travel or waiting time creates lower demand for medical care.

APPENDIX TO CHAPTER 5

An Example of Medical Decision Theory

The problem of using a diagnostic study has received considerable attention in the medical literature.[16] Even in its simplest form, the problem has some important complications, making it a good example of how formal decision theory can help clarify medical judgment. To set the problem up usefully, we need some notation. Let

$$f = \text{probability that patient is sick}$$
$$(1 - f) = \text{probability that patient is healthy}$$

This problem focuses on the use of diagnostic devices, so we need a simple way to characterize their capabilities. All diagnostic devices are imperfect, sometimes giving the wrong answer. We can follow the standard approach by measuring rates of correct and incorrect diagnosis as:

$$p = \text{probability of true positive (if sick)} = \text{SENSITIVITY}$$
$$(1 - p) = \text{probability of false negative (if sick)}$$
$$q = \text{probability of false positive (if healthy)}$$
$$(1 - q) = \text{probability of true negative (if healthy)} = \text{SPECIFICITY}$$

We describe benefits to patients (utilities) as U, and costs as C. These are the patient's own utilities.[17] Our simple world contains only two treatment choices: treat (T) or not treat (N). Thus, utilities and costs have a dual-state dependence, U_{ij} and C_{ij}, where i denotes the true state of health and j denotes the treatment. Thus:

$$U_{ST} = \text{utility of sick person, treated}$$
$$U_{SN} = \text{utility of sick person, not treated}$$
$$U_{HT} = \text{utility of healthy person, treated}$$
$$U_{HN} = \text{utility of healthy person, not treated}$$

Presumably, $U_{ST} > U_{SN}$ if the treatment works. Similarly, $U_{HT} < U_{HN}$—for example, due to side effects of the therapy. Actually measuring these utilities is a complicated problem, about which a considerable amount is now known.[18]

---

[16]The landmark study was by Pauker and Kassirer (1980).

[17]Indeed, some standard techniques help elicit these utilities from patients and use them in analyses such as this one.

[18]The techniques use time trade-off methods, "standard gambles," and rating scale. For an excellent summary review of this work, see Torrance (1986). Torrance (1987) offers a less technically intense summary.

In parallel notation, the associated costs are

$$C_{ST} = \text{cost of sick person, treated}$$
$$C_{SN} = \text{cost of sick person, not treated}$$
$$C_{HT} = \text{cost of healthy person, treated}$$
$$C_{HN} = \text{cost of healthy person, not treated}$$

We can now define some differential costs and utilities, comparing in each case the value (or cost) associated with treating people correctly, in accord with their true condition, compared with the incorrect action. Call these incremental utilities and incremental costs. Thus,

$$\Delta U_S = U_{ST} - U_{SN} = \text{utility gain by treating sick person}$$
$$\Delta U_H = U_{HN} - U_{HT} = \text{utility gain by not treating healthy person}$$
$$\Delta C_S = C_{ST} - C_{SN} = \text{change in cost by treating sick person}$$
$$\Delta C_H = C_{HN} - C_{HT} = \text{change in cost from not treating healthy person}$$
$$\text{(probably negative)}$$

With this notation, we can evaluate the net gains from use of a diagnostic device. To do this, we need to answer several specific questions: Without additional testing, what treatment (if any) should the clinician recommend? Should diagnostic tests be used? If so, how should the clinician best interpret them? If the diagnostic test is used, how will the patient's outcomes change, and how will the benefits of any such change compare with the costs? Answering these questions provides the basis for evaluating the benefits and costs of a diagnostic technology and for deriving the patient's demand for the diagnostic test.

If the probability of disease is f, the expected utility from treating is $[f \times U_{ST} + (1 - f) \times U_{HT}]$ and the expected cost is $[f \times C_{ST} + (1 - f) \times C_{HT}]$. The alternative action is not to treat, with expected utilities and costs $[f \times U_{SN} + (1 - f) \times U_{HN}]$ and $[f \times C_{SN} + (1 - f) \times C_{HN}]$, respectively. The incremental expected utility from treating versus not treating is the difference between these,

$$[f \times U_{ST} + (1 - f) \times U_{HT}] - [f \times U_{SN} + (1 - f) \times U_{HN}]$$
$$= f \times (U_{ST} - U_{SN}) + (1 - f) \times (U_{HT} - U_{HN})$$
$$= f \times \Delta U_S - (1 - f) \times \Delta U_H \qquad (5A.1a)$$

This is really a simple idea. The expected gain from treating everybody is the gain for those correctly treated (ΔU_S) times the probability that the person is sick (f), minus the value of correctly not treating those who are healthy (ΔU_H) times the probability of that occurring ($1 - f$). Similarly, we can define expected difference in cost from treating everybody (versus not treating everybody) as

$$f \times (C_{ST} - C_{SN}) + (1 - f) \times (C_{HT} - C_{HN})$$
$$= f \times \Delta C_S - (1 - f) \times \Delta C_H \qquad (5A.1b)$$

We can convert this to a simple decision problem *if* we know how much the consumer values in dollars a unit of utility. That is, we need something to allow us to convert "utils" to dollars or vice versa. Although the process to do this can be somewhat complicated, it can be done. For example, the outcomes (the *U*s) can be expressed in quality adjusted life–years (QALYs), and we can ask or infer how much people are willing to pay for a QALY. Another approach, valuable in some settings such as cancer therapy, uses as an outcome the increased probability of survival. We can learn from studies of people's own choices how much they are willing to pay to increase their chance of survival.[19]

We will use the label *g* to specify how much people are willing to pay for a unit of the health outcome. If the outcome is a QALY, for example, they may value the outcome at $100,000. If so, then $g = 1/100,000$. Now we can convert the decision problem into a simple question: Which choice (treat or not treat) has the higher *net* expected utility, subtracting the utility value of all associated costs? That's where the *g* factor comes in. Using that multiplier (if you will, an exchange rate between dollars and utils), the decision rule says to treat if the expected utility of treating exceeds that of not treating:

$$f \times (\Delta U_S - g \times \Delta C_S) > (1 - f) \times (\Delta U_H - g \times \Delta C_H) \qquad (5A.2)$$

We can reorganize the same information to tell what probability *f* determines the choice of treat versus no treat. To find the point of indifference between the two choices, we make equation (5A.2) an equality and solve for *f*, yielding the critical probability of disease:

$$f_c = \frac{(\Delta U_H - g \times \Delta C_H)}{(\Delta U_H - g \times \Delta C_H) + (\Delta U_S - g \times \Delta C_S)} \qquad (5A.3)$$

If the probability of disease *f* exceeds f_c, treatment is the correct choice, and conversely if *f* falls below f_c. We can call this choice the fallback strategy. It provides the best advice for the patient if no further information is available—that is, if there are no more diagnostic tests that might be used.

The choice of a fallback strategy sets the stage for analyzing the desirability of using diagnostic information. It turns out that the expected value of a diagnostic test to the patient depends upon the fallback strategy and the accuracy of the test. Intuition gives good guidance here to the formal concepts that follow. If the doctor would treat anyway (fallback = treat), then

---

[19]The most common methods look at the wages people earn in the labor force and the risks of their jobs. The higher wage people get for working in riskier jobs allows us to infer how much people value a decrease in the probability of dying. For a summary of earlier work, see Graham and Vopel (1981). Using this approach, a recent study puts the value of a "statistical" life saved at more than $5 million (Moore and Viscusi, 1988a).

the expected value of a test is very high if the patient's true probability of disease is low because the test will probably reveal that the doctor would be making the wrong choice (treating a patient who isn't sick). Similarly, if the patient has a high probability of being sick, then the test isn't worth much because it will just confirm the doctor's fallback strategy of treating.

Exactly the opposite pattern holds if the fallback is not to treat. The test is most valuable to a patient who is truly sick, and not so important to the patient who is healthy. The test should be used whenever the expected value of diagnostic information (EVDI) exceeds the cost of the test, C_t. The EVDI depends upon the fallback strategy. If the fallback is to treat, then

$$\text{EVDI}_T = -(1-p) \times f \times (\Delta U_S - g \times \Delta C_S) \\ + (1-q) \times (1-f) \times (\Delta U_H - g \times \Delta C_H) \quad (5A.4)$$

Similarly, if the fallback is to not treat, then the EVDI_{NT} is

$$f \times p \times (\Delta U_S - g \times \Delta C_S) - (1-f) \times q \times (\Delta U_H - g \times \Delta C_H) \\ (5A.5)$$

and the test should be used if $\text{EVDI} > C_t$ in either case.

These two equations, combined with the cost of the test, define the correct decision among the three alternatives of testing, treating right away, or doing nothing. Figure 5A.1 shows these two EVDI curves plotted against the probability of illness (f). The right-hand (downward-sloping) curve is relevant when the fallback is to treat, and the left-hand (upward-sloping) curve is

FIGURE 5A.1

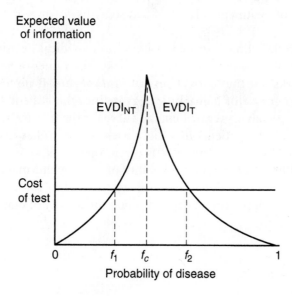

relevant when the fallback is not to treat. The test should be used whenever the EVDI exceeds the cost of the test (converted to utils with the multiplier g), so the relevant decision is to test if the probability of disease lies between f_1 and f_2. If the patient has a best-guess probability of disease that is less than f_1, then nothing should be done; if the prior probability exceeds f_2, the doctor should treat the patient without bothering with the cost of the test. It turns out that the highest possible value of information from a diagnostic test occurs when $f = f_c$. This makes good sense, because that's the point at which the patient would be indifferent between choosing "treat" or "not treat." If you will, f_c is the point of maximum uncertainty, which must be the point at which information has the greatest possible value.

The patient's individual demand curve depends on the probability of disease (and, of course, the utilities, costs of treatment, and the conversion factor g). We can see easily that the desirability of testing increases as the cost C_t falls. The range at which testing is a good idea (between f_1 and f_2) gets wider as C_t gets smaller.

The aggregate demand curve for a "society" simply adds up all the demands of individuals. In any society, there will be a distribution of prior probability of disease when person i in the society has illness risk f_i. Some of the patients (those with f_i near f_c) will have a high expected value for the test, and they create the top part of society's demand curve for the test. Others (at very high or low values of f_i) will have only a low expected value from the test. They form the bottom part of the demand curve for the test. Filling in each person's expected value of diagnostic information gives the demand curve for the test for the entire society. This demand curve shifts upward if the willingness to pay for a QALY increases (for example, because of increased income) or if the costs of treatment fall and, of course, shifts downward if the opposite happens.

This "simple" clinical problem shows how medical decision theory is linked to the demand for medical care. It takes the values of *health* as given and then works out the "correct" use of *medical care.* If no tests are available, then the choice of fallback strategy defines the patient's demand for medical care, and an aggregate demand curve for the treatment just adds up the values of all the patients in society, each of whom has his or her own probability of disease f_i. If the test is given, then it "updates" the doctor's and patient's belief about the probability of disease and makes a different treatment recommendation. Thus, for example, the "informed" demand curve for a medical treatment depends upon the quality of diagnostic information available.

CHAPTER 6

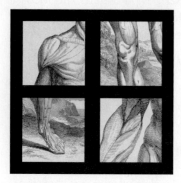

The Physician and the Physician Firm

The physician stands as a central actor in production of medical care and health. Far out of proportion to the dollars actually paid to them, physicians guide and shape the allocation of resources in medical care markets, beginning with the smallest details of caring for a patient and ending with the capital allocation plans of hospitals and even the biomedical research undertaken in the National Institutes of Health; universities; and companies making drugs, equipment, and supplies for the medical care sector.

This chapter studies the physician as an economic agent. To do this well, we need to distinguish carefully among the various roles the physician can and does play in the production of medical care and health. The key we need to keep in mind is the distinction between physicians as *inputs* into a productive process; physicians as *entrepreneurs;* and the final product of *physician services,* the actual event that involves patients.

Almost every idea in this chapter applies equally to other types of medical care providers and healers, including dentists, podiatrists, social workers,

LEARNING GOALS

- Differentiate between a *physician* and a *physician-firm.*
- Apply the concept of substitution in production to physician-firm activities.
- Delve into the detail of what economic "goods" are produced during a physician visit.
- See how different organizational structures of physician-firms matter (size, complexity, etc.).
- Track the common threads in understanding the economic forces behind people's decisions to become doctors, and their specialty choices.
- See how "international trade" (doctors trained in other countries) affects the U.S. market.

165

clinical psychologists, optometrists, nurse-practitioners, Christian Science healers, chiropractors, and many other specialized types of persons engaged in healing arts. Thus, although this chapter describes physicians and focuses on the particular work they do, nothing differs meaningfully (except the labels on some of their inputs) when other types of healers are considered.

THE "FIRM"—INPUTS, OUTPUT, AND COST

Rationale for the Firm

Before beginning the actual study of the supply of physician services, a brief review of the economics of "the firm" will prove helpful. "The firm" is an economic entity designed to make decisions. "The market" also makes decisions, often the same types of decisions as an individual firm makes. The boundaries between when markets make decisions and when firms make decisions are often fuzzier than one might expect. For example, a steel foundry might buy its coal from an independent supplier (in which case the market sets the price of coal) or might produce its own coal from a mine it owns. In the latter case, the production is managed internally. The extent of "vertical integration" for a firm is one of the important decisions its managers must make.

While economists are fond of saying that "the market" is the most efficient allocator of resources available, this is not always true. "The market" is really a collection of economic agents engaging in contracts with one another. Firms emerge precisely because it is more efficient to manage a particular productive process by command and control rather than through a series of external (contractual) relationships.[1] In most markets, we observe more than one firm, and economists believe that any attempt to organize the entire market through command and control would reduce the efficiency of production.[2] In many areas of resource allocation in medical care, we have drawn away from an unfettered market, for better or for worse, toward more centralized control (via regulation). In the market for physician services, this has happened much less than elsewhere in the medical care sector, with "firms" serving a much more important role in resource allocation, together with the invisible hand of the market, rather than through central command and control or regulation.

---

[1] The classic discussion of this problem appears in Ronald Coase's article, "The Nature of the Firm," 1937.

[2] The widespread inefficiency of the former Soviet economy stands as a classic example of what happens when an economy relies too much on command and control and not enough on markets.

Firms hire and control the use of resources. The way they make those decisions determines the profitability and survival of the firm. The decision makers in a firm face two separate constraints in their decision making: the production process available to them and the market demand for their final product. We can presume that these decision makers seek to maximize some objective function, subject to the relevant constraints. The normal "theory of the firm" includes only profits of the firm in the objective function. Most discussion of physician-firms has extended that objective function at least to include the leisure of the firm's director (and the only physician, if the firm is a solo practice) and sometimes the health of the patient. This last issue creates a strong separation between groups of economists studying the health care sector. Some believe it is at least unnecessary and possibly heretical. Others view it as an important addition to the careful study of the economic behavior of physicians.

These issues highlight the interaction of the physician and patient, which we consider in more detail later. As a brief introduction to the issues, we can note here that the question revolves around the market's response to a major type of uncertainty in health care—namely, the diagnosis and recommendation of proper treatment for patients. Inherently, doctors know much more than patients about such matters due to their professional training. With this advantageous position, they have the opportunity to deceive patients into buying more medical care than is "optimal" in an objective sense. Defining a utility function for physicians in terms of labor and leisure alone leads to a set of conclusions about how the market might function, and (in turn) how the government might wish to intervene in the market (e.g., to protect the patient). However, if one includes the patient's health in the physician's utility function, it is easy to see that a balancing automatically occurs, whereby the physician's interests in protecting the patient's health limit any incentives for deceiving the patient that might otherwise lead to higher physician profits.

THE PHYSICIAN AS ENTREPRENEUR

The physician directing a physician-firm serves two roles, one as a labor input in the firm and the other as entrepreneur. We can infer the value of labor by asking what other opportunities the doctor might have elsewhere, for example, on salary in a group practice of other doctors or as an employee of some other organization. Any other financial returns the doctor receives as physician-entrepreneur are due to the management of the firm and the returns (for better or worse) from the decisions that guide the firm. Those decisions include location, staffing, the product line of the firm (e.g., specialization, degree of vertical integration), pricing, and other similar choices.

THE PHYSICIAN-FIRM AND ITS PRODUCTION FUNCTION

The product of the physician-firm is "physician visits." Of course, this is as misleading about the physician-firm as saying that "hospital admissions" are the product of hospitals. Just as the hospital is a multifaceted "job shop," so is the physician-firm. The product of a physician-firm is really an array of diagnoses, referrals, and treatments for patients with a mix of disease and illness, each unique in at least some ways but having common characteristics about which the physician and other participants in the physician firm are knowledgeable.

The typical physician-firm is better known as an office practice because it is carried out most predominantly in that setting.[3] (The physician also works in the hospital and may, in unusual circumstances, treat patients in their own homes.)

The physician-firm must involve at least one physician. By law, the firm's activities must come under the direct supervision of a licensed physician. Other labor inputs include those of nurses; receptionists; bookkeepers and accountants; lawyers; laboratory technicians; and, sometimes, X-ray technicians; therapists; and other specialized personnel. Nonlabor inputs include the physical office itself, office equipment, medical equipment, computers, supplies, electric power, and insurance (including, most importantly, medical malpractice insurance).

This list of inputs to the physician-firm does not reveal much about the economic behavior of the organization. We can ask, for example, how the combination of inputs is selected to produce a given set of outputs—that is, the mix of physician visits provided. To understand how these choices might work, we need to inquire about the production process itself.

As with all productive activities, the production of physician services allows some substitution of one type of input for another. Some types of substitution are obvious. For example, a receptionist can replace some functions of a "general purpose" nurse. An accountant can replace some of the activities of the (physician) owner, but one hopes not those involving surgical procedures. Disposable supplies can substitute for labor and capital (the time and equipment needed to sterilize instruments). Other types of substitution are less obvious, but equally available. Careful record keeping by the doctor may substitute for the use of legal services (by avoiding malpractice suits). Either

---

[3]This is sometimes called *ambulatory care* because the patients walk in. An alternative designation is outpatient care, as opposed to inpatient care in the hospital. Of course, ambulatory care and outpatient care involve not only the office practices of physicians but also the services of hospital outpatient clinics and emergency rooms, as well as other specialized treatment settings.

nurses or doctors can garner routine history and physical examination information, providing the opportunity for substituting lower cost nurse labor for
higher cost physician labor. Indeed, computer-based systems now exist that
"take a history" from a patient, sometimes without the presence of either a
physician or a nurse.

The extent of substitution in production is constrained both by technical
and legal factors. In some cases, the technology does not permit substitution.
For example, we do not have (as yet) robots that can perform surgery successfully. Physician-firm entrepreneurs *cannot* make such substitutions. In other
cases, the law does not permit it. Entrepreneurs *may not* make these types of
substitution. Only licensed medical doctors may perform surgery, for example, although the anesthetic for surgery may legally be administered either by
a medical doctor or a registered nurse.

THE PHYSICIAN AS DIAGNOSTICIAN

The "core business" of a physician-firm is the diagnosis and treatment of
patient illnesses. Diagnosis is the hard part; treatment choices follow diagnosis more readily, albeit not perfectly, as we saw in Chapter 3 in the discussion
of medical practice variations. But let's consider the diagnostic problem more
fully.

Patients come into physician offices with a multitude of ailments and
complaints, some with visible consequences (rash, broken arm), and others
with no visible or measurable component (headache). Some have related
physical symptoms that could have multiple etiologies: A stiff back, for example, could come from a muscle strain or a pinched nerve. A rash could have
psychological sources or viral sources. Stomach pain can come from ulcers,
food poisoning, bacterial or viral infections, or cancer. Many symptoms have
both benign and serious possible causes. And the list of possible symptoms
extends readily into the multiple hundreds, if not thousands, and they often
come in combinations (headache and rash) that may or may not have a common biological cause. The book classifying these diseases, the *ICD-10*, has
thousands of entries. The current book describing possible treatments, the
CPT- 2009, also has thousands of entries.[4]

---

[4]*ICD, the International Classification of Diseases,* published by the World Health Organization
(WHO) is in its 10th edition. Work on *ICD-11* is underway, with drafts expected in 2009 and
operational status several years later. See www.who.int/classifications/icd/en/. *CPT, the Current Procedural Terminology,* is published regularly by the American Medical Association. See
www.ama-assn.org/ama/pub/category/3113.html.

Physicians first approach this problem as diagnosticians. Following classical medical training, the physicians begin with a "differential diagnosis" that lists possible causes of the symptoms, sometimes with explicit or implicit probabilities attached to them, and then begins to sort through the list and rule out some (or most) of the list based on further history, diagnostic tests (blood and urine samples or images from CT, MRI, X-ray or ultrasound), or physical examination (which may include manipulating a part of the body to determine what motion elicits pain, for example). Sometimes two diagnostic possibilities remain after this process. Often in such cases, doctors will treat as if one (usually the more serious) is the "true" disease (e.g., prescribing a drug), and if the treatment fails, turn to the next on the list.[5] Thus, a failed treatment can itself be diagnostic.

Like other parts of the patient-physician encounter, this problem has also become a focus of attention for people studying health care delivery. This line of inquiry suggests (in the same spirit as the economic field known as "constrained rationality") that the complexity of the problem leads to physicians building up a list of "shortcuts" that assist in the diagnostic problem. According to some of this research (Mauksch et al., 2008), physicians develop "stories" that fit patients with certain diseases. These stories are common patterns of symptoms and their evolution through time. When a patient's symptoms approach those of one of the standard stories sufficiently closely, the doctors seem to "lock in" on that story and announce a diagnosis connected to it. Then they treat accordingly.

This problem of diagnosing a patient's illness is closely associated with one of the most complicated computer problems known to science: pattern recognition. Humans are astonishingly good at recognizing patterns, yet few computer scientists and software engineers have succeeded in approaching human capabilities in pattern recognition using computers. To put it in a slightly different way, we really have no good understanding of how good diagnosticians achieve their results. Some are very good at it. The very best become "the doctors' doctor" because most doctors recognize excellence in this activity even if they are not good at it.

We can also return to the discussions of medical practice variations in Chapter 3 and their economic impact (in Chapter 5) with this complex diagnostic problem in mind. Given the immense array of clinical problems confronting the typical doctor and the even-larger array of possible treatment strategies, it would seem astonishing if doctors solved each of these problems perfectly. In a world constrained by time (remember, as Nobel Laureate Gary

---

[5]The television series *House,* starring Hugh Laurie as the brutally frank but brilliant diagnostician Gregory House, is filled with examples of such strategies.

Becker noted (Becker, 1965), "time is the ultimate source of all utility"), physicians are likely to adopt time-saving heuristics to assist in this diagnostic problem. One source of help—low in cost and readily available to all doctors—is the observed practice styles of partners, colleagues, and fellow doctors on the hospital medical staff where the doctor practices. This helps explain why regional geographic patterns of practice persist—the doctors' own information-gathering strategies will reinforce existing patterns of practice as each doctor comes to conform with the prevalent practice style in his or her community (or group of partners).

As one looks at the cost-effectiveness data in the literature (e.g., as in Table 3.2), it also becomes clear that the treatment recommendations along the extensive margin are mainly responsible for widespread medical practice variations. Even with the same diagnosis in mind, different doctors will treat more or less aggressively, thus leading to different practice styles. All of this, of course, can also be influenced by other economic phenomena such as induced demand, which is itself mediated by the method of compensation for the doctor and the degree of competition in the medical community.

Physician-firms employ many nonphysician assistants. In earlier studies, Reinhardt (1972, 1973, 1975) found an average of about two aides per full-time equivalent (FTE) physician, and he found (using operations research techniques) that the optimum would be nearer to four (double the sample average). Times have changed: recent data (Bureau of Health Professions, 2006) show that the average family practice physician-firm employs about 4.5 para-professionals per FTE doctor, and multispecialty groups about 5. Cynics (perhaps accurately) will state that most of this increase comes from people attending to the billing process for patients—dealing with insurance plans and Medicare—so this increase may or may not reflect a shift to a more optimal support staff than Reinhardt found many decades ago. An analysis by Woolhandler, Campbell, and Himmelstein (2003) found that "between 1969 and 1999, the share of the U.S. health care labor force accounted for by administrative workers grew from 18.2 percent to 27.3 percent." They found that in 1999, administrative and clerical workers accounted for about 4 out of 9 workers in physician offices, about a 50 percent increase from three decades earlier.

Costs of a Firm

As firms assemble the final product (here, "physician visits"), they generate a *demand for inputs* that varies inversely with the price per unit of those inputs (i.e., a typical demand curve) and directly with the scale of the firm. By combining these inputs, using whatever substitution is legally and technically possible, the firm produces its product or service. The payments made to these input factors are summarized in Box 6.1, using data from the most

BOX 6.1 PHYSICIANS' COST STRUCTURE

Physicians' cost structures differ considerably by type of practice. The table on the opposite page portrays the structure of physician costs in 2000, using data from a survey conducted by the American Medical Association.

The structure of primary-care doctors' costs (general practice, internists, pediatricians) all look quite similar. Surgeons and obstetricians/gynecologists have similarly appearing "office" costs, but higher malpractice insurance. Psychiatrists and anesthesiologists both have low total costs, but it is a very different structure of costs. The typical psychiatrist's practice would have mostly space rental with little specialized medical equipment and probably only a part-time receptionist/bookkeeper. The anesthesiologist spends no time in "an office" with patients but rather has all contacts with patients in the hospital, thus incurring office rental space only for clerical-secretarial assistance and so on. However, anesthesiologists' professional liability insurance is the highest of any speciality listed, reflecting the risks associated with participating in surgical activities. Chapter 13 discusses medical malpractice issues in more detail. A more detailed study of medical costs appears in Becker, Dunn, and Hsiao (1988, pp. 2397–2402).

recent survey of practices in calendar year 2000 made available by the American Medical Association (AMA).

Several things are worth noting about these data. The first comment clarifies the distinction between "per physician" data and "contract physicians." These data are all normalized on the number of *partners* in the physician practice. (The median is about 3 physician-partners across all specialties, but the mean is about 20, which requires some very large practice groups in the survey.) Thus (for example), $31,000 in contract physician expense means that only a fraction of 1 physician (about one-sixth of an FTE) works on contract per physician-partner.

The second observation is that "other expenses" include personnel (nurses, aides, receptionists, bookkeepers, etc.), equipment and supplies, and office rental costs. Previous surveys from the AMA broke these down into more refined categories, but the most recent survey aggregates them.

The third observation is that medical liability premiums are both small as a fraction of total practice expenses (under 4 percent for all practices) and falling in comparison with older surveys. For example, the comparable survey using 1992 data (AMA, 1994) showed malpractice premiums at about 7.5 percent for all practices. Even for the highest-risk specialties (OB-Gyn, and anesthesia, which is not included in the table), the malpractice premiums are under

DATA FOR BOX 6.1

		Distribution of Physician Practice Expenses (thousands of $)			
Specialty	Contract Physicians	Medical Liability Premiums per Physician	Other Expenses Expenses per Physician	Net Income per Physician	Practice Revenue per Physician
All practices	31	18	247	205	484
General/ Family	20	14	206	145	358
Internal medicine	27	14	244	196	445
Surgery	28	24	298	275	591
Pediatrics	36	12	209	138	375
Radiology	73	19	299	310	689
OB/Gyn	24	39	309	227	577
Other	31	12	212	192	443

Source: AMA (2003), Tables 22, 23, 24, 26, 29 and 35.
Note: Final column is not sum of previous columns.
Data from survey reflect 2000 medical practice costs.

7 percent in the 1992 data. Thus (a topic to which we return in Chapter 13), it is difficult to "blame" either high medical costs or rising medical costs in medical liability insurance directly.[6]

Finally, we can see that personal income per physician is only about 40 percent of the overall practice revenue in the 2000 data, and ranges from about 35 percent (pediatrics) to about 45 percent (radiology). Comparison across time is also illuminating: In the comparable 1992 data, physician income was almost exactly half of total practice income. In the intervening years, "other costs" have increased in share from 50 to 60 percent. Because physician incomes grew only from $177,000 in 1992 to $205,000 in 2000, this requires that "other costs" grew from about $180,000 to $280,000 (annual growth rates of 1.8 percent and 5.8 percent, respectively). Because malpractice costs have fallen as a percent of earnings over this period, the most likely candidate for the increased expenses is either wage compensation to key staff (e.g., nurses) or increased staffing to deal with managed care contracts (a topic we explore more in Chapter 11). Alas, these data do not allow effective identification of the sources of increased costs.

---

[6]This does not take into account "defensive medicine" issues that Chapter 13 discusses in more detail.

The cost curve of a firm combines two ideas. First, it summarizes the costs of the resources actually used by the firm. These reflect the accounting costs that would typically appear in the financial records of the firm. A cost curve also reflects the technical relationship between inputs and outputs, something that an accountant cannot describe or measure. A good engineering or operations research study might reveal these relationships, but in general, such studies show that as a firm expands the scale of its activity (and hence its use of various inputs), its average costs first decline (with economies of scale) and then increase (with eventual diseconomies of scale).

If we were to draw the cost curve for a physician-firm (assuming for the moment that we knew what its output was), we would do what we would do for any economic entity with traditional production techniques, namely, to use a U-shaped curve showing how average costs fell with increasing output at first and then increased as the scale of the firm increased. At one particular output, the firm has the lowest possible (minimum) average cost, at the bottom of the U. This is the output rate sought by purely competitive firms, but, as we shall see, it seems unlikely that physician-firms operate at this point.

We could also draw the marginal cost of the firm, the rate that total costs change as output changes. Except in technologies consistent only with natural monopoly (persistent increasing returns to scale), marginal cost curves *always* rise and fall more steeply than average cost curves and *always* go through the average cost curve at its precise minimum.[7]

This cost curve would shift up and down as the cost of any input shifted up and down. For example, if nurses' wages increase, then the average cost *curve* for a doctor's office will shift up. At every possible output, it will cost more to produce "doctor visits" than it would at a lower wage for nurses. This relationship between input prices and output costs should also translate directly into a higher product price, although not necessarily on a one-for-one basis. The appendix at the end of this chapter shows the effects of an input price increase on product price in several settings. The results appear as follows: In a long-run equilibrium in a competitive market, each $1 increase in the marginal cost of production of a good or service leads to a $1 increase in product price.

In any "short" run, the price increase will be less than the costs. In particular, the percent of passthrough (P) in any competitive market will be

---

[7]Problem 1 at the end of the chapter asks you to prove this statement.

$P = \epsilon/(\epsilon - \eta)$, where ϵ is the elasticity of supply of the final product and η is the demand elasticity at the market level. This provides a nice characterization of the "long run" as well. When all inputs are free to vary, the elasticity of supply in a competitive industry should become very large. As ϵ approaches infinity, the passthrough rate P approaches 1 for any finite demand elasticity. Thus, the previous statement about dollar-for-dollar passthrough in the long run is just a special case of this more general model. By contrast, in a pure monopoly, an increase in the marginal cost of production of $1 will lead to an increase in price that can be either more or less than $1. The appendix proves both of these assertions about cost passthrough. Chapter 7 elaborates these ideas in a monopolistic-competition framework.

Steinwald and Sloan (1974) studied fees charged by physicians throughout the United States, including the effects of wages of office workers on fees. They used a composite measure of the wage rates for five "typical" office workers in physician offices to measure wages. Their results showed that fees always increased proportionately with wage costs, in a way quite close to that expected in a competitive (or monopolistically competitive) industry. For example, for fees of general practitioners, a 1 percent increase in wage costs led to a 0.84 percent increase in fees. For general surgeon office visit fees, a 1 percent increase in wage costs led to a 0.93 percent increase, and for pediatricians, a 1 percent increase in wage costs led to a 0.48 percent increase. In a purely competitive market, the proportionate increase would always be less than 1.0 percent unless the firm was experiencing pronounced diseconomies of scale.[8] The elasticities for several specific in-hospital procedures are also available from the Steinwald and Sloan study. For appendectomies, the elasticity is 0.85; for a normal delivery by obstetricians, the elasticity is 0.75. Recall that these estimates come from an era preceding managed care insurance, which (as Chapter 11 discusses in detail) generally increases demand elasticities facing individual providers. Thus, these estimates probably overstate what one would find on more current market conditions, although no more recent estimates are available.[9]

---

[8]To a first-order approximation, the elasticity of price with respect to the cost of an input L (for "labor") would be $[\epsilon/(\epsilon - \eta)] \times$ (cost share) $\times$ (%dL%dQ), where %$dL = dL/L$ and % $dQ = dQ/Q$. The term involving elasticities of supply and demand must be less than 1.0, as must the cost share. Thus, the elasticity of fee with respect to wages must be less than 1.0 in a competitive industry unless %dL/%dQ is larger than 1 by enough to offset the other two factors that are less than 1. This would occur only if the firm experienced significant diseconomies of scale in labor.

[9]Or at least none are known to the author.

NONPHYSICIAN PRIMARY-CARE PROVIDERS

Many of the overall physician visits each day involve relatively simple medical conditions, and the practice of medicine that deals with these events is commonly described as primary care. The medical practices of general practitioners, specialists in family practice, internists, pediatricians, and obstetricians/gynecologists contain much of this sort of activity. For these primary-care visits, even more extreme substitution in the production of health may be possible than Reinhardt suggested, by breaking out of the model requiring a physician as the central actor in face-to-face patient visits. Although state licensure generally requires the presence of physicians in such a setting, some evidence suggests that other ways to produce primary-care visits may be at least as good, and at lower cost.

One organization that *may* use different models of production of primary care is the military health care system of the United States. Each of the major uniformed services (Army, Navy, and Air Force) operates its own health care system, responsible not only for the care of active duty personnel but also for the dependents of such personnel and any retirees from the military. Because the federal government operates these programs, state licensure laws do not apply to them. They can set aside legal *may-not* concerns and concentrate on finding the boundaries of *can-not* in the production function.

During the 1970s, the U.S. Air Force instituted an experimental model of primary patients' visits in a number of its clinics in which the patient saw only a trained paramedic. Although a physician was "in the vicinity" for consultation, the paramedic determined when to call the physician for assistance.

Studies of this alternative way of producing office visits revealed three clear features (Buchanan and Hosek, 1983). First, the cost was obviously considerably less; the paramedics earned about a quarter of what the physicians earned. Second, the quality of care, as rated by panels of physicians reviewing the medical records, was at least as good by the paramedics as by the physicians. Third, patients were at least as happy with the paramedic visits as with the doctor visits (Goldberg et al., 1981).

Several states now allow paramedics to practice under the relatively loose supervision of physicians, but none allows freestanding practice by paramedics, for example, that includes the prescription of drugs.

Another new model of production of health visits uses the nurse-practitioner as the entrepreneur. The evolution of this approach to provision of primary care depends in part on legal rules, which vary by state. One increasingly common area for independent nurse-practitioners is in the role of midwives. Many normal deliveries are now carried out by midwives in the United States, almost all of whom are trained as nurses, usually with advanced (master's degree level) training in their specialty. Some of these nurse-midwives work in independent practices, and some work in groups with physicians (obstetricians). Many surgical procedures are also carried out with a nurse-anesthetist instead of an M.D. trained in anesthesiology.

The quality of care and costs of care by nurse-practitioners continue to be areas of active inquiry. Very few randomized trials compare outcomes, for example, of infants born in birth centers (under the direction of nurse-midwives) with those of infants born in hospitals (under the direction of obstetricians and other physicians). One large national study (Rooks et al., 1989) studied birth outcomes of nearly 12,000 women admitted to 84 different birth centers around the country between 1985 and 1987 and compared those outcomes with several previously published studies of in-hospital deliveries of (hopefully) comparable low-risk women. (Making such comparisons can lead to erroneous conclusions if standards of care change through time or if the risks of the historical "control" populations differ meaningfully from those in the birth centers.) This study found birth center outcomes at least as good as those in the hospital, as measured by rates of eventual Caesarian section delivery (4 percent versus 8–18 percent in historical controls) and perinatal mortality rates (10 deaths out of 12,000 deliveries, or a rate of 0.8 per 1,000, as compared with rates of 1.0 to 2.6 percent in the historical hospital comparison groups). Costs are typically lower for birth centers as well, although evidence on this is less reliable.

The comparison of nonphysician primary care providers to physicians raises the obvious question: Just what does take place during a typical physician visit? The answer is that "an office visit" is an extremely complex matter, and research is coming only now to understand the true micro-micro-economics of physician visits. This issue is now studied in quite scientific ways, including tapings of individual doctor-patient visits, transcribing the discussion, and characterizing what occurs (Roter and Hall, 1992, Seale, McGuire, and Zhang, 2007). The topic has even become the subject of randomized controlled trial studies (Epstein et al., 2007) using trained actors to behave as real patients in real doctors' offices.

Several things immediately become obvious when one begins to look inside the black box of physician visit (Testa-Wojtekczko, 2008). First, two time constraints loom over the shoulder of the doctor: how far into "the day's work" the visit occurs (and how far behind schedule the doctor has become) and how many minutes have elapsed in a specific visit. Economists call these the "shadow prices" of time. Not all minutes are created equal in this world. If a patient brings up a topic late into (say) a planned 15-minute "visit," the response will be quite different than if the same topic emerged (say) 5 minutes into the visit. Similarly, the response could differ for a last-minute issue[10] depending on whether the visit is the first in the day or near the end of the day, and how large the patient backlog is in the waiting room.[11]

Researchers studying the micro-content of physician visits tend to classify the discussion in terms of identifiable "actions" (perhaps thought of in economics terms as "intermediate products" produced within the physician visit):

Physical examination of the patient

Gathering of medical history from patient

Specific diagnostic tests (e.g., urine dip stick) performed

Physical specimens for later diagnostic tests (e.g., blood and urine samples) gathered

Information flow to the patient

Reassurance of the patient

Empathy for the patient (sometimes, for the doctor too!)

Request by the patient for some specific action (e.g., prescribing a drug)

Response by the doctor to a patient request, such as

- deciding to gather more information (a new diagnostic test)
- recommending a specialist visit
- writing a prescription
- assuring the patient that the symptom is trivial and does not require intervention

Bioethicists Emanuel and Emanuel (1992) identified four idealized, abstract models of physician–patient relationships. These relationship types included the *Informative, Interpretive, Deliberative,* and *Paternalistic* models, each of which varied by its embedded definitions of patient values and physician responsibilities, as well as conceptualizations of the extent of

---

[10]Some doctors call these "doorknob" questions, the implication being that the doctor is literally walking out of the examining room when the patient says something like "Oh, I almost forgot, doctor, but I've been having some pretty bad headaches recently. Could that be serious?"

[11]A hint from the author: Schedule physician visits first thing in the morning or first thing after the lunch break if possible. You are less likely to have to wait to see the doctor (because the doctor cannot have fallen far behind schedule), and the doctor will be more willing to spend extra time with you if you need it (because a lot of time remains in the day to catch up to the schedule if you take extra time in your own visit.) If you can't schedule such visit times, bring along some good reading—preferably this textbook to study fervently if the visit occurs before your final exam.

patient autonomy and the physicians' proper role. *Paternalistic* providers recommend (sometimes strongly) the therapeutic pathway deemed most appropriate by the selfsame provider. In other words, the provider's preferences (utility structure) become part of the recommendation; the provider acts in some way as the patient's guardian, in much the same way parents do for their children.[12] *Informative* providers (the prototypical economist's "perfect agent") convey technical information to assist patients in finding the best course of action as defined by patient preferences. Patient values remain unexamined, and patient autonomy is maximized. *Interpretive* doctors do much the same as *informative* doctors, but also engage in dialog with patients to elicit and clarify (and sometimes form) values. The *deliberative* physician does all the things an *interpretive* doctor does, but also invokes moral persuasion to emphasize certain moral values and their benefit to the patient—somewhat of a combination of the *interpretive* and *paternalistic* doctor.

No matter what the style, economic analysis suggests that the response a patient receives will systematically depend on the time pressures (the shadow price of the physician's time). A request for a prescription drug early in a visit may lead to a discussion about the symptoms, perhaps a specific physical examination, or a discussion about lifestyle habits the patient has that might be related to the symptom. However, late into the scheduled time for a visit (or if the patient backlog in the waiting room has become long), the response could more likely be that the doctor writes the requested prescription and says "get back to me in a couple of weeks if these aren't making you feel better."

In this light, one can envision how patients might readily view a longer visit with a paramedic as being higher in quality than a short visit from a busy physician. The production of empathy, for example, takes time, so busy doctors may do less of that than less tightly scheduled paramedics. Some doctors, particularly surgeons, have turned over some of these activities to nurse practitoners or other paraprofessionals.

It is also clear from ongoing research that the patient's preparation for the "visit" changes this discourse. In particular, the advent of the Internet (allowing patient searches for specific therapies, for example) and the advent of Direct-to-Consumer (DTC) advertising by pharmaceutical companies to patients ("ask your doctor if the Purple Pill is right for you") alter the doctor–patient exchange.

---

[12]For a stunning portrayal of this phenomenon, see the movie *Who's Life is It, Anyway* starring Richard Dreyfuss as the patient and John Cassavetes as the well-intentioned but paternalistic doctor.

THE SIZE OF THE FIRM—GROUP PRACTICE OF MEDICINE

Physician-firms can obviously contain more than one physician. Indeed, most doctors now practice in multidoctor groups. These groups can include doctors of only a single specialty (such as pediatrics) or of multiple specialties. The extent to which such groupings are desirable depends on the economies of scale and the economies of scope of medical practice.

Economies of scale in physician-firms, as with those for hospitals (and any other productive firm), occur when the average costs fall as the scale of the firm rises. It is possible for both average *variable* costs and average *total* costs (including fixed costs) to fall, and finally to rise, with the firm's scale. People commonly assume that average costs must fall with size. For example, people observe the cost-saving possibilities for grouping doctors together to share "overhead" items (such as telephone and secretarial staff) that might not be fully utilized in a single-doctor office. The idea that average costs might rise as the size of the group increases is less intuitively obvious.

One way in which groups can eventually confront increasing costs (decreasing returns to scale, or diseconomies of scale) arises through problems of coordination, control of costs, and monitoring of work effort, which in turn depend on how the doctor is paid within the group.

Suppose at one extreme that each doctor in a group is paid on a flat salary. This is a common arrangement in large multispecialty groups and is often true for junior members of smaller single-specialty groups. The product of each doctor (patients' health) is somewhat difficult to observe directly so any attempt to monitor the work level of a doctor within the group usually falls back on some intermediate measure, such as visits by patients per hour or per day. Some groups control this by tightly scheduling the patients' visits for each doctor.[13] Of course, the doctor's total workload depends in part on the complexity of patients seen, so one possible response is to try to get the patients to return more often for an easier "repeat" checkup.[14]

Salaried doctors also have little incentive to control the use of costly resources within the group because their earnings are independent of the group's other costs. If they can make their own work easier (for example, by using more R.N. or secretarial time), they can be expected to do so.

---

[13]The military health care systems use this technique to the extreme. See Phelps et al. (1984).

[14]In the military health care system, in which doctors are on salary, this "quota-meeting" behavior produces some very unusual patterns of physician visits. For example, when a normal private-practice doctor might see a diabetic patient three to four times per year for routine visits, the same patient might return monthly in the military setting. Doctors can enforce this by giving prescriptions that last only 1 month. The patients, relatively captive in this system, are thus forced to cooperate with the doctor's activities designed to minimize total daily work effort, subject to the constraints imposed by the system.

The difficulty in monitoring such behavior by the group stems from the job-shop nature of medical practice. Each patient is unique, at least partly, so it becomes more difficult to monitor excessive use of resources or other costly activities with great precision. Sometimes, it is difficult to tell whether a particular activity is patient related or merely goofing off, as Figure 6.1 suggests. Obviously, a serious shirker can be fired from the group, but within some bounds, the problem is difficult to detect and control.

One way to help reduce these problems is to pay all doctors within the group on a profit-sharing basis, so that their use of costly resources cuts (at least partly) into their own pockets. Newhouse (1973) showed how this works. If each of N doctors in the group has $1/N$ of the patients, then each of the doctors has to worry about $1/N$ of the costs. In a totally noncooperative situation, a large group looks more and more like a group paying doctors on salary, with each having little concern about the costs of the group. Of course, many management methods exist to help control such behavior (i.e., shirking and resource waste), but these are also costly to undertake, in terms of both the direct management activity and the corresponding added work of the doctors in the group (filling out forms, attending meetings, etc.).

Gaynor and Gertler (1995) studied a parallel question: the effect of changing compensation methods so they are based on the work effort of physicians. For example, paying physicians a flat salary but giving them strong incentives to share in cost savings or paying them on a fee-for-service basis but ignoring the costs they incur while practicing medicine creates a mixed incentive system. That is, incentives can affect either work effort or

FIGURE 6.1 The problem of detecting shirking in large organizations.

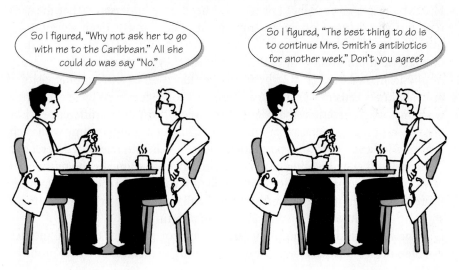

cost consciousness. Newhouse focused more on the costs; Gaynor and Gertler focused more on the compensation question.

Gaynor and Gertler used data from a survey of physicians' practices that described payment arrangements within the group, ranging from flat-salary arrangements at one extreme to complete fee-for-services performed on the other, with mixed payments (guaranteed salary of x plus y per office visit, etc.), the size of the group, the number of patients seen by the surveyed doctors per week ("office visits"), and a measure of risk aversion (asking doctors how important a steady income was to them). They posited that those doctors with greater distaste for fluctuating incomes would choose groups with stable (salarylike) payment methods. The key question is how the payment plan affected the work effort of the doctors.

Gaynor and Gertler's results showed a strong link between payment schemes and work effort by physicians, and that link is even stronger in larger groups, in which it is harder for doctors to separate slackards from hard workers. In small groups, doctors with the most salarylike compensation worked only two-thirds as much as those with the most fee-for-service-like compensation. In medium-sized groups, the relative work effort was barely more than half (comparing those with weakest incentives against those with the strongest), and in large groups, the relative work effort was barely 40 percent. This study shows not only that incentives affect work effort, but also that the magnitude of response by physicians to changes in payment incentives can be very large.

Another piece of evidence on the role of incentives in work effort of physicians emerges by comparing the rate of patients' visits produced by physicians in private (fee-for-service) practice and in a fee-for-service payment plan (independent practice association, or IPA) with the rate for those on straight salary in a "staff model" HMO setting. (Chapter 11 discusses the IPA and HMO concepts more fully.) For now, we need only understand that the staff model HMO doctors receive an annual salary, not directly dependent on the number of patient visits they produce, whereas IPA and fee-for-service doctors receive more money for each patient visit they produce. In a 1980 survey of physicians, salaried HMO physicians produced office and hospital visits at only about 80 percent of the rate of their IPA colleagues (see Table 6.1) while working for 93 percent as many hours per week. Most of the difference arises because HMO physicians apparently spend a longer amount of time with each patient. However, the "time per patient" was not directly measured here, but rather arrived at by dividing hours spent in office-visit time by the number of visits. Thus, the larger time per visit calculation could also reflect, for example, more trips to the water cooler, chatting with colleagues, or other forms of shirking difficult to monitor in a professional setting.

The eventual diseconomies of large groups of physicians are yet another manifestation of the pervasive role of uncertainty in medical care. The problem

TABLE 6.1   PHYSICIAN PRODUCTIVITY IN ALTERNATIVE PRACTICE SETTINGS

	Hours per Week	Patient Visits		Minutes/Visit	
		Office	Hospital	Office	Hospital
Salaried HMO M.D.s	46.4	67.2	24.5	23	40
IPA M.D.s	50.6	83.0	30.0	20	33
All doctors	49.6	78.7	33.1	20	30

Sources: HMO and IPA data from Wolinsky and Corry (1981); data for all doctors from same publication, "Part III—Selected Tabulations," Tables 12, 13, 19, and 20.

extends not only to cost control but also to the monitoring of a doctor's quality of care. Because the final output of each doctor is difficult to observe, even a poor doctor can exist for a long time within a group before it becomes apparent. A series of bad outcomes might easily appear as a run of bad luck. As with quality, similar difficulties occur with detecting doctors' using resources excessively. A doctor might successfully hide excessive use of a group's resources for some time because of the difficulty in knowing what "should" be used for a given set of patients.

The problems of shirking exist within any organization, but they diminish rapidly in small firms because detection is easier. They are more difficult to control and monitor within an organization that produces services rather than physical products because the tasks are more difficult to measure. The job-shop nature of the physician-firm compounds the problem. These issues eventually lead to increasing costs as the size of the physician-firm increases, and they ultimately limit the firm's optimal scale.

Another important limitation on the scale of the physician-firm is a cost that does not appear on the firm's books: patients' travel time. As with any service requiring the participation of the client-patient, travel time ultimately limits the sphere in which the physician-firm's market can meaningfully operate, providing yet another diseconomy of scale. This particular diseconomy of scale is not directly apparent from physicians' cost accounting because patients provide their own travel to the doctor's office. However, an equally feasible arrangement technically would have the doctor provide transportation to each patient, in which case the costs of expanding the scale of the doctor's office would soon become apparent.

Referrals Among Doctors—"Subcontracting" in Medicine

Often, a patient comes to a doctor who then determines that the patient's illness will be best treated by a physician of another specialty or subspecialty.

Typically, the primary-care doctor will then suggest a referral to a more specialized doctor, who treats patients for that particular illness only. This is one natural consequence of specialization by physicians. Thus, one of the particular assets of the primary-care physician-firm is the set of specialists to whom it refers.

The networks of referral doctors maintained by a primary-care doctor arise through a variety of ways. In a sense, the primary-care doctor takes the place of the patient in searching for another doctor. This aspect of a doctor's activity is considered further in Chapter 7, in which we more fully discuss search in physician markets.

One feature of the referral market—the prospect of fee splitting—particularly draws the attention of economists. Fee splitting simply means that the doctor making the referral receives part of the fee received by the specialist as a reward for sending the patient to the specialist. Medical ethics strongly discourages the practice of fee splitting. One reason why medical ethics views this practice as a problem (again, further discussed in Chapter 7) is that it could distort the physician's judgment about the "best" referral to make for a particular patient. If the doctor is supposed to act on the patient's behalf in selecting the specialist for consultation, then any fee-splitting arrangement can only distort that choice. As such (for example), it could violate the Hippocratic oath's requirement to do the best possible for the patient.

Fee splitting does have a potential good side. For example, some procedures can be carried out either by a first-contact generalist or a referral specialist. If the specialist offers higher quality (e.g., lower chance of side effects or iatrogenic illness), then something that increases the rate of referral may be desirable for the patient. (Notice that we can't say "will be desirable" because the patient may prefer to pay less for lower quality.)

The actual extent of fee splitting is almost impossible to measure because no doctor will readily admit to it.

Multispecialty Firms

Some doctors work in multispecialty groups, usually with a large number of physicians. Several of these groups have become quite famous nationally,[15]

---

[15]The Mayo Clinic in Rochester, Minnesota, is probably the most famous. Few people know the correct origin of the name, incorrectly attributing it to the name of the founding doctors, two of whom were brothers named Mayo. Actually, the group's fame arose from a large picnic in the town one summer, at which the mayonnaise in a chicken salad went bad, creating widespread stomach illness. The doctors' success in treating that event eventually led to the formation of the "Mayo" Clinic.

despite their relatively rare nature. An advantage of these multispecialty groups from the patient's perspective is "one-stop shopping" for a wide variety of medical diagnosis and treatment alternatives, with (presumably) closer coordination of care. The physical proximity of all doctors within a multispecialty group also offers an advantage to patients, reducing travel time and costs, compared with other arrangements. The location of many physicians in a single office building offers the same advantage and may help explain why doctors "bunch up" so much in the same area. Of course, doctors' office buildings also are usually near hospitals, so the doctor can go to see patients within the hospital easily.

From the group's perspective, the guaranteed "referrals" within the group may increase profitability by reducing reliance on outside referrals. However, the overall scale of the group usually must be quite large to make this work well, particularly in rarely used subspecialty areas. The problem can arise when the multispecialty group hires, for example, a neurosurgeon, but then the number of illnesses requiring that type of care may be too small to carry the doctor's salary.

Most likely because of the large volume of patients required to maintain a proper balancing act, most multispecialty groups have arisen in combination with an insurance plan that inherently attracts many patients. These combinations—health maintenance organizations and similar arrangements—are discussed in Chapter 11, after we have discussed the insurance market more completely.

THE PHYSICIAN AS LABOR

The previous discussion illuminated issues decided by physicians acting as entrepreneurs. They must also act as workers in a labor force. Thus, we can now turn to the questions of how the physician decides to supply labor into the market. Undoubtedly, many people decide to enter medical school for reasons not wholly related to the financial rewards. Indeed, as we will see later, some of the decisions about specialty training appear to involve important factors in addition to "dollars." However, there are also systematic financial questions associated with the practice of medicine that deserve study.

The three major decisions we can study are (1) the initial decision to become a physician, (2) the decision to specialize, and (3) the decision about how much to work (hours per year) once the physician has completed training. All of these have systematic economic components.

The Decision to Become a Physician

Entering medical school is an important investment. The physician-to-be invests the tuition payments and other costs of schooling (more than $40,000 per year currently for private medical schools, and about half that in public medical schools) for 4 years. More importantly, in addition to the 4 years in medical school, the physician-to-be invests 3 or more years in specialty training, which could be used in some alternative work. Thus, the *opportunity cost* of entering medical school is the forgone earnings from some other career that would be relevant for a person with a college degree. Much of this investment is financed in exactly the way we would expect: Medical students borrow extensively to finance their educations. By 2000, the average graduate from medical school carried nearly $100,000 in debt, growing at 5–7 percent per year (Association of American Medical Colleges, 1999).

Applications to medical school follow normal economic trends. The United States has about 16,000 positions open for new physicians every year in 130 medical schools. Although achieving an M.D. degree has long been both a prestigious and profitable endeavor, recent trends in health care (and competing alternatives elsewhere in the economy) have changed the particulars of this story to some degree.

Applications to U.S. medical schools have shown several major periodic swings through time. Introduction of the Medicare program in the United States in 1966 (and concurrent expansion of private health insurance) made the practice of medicine significantly more lucrative than in previous years, as millions of elderly Americans suddenly acquired much stronger health insurance than they had previously held. This led to a rapid growth in both the demand for medical education and the supply of new positions, with an approximate doubling of available positions in the United States in the decade following Medicare's beginnings. From the mid-1970s until the late 1980s, applications to medical school overall experienced a decline that is only partly understood. Price controls (see Chapter 15) entered the U.S. economy, perhaps triggering fears that the economic returns of an M.D. degree would decline. However, beginning in the late 1980s through 1996, applications for medical school steadily increased, so by 1996 (the peak year) nearly 47,000 persons applied to U.S. medical schools to become physicians, nearly triple the number of available positions (AAMC, 2008). Since 1996, the number of applicants has declined steadily, until (in 2001, the most recent year for which data are currently available) just under 35,000 persons applied to medical school, a decline of 21 percent from the peak a mere 5 years previously. Current commentary lays the blame on the emergence of managed care (see Chapter 11) and its consequences on physicians' incomes and ability to practice medicine freely.

Strictly as an investment, one can evaluate the desirability of medical school by comparing it with alternative investments the physician-to-be might make. The medical school investment has heavy front-end costs and higher earnings in later years. The "college" investment has higher initial earnings and lower average earnings in later years. The desirability of one or the other investment hinges on the *time preferences* of the physician-to-be. Those with relatively strong preferences for current consumption will be less likely to become physicians. Those with relatively similar preferences for current and future consumption will gladly give up some current consumption now for substantially larger consumption opportunities (earnings) in the future.

The most compact way to summarize the desirability of an investment is to use the internal rate of return (IRR). In its simplest terms, the IRR asks, "If I put the same amount of money into a bank account as in this investment, what rate of interest would the bank have to pay to make me indifferent in choosing between the bank account and the alternative investment?" When studying the economic returns to postcollege education, studies commonly use the "typical" college student's economic opportunities as the basis of comparison. A study by Burstein and Cromwell (1985) has made just such a calculation for physicians, dentists, and lawyers, comparing each case with the alternative of going to work directly after college.

This study adjusted for the average costs of tuition, the wages received during training after medical school (residency), and the average hours worked by physicians in their posttraining years. Physicians work many more hours per week than the average college graduate, the reasons for which are discussed here. If one ignored this larger work effort, the apparent returns to schooling would be overstated.

Table 6.2 shows these economic returns. As is commonly perceived, the financial returns to becoming a physician are considerable. An IRR of 12 percent

TABLE 6.2 RATES OF RETURN TO PROFESSIONAL TRAINING

	All Physicians, Hours Adjusted (%)		Dentists, Hours Adjusted (%)		Lawyers, Hours Adjusted (%)
	Yes	No	Yes	No	No
1980	12.1	14.0	—	—	7.2
1975	11.6	14.2	12.3	16.7	7.1
1970	11.8	14.7	12.1	16.8	7.0
1965	—	24.1	—	—	—
1955	—	29.1	—	—	—

Sources: Burstein and Cromwell (1985) for 1970–1980; Sloan (1970) for 1956–1965.

means that you would have to find a bank paying 12 percent *real* rate of interest (i.e., 12 percent above the inflation rate) to make it comparable. By contrast, the real rate of return on low-risk investments in our economy has over this century fluctuated nearer 3 percent or so.

Some of the higher incomes physicians earn reflect their long hours of work. When that is not adjusted for, the apparent rate of return for physicians exceeds 14 percent in most of the years studied by Burstein and Cromwell. On average, adjusting for work effort reduces the rate of return calculated by 2 to 3 percent. Nevertheless, the return on the investment in education for physicians is considerable and exceeds that available in most alternative investments.

The Decision to Specialize

Most physicians in the United States continue their training beyond that required by law to obtain a license to practice medicine. Licensure requirements vary from state to state, but they invariably include (1) graduation from an approved medical school and (2) 1 year of training in an approved internship or residency program.[16] Most doctors continue further training to become eligible to take voluntary certification examinations offered by specialty boards, that is, organizations that administer advanced tests in special areas of medical competence. Those doctors who pass "the boards" may indicate that they are members of the appropriate specialty board. These specialty boards exist for virtually every area of medicine and, indeed, comparably for many nonphysician providers of health care as well. For physicians, specialty boards exist for internal medicine, surgery, obstetrics/gynecology, family medicine, pediatrics, psychiatry, radiology, pathology, and many "subspecialty" boards.[17]

Board certification adds many years to a doctor's period of training. Almost all specialty boards require at least 3 years of training beyond the 4 years of medical school. Some complicated surgical specialties (such as neurosurgery) have requirements extending for 7 or more years beyond medical

[16]Until recently, all of these first postgraduate programs were called *internships*. They then became specialized as medical internships or surgical internships or pediatric internships. Now such programs are almost all part of a multiple-year program and are just called *first-year residencies*.

[17]For example, in pediatrics, subspecialty certification is available in such areas as pediatric allergy, cardiology, surgery, and newborn intensive care. In surgery, specialty boards exist for orthopedic surgery, cardiac surgery, thoracic surgery, plastic surgery, neurosurgery, and many other portions of the anatomy. For a good picture of the distribution of such surgeons, open up the Yellow Pages of any major city in the United States to the heading of "Physicians and Surgeons—MD" and you will get a good sampling of the number of various specialty areas and the number of doctors in such a community with specialty training.

school. Some doctors seek still further training in fellowships to learn specific techniques or to become more adept in an area of research.

This specialty training takes place in residency programs in hospitals throughout the United States. Almost all of these residency programs have some affiliation with a medical school, although in many programs the affiliation is quite weak and the residency training is provided "on a voluntary basis" by the doctors on the hospital's medical staff, rather than by full-time medical school faculty. Each specialty board approves the corresponding residency programs, and successful completion of such an approved residency is a prerequisite to taking the final specialty board qualifying examination.[18]

Several studies have measured the rate of return to physicians' specialty training through time, one for the period 1955–1965, another for 1967–1980, a third for 1987, and most recently for 1994. The earliest three of these studies analyzed four subfields of medicine: internal medicine, general surgery, obstetrics and gynecology, and pediatrics. It is important to adjust the dollar incomes of physicians for hours of work because physicians typically work a much more time-intensive "week" than many workers in the U.S. economy. All of the studies cited here do adjust for hours of work because, as noted previously, the failure to adjust for hours of work per year would bias upward the apparent returns to the training. The results of these studies appear in Table 6.3.

TABLE 6.3 RATES OF RETURN ON SPECIALTY TRAINING
(Hours Adjusted)

	Internal Medicine (%)	General Surgery (%)	Obstetrics and Gynecology (%)	Pediatrics (%)
1987	12.7	22.1	25.9	1.5
1980	9.8	13.6	14.8	—
1975	12.5	11.6	12.1	—
1970	9.3	11.2	11.8	2.4
1967	8.3	7.4	7.5	1.6
1965	1.5	5.2	4.8	<0
1955	<0	5.7	6.7	<0

Sources: Marder and Wilke (1991) for 1987 estimates; Burstein and Cromwell (1985) for 1967–1980, Sloan (1970) for 1955–1965.

---

[18]A doctor who has completed the requisite training program is usually called *board eligible.* Upon successfully taking the examination, the doctor can use the title *board certified.*

These three studies systematically reveal three phenomena. First, the rate of return on specialty training has been large, and second, the returns seem to have been increasing through time, particularly after the advent of Medicare. Third, the only counterexample to this is the return on specialization in pediatrics. Doctors who choose to enter this field clearly forgo significant economic returns to carry out their specialty training. In every study that has identified pediatrics as a specific subfield, the rate of return has either been negative or well below the borrowing costs of money at any time during this period.

A fourth study with much more recent data compared the return to "primary care" physicians and procedurally oriented specialties. This study [Weeks et al. (1994)] is important because it used data showing incomes of physicians in an era when managed care has been in place for a considerable time and is widely dispersed across the nation. (See Chapter 11 for a more complete discussion of managed care. Suffice it to say at this point that most observers feel that managed care squeezes the incomes of physicians compared with traditional insurance programs.) Again adjusting for hours of work, Weeks et al. found the rate of return to specialist physicians was 20.9 percent, and only 15.9 percent for primary-care doctors. The same pattern emerges here as in earlier studies—speciality training is more economically rewarding than primary-care training. However, for the first time in nearly half a century, the trend has been reversed in terms of the growth of the rate of return. Primary-care doctors (compared with internal medicine in the earlier studies) show a modest growth in the rate of return, but specialty training shows a lower return on the investment than did the 1987 study (Marder and Wilke, 1991).

It is probably too soon to state as a formal conclusion that the rates of return on specialty training have fallen from their 1980s highs—that will require additional data and new studies to confirm this trend—but the warning light has come on that the economic returns on medical training may have begun to decline. It may just be coincidence, but the decline in applications to attend medical school from the peak in 1996 could easily be interpreted as a market reaction to the declining returns (and other changes in the nonmonetary aspects of medical practice).

The Weeks et al. study also estimated rates of return on other professional educational opportunities, namely business, law, and dentistry. The study found the internal rate of return for business to be 29.0 percent, for law 25.4 percent, and for dentistry 20.7 percent. Thus, it appears on the basis of their analysis that medicine is now far from the most "profitable" career to enter when taking only the economic value of the future income stream into account.

THE AGGREGATE SUPPLY CURVE: ENTRY AND EXIT

The aggregate supply of physicians in the labor market and of physician-firms in the final product market is composed of the horizontal summation of all supplies (at various prices) of each doctor or firm participating in the market. In the case of the physician labor supply, the physician may decide to retire, thus withdrawing his or her services from the labor market. This does not necessarily change the final product market. If the physician is employed in a group, the group may simply hire another doctor. If the physician has been an entrepreneur directing a physician-firm, the firm may be sold to another physician. An active market exists for the latter type of exchange, including a number of brokerage firms that advertise weekly in widely read medical journals such as the *Journal of the American Medical Association*, the *New England Journal of Medicine*, and numerous specialty journals.

THE OPEN ECONOMY: U.S.- AND INTERNATIONALLY TRAINED PHYSICIANS

The supply of physicians' services at any time comes from all of those who have entered practice but not yet retired. To change the stock of physicians takes time because the annual *flow* of new physicians moves slowly relative to the stock. On average, medical schools in this country graduate only a number matching (at most) several percent of the aggregate stock.

In the U.S. economy, where overall demand for medical care is growing (and has been for the last several decades), two sources can supply new doctors to the U.S. market: U.S. medical schools and foreign medical schools. In an open economy (that is, one that involves foreign trade), a large increase in demand (as accompanied the introduction of Medicare and Medicaid in the United States in 1965) should generate a rapid increase in supply from all available sources. The most elastic supply is the rest of the world because we can draw physicians not only from other countries' medical school output but also from the stock of practicing physicians in other countries.

At least some sources allege that U.S.-trained physicians are of higher quality than foreign-trained physicians. Rates at which international medical graduates (IMGs) pass licensure examinations are below those for U.S. medical graduates, for example.

Figure 6.2 shows the proportion of newly licensed physicians in the United States since World War II attributable to foreign competition. The large demand stimulus associated with Medicare clearly created a massive

FIGURE 6.2 International medical graduates (IMGs) as a percentage of new doctors, 1945–1992.
Source: Noether (1986) for data through 1985; American Medical Association for subsequent years.

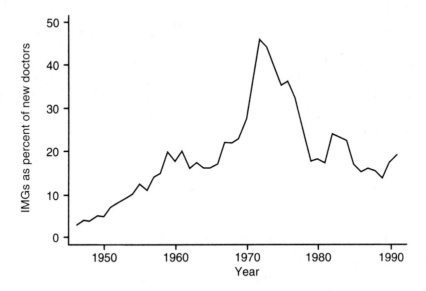

influx of foreign-trained physicians.[19] At the peak in 1972, nearly half of all newly licensed physicians came from foreign medical schools.

This increase in immigration of IMGs could not have taken place without changes in U.S. immigration rules. Partly in response to a perceived doctor shortage, these rules were greatly relaxed in 1968, particularly allowing for almost unrestricted immigration of physicians from the Eastern Hemisphere and allowing any physician admitted into the United States on a training visa (e.g., for a residency program) to apply immediately for permanent citizenship. Increasing restrictions in immigration laws, particularly as part of the Health Professional Educational Assistance Act of 1976, reversed many of these liberalizations in immigration policy, precipitating the decline in new IMGs shown in Figure 6.2 after 1976.[20] As Figure 6.2 shows, the proportion of newly licensed physicians who graduated from foreign medical schools stabilized in the early 1980s at about 15 percent.

---

[19]One rumor during the early 1970s held that the entire graduating class of a medical school in Thailand had chartered a Boeing 747 to fly en masse to the United States after their graduation from medical school.

[20]For an extended analysis of the roles of immigration and the U.S. government's support of medical schools as another source of competition for existing doctors, see Noether (1986).

In the past decade, the role of IMGs has stabilized, but still shows small trends upward in importance in the overall supply of physicians. In the most recent data available (1997), 26.3 percent of all residents in their first year of training are IMGs, and 25.7 percent of all residents in training are IMGs. In 2000 (the most recent official data available), the aggregate supply of active physicians in the United States (814,000 total) had 24.0 percent IMGs, a proportion that has slowly increased over the past 15 years from 21 percent in 1980 and 1990 to the current 24 percent (Bureau of Health Manpower, 2006). The current mix of IMG and domestic residents in training suggests that (at least for now) the system has approximately stabilized, baring changes in U.S. immigration law or federal funding for IMGs through Medicare (see Chapter 12).

SUMMARY

Physicians control much of the flow of resources in the U.S. health care system. We can think about physicians in separate roles, first as the entrepreneurs of physician-firms and second as labor input into the production function of physician-firms. In the former sense, physicians make the same sorts of decisions as any entrepreneur—which input to use, how much to produce, how to price one's product, and so on. In the latter sense, physicians behave much as other skilled labor behaves. We can think about the economic returns on specialization, for example, as a rational investment in education, much like any other worker's decision. Physicians as workers also have decisions to make about labor supply to the market and (unless protected by legal barriers) will likely face competition from foreign sources of supply.

RELATED CHAPTERS IN *HANDBOOK OF HEALTH ECONOMICS*

PROBLEMS

1. Prove that average cost and marginal cost are equal only at the point of minimum average cost. [*Hint:* Define $TC(Q)$ = total cost, $AC(Q) = TC(Q)/Q$, and $MC(Q) = dTC(Q)/dQ$ = marginal cost. To find the point at which average costs are at a minimum, take the derivative of AC with respect to Q and set it equal to zero. When you do this, you will find that $AC = MC$.]

2. (The result from this problem becomes useful in the next chapter.) Suppose that the cost curve of a physician-firm has the form $TC = a_0 + a_1 Q + a_2 Q^2 + a_3 Q^3$.
   a. What is the average variable cost (AVC) curve?
   b. What is the marginal cost (MC) curve?
   c. Find the level of output at which AVC reaches the minimum. (*Hint:* Take the derivative of the AVC curve, set it to zero, and solve for Q. Call this result Q^*.)
   d. Find the level of output at which MC reaches its minimum. (*Hint:* Use the same strategy, but use the MC curve.)
   e. Express the output at which marginal cost reaches its minimum relative to Q^* (where AVC reaches a minimum).

3. What features distinguish the physician-firm from physicians themselves?

4. "Physicians earn above-competitive wages, and the best evidence of this is the very high annual incomes that some doctors earn." Comment.

5. "The increasing costs of medical care can all be directly attributed to increased medical malpractice insurance costs." Comment.

6. When one thinks casually about economies of scale, one might conclude that physician-firms should be very large. What economic forces outside the physician-firms might cause them to limit themselves to relatively small sizes? (*Hint:* What would happen to firm size if doctors went to patients' homes rather than patients coming to doctors' offices?)

7. If the demand for physician services increases dramatically (as happened in the 1960s), what are the potential sources of increased supply of physician labor?

8. Discuss at least two distinct reasons why studies might show that physician-firms might use "too few" nurses and other aides relative to a profit-maximizing amount of those types of inputs.

9. People often think about "economies of scale" in firms because of the presence of fixed costs that can be spread over larger amounts of business to reduce average costs. Discuss two sources of potential *diseconomies* of scale in physician groups. (*Hint:* One source comes from an incentive to overuse costly resources within the group. The other comes from incentives to work hard on the part of individual doctors.) What evidence do you know that speaks to these issues?

APPENDIX TO CHAPTER 6

Cost Passthrough

I. *Competitive Markets.* The behavior of prices in a competitive market follows a simple rule: Cost increases are passed through to consumers as higher prices by a ratio that depends upon both the supply and demand elasticity in the market. The change in price (dP) for a given change in marginal cost of production (dMC) is

$$dP/dMC = \epsilon/(\epsilon - \eta)$$

The proof follows, using linear demand and supply curves, although the proposition holds generally:

Let the inverse supply curve (supply price curve) be of the form

$$P_s = \alpha + \beta Q$$

and the inverse demand curve be

$$P_d = \gamma + \delta Q$$

The intercepts of the supply and demand curves are α and γ ($\gamma > \alpha$), and the slopes of each curve are β and δ, respectively ($\beta > 0$ and $\delta < 0$).

In competition, $P_s = P_d$, so we can set these two equations equal to one another and solve for the equilibrium quantity Q^*:

$$Q^* = (\gamma - \alpha)/(\beta - \delta)$$

Note that Q^* must be positive because $(\gamma - \alpha) > 0$ and δ is negative because it is the slope of the inverse demand curve.

Once we know Q^*, we can find the equilibrium price P^* using either the supply or demand relationship. Insert Q^* into, for example, the supply curve, giving

$$P^* = (\beta\gamma - \alpha\delta)/(\beta - \delta)$$

Now we can find the effect of changing marginal cost. The simplest way to change marginal cost is to shift that whole cost curve upward—that is, change α. To see the effect on P^*, take the derivative of P^* with respect to α, giving

$$dP^*/d\alpha = (-\delta)/(\beta - \delta)$$

Now if we multiply both the numerator and denominator of this expression by Q/P, we get

$$\frac{dP^*}{d\alpha} = \frac{(-1/\eta)}{(1/\epsilon) - (1/\eta)}$$

where $\epsilon = \%dQ_s/\%dP$ = the elasticity of supply and where $\eta = \%dQ_d/\%dP$ = elasticity of demand. Again, after a bit of algebraic manipulation to complete the proof, this becomes

$$\frac{dP^*}{d\alpha} = \frac{\epsilon}{(\epsilon - \eta)}$$

II. *Monopoly Markets.* In a monopoly market, the monopolist selects the quantity of output so that marginal revenue equals marginal cost and then chooses the price from the demand curve to clear the market at that quantity.

Depending on the shape of the demand curve and marginal cost curve, the monopolist's passthrough of increases in marginal cost can in some occasions exceed 1.0, whereas the competitive market passthrough rate is always between 0 and 1.0. To find a circumstance in which the passthrough exceeds 1.0, consider the case of a constant-elasticity demand curve. The monopolist's profit-maximizing rule says that $MR = MC$, or, with a slight reformulation, $P = \eta MC/(1 + \eta)$, where η is the demand elasticity. Because no monopolist would willingly operate in an environment in which demand is inelastic (one could always increase profits by lowering output and raising price), the ratio $\eta/(1 + \eta)$ exceeds 1.0. When the demand elasticity is constant, that price is always MC "marked up" by that ratio.

In other settings, the passthrough rate is less than 1.0 for a monopolist. In the case of a linear demand curve with constant marginal cost, for example, the passthrough rate is always 0.5. To prove this, work through the following exercise: Set $MC = a$, and the inverse demand curve as $P = c - dQ$. Then $MR = c - 2dQ$. Set $MR = MC$, and solve for Q. Then put that expression back into the inverse demand curve, yielding the expression $P = (c + a)/2$. Obviously, changing MC (a here) results in a change in price one-half the amount of the change in a.

CHAPTER 7

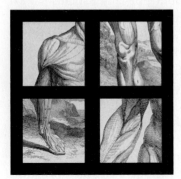

Physicians in the Marketplace

Chapter 6 described physician-firms without considering much how these firms interact with one another and with patients. This chapter analyzes the market for physician services further, emphasizing the interactions between producing firms and the interaction between firms and consumers.

This chapter first deals with the most general long-run question confronting doctors: Where should a practice be located? The answer to this question not only contains important economic information but also represents a long-standing issue in public policy. For decades, public policy discussions have concerned themselves with getting more doctors into "underserved" rural and low-income urban areas. Any mechanism to achieve this in the United States (and any other country with a moderately decentralized health care system) must operate within a market structure in which doctors can freely migrate and select the location of their medical practice.

LEARNING GOALS

- Identify how doctors choose to locate their medical practices in a spacial equilibrium.
- Master the concepts of monopolistic competition as a way of understanding medical service markets, and understand how prices and output of each physician-firm are set in such markets.
- Follow the role of consumer search and how it affects physician-service markets.
- Understand how advertising and licensure affect these markets.
- Grasp the distinction between the market-level demand curve and the demand curve facing specific physician-firms.
- Explore the world of "induced demand" for medical care and its consequences.
- Examine various studies showing the extent of induced demand in various settings, and critique the quality of this evidence.

197

This chapter next deals with the second question, the intermediate-run process by which individual patients and doctors are matched with one another. This process of search and matching of doctors and patients plays a prominent role in how well the market functions in matters of medical care and health. As we shall see, it also speaks importantly to the third question we study in this chapter: how the episode-by-episode relationship between doctors and patients actually works.

This third question centers on the interaction of physicians and patients and the role of information in that interaction. Physicians have more knowledge—arguably, massively more knowledge—than patients in the interchange between them. A broad line of inquiry in health economics seeks to know how doctors use this informational advantage. Some believe that doctors use it to create more demand for their services, possibly stopping only when they have reached a "target income." Others believe that although such demand creation might happen, it is not an important part of the interchange between doctors and patients and is surely self-limited by market forces. Still others deny the existence of demand generation. We study the logic and evidence behind the phenomenon of induced demand in some detail. As a phenomenon or concept, induced demand represents yet another of the important areas in health care in which uncertainty and information centrally affect the way the market functions and the ways in which we should think about the medical care market.

These three questions form the basis for our discussion of physicians in the marketplace. We begin with the long-run decision of geographic location, continue to the shorter-run question of matching patients and doctors, and conclude with the question of demand inducement.

PHYSICIAN LOCATION DECISIONS

A general phenomenon of markets is the spreading of suppliers across demanders. The process was first described by Hotelling (1929). A simple model to think of is ice cream vendors on a beach with people (potential ice cream customers) uniformly distributed along it. (This simplifies the problem because the "world" is linear rather than two dimensional like a map.) If only one vendor exists, the optimal location for that vendor is in the center of the beach, with equal numbers of customers on each side. This minimizes the average travel cost of the customers and hence maximizes the demand confronting the seller. If more than one vendor exists, the new ones will try to compete for location by situating themselves between the existing vendor(s) and the largest possible set of customers because (by presumption) customers will shop at the closest possible vendor.

The key idea with this type of spatial competition is that every seller confronts the same expected number of customers. If new sellers find it profitable to enter, the long-run allocation of sellers to locations must adjust to make the number of customers equal for each. Of course, if some of the customers have more income than others, they "count" more in this process because they will buy more of the sellers' goods. Thus, more precisely, each seller should face the same effective demand when a process of spacial competition occurs.

In markets for physicians, we can understand this process unfolding by thinking of a number of cities with various populations. Table 7.1 shows a small society with three cities having a total population of 125,000. If the total doctor/population ratio is slightly less than 1/10,000 (12 doctors total in this small society), Cities A and B will have the same ratio of doctors per person but City C will have none because with a population of 5,000, it cannot compete with either City A or B to attract a new doctor. Even if the total number of doctors increases to 23, each physician will find it more profitable to enter Cities A or B than C because the effective demand per doctor would be higher there.[1] Only when the total number of doctors exceeds 24 will City C finally attract a doctor. (The twenty-fourth doctor will just drop the equilibrium doctor/patient ratio to 1/5,000 in both City A and City B.)

We can observe this process in action because of a natural experiment conducted by U.S. medical schools during the 1970s. Following the doubling of medical school enrollment, plus the influx of foreign-trained physicians, the number of active doctors per 100,000 persons actually increased by almost 50 percent (from 146 to 214 per 100,000). Thus, we can actually examine where doctors chose to practice medicine and how that changed in response to this large outpouring of new graduates.

Under one extreme model, the new physicians would select the most desirable locations for practice, establish themselves, and "induce" enough demand to keep themselves content. This requires almost unlimited ability to induce demand in the extreme case. Under the other extreme model (pure

TABLE 7.1 HYPOTHETICAL DISTRIBUTIONS OF DOCTORS ACROSS TOWNS

City	Population	Number of Doctors (1 per 10,000)	Number of Doctors (1 per 5,000)
A	100,000	10	20
B	20,000	2	4
C	5,000	0	1

[1]This simple example obviously ignores the possibility of monopoly pricing, which would change the picture somewhat, but not the general idea. Thus, we can proceed with the simplified belief that every doctor will charge the same price, no matter which city is selected.

spacial competition), doctors would resettle themselves in a way correspon-ding to that shown in Table 7.1 comparing the last two columns. This sort of change would manifest itself in the emergence of doctors in small cities where none had previously been in practice.

In most cities and even most small towns, at least one doctor is present, but the same ideas of "spacial competition" should appear as well in terms of location of doctors within individual specialties. Once having selected a spe-cialty, doctors must also make a choice of location. How much does econom-ics play a role in this decision?

The results correspond closely to that expected by spacial competition models (Schwartz et al., 1980; Newhouse et al., 1982a, 1982b). As Table 7.2 shows, drawn from their work, the diffusion of specialists into small towns occurred only when the total doctor/population ratios became sufficiently high to make the small towns effective competitors for a new physician. Moreover, the aggregate ratio of doctor/population of each of these special-ists corresponds closely to the size of the town that can effectively compete for a doctor within that specialty. For example, in 1979 there were about 9 pediatricians per 100,000 population in aggregate, or about 11,000 people per pediatrician. The spacial competition model indicates that towns smaller than that should not be able commonly to attract a pediatrician. Indeed, as Table 7.2 shows, only a small fraction of towns with 5,000 to 10,000 people had a pediatrician, even in 1979. More than two-thirds of the towns of 10,000 to 20,000 citizens had attracted a pediatrician by then, and nearly all larger towns had one.

Similarly, there were about 65,000 patients per neurosurgeon in 1970 overall in the United States (1.5 per 100,000). As Table 7.2 shows, only cities in the 50,000–200,000 population size regularly contain a neurosurgeon. Indeed, the same general phenomenon is true in all specialties studied, although one can often see significant numbers of cities in the next size down with the relevant specialist, for example, cities of 30,000–50,000 for neuro-surgeons. The overall population/doctor ratio for any given specialty in the country as a whole provides a good prediction of the size of city needed to attract a doctor in that specialty.

These studies clearly demonstrate how powerful economic forces direct the location of doctors. Doctors respond to effective demand by locating in regions with the highest population/doctor ratio yet available. As the out-pouring of doctors from medical school and immigration increased the over-all doctor/population ratio (and similarly in each specialty), doctors diffused across the country into increasingly small towns, just as spacial competition requires. By the end of the period (1970–1978) discussed in these studies, the ratio of patients to doctor had fallen considerably, so smaller towns became more likely to have a specialist that fit into their size category.

TABLE 7.2 PERCENTAGE OF COMMUNITIES WITH NONFEDERAL PHYSICIAN SPECIALTY SERVICES IN 1970 AND 1979[a]

Specialty	Number of Full-Time Equivalent Physicians in 23 Sample States[b]	Population in Thousands (%)						
		2.5–5	5–10	10–20	20–30	30–50	50–200	200+
Group 1								
General and family practice								
1970	11,514	89	96	99	100	100	100	100
1979	11,869	86	96	99	100	100	100	100
Group 2								
Internal medicine								
1970	5,242	17	40	69	96	100	100	100
1979	9,467	23	52	84	97	100	100	100
General surgery								
1970	5,214	42	79	97	100	100	100	100
1979	6,071	44	77	96	100	100	100	100
Obstetrics-gynecology								
1970	2,928	13	32	74	96	100	100	100
1979	3,978	15	35	77	97	100	100	100
Psychiatry								
1970	1,990	3	12	28	46	91	100	100
1979	3,203	9	17	40	59	96	100	100
Pediatrics								
1970	2,263	6	17	57	92	100	100	100
1979	3,429	12	25	68	92	100	100	100
Radiology								
1970	1,823	5	22	60	88	100	100	100
1979	3,042	9	30	73	97	100	100	100
Group 3								
Anesthesiology								
1970	1,527	11	19	34	65	90	97	100
1979	2,303	11	19	40	83	100	100	100
Orthopedic surgery								
1970	1,380	2	6	29	67	91	100	100
1979	2,409	7	17	47	88	100	100	100
Ophthalmology								
1970	1,539	4	15	54	87	100	100	100
1979	2,147	4	14	62	89	100	100	100
Pathology								
1970	1,073	1	8	36	71	95	100	100
1979	1,840	4	15	50	85	95	100	100
Urology								
1970	950	1	7	29	62	98	100	100
1979	1,340	2	10	47	89	100	100	100
Otolaryngology								
1970	902	2	9	38	85	95	100	100
1979	1,127	2	6	29	79	98	98	100

(continued)

TABLE 7.2 PERCENTAGE OF COMMUNITIES WITH NONFEDERAL PHYSICIAN SPECIALTY SERVICES IN 1970 AND 1979[a] (continued)

Specialty	Number of Full-Time Equivalent Physicians in 23 Sample States[b]	Population in Thousands (%)						
		2.5–5	5–10	10–20	20–30	30–50	50–200	200+
Dermatology								
1970	528	1	3	10	31	79	100	100
1979	795	1	3	15	59	96	98	100
Group 4								
Neurology								
1970	365	1	4	6	25	48	73	100
1979	724	0	4	13	24	70	98	100
Neurosurgery								
1970	349	0	1	2	8	28	78	100
1979	523	0	1	2	18	56	88	100
Plastic surgery								
1970	210	0	1	1	2	16	51	97
1979	430	1	1	8	20	46	83	100
Any physician								
1970	41,325	92	97	99	100	100	100	100
1979	58,911	92	98	100	100	100	100	100
Number of towns in each population range								
1970	—	615	352	182	52	58	37	33
1979	—	644	379	206	66	57	40	34

[a]Population of towns is specific to the relevant year. Data are from the following 23 states: Alabama, Arkansas, Colorado, Georgia, Idaho, Iowa, Kansas, Louisiana, Maine, Minnesota, Mississippi, Missouri, Montana, Nebraska, New Hampshire, North Dakota, Oklahoma, South Dakota, Tennessee, Utah, Vermont, Wisconsin, Wyoming.
[b]These values include physicians in towns with populations of fewer than 2,500.
Source: Newhouse et al. (1982a).

A study of the migration of physicians and dentists (Benham, Maurizi, and Reder, 1968) provides a different but supporting portrait of the same market forces. That study looked across states (not towns) and found that doctors and dentists tended to move *from* states with relatively low economic returns *to* those with relatively high economic returns. Thus, direct study of the movement of physicians across states also supports the importance of market forces in determining the location of physicians and other healing professionals.

The Health Service Corps

Given these strong economic forces to equalize "effective demand" per doctor across geographic regions, it should come as no surprise that programs intended to cause doctors to locate in low-density rural areas typically have little effect. The most prominent of these programs, the Health Service Corps (HSC), gives significant financial inducements to doctors to locate in "underserved areas" through loan forgiveness programs after medical school.[2] Repeated studies have shown little long term equilibrium effect. Held (1976) showed that rural areas with and without prior HSC placements were equally likely to have a primary care doctor. Cullen et al. (1994) measured a 20 percent retention at the original site and 20 percent at another rural site. Pathman, Konrad, and Ricketts (1992) found only 12 percent retention on site after 8 years. Davidson et al. (1996) show only 1 in 6 HSC doctors remaining on site after five years.

Similarity to Decision to Specialize

The decision about location of a medical practice has considerable similarity to the decision to select a specialty. In both cases, economic forces direct the aggregate patterns, while individual preferences may well influence individual choices. Whether we think about a choice between neurosurgery and radiology or a choice among Spokane, Washington; Washington, D.C.; Washington, Iowa; and Phelps, New York, the same economic forces affect the choices of doctors. In the case of a choice of specialty, as we have seen previously, one must consider the present value (at the time of decision) of the future income stream because the decision to specialize represents a time-consuming investment. Although a geographic locational choice has lower costs and is easier to adjust, the general proposition remains the same: Doctors respond to economic forces in systematic and predictable ways.

Another similarity occurs in terms of potential barriers to entry. In the case of specialty choice, there is the possibility of a specialty training organization (particularly if granted quasi-official status through licensure mechanisms) to restrict entry into a particular field. Signs of such a restriction would include either persistent large returns to the investment of time (rate of return) and the appearance of major queueing or excess demand to get into specialty training programs. One commonly finds, for example, that certain residency and postdoctoral fellowship programs are committed years in advance, a sign of excess demand for the training (and hence an indicator of restrictive supply conditions.)

In the realm of choice of location, particularly for physicians with a heavy use of the hospital, the ability to gain admitting privileges to a hospital staff loom large in location choice. In earlier times, but seldom now, medical staffs

---

[2] See nhsc.bhpr.hrsa.gov/.

of hospitals (see Chapter 8 for a more extended discussion) would declare themselves "closed," meaning that no new physicians could admit patients to the hospital. In areas in which most or all of the hospitals were "closed," entry of physicians was effectively stifled, at least for specialties such as surgery and obstetrics.

CONSUMER SEARCH AND MARKET EQUILIBRIUM

Having studied how doctors select a location, we can turn to the next question in our analysis of physician-service markets of how doctors and patients "match up" and how the price is determined.

In a classic textbook competitive market, several clearly distinguishable features would appear. First, we could unambiguously determine the market supply and demand curves by adding up the supply and demand curves from all participants in the market. The quantity and price that we observe in the market would be determined by the intersection of these market supply and demand curves. We could also readily calculate the effect of changes in cost on the equilibrium quantity and price (see the appendix to Chapter 6). Each consumer and provider would of necessity take the market-determined price as given and would respond accordingly. Suppliers would select the amount to produce, and consumers would select the amount to consume, based on this market price. Their collective choices would lead to the "right" quantity being produced and consumed. Finally, if we could cleanly and clearly measure the quality of care, only one price would prevail in the market for each level of quality observed. This would be "the" price of an office visit to a physician in the market.

The contrast with what we observe in actual data seems remarkable, as Box 7.1 shows. For the most part, many prices prevail in a given market area. The dispersion of prices seems far too large to correspond to quality differences. Indeed, several studies have shown substantial price dispersion for identical goods in the same geographic area (see, for example, Pratt, Wise, and Zeckhauser, 1979).

Second, doctors seem to face a downward-sloping demand curve for their services. There is a widespread belief (albeit poorly documented) that doctors use price discrimination—that is, they charge different people different amounts for the same service.[3] Such discrimination is impossible in a purely competitive market. (Box 7.2 describes monopoly pricing and price discrimination in more detail.)

---

[3]The classic article on this topic (Kessel, 1958) describes the pervasiveness of the phenomenon. However, the logic used by Kessel blurs the distinction between a monopoly in an input market (physician labor) and the way the output market functions (physician services).

BOX 7.1   PRICE DISPERSION IN MEDICAL MARKETS

In medical markets, dispersion of prices is very common. Although some of the differences in price are surely related to quality, it seems hard to accept that all of these differences are quality related. For example, in the city of Dayton, Ohio, in 1975, the average difference in price for a "standard office visit" between general practice doctors and internal medicine specialists was only $1.50, while the spread in prices was much larger. The specialists on average received only 10 percent more for an office visit than the G.P.s (Marquis, 1985).

Figure A shows distributions with the same averages and standard deviations as the distributions of prices in Dayton. The averages in this figure are general practice (G.P.), $15.30; internists, $16.90; other, $15.80. The range of prices for G.P.s extends from less than $9 to more than $21. For internists, the range extends from less than $10 to nearly $23. Thus, while the average difference between specialists and G.P.s was only 10 percent of the price, the dispersion of prices within each specialty group was such that the high price was more than twice the low price.

FIGURE A

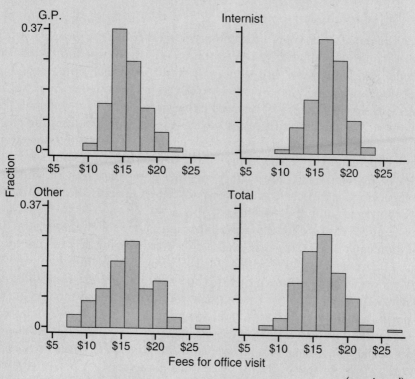

(continued)

BOX 7.1 PRICE DISPERSION IN MEDICAL MARKETS (continued)

The same phenomenon appears pervasively in other markets and for other medical services. In Seattle, for example, the same study showed a slightly bigger difference between specialists and G.P.s, but an even larger within-specialty dispersion. In dental markets, insurance data commonly show that the dispersion in prices for "routine" services such as cleaning, extractions, and fillings has similar characteristics.*

Surely, some of these differences are due to quality differences perceived by patients but not measured by the researcher. Tautologically, one could say that *all* of these differences in price are due to such unobserved quality differences, and there would be no way to refute that. However, given the small difference between the average price charged by G.P.s and specialists, it seems difficult to believe that the entire dispersion is quality related.

*The same thing occurs in other markets as well. Auto insurance companies commonly require that you get three quotes on any auto repair job and then pay for the lowest of those three. A rule of thumb says that when you get three quotes, the highest price will be twice as high as the lowest price for body work.

The model of monopolistic competition describes the physician service market quite usefully. The basic idea of monopolistic competition is that each producer faces a downward-sloping demand curve that shifts inward (or outward) as the number of other producers in the market increases (or decreases) or as the market demand curve shifts inward (or outward). The number of other sellers increases or decreases as opportunities for profits change. The "monopolistic" part of the name comes from the downward-sloping demand curve. The "competition" part of the name comes from the idea of free entry into the market by other competitors. In monopolistic competition, entry occurs until everybody is just making a competitive rate of return (zero monopoly profits).

Figure 7.1 shows how the typical firm appears in the monopolistic competition equilibrium. The firm faces a downward-sloping demand curve and has an average cost curve with a typical U shape. In equilibrium, *entry by other firms will have occurred until the demand curve for each firm is just tangent to its average cost curve.* At this point, each firm just covers its cost, it faces a downward-sloping demand curve, and no further entry into the market is economically attractive. Price equals average cost ($P = AC$), but production does not take place at a minimum average cost (i.e., not at P_{min}). As Chamberlin (1962), the originator of the idea, described it, there will be persistent excess capacity in the market in the sense that every producer could expand output and obtain lower costs.

FIGURE 7.1 Typical firm in monopolistic competition equilibrium.

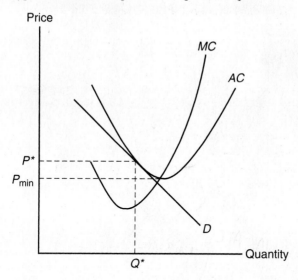

The physician's decision about geographic location described in the previous section precisely describes this type of entry-exit decision. When a market has above-average economic potential, physicians will enter. Otherwise, they will disperse themselves uniformly around the effective demand in all other markets.

BOX 7.2 MONOPOLY PRICING AND PRICE DISCRIMINATION

A monopolist is the only seller in a market, and thus the demand curve facing the seller is identical to the market demand curve. If the monopolist wishes to maximize profits, the best solution is to reduce output below the competitive level and raise the price in parallel.

For each intended increase in the volume of sales, the monopolist must lower the price on *all* units sold. Thus, the addition to total revenue ("marginal revenue") coming from one more unit of sales is the revenue on that sale *minus* the reduction in price on all other units sold. Because the monopolist confronts the demand curve of the market, the amount the price must fall can be determined from the market demand curve.

The marginal revenue curve in Figure A shows the additions to total revenue associated with the market demand curve. (For straight-line demand curves, the *MR* curve just bisects the angle between the demand curve and the axis of the price-quantity diagram.) Intuitively, what the monopolist wants to do is expand production until marginal revenue just equals marginal cost of production. At that point, any further additions to output create less

(continued)

BOX 7.2 MONOPOLY PRICING AND PRICE DISCRIMINATION (continued)

FIGURE A

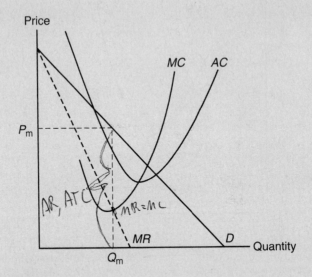

incremental revenue than the incremental costs of production. Profits reach a maximum when $MR = MC$. A monopolist picks this quantity of output and then sets the price *by moving up to the demand curve* at that level of output. Thus, in the monopoly market, output is lower and price is higher than in a competitively priced market with the same demand curve and marginal cost curve.

The marginal revenue function can be described formally in terms of the demand elasticity. $MR = P(1 + 1/\eta)$, where η is the demand elasticity. Note that MR is negative if the demand curve is *inelastic* ($-1 < \eta \leq 0$). Thus, no monopolist will willingly operate in the realm of inelastic demand. It always would pay to reduce output and raise price. The general pricing rule for a monopolist is to set $MR = MC$, so $P(1 + 1/\eta) = MC$. Another reformulation of this says that $P = MC\eta/(1 + \eta)$. Because $(1 + \eta)$ is negative when demand is *elastic*, $P > MC$ at all points at which a monopolist will operate. For example, if $\eta = -1.5$, $P = 3 \times MC$. If $\eta = -2$, $P = 2 \times MC$. If $\eta = -20$, $P \approx 1.05 \times MC$. Thus, although it is strictly correct to describe a firm as a monopolist if $\eta = -20$, it's not very interesting, because we can't measure MC of firms within a 5 percent accuracy. The general rule is that the larger the demand elasticity confronting the monopolist, the closer the price will be to marginal cost.

Discriminating Monopoly. In a price-discriminating monopoly, the monopolist can identify different segments of the market with different demand elasticities and sets a price to each of them according to the price rule just described. Those with more elastic demands get lower prices, and conversely.

ATC = AR → Economic Profit = 0
Normal " > 0

> To maintain a successful discrimination, the monopolist must be able to prevent resale of the product from those getting the low price to those getting the high price. Medical care is ideally suited for this. It's hard to buy a few extra appendectomies and resell them to your friends. For further discussion, see Newhouse (1970a).

A More Refined Model

Recent advances in the modeling of physician behavior in monopolistic competition have turned to a more refined approach to thinking about the physician—patient interaction. This new approach emphasizes the ability of the doctor to set the amount of care the patient consumes, even if the price is determined separately by insurance, government, or market forces. In this approach, McGuire (2000) has brought together several issues previously considered separate manifestations of the physicians' superior-information position.

In the McGuire approach, the patient has some minimum net benefit desired for any medical encounter (similar to consumer surplus, but for technical reasons, not quite the same). The doctor will attempt to maximize profits from each patient, but limited by the minimum net benefit that the patient expects (or "requires"). This net benefit can be thought of as the patient's best approximation of the best net benefit from seeking treatment elsewhere (or deciding to forgo treatment). This puts a natural cap on the ability of the physician to extract consumer surplus from the patient, but the limits rest entirely on profit-maximizing motives of the doctor, rather than on altruistic or other considerations.

The idea can be captured in a simple diagram (Figure 7.2), taken from McGuire (2000). The patient comes to the doctor with some dollar value of *NB* that must be reached (NB^0 in McGuire's notation and in the figure). The doctor picks a price and quantity that maximize profits, while preserving the minimum *NB* for the patient. This is done by a combination of raising the price (to p, when the cost is a lower amount c per unit), and then "requiring" that the patient consume x^* quantity. Just as the case in the analysis of regional variations in medical practice, the consumer loses some surplus because of the extra consumption. (The consumer would prefer a smaller quantity than x^* at a price p, but the doctor does not offer the choice.)

A key issue is how doctors would set quantity consumed for each patient (or more particularly, each episode of illness for which the patient comes to the doctor). In part, this simply reflects the immense informational advantage the doctor has. "I'm going to prescribe some medicine for you, but I want to see you in a week to follow up and make sure it's working right." The

FIGURE 7.2 Setting price and quantity with net benefit constraint.

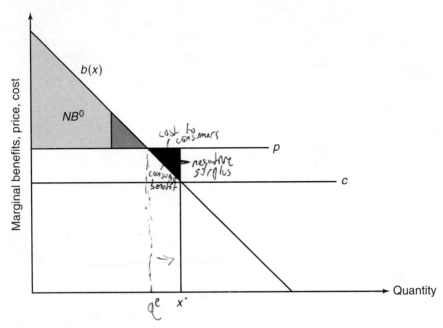

doctor can also imply that if the patient doesn't wish to follow the prescribed protocol, then perhaps treatment should be sought elsewhere.

This approach has valuable implications for many aspects of physician behavior. A bit later in this chapter, we encounter the idea of "induced demand" more formally, an obvious issue for which this model provides insight. In later chapters on managed care and government programs such as Medicare and Medicaid, we will see how the insurance programs alter the incentives to physicians precisely to deal with the quantity-setting choices physicians have available.

McGuire's approach also has interesting implications for what is widely described as the "doctor–patient relationship." Physicians (and their professional organizations) often emphasize the importance of this relationship.[4] These "doctor–patient relationships" are quite real and can be quite important in the doctor's ability to diagnose and treat a patient. Doctors can recognize changes in a patient's appearance, overall sense of well-being, happiness or depression, and so on that cannot meaningfully be codified in a medical record and passed on to other physicians. Similarly, the doctor may know

---

[4]The adjective "sacred" was often attached to the phrase in political discussions during the time of Medicare's implementation, meant to limit the government's ability to intrude upon this relationship.

things about the patient's willingness to abide by treatment regimens that can alter the treatment choice in a way that enhances the patient's chances of cure. In the context of a "net benefit" model, one implication of having an ongoing doctor–patient relationship is that the patient-specific knowledge held by a given doctor will be higher the longer the patient has used that doctor. As this relationship builds, the net benefit for each encounter grows, and (in the McGuire model), the doctor should be able to extract much if not all of that increasing net benefit through combinations of higher price and higher quantity.

Perhaps the most important aspect of McGuire's approach is that it sets aside widespread concerns about our ability to use demand-curve information in health care to make statements about consumer well-being (consumer surplus). The concern spreads wide among health economists: If doctors can willy-nilly shift patients' demand curves, then it becomes difficult, if not impossible, to draw any conclusions about patient well-being based on standard demand-curve-based welfare economics models. Without the anchor of solid patient preferences, the meaning of "value curves" (recall this as the alternative name for demand curves in Chapter 4) becomes vague. McGuire's approach restores our ability to draw consumer-surplus conclusions from observed behavior, although in most cases it requires additional modeling compared with a simple competitive equilibrium approach. Because McGuire's structure predicts virtually every observed "induced demand" phenomenon, it allows us to understand induced demand and at the same time carry out welfare-analysis calculations. Although this may seem more or less incidental to the entering student of health economics, the problem of how to do welfare analysis in the face of induced demand theory (and evidence) has perplexed many health economists. McGuire's model allows us again to use consumer surplus models without apology.

Quality Added to the Picture

Dranove and Satterthwaite (2000) present a more complicated model of equilibrium cost-passthrough that incorporates the effects of both quantity and quality on supply and demand (and hence equilibrium price), where "quality" has two characteristics: clinical quality (e.g., length of visit) and patient amenities, each of which can be produced with its own marginal cost structure. They define the cost of producing a medical visit as $C(q, x, y)$ where q is the number of visits produced, x is the clinical quality, and y is patient amenities. In a simple world where the marginal cost of producing a physician visit is a simple linear function $MC = a + bx + cy$. In other words, it costs a per visit with minimal quality, with linear additions of b per unit of clinical quality (e.g., time spent with the physician) and c per unit of patient amenities (e.g., shorter waiting time, more current magazines in the waiting room, an exotic fish tank in the waiting room). Dranove and Satterthwaite also define elasticities of demand (quantities) for visits to a doctor's office similar to the standard price elasticity: η_p is the traditional price elasticity of demand, η_x is the clinical quality elasticity, and η_y is the patient amenity elasticity. This is the same idea as appears in Chapter 4 showing how demand curves shift as quality of treatment changes.

The Dranove and Satterthwaite model uses a monopolistic competition framework, not the standard competitive equilibrium, and assumes that each physician firm faces a downward-sloping demand curve (as discussed earlier) with respect to price. This allows for a world where patients are immunized from price (e.g., with excellent health insurance) and hence relatively insensitive to price, or are more sensitive to price (e.g., with no insurance). The "markup" rate in this world is defined by $\mu = \eta_p/(1 + \eta_p)$. The equilibrium price is $P^* = \mu$ MC. Thus, for example, if the elasticity of demand facing a single provider is -2.5, then $\mu = -2.5/-1.5 = 5/3 = 1.6666\ldots$ and $P^* = 1.6666$ MC.

The most interesting part of the Dranove and Satterthwaite work defines how equilibrium quality characteristics come into being. Equilibrium qualities levels are defined as $x^* = (\eta_x/\eta_q)/(b/P^*)$ and $y^* = (\eta_y/\eta_q)/(c/P^*)$. A little algebraic manipulation of these equilibrium amounts gives a more interesting picture. For example, with x (clinical quality), $bx^*/MC = \eta_x/(1 + \eta_p)$, where bx^*/MC is the proportion of total marginal cost accounted for by clinical quality. A similar formula holds for amenities (y). This result has strong intuitive appeal: The more consumers respond to quality and the less they respond to price, the more emphasis the physician firm will place on high quality.[5] Similarly, if consumers don't respond much to quality, in equilibrium, a rational physician-firm will devote relatively little effort to provide quality.

These notions have at least an important conceptual force in thinking about optimal insurance design. Recall from Chapter 4 that traditional health insurance makes consumers relatively insensitive to price. Second, as we shall see in Chapter 11, managed care insurance essentially replaces the consumer's search efforts with "centralized" insurance-company search for low prices.

---

[5]A couple of quick caveats here: First, remember that demand elasticities are negative, so this makes sense only in a world where the demand elasticity exceeds 1.0 in absolute value. Second, remember that these are demand elasticities facing a single physician-firm, so we cannot use work (say) from the RAND Health Insurance Experiment for these data (the number would be something like $\eta = -0.3$ at the market level) but use the demand facing individual firms [e.g., such as estimated by McCarthy (1985) at about $\eta = -2.5$]. These are conceptual ideas; no good measurements exist for parameters such as η_x or η_y.

The Dranove and Satterthwaite model thus directly predicts that physician-firms will put less effort into producing quality under managed care than they would in a traditional fee for service market.

Probably the most important aspect of "quality" is time spent with patients.

Finally, as we will also see in Chapter 11, some new models of physician compensation directly incorporate quality in the price offered (so called pay for performance, or in text-messaging style, P4P). This new approach will presumably offset the downward pressures on quality that managed care insurance creates.

Search in Monopolistic Competition

The most powerful analyses of market behavior have employed the concept of consumer search in tandem with the monopolistic competition model. To understand the role of search, we can begin with an extreme case. Suppose *no* consumers in a market ever engaged in search for a "better" doctor (improved price, quality, or both). Patients and doctors would be matched at random or on some other basis that did not correspond to price or quality. Each firm's demand curve would be a scaled-down replica of the market demand curve. If the market demand curve had an elasticity of −1.5, so would each firm's demand curve. Each would price according to the pure monopoly model because each would know that the consumers who arrived at the firm were "theirs."

Now consider a consumer who engages in search. Suppose, for example, that the consumer decides (by some process) to search three firms and take the firm with the lowest price (or most desirable price-quality combination). Now the firm faces a dilemma when setting price. At higher prices, it gets more profits from the sales it makes, but it increases the risk that a comparison shopper will find a lower priced firm, and, thus, the higher priced firm will lose business. Lower prices obviously do just the reverse. Selecting the firm's best price requires a balancing act between these two forces.

It should seem clear (and can be proven) that as more and more of the consumers in a market engage in search, the closer the market comes to being purely competitive. The fewer consumers who search, the higher the price that can be expected, with monopoly prices as the extreme outcome when nobody engages in search.[6]

---

[6]The most comprehensive study of this (Sadanand and Wilde, 1982) is highly technical and not recommended for the novice economist. A more accessible version of this work appears in Schwartz and Wilde (1979), written for lawyers, or Schwartz and Wilde (1982b).

The other useful feature of this model is that it allows different prices for different producers, depending on their cost structure. For example, differences in fixed costs of each firm lead to different optimal prices for each firm. Thus, at least when a "small" proportion of the consumers in a market engages in price searching, the market should have a distribution of prices (rather than everybody charging the same price), even if everybody's quality is the same. Those with higher fixed costs have higher prices, and conversely. Of course, when a "large" fraction of consumers shops around, the distribution of prices collapses to the competitive price.

Health insurance plays two roles in this story. The first is a technical matter in the mechanics of the monopolistic competition model. As the demand curve becomes less elastic (less price responsive), the price dispersion increases and average prices become higher. Intuitively, we can see how this happens by noting that demand curves become more vertical (less elastic) with insurance (see Figure 4.9 and the related discussion). Hence, the point at which the demand curves become tangent to any firm's AC curve *must* be higher up to the left, rather than lower down near the bottom of the U shape of the curve. This is one effect we can expect from health insurance on the equilibrium dispersion of prices on physician markets.

Second, at least with some forms, insurance may also change the incentives for people to shop. The obvious effect, for example, of full-coverage insurance is that it reduces the incentive to shop for price. Some forms of insurance preserve at least some of the incentive to search for price, but at the extreme, a person with full coverage has no incentive to search for price. As one study has pointed out, however, insurance can also *increase* the amount of comparison shopping. By eliminating much of the financial cost of "trying out" a different doctor, insurance might actually increase search (Dionne, 1984). Particularly if some consumers wish to sample the "quality" of a different provider, insurance can promote search. Given the relatively wide dispersions in prices, it would be difficult to *presume* that quality and price are strongly correlated in this market, even though they are clearly connected.

There is growing evidence that doctors create a "style" of practice that best matches their own preferences and then attract patients who also prefer that style (Boardman et al., 1983). One "style," for example, might be the "busy office practice" with "standard" amenities. Another might be "Medicaid patients," which would probably decrease the amenities and increase the rate at which patients were seen in the practice.[7] A third style might be called "Beverly Hills Doc," with a low patient volume and extended physician contact time (and high prices) for each patient visit.

---

[7]The pejorative term *Medicaid mills* has been applied to some doctors and clinics. Clearly, not everybody who adopts a Medicaid-intensive style necessarily practices medicine deserving of scorn.

Several studies have characterized the search process patients might undertake in a specific way [see, for example, Pauly and Satterthwaite (1981) and Satterthwaite (1979, 1985)] and concluded that there is *less* search in markets with a high density of doctors. Their logic is that it is difficult for any individual person to find anybody else who uses a particular doctor when there are large numbers of doctors in the city. The style of search in this analysis is exemplified by a patient's expressing an interest in Dr. Johnson and then starting to ask friends, "What do any of you know about Dr. Johnson?" In a small city with only a few doctors, somebody to whom the patient speaks will surely know Dr. Johnson, and the search will be successful. In a larger city with many doctors, the answer will probably be "nothing," in the sense that no single patient is likely to know much about a randomly named doctor.

Two problems appear in this search model, however. First, if the search concentrates on prices, then it seems no more costly to acquire price information from a sample of five doctors, regardless of whether there are five or five hundred doctors in the city. Each requires only a phone call to determine how much, for example, is charged for a physical examination. Thus, the Pauly–Satterthwaite type of search would be most relevant for gathering information on quality.

The second issue is how patients actually conduct their searches. In a search process that is an alternative to the one embedded in the Pauly–Satterthwaite model, a person would begin by asking several friends who their doctor is, how well they like the doctor, and something about the doctor's "style." By selecting friends with similar preferences, the person could gather at least some useful information about some doctors in town quite readily. The costs of gathering such information seem about the same, no matter how many doctors are in the city. If so, then search costs should be about the same in any city. Box 7.3 extends the discussion of patient's searches.

The main motivation for the analysis by Pauly and Satterthwaite is to explain a common empirical phenomenon—namely, that prices for doctors are higher in big cities than in small cities, even after adjusting for costs of inputs. They explain this with the logic that search is more costly in the bigger city. The debate among economists (as with the debate on the evidence for "induced demand" that we review shortly) hinges on numerous technical issues and has not been resolved clearly.

We should be careful not to embrace any economic model just because the data are "consistent" with it. Other equally plausible models also may match a particular empirical finding, but those models might disagree on other important dimensions. Key tests among models occur when they make different predictions about the world, and then critical data can be found or produced that focus precisely on the differences in predictions, rather than on their similarities.

In the case of Pauly and Satterthwaite's model, for example, another very simple economic model predicts precisely the same phenomenon (higher prices when higher physician density occurs). This study, by DeVany, House, and Saving (1983), emphasized the trade-off between price charged and the rate at which patients can be served by doctors. In their model, a community in which patients have a relatively high value of time leads physician-firms to establish a practice style with relatively short waiting times for patients, but at higher costs (and hence higher price). The reverse is true in communities with a low value of time. The researchers concluded that "we must observe a positive association between money price and firm density." Thus, the empirical finding that prices are higher when physician density is higher can appear without any of the differences in search cost that Pauly and Satterthwaite depended upon.

ACTUAL SEARCH BY PATIENTS

One study shows how often (and for what reasons) patients actually do search for a new doctor (Olsen, Kane, and Kastler, 1976; Kastler et al., 1976). In a survey of 632 households in the Salt Lake City region in 1974, residents were asked about their use of doctors, including whether they had ever changed doctors. About 60 percent of the respondents had changed doctors at some time [at about the same rate for both low and high socioeconomic status (SES) groups], and about another 10 percent wanted to change doctors but were deterred in some way (e.g., due to fear of offending the current doctor). The reasons given for changing doctors appear in Table 7.3. Note that the most prominent reasons are all the "right" kind from the point of view of economic search models. For example, patients switched doctors because the

TABLE 7.3   REASONS FOR DOCTOR SHOPPING BY SOCIOECONOMIC STATUS (SES)

	Percentage of Shoppers	
Reasons for Shopping	High SES ($n = 234$)	Low SES ($n = 153$)
Appointment not available within week	53%	51%
First doctor not helping patient	49	44
Verification of a diagnosis from first doctor	38	34
Another doctor recommended by friend	26	26
Nontraditional healer sought because doctor wasn't helping	19	16
Care too expensive or could do with less expensive care	12	22
Personal friends with doctor	16	5
Member of same club or church as doctor	6	5
Doctor of different gender than first doctor preferred	3	3

Source: Olsen, Kane, and Kastler, 1976.

delays in getting an appointment were too long, they didn't like the quality of care, they sought verification of a diagnosis, or the price was too high. Note also that about one-quarter of those who switched used the recommendation of a friend (see discussion below about search in Pauly and Satterthwaite's model).

BOX 7.3 CONSUMER SEARCH AND PRICES

The technical debate between economists about the role of consumer search and prices can get quite complicated, but some key ideas appear throughout this work. The following contains some selected sections from a discussion by Mark Satterthwaite, telling why he believes that consumer search is more difficult in a market with many doctors, and a response by Jeffrey Harris, offering an alternative explanation for the same phenomenon. The discussion revolves around two pervasive phenomena, as characterized by Satterthwaite (1985, pp. 245–247):

1. At any time, physicians in communities that are well supplied in terms of physicians per thousand population are likely to charge higher fees than physicians in communities that are less well supplied.
2. Increasing the aggregate supply of physicians per thousand has had no obvious downward effect on physician's prices.

Satterthwaite offers the following:

Consumers when they are seeking a new physician . . . generally rely on the recommendations of trusted relatives, friends and associates. . . . If the cost of eliciting detailed and useful recommendations from trusted relatives and friends is low, then the problem of finding a new physician is easier than if the subjective cost is high. . . . The ease with which a consumer searches for a new physician . . . depends on two factors: the number of people in the community from whom he or she feels comfortable seeking recommendations, and the level of relevant knowledge possessed by those whose recommendations are sought. Both of these levels are likely to be low in communities that are experiencing rapid growth, that have a great deal of population flux, and that do not have a high level of social cohesion. . . . In addition to these straightforward social and demographic determinants of the cost of search, the number of physicians in the community, N, may by itself affect the ease or difficulty of consumer search. . . . Because so many physicians practice in a large city and their practices overlap geographically to a greater degree, every urbanite hears stories about a large number of different doctors. Except for those blessed with unusual memories, the stories [heard from friends about doctors] become a jumble; people do not remember which story is about which physician. Therefore, when a person is asked for a recommendation, oftentimes they can only report on their own personal physician, because they cannot remember any specific information about any other physician. This makes search more difficult and means, in conclusion, that [other things being equal] the more physicians serving a community, the poorer consumer information is likely to be.

BOX 7.3 CONSUMER SEARCH AND PRICES (continued)

In a discussion of this article (which followed Satterthwaite's 1985 article, beginning on p. 271), Jeffrey Harris, who is both an economist (at MIT) and a physician (at the Massachusetts General Hospital) offered the following ideas:

> In the Chamberlinian story of monopolistic competition, an expansion in the size of a market is ordinarily accompanied by an increase in the extent of product differentiation. At the start, microcomputers offered a few basic packages. As the market grew, specialized home computers, scientific computers, and computerized games appeared. At the start, Camels, Chesterfields, and Lucky Strikes were the three main brands of cigarette. As the market grew, menthol cigarettes, filter cigarettes, 120 mm cigarettes, and low-tar cigarettes emerged.
>
> The same phenomena are taking place in the physicians' services market. Starting in the 1960s, the U.S. government markedly increased its subsidy of both the cost of medical care and the cost of medical education. The resulting growth of physician supply has been accompanied by a proliferation of "physician brands." This product differentiation has not been confined to the emergence of new subspecialties based on new medical techniques. The emergence of new residency programs in primary care and family medicine were also manifestations. Physicians moved increasingly into . . . group practices. New practice styles, with enhanced use of paramedical personnel, have evolved. . . . We are seeing more physician-managed diagnostic centers, emergency care centers, and ambulatory surgical centers. . . . We have no unequivocal economic basis for proclaiming that the proliferation of new styles is beneficial or deleterious. . . . My guess, in any case, is that the welfare consequences of such increased product differentiation overshadow the consumer search effects that Professor Satterthwaite has identified. To me, the issue is whether surgicenters offer better medical care, not whether the proliferation of such centers makes it more difficult to pick a surgeon.

In a separate study of physician practice styles and prices, Boardman et al. (1983) discussed the positive association of physician fees and the number of physicians, noting that Satterthwaite explains this in terms of search costs. On the basis of their study, however, Boardman et al. offered another idea—namely, that the association rests on the link between the scale of the market and the degree of specialization that one would expect to find:

> There are other possible explanations. In towns with few physicians there would be tremendous pressure for . . . physicians to "compete at the median" and adopt [a busy, successful ambulatory practice style]. In larger cities with many patients with different tastes and many physicians willing to meet these diverse needs there would be greater opportunity to segment the market. In particular, we would expect some physicians to see fewer patients, but charge higher fees.

Their empirical studies support these ideas. The propensity for a doctor to adopt a few-patient, high-fee ("Beverly Hills Doc") practice was strongly increased with the physicians per square mile, while the propensity to adopt the "standard" practice fell. Of necessity, this increases the average price in a community as physician density increases. This corresponds closely to the model of DeVany, House, and Saving (1983).

ADVERTISING AND THE COSTS OF INFORMATION

One way to increase the amount of search in a market is to reduce the cost of information. Having consumers search is intrinsically desirable because it moves the market closer to the amount of medical care delivered (and hence received) that is "correct" from an economic standpoint. (The "right" level occurs when the marginal value to patients of X amount of care just equals the marginal cost of the same amount. This maximizes total social well-being, which is the economists' usual definition of "right.")

Many states prohibited advertising for professional services for years. These prohibitions have been struck down by many states recently as anti-competitive, but there still remains strong pressure from most professional groups against advertising. Advertising, like "The Force" in the *Star Wars* science fiction movies, has both good and bad sides to it. Certainly it has the capability of distorting patients' choices, and it is this "dark side" of advertising that professional groups emphasize in their opposition to it. The word *quack* commonly appears in such discussions, and the prohibition against advertising allegedly protects consumers from quacks.[8] Some people even fear that advertising, by increasing the demand for a product, might cause higher prices to appear. (Of course, when advertising is common in a market, the costs of that advertising form part of the cost structure of the firm, and hence are part of its pricing strategy.)

The other thing advertising might do, however, is to reduce the costs of providing information to consumers. In the monopolistic competition-search model, more consumer search leads to lower prices and a smaller dispersion in prices. In a classic study of the effects of advertising, Benham (1972) used survey data to measure the price paid for eyeglasses by consumers throughout the country and repeated the study with more sophistication 3 years later on another data base (Benham and Benham, 1975). Some of the states prohibited advertising, while others permitted either limited or unlimited ads. Their study found that the price paid for a pair of eyeglasses in states that permitted advertising was about 25 percent lower than in states that prohibited advertising (a difference of about $8.50 in 1970, corresponding to about $50 currently), even after controlling for other factors that might affect price. In states with advertising, the average size of firms selling eyeglasses considerably exceeded that in the nonadvertising states. Apparently, one effect of advertising was to allow some firms to attract enough customers that they could take advantage of existing economies of scale.

---

[8]Despite the connotation of the sound of a wild fowl, the word *quack* comes from elsewhere (although not the Greeks, this time). *Quack* is a short form of the German for *quacksalver*, a person who attempts "quickly" to heal with salves, but without any scientific basis for the cure.

Subsequent studies have extended the ideas contained in Benham's original work. Cady (1976) has shown the same phenomenon for prescription drugs, but with a smaller proportional effect. (Results showed about 4 percent higher prices in restrictive states.) Benham and Benham (1975) showed that the higher prices that correlated with advertising restrictions also reduced the quantity of the product consumed. Feldman and Begun (1978) held quality of the product constant and compared prices across states, finding prices on average to be 16 percent higher in those states without advertising for eyeglasses. Kwoka (1984) measured the quality of service provided and found that one way advertising reduced the cost of eyeglasses was a parallel reduction in quality of service. Apparently, when firms could not advertise with price, they resorted to quality-based competition that led to quality that was "too high" from a market perspective (in the sense that when advertising was allowed, the market reverted to a lower price and lower quality combination).

Some interesting puzzles involving the question of professional advertising remain. For example, advertising by dentists appears much more common than advertising by physicians. Inspection of the weekly television guide in the newspaper of many cities commonly reveals ads for dentists, but almost none for physicians. The Yellow Pages telephone directory shows the same phenomenon, although advertisements by physicians are now much more common than they were, for example, 10 years ago. For the most part, when physicians do advertise, they either do so because they are in direct competition with nonphysician firms for a similar service (quit-smoking or weight-loss clinics) or because they have a new service to offer of which few people are aware.

Perhaps the most widespread example currently involves laser surgery to correct refractive vision problems. This new approach to vision correction has spawned widespread advertising in most regions of the country, touting the benefits of the procedure and the experience of the actual physicians doing the procedures. Other specific medical procedures with frequent direct-consumer advertising often involve plastic surgery of various sorts, often designed to enhance the consumer's sexual appeal (or at least the promise thereof). Interestingly, most of the procedures for which widespread mass media advertising occurs are those precluded from coverage by most health insurance companies. This is most likely not just a coincidence: Those procedures for which demand is most susceptible to influence by advertising are those least likely to be good candidates for insurance coverage, as Chapter 10 will illuminate in more detail.[9]

---

[9]A separate topic—direct-to-consumer advertising of prescription drugs—is discussed more fully in the section on pharmaceuticals in Chapter 15.

One of the more puzzling and interesting mass-marketing advertisements appeared recently on radio in New York City. There were one-minute radio "spots" for *brain surgery,* touting the quality of care by a particular hospital and neurosurgical group. This sort of direct advertisement for an apparently rare and highly sophisticated surgical intervention stands as an unexplained puzzle because the most common way to choose such a surgical subspecialist is either through one's own primary-care provider or through an approved referral program from the insurance provider for a given patient.

THE ROLE OF LICENSURE

Licensure by the state for professionals has a long if occasionally checkered history. Our governments (at various levels) license physicians, registered nurses, dentists, and those in many other healing professions. Governments also require licenses for barbers and beauticians, airplane pilots, automobile drivers, and civil engineers, but not college professors, hockey players, financial advisors, rock musicians, or economists. It is not readily apparent that in the absence of licensure, the licensed groups (e.g., beauticians) would be intrinsically more dangerous to society than the unlicensed group (e.g., rock musicians), but licensure is commonly supported in the belief that it protects the safety of the public from incompetence by practitioners of a profession. Interestingly, licensure commonly occurs for *inputs* into a productive process, but seldom for the firm responsible for the *output.* In the case of medical care, for example, doctors and nurses not physician-groups, receive licenses. Although hospitals receive safety inspections, these relate more to fire hazards and food safety than to the quality of the actual product. In air travel, pilots and airplanes are both rigorously certified, but not airline corporations.

As with advertising, licensure has both potential good and bad features. The obvious "good" is the maintenance of quality and the prevention of harm to patients, which loom particularly large if patients have difficulty in assessing the quality of a provider of care. Licensure can provide a "floor" on quality of care upon which consumers can rely without any investigation of any particular provider. To the extent that it succeeds in this, licensure can also increase search, by making price information seem more useful (in the sense that a low price would not imply too-low quality).

As one of its "bad" features, licensure also can stand as a barrier to entry, decreasing competition and creating monopoly rents to those who obtain a license. Taxicab licensing in some cities has clearly done this, for example, as evidenced both by the presence of unlicensed taxicabs (despite the risks of conviction) and, more importantly, by the resale price of a taxicab medallion, the actual license that is attached to the vehicle (Kitch, Isaac, and Kaspar, 1971).

In a classic study of physician markets, Kessel (1958) argued that licensure restrictions on entry into the medical profession led not only to monopoly pricing by physicians but also to price discrimination. (See Box 7.2 describing monopoly pricing.) Although Kessel's evidence on price discrimination may be accurate, the imputation of cause to medical licensure cannot be correct. Licensure might create a barrier to entry of an *input* in the production of physician services, but it has nothing to do with the production or market organization of the *output* market. If licensure does create an economically important entry restriction in the input market, it will raise the cost curve of every firm producing physician services. Licensure cannot, however, create the opportunity for such firms to price monopolistically because (1) physicians can and do migrate (see Benham, Maurizi, and Reder, 1968) and (2) physician-firms can (and do) substitute other inputs for those of physician labor (see Reinhardt, 1973, 1975). Other economic phenomena, primarily including the extent of search by patients, determine whether physician-firms act as monopolists or competitors.

On net, licensure can have both economically desirable and undesirable features. The capability for limiting entry obviously has some economic liabilities associated with it. However, the quality control capabilities of licensure are probably positive. On net, one cannot say that licensure is necessarily a benefit or a harm to consumers. The potential gains in quality information may outweigh any costs from monopolization.[10] Indeed, it may even be that the market operates more competitively because the "minimum quality" guarantee that licensure produces may increase consumer willingness to search for lower prices.

Medical specialty boards have aspects about them that are similar to licensure, except that they are voluntary rather than mandatory. Thus, although every doctor is supposed to have a license, specialty certification is completely optional. Of course, because specialty boards cannot limit entry into the medical profession, they primarily serve as indicators of quality. It would be difficult to construe them as barriers to entry because one can practice a specialty without having board certification (although a doctor cannot claim that he or she is certified by the board unless that is true). In addition, occasionally multiple (competing) organizations provide certification for the

---

[10]The earliest proponents of the monopoly restriction hypothesis were Friedman and Kuznets (1945), Kessel (1958), and M. Friedman (1962). The importance of licensure for quality control was emphasized by Arrow (1963) and, more recently, by Leffler (1978).

same area of medical practice, although, in general, only a single specialty board exists in any given area of medical practice.[11]

ESTIMATES OF THE DEMAND CURVE FACING PHYSICIAN-FIRMS

The various concepts discussed previously all have some effect on the scope of physician practices and where they locate. Given all of these factors, we know that doctors disperse themselves into various regions. What market conditions do they face then? One study has estimated the demand curve confronting primary-care physician-firms using survey data from the American Medical Association (McCarthy, 1985) for firms located in large metropolitan areas (defined as those with a population of more than 1 million). The results support much of the previous discussion and add empirical specificity to the concepts previously discussed. Perhaps of most importance, the price elasticity of the demand curve facing a typical large-city primary-care physician is quite large. In all of the various forms estimated, this study found the *firm's* demand curve to have an elasticity of −3 (or larger, in absolute value). We should be careful not to confuse this with the elasticity of the *market* demand curve, which (according to the RAND HIS results—see Table 5.3) is about −0.2 to −0.3. The difference, of course, is that the individual firm loses customers to other firms by raising prices, where "the market" as a whole loses customers only when they drop out totally due to higher prices. An elasticity of −3 certainly confirms the validity of using something other than a "perfectly competitive" model to explore physician markets, but it also shows that the departures from purely competitive markets cannot be huge.[12]

The estimates in this study also showed the effects of waiting time on prices just as one might expect. Longer waiting times in the office reduced

---

[11]In some areas of the economy, multiple certification is common. For example, in scuba diving instruction, three common certification bodies include the National Association of Underwater Instructors (NAUI), the Professional Association of Diving Instructors (PADI), and the YMCA. In the area of medical care, certification for people prescribing eyeglasses has arisen at least in three separate areas: for physicians, the Board of Ophthalmologists; for optometrists (who have different training in separate schools); and, most recently, for "prescribing opticians," that is, a group of people who formerly specialized in making lenses, but who now also prescribe them.

[12]The optimal price for a monopolist is inversely related to the demand elasticity confronting the firm. In general, where MC = the marginal cost of production, the optimal price is found by setting $P = MC/(1 + 1/\eta)$, where η is the demand elasticity facing the firm. If $\eta = -3$, then $P = MC/(1 - 1/3) = (3/2) MC$. Put differently, there would be a 50 percent "markup" of price above marginal cost.

demand for physician visits, holding price constant. The estimated waiting-time elasticity confronting physician firms ranged from −0.4 to −1.1 in various versions of the model estimated.

In the context of the monopolistic competition and search models, another interesting result emerged. Contrary to previous empirical findings (which show higher fees with higher density), this study, which used data on individual firms rather than data at the county or standard metropolitan statistical area (SMSA) level, found that higher physician density in a region *reduced* the demand confronting a physician. This finding corresponds precisely to the standard monopolistic competition model, in which more firms in a community imply fewer customers per firm. This, of course, shifts inward the demand curve facing any firm, thus reducing the price it can charge. This finding helps strengthen the belief that something other than "difficult search" makes prices higher in markets with more doctors.

Excess Capacity

A final aspect of the monopolistic competition model is the predicted presence of "excess capacity" in the market. This sort of excess capacity is most likely to arise in areas in which the demand curve facing a single physician-firm is least elastic. (See Figure 7.1, and imagine the output rate at which the tangency exists with the U-shaped *AC* curve, compared with the output producing minimum *AC*. The steeper the demand curve, the further the actual price is above the minimum *AC*.) Markets in which search is least likely to take place and where insurance coverage is greatest offer likely targets to find considerable excess capacity. In one study, Hughes et al. (1972) examined the actual working hours and practices of surgeons. They found persistent excess capacity among surgeons, often with as much as 40 percent "slack time" in surgeons' practices.

Excess capacity is more likely to surface in other ways now that "managed care" has become more prominent (see Chapter 11). Managed-care plans now either hire surgeons directly on salary (limiting the number hired to ensure that they maintain a "full" schedule) or else arrange for "selective contracting" with a narrow range of surgeons who (in exchange for a lower fee) get a considerable volume of business referred to them by the insurance program. In either case, one finds that *some* surgeons appear "very" busy while others may actually become unemployed, as has been observed with increasing frequency in California and other markets with substantial numbers of people selecting managed-care programs rather than traditional insurance.

INDUCED DEMAND

Lather. Rinse. Repeat.
[Common attempt to induce demand by manufacturers of consumer product]

It is probably fair to say that the question of induced demand separates "academic" study of health economics from "policy-related" questions more than any other topic. Academics find the topic fascinating and spend nearly endless resources devoted to its study.[13] By contrast, probably few members of Congress could even define the topic, although perhaps they should learn what it is. The three key political issues (and the government studies evolving from those interests) are cost control, cost control, and cost control (to paraphrase the standard statement about real estate).[14] However, if the proponents of the induced demand concept are correct, perhaps political issues should at least also contain the concept of induced demand.[15]

The idea of induced demand is not limited to the provision of medical care. Almost any person who has ever owned an automobile has probably felt at some time that he or she had been sold a repair service that was possibly not needed. From the consumer's point of view, however, it's sometimes just not worth the trouble to check up on a mechanic (Darby and Karni, 1973). In medical care, the large differences in knowledge between the doctor and the patient certainly suggest the possibility that doctors could use their position of superior knowledge for their own financial benefit.

Let's be precise about what we mean by "induced demand." McGuire (2000) carefully specified provider-induced demand as occurring "when the physician influences a patient's demand for care against the physician's interpretation of the best interest of the patient." Left implicit in this definition is the "why" question. Unless guided by pure meanness or dislike for a particular patient, the obvious answer is that the influence financially benefits the physician. This economic aspect is crucial. For example, physician disagreement about the proper treatment strategies across geographic regions (see

---

[13]The editor of the *Journal of Health Economics,* Joe Newhouse, once said that he had considered renaming the journal the *Journal of Induced Demand* because he had so many articles submitted for publication on this topic.

[14]Location, location, and location.

[15]Recent changes in Medicare payments to physicians actually did take account *in advance* of a presumed increase in quantity of services in response to a reduction in physicians' fees. Thus, demand inducement has, in some ways, entered health policy. See Chapter 12 for a further discussion.

discussion in Chapters 3 and 5) would *not* constitute induced demand in general because we see no systematic differences in the way physician incentives differ across regions in ways that would explain geographic practice variations.

The idea of "demand inducement" by doctors was given its most prominent boost by studies of Robert Evans (1974) and Victor Fuchs (1978). Since then, literally dozens (perhaps hundreds) of studies that have appeared in professional economics journals discuss aspects of the question.[16] The central idea stems from the observation that (with hospitals) areas that had a larger hospital bed supply had more hospital utilization (Roemer, 1961). Economists were quick to dismiss the relevance of such simple data with the observation that a competitive market would produce such results, with supply *following* demand into areas of high demand.

Fuchs's study offers a good example of the type of evidence available on the extent of inducement. He estimated the demand for surgical procedures in a number of SMSAs, holding constant price, income, and other relevant variables and using the physician supply *predicted* to be in a region from economic forces that could be measured.[17] He found that as that predicted supply increased by 10 percent, the number of surgical procedures increased by 3 or 4 percent. This type of result was more disquieting to neoclassical economists because it dealt with the earlier refutation and still produced the result that supply could apparently create its own demand, at least to some extent. Box 7.4 provides examples of the existing disagreement on the subject.

The debate in the health economics literature has become arcane and complicated, with various alternative explanations offered by economists showing how the positive association between supply and quantity demanded could sustain itself in a competitive structure: One argument is that perhaps more doctors (through their increased density) lower the time

---

[16]For the student truly fascinated by the topic, the list contains (in alphabetic order, but not comprehensively) Auster and Oaxaca (1981); Boardman et al. (1983); Cromwell and Mitchell (1986); DeVany, House, and Saving (1983); Dranove (1988a); Evans (1974); Evans, Parish, and Scully (1973); Farley (1986); Feldman (1979); Fuchs (1978); Fuchs and Kramer (1972); Green (1978); Hadley, Holohan, and Scanlon (1979); Hay and Leahy (1982); McCarthy (1985); McCombs (1984); Newhouse et al. (1982a, 1982b); Pauly (1980); Pauly and Satterthwaite (1981); Reinhardt (1985); Rice (1987); Rice and Labelle (1989); Rossiter and Wilensky (1983); Satterthwaite (1979, 1985); Schwartz et al. (1980); Stano (1985, 1987a, 1987b); and many others. Space limitations argue against providing a complete listing of relevant citations.

[17]This technique involves the simultaneous estimation of supply and demand curves for a product. In econometric terms, one uses two-stage least squares (TSLS) or some nonlinear equivalent.

cost to patients, thereby increasing the quantity demanded. Another suggests that perhaps there are hidden flaws in the statistical analysis.[18] One model showed how increasing physician supply could lead to both more office visits and fewer hospital admissions through a profit-maximizing substitution of outpatient for inpatient care (McCombs, 1984), but without any inducement. This model of the market has the distinction of actively predicting a phenomenon (reduced hospitalization) that has been observed in parallel with the increasing physician supply, rather than merely being another "non-inducement" explanation of the phenomenon originally ascribed to inducement (the positive association of physician supply and doctor visits). Not uncommonly, the studies focused on prices, which (in the pure classical sense) should decline as supply shifts outward but are commonly found to be higher in areas with higher per capita supplies of physicians. Several studies (including DeVany, House, and Saving, 1983; Boardman et al., 1983) offered explanations for the positive association of price with supply in a "classical" framework, without resorting to inducement. However, none of these studies could show that inducement *was not* occurring, only that an alternative explanation existed for the phenomena said to arise from inducement.

Several conceptual ideas emerged with nearly unanimous support. First, if inducement could occur, some limit to inducement had to take place, or doctors would own the entire world. Some analysts posited a "target income" for doctors (Newhouse, 1970a; Evans, 1974), while others posited a doctor who felt more and more guilty with greater inducement (Sloan and Feldman, 1978; Gruber and Owings, 1996). Pauly (1980) and others noted that under any of these models, any doctors who would induce at all would induce "to the max," or as much as any constraint present would allow, and this idea has received widespread support (although some people believe that the constraints are totally binding, so that there is no inducement). Dranove (1988a) developed a model in which patients' wariness about inducement would create natural limits to inducement, even for a profit-maximizing doctor.

Recently, a remarkable study cast considerable doubt on the underlying methodology used for many of the previous studies of induced demand. Without delving into the statistical issues in great detail, let's consider the fundamental issue. If one looks in different regions of the country, one finds a positive association between the number of, for example, orthopedic surgeons per capita and the number of orthopedic operations performed per capita. One would expect this, of course, in a competitive market environment in

---

[18]One empirical foray in this literature (Cromwell and Mitchell, 1986) dealt with most of these issues. Even then, complicated statistical problems remained (Phelps, 1986a). Some natural experiments provide further evidence (Rice, 1987).

BOX 7.4 ECONOMISTS' PERSPECTIVES ON DEMAND INDUCEMENT

The idea of demand inducement creates strong feelings among economists, some of whom accept it as a simple matter of course, and others of whom adamantly deny its very existence. The reasons for worrying about it are not trivial. Demand inducement complicates the use of inverse demand curves as measures of consumer's private valuation of medical care. In turn, this makes welfare-economic applications in health care somewhat suspect. Demand inducement also means that "markets aren't working," and this intrinsically bothers many economists as well. Thus, the idea of demand inducement and research surrounding it seems to evoke strong passions among health economists. Two commentaries from the literature on this issue follow. The first, from a study by DeVany, House, and Saving (1983, pp. 669–670), discusses their own research on this issue:

> Proponents of the "supplier induced demand model" argue that physicians inflate demand whenever the supply of medical manpower is expanded. This interpretation has gained attention because it appears to offer an explanation for the observed cross-sectional positive relationship between fees and the density of health care providers. . . . We explain the positive association of fees and density using an expanded version of standard competitive market theory and offer some interesting empirical support collected from dental markets. . . . The cross-sectional pattern of fees and density reflects the willingness of patients to pay higher fees in exchange for lower time cost. This positive relation between high density and low time cost gives rise to the observed cross-sectional relation between fees and provider density. . . . We believe that our results clearly indicated that the observed cross-section positive relation between fees and provider density is not the result of demand creation. Rather, this seemingly perverse relation is simply a reflection of the preferences of patients for times supplied to the dental practice.

Victor Fuchs (1986), commenting on a particular study of demand inducement (which estimated that an important amount of demand inducement existed), offers the following:

> Whether the shortcomings [of this study] lead to an over-estimate or an under-estimate of the "inducement effect" is not certain. What is certain, however, is that many economists will react to the study . . . as they have in the past on this issue, with the fervent hope that maybe there is no inducement.
>
> This reaction has always reminded me of the story of the Frenchman who suspected that his wife was unfaithful. When he told his friend that the uncertainty was ruining his life, the friend suggested hiring a private detective to resolve the matter once and for all. He did so, and a few days later the detective came and gave his report: "One evening when you were out of town I saw your wife get dressed in a slinky black dress, put on perfume, and go down to the local bar. She had several drinks with the piano player and when the bar was closed they came back to your house. Then they sat in the living room, had a few more drinks, danced and kissed." The Frenchman listened intently as the detective went on: "Then they went upstairs to the bedroom, they playfully undressed one another, and got into bed. Then they put out the light and I could see no more."
>
> The Frenchman sighed, "Always that doubt, always that doubt."

which higher demand (e.g., due to higher income) attracts more supply. The question one can't tell from the association itself is whether the supply followed the demand (the classic market response) or the supply *created* the demand (the induced demand hypothesis). Various sophisticated statistical techniques have been employed in much of the literature on induced demand to attempt to untie this conceptual knot.

Do these methods work well? To answer that question, Dranove and Wehner (1994) used the same statistical approaches that others had used, but they attempted to explain "physician-induced demand for childbirths." Now, the very idea that physicians could induce demand for childbirths strikes most observers as unusual, to say the least, and perhaps ludicrous. (The language Dranove and Wehner used was "where there is at most only a trivial amount of demand inducement.") Their analysis showed that the standard approach to this problem "leads to the absurd conclusion that obstetricians induce demand for childbirths." Because nobody believes that this could actually occur, the only other logical conclusion to draw is that the methods themselves may be faulty, leading to inaccurate conclusions.

We can return here to the ideas set out by McGuire (2000) and those he cites, summarized earlier in this chapter, and look at the consequences for "demand creation" with a regulated price. As he notes, the general tests of demand inducement most often follow one of two approaches. In one approach, some exogenous shift in aggregate demand occurs that causes physicians to respond. For example, if a new drug is invented that would take away "business" from a surgeon, the induced-demand model predicts that the physician would attempt to generate more demand to offset the income loss, presumably by altering the advice given to patients about the value of the treatment in their own case. The second approach studies what happens when regulators or insurance plans (government or private) reduce the price for a specific service. The following sections explore some of these issues in more detail.

Exogenous Shifts in Aggregate Demand

A class of induced-demand tests looks carefully at what happens when something changes in the market to shift (usually to reduce) aggregate demand for a physician's service. The classic target income studies often looked at such changes. One very elegant and recent introduction to this literature shows this approach at its best. Gruber and Owings (1996) studied state-by-state differences in the reductions in birth rates in recent decades. For obstetricians in particular, reductions in birth rates present a classic exogenous downward shift in demand for their services. One response studied by Gruber and Owings looks at the frequency with which the birth takes place by Caesarian section (C-section) rather than by normal delivery. Overall in the 1970–1982 period, birth rates fell by 13.5 percent. (Recall that physicians per capita were also increasing in general during this period, exacerbating the problem for obstetricians.) Gruber and Owings took advantage of differences from state to state in the timing and magnitude of the decline in birth rates to learn the effect on recommendations for C-sections. They found that a 10 percentage point fertility drop led to 0.6 percentage point increase in the C-section rate. Although this is not a huge effect, their research showed it to have strong statistical reliability. Because the average C-section rate is about 20 percent, this means that a 10 percent change in birth rates created (relatively) about a 3 percent change in the rate of C-sections.

The Physician as "Agent" for the Patient

A conceptual approach that has proven quite fruitful in these discussions relies on the game-theory concept of "agency," in which a principal (the patient) delegates authority to an agent (the doctor) to make crucial decisions. The problems between principals and agents arise when the principal cannot fully monitor the behavior of the agent, and yet the agent may sometimes confront situations in which the goals of the principal conflict with those of the agent. Various arrangements (contracts, agreements, and rules) emerge to try to "make" the agent do what the principal wants, but these are difficult to enforce in many settings. Dranove and White (1987) provide a good discussion of the role of agency in health care delivery.

The Doctor/Agent Making Referrals

In the previous chapter, we discussed how doctors make referrals for some treatments and how fee splitting might alter the decisions of the doctor about such arrangements. Within the context of a principal-agent model, the potential importance of fee splitting is easy to understand. When Dr. C (a cardiac surgeon) agrees to split any surgical fee with Dr. A (a referring cardiologist) or Dr. B (a referring internist) for any surgery undertaken, the advice from Drs. A and B will be distorted. Particularly if the patients of Drs. A and B do not know about the arrangement, they will be too willing to consult with Dr. C and, therefore, too willing to undergo surgery at the recommendation of Dr. C.

By the same token, an "honest" principal-agent relationship between patient and doctor can go a long way toward solving the inherent problem of asymmetric information. If the agent (the doctor) really does provide unbiased advice about medical treatments, particularly those regarding referrals, then it really wouldn't matter how uninformed the patient was because the agent (the doctor) would always provide good advice. Alas, we have not yet discovered a contractual agreement that turns all doctors into perfect agents. One important role of "medical ethics" may be to encourage such honest agency performance. (See also Pauly, 1979.)

"Self-Referral"—Doctors' Referral to Self-Owned Facilities

A separate type of referral brings the question of demand inducement into a more prominent light: self-referral by doctors to "independent" facilities in which they have a financial interest. Such facilities can include diagnostic radiology facilities, radiation therapy facilities, medical laboratories, physical therapy clinics, and the like. Jean Mitchell has carried out an illuminating series of studies on this matter, often in collaboration with others. The key financial arrangements are known as "joint ventures," wherein a physician becomes a financial partner in an enterprise producing medical services that the doctor can prescribe. Critics of this practice argue that the arrangement provides a hidden form of kickbacks, illegal in Medicare and Medicaid and under specific laws of 36 states. Proponents of the arrangement claim that because doctors may invest in facilities that might otherwise not meet a market test, they may increase access to care and, separately, may lead to improved quality of care because of the physician's participation.

The practice appears to be quite common now. In a study of Florida physicians, Mitchell and Scott (1992a) found that at least 40 percent of surveyed doctors involved in direct patient care have an investment in a health care facility to which they can refer their patients. About 40 percent of these investments occur in diagnostic imaging centers, to which many types of physicians can make referrals. What are the consequences of such ownership?

One study (Hillman et al., 1990) compared the frequency and costs of radiologic imaging tests (X-ray, CT, and MRI) among doctors who referred to independent providers (with no financial gain) versus those who provided those services themselves. Based on a study of more than 65,000 insurance claims, these analysts found that doctors who own imaging machines ordered more than four times as many imaging tests as those referring to independent radiologists. Furthermore, they charged more than independent radiologists for similarly complex procedures. (For a discussion of a similar issue with prescribed drugs in Japan, see Chapter 16.)

In a study of the use of radiation therapy facilities, Mitchell and Sunshine (1992) found that joint ventures served none of the possible positive goals alleged by their supporters. They did not increase access, but they did increase the amount of service used and costs of care, and, if anything, that care was of lower quality than it was in facilities that were not joint ventures.

In a similar vein, Mitchell and Scott (1992b) studied the use, costs, and quality of physician-owned physical therapy centers. Visits per patient in such centers were 39 percent higher than in independent facilities, and gross revenue, net revenue, and markups were all similarly higher in the physician-owned ventures. Licensed physical therapists spent about 60 percent more time per visit treating patients in independent facilities than in physician-owned facilities. The physician-owned ventures also generated more of their income from well-insured patients.

These and related studies point in the same direction: Of competing hypotheses about joint venture ownership, the profitability hypothesis seems the more likely than either of the "altruistic" hypotheses (improved access to care or improved quality). Perhaps most importantly, these studies all show the potential importance of induced demand in settings in which the doctor has both the informational "power" to recommend treatment to patients and a direct financial reward from doing so. These outlets for demand inducement may prove (in the modern world of complex medical care) more important measures of induced demand than simple measures such as the amount of surgery performed.

The Role of Consumer Information

Several studies also attempted to measure the role of consumer information by comparing the rate at which *doctors and their families* received medical treatment with the rate for a more general population. The general idea of these studies is that doctors could not "fool" other doctors into accepting "unnecessary" care. Bunker and Brown (1974) made the first of such studies, using other professionals (teachers, ministers, etc.) as controls. They found that doctors and their families received *more* care than the controls. Unfortunately, for a variety of reasons, the comparison was flawed.[19] A later study (Hay and Leahy, 1982) used national survey data to make a similar comparison but controlled for the extent of insurance coverage and other relevant economic factors, using the techniques of multiple regression analysis. Hay and Leahy found the same thing that Bunker and Brown did—namely, that if anything, doctors and their families received more care than others. This tends to cast doubt on the extent to which consumer ignorance plays a strong role in inducement, although the studies still cannot directly correct for the role of professional courtesy (free or discounted care), which should create larger

---

[19]Most importantly, doctors had higher incomes and probably better insurance coverage than the comparison groups. Doctors also often receive professional courtesy from other doctors, thereby reducing the out-of-pocket price to zero. This would normally make the doctors' use higher than that of others if the other groups faced any positive price. If a study found the same rate of use (which Bunker and Brown did), this might imply that doctors had resisted some inducement.

demands by physicians and their families, other things being equal, than by otherwise comparable persons. The practice, widespread and widely acknowledged in earlier times, is apparently still widespread. A 1993 study of U.S. physicians revealed that 96 percent of surveyed doctors offered professional courtesy to physicians and their families, most commonly billing only the insurance plan (75 percent of doctors), sometimes providing free care (49 percent), or offering partial discounts (23 percent). (See Levy et al., 1993, for details.)

THE ROLE OF PAYMENT SCHEMES

The idea of providers altering their treatment recommendations on the basis of financial reward is at the heart of the concept of induced demand. One analysis specifically developed the ways in which payment methods could alter the treatment recommendations of "ethical" physicians who knew what the "right" standard of care was and who had a utility function that included leisure and the provision of appropriate care to their patients (Woodward and Warren-Boulton, 1984). This study considers three types of payments to physicians: an annual salary, a time-based wage payment, and a payment based on the number of procedures performed (such as the usual fee-for-service system). This model unambiguously predicts that physicians paid by the first two methods will deliver less than the "right" amount of care, and physicians paid on a fee-for-procedure system will deliver *more* than the "right" amount of care.

Remarkably, a randomized controlled trial exists that tested precisely this idea (Hickson, Altmeier, and Perrin, 1987).[20] Using the residents in a continuity care clinic at a university hospital, this study randomly selected half of the doctors to receive a fee-for-service payment and half to be paid by flat salary. Patients coming into the clinic were also randomized as to the type of doctor they would see. Once assigned to a given doctor, the patients continued with that doctor for all their care (hence the name "continuity care"), unless the doctor missed an appointment, in which case another doctor would see the patient. The payments were set so that, on average, every doctor would receive about the same income from this activity and the "profit" per patient corresponded to that achieved by physicians in private practice in the community (about $2 per patient).

---

[20]This study is not well known in the economics community because it was reported in *Pediatrics,* a journal to which few economists subscribe and which is not cross-indexed in economics literature databases. The only solutions available for an economist who is interested in health care are (1) to read medical journals or (2) to marry a doctor who reads medical journals.

This study directly supported the model of Woodward and Warren-Boulton. Physicians paid by a fee for service scheduled more visits for their patients (4.9 visits per year versus 3.8 visits per year) and saw their patients more often (3.6 visits versus 2.9 visits).[21] Almost all of the difference in behavior was due to well-care visits (1.9 visits versus 1.3 visits).

The American Academy of Pediatrics has a schedule of recommended treatment for children (well-care visits for routine examination, vaccinations, etc.), corresponding to the idea of a standard of "correct" care. Doctors on the fee-for-service payment system missed scheduling any of these recommended visits only 4 percent of the time, whereas doctors on the salaried group missed scheduling recommended visits for their patients 9 percent of the time. (The difference is strongly statistically significant.) Thus, the prediction about salary-paid doctors providing "too little" care is supported.

In addition, the fee-for-service doctors scheduled excess well-care visits beyond those recommended for 22 percent of their patients, while the salary doctors did this for only 4 percent of their patients. (This difference is also very significant statistically.) Thus, the prediction about "too much" care for fee-for-service doctors is also supported.

Changes in per Procedure Reimbursement

Just as the study of pediatric practices reveals the importance of the way physicians are compensated, we can also learn from the response of doctors to changes in fees paid for specific procedures. Two recent studies, as an example of this class of work, looked at the effects of Medicare fee reforms for physicians that took place in 1990. The full model (McGuire and Pauly, 1991 and Gruber and Owings, 1996, provide good expositions of this approach) posits that a reduction in fees has two possible consequences: an "income effect" and a "substitution effect." (These are close intellectual cousins to the income and substitution effects found in the usual discussion of the backward-bending labor supply curve, a standard phenomenon in labor economics.) The idea starts with a physician who prefers more income to less (marginal utility of income is positive) but who dislikes inducing demand. (One can also think of this as having a guilty conscience that nags more and more as demand inducement increases.) The reduced fee causes income to fall, putting more pressure on the "earn more income" side of the utility function. The guilty conscience side of the utility function puts a brake on

---

[21]Doctors missing a patient's visit and turning the patient over to another doctor on duty accounts for the difference between scheduled visits and actual visits.

things. In concept, either can carry the day in terms of net observed change in behavior.

In a refined study of the effects of the 1990 Medicare physician reimbursement changes, Nguyen and Derrick (1997) looked at the "over priced procedures" for which Medicare reduced fees significantly, and (in the nice part of their work) added all of the effects on individual doctors' practices using Medicare claims data. Thus, they could tell who was hit hardest in their income stream by the Medicare changes. Overall they found no significant volume changes, but for those 20 percent of doctors hit hardest by the changes, they found a small but significant volume increase (0.4 percent total). In a related study, Yip (1998) looked at the Medicare fee changes on thoracic surgeons, who were predicted to lose over a quarter of their incomes if volume remained unchanged. She found that the Medicare fee cuts led to volume increases to both Medicare and private pay patients (as one would expect) to the extent that 70 percent of the fee loss from Medicare was recaptured by enhanced volume.[22]

SUMMARY

Economic forces direct many of the important decisions doctors make and how they interact with patients. In particular, we have seen (in the previous chapter) how economic forces guide the choice of physician's specialty and even the decision to enter medical school. In this chapter, we expanded the discussion to show how economic forces affect the locational decisions of doctors, in a way actually similar to the choice of specialty at a conceptual level.

We next investigated the way in which prices are set in markets such as those for physician services. A model of monopolistic competition with incomplete search seems to fit this market well: Rather than a single price, a dispersion of prices exists, often quite wide. Although some patients change doctors, many do not, and some would not consider it, not wishing to offend their doctor. Thus, search is probably incomplete, and each doctor has some price-setting power.

The price-setting power also interacts with the possible ability of doctors to "induce demand" by their patients—that is, to shift the demand curves outward, thereby increasing economic opportunities.

---

[22]The arithmetic here can be a bit tricky. Begin with a price decline of 26 percent, the estimated loss in income if volume remained unchanged. The analysis showed that the actual income loss was only about 8 percent, meaning that volume increased enough to offset 70 percent of what would otherwise be the income decline. It takes about a 25 percent increase in volume to achieve this result.

The most recent modeling of induced demand looks at the ability of the physician to alter the quantity consumed by posing an "all-or-nothing" demand choice on consumers. This model leaves the consumer's demand preferences intact (rather than having them shifted by the physician, as in the earlier descriptions of this behavior) but allows the physician to limit the quantity choices of the consumer in a way that increases the physician's income.

Numerous studies of demand inducement exist, many with statistical difficulties or flaws. Nevertheless, a controlled trial in a pediatric clinic conclusively demonstrates that the mechanism of payment alters the number of visits both recommended to patients and the number of such visits actually undertaken by the patient. In a separate line of analysis, numerous studies have shown that physician ownership of medical service-facilities (X-ray, lab tests, physical therapy, etc.) markedly increases the rate at which doctors prescribe these services to their patients, as well as increases the price and lowers the apparent quality of care at least sometimes. Market forces apparently limit actual demand inducement, however, so that many observable phenomena (such as a physician's location) correspond closely to those that would occur without inducement. As with other matters in health economics, this seems a case in which consumer information could play an increasingly important role.

RELATED CHAPTERS IN *HANDBOOK OF HEALTH ECONOMICS*

Chapter 9, "Physician Agency" by Thomas G. McGuire
Chapter 19, "The Industrial Organization of Health Care Markets" by David Dranove and Mark A. Satterthwaite

PROBLEMS

1. "Physicians will never go to work in rural areas because they can always generate more demand for their services in big cities, where they prefer to live." Comment.
2. The AMA has had a long-standing effort to suppress advertising by physicians, asserting that it was "unethical." What effects might advertising have on consumer search? What effects does consumer search have on the elasticity of demand confronting individual firms? In a monopolistic market, what happens to the optimal price (and returns to the monopoly) as the demand elasticity becomes large in absolute value? Do these ideas help explain the AMA's position on advertising?

3. Suppose a society consists of three cities (A, B, and C), with populations of 99,000, 51,000, and 6,000 people, respectively. Suppose also that the society has a total of 15 doctors.
   a. What cities will have how many doctors?
   b. If the number of doctors doubles, how many will live in each city?

4. What experimental and nonexperimental evidence can you cite about the extent of induced demand? Is there any? Is it unlimited in extent? Does the experimental evidence also reveal anything about the tendencies for shirking in a physician-firm that pays doctors a flat salary rather than on a piecework basis? On net, what can we say for sure about whether a salary or fee-for-service arrangement is better for patients?

5. Why do discussions about induced demand always focus on doctors, rather than on, for example, nurses?

6. Physician organizations often tout the importance of the doctor–patient relationship. Discuss important economic aspects of such a relationship, using economic, not psychological, concepts.

7. Evidence in Chapter 5 places the best estimates of the elasticity of demand for physicians' services at the market level at about −0.2. Data in this chapter show that the elasticity of demand confronting a typical physician-firm is about −3.0. How do you account for this important difference?

8. Suppose you saw the following data on average doctor visits per year (these are hypothetical):
   a. Physicians and their families: 5.0 doctor visits per person per year.
   b. Matched sample of nonphysicians and their families: 4.5 doctor visits per person per year where "matched" meant the same age and gender mix, incomes, geographic location, and race.

   Taking into account what you know about the actual prices paid by doctors and their families for doctor visits (see discussion in this chapter), and the effect of price on demand for care (see Chapter 5 for relevant evidence), what (if anything) would you conclude about demand inducement using these data? (*Hint:* You may need to make some assumptions about the nature of insurance coverage held by typical families in the United States.)

CHAPTER 8

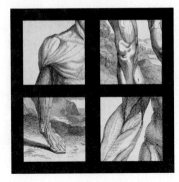

The Hospital as a Supplier of Medical Care

The hospital stands as the center of modern medicine, for better or for worse. Almost all people who become seriously ill will find themselves in the hospital, and $3 out of every $8 spent on health care in the United States is spent on hospital care. Remarkably, most of the decisions made about the delivery of medical care in hospitals—whom to admit, which procedures to use, which drugs to give to the patient, how long the patient should stay in the hospital, and where the patient should go upon discharge—are made by persons who are neither employees of the hospital nor under its direct control or supervision. In this chapter, we examine the organization of the hospital and study the various forms of ownership of the hospital (not for profit, for profit, government) and the effects of such ownership on the behavior of the hospital.

LEARNING GOALS

- Grasp the unique nature of the typical hospital, where most of the activity is directed by somebody who is not employed by the hospital (the private doctor!).

- Follow the discussion about "who owns the hospital" and its consequences (doctors, administrators, etc.).

- Pursue the importance of the governing board ("board of trustees") for a hospital, understand the "political" model of governance, and apply this approach to understanding hospital behavior.

- Understand the nature of the costs of operating a hospital, and how the world of hospitals has changed over recent decades.

- See how ownership (for profit versus not for profit) matters.

- Come to understand the difference between the market-level demand curve for hospital care versus the demand curve facing a single hospital.

238

THE HOSPITAL ORGANIZATION

It may seem odd to begin the discussion of the economics of the hospital with an organizational chart (Figure 8.1), but indeed we must in order to understand the hospital meaningfully. As we shall see, it may be more appropriate to draw two organizational charts for the same hospital, although drawing appropriate links between them has proven almost beyond the capabilities of most artists or chartists.

This discussion focuses on the typical not-for-profit hospital that dominates the market in the United States (and some other countries). Important distinctions between this type of hospital and others (such as for-profit hospitals) appear throughout the discussion. To begin with, we need to understand just what a not-for-profit hospital is and is not, and what it may and may not do. Not-for-profit hospitals may, can, and do earn profits. However, because of their form of organization, they may not, cannot, and do not distribute such profits to shareholders (as for-profit organizations of all types commonly do). In a typical for-profit organization, the shareholders are the residual claimant, receiving any revenues of the organization after it has paid *all* costs, including labor, materials, supplies, interest on bonds, taxes, and so on—the "profits" of the organization. The not-for-profit organization has no shareholders and, hence, no legally designated residual claimant.

FIGURE 8.1 Hospital organizational structure.

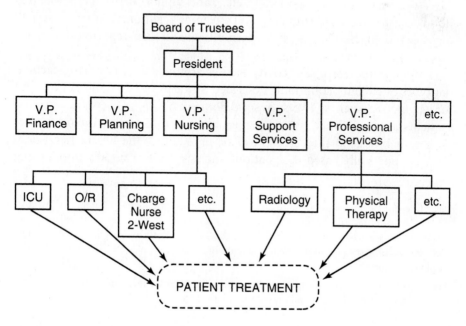

Not-for-profit hospitals differ importantly from standard corporations. In the absence of a residual claimant, their profits must be distributed to somebody else. How and to whom they do this affects the product mix, the costs, the input mix, and possibly the size of the hospital.

Numerous models of the not-for-profit hospital have sprung up, depicting various ways this might happen, which we review momentarily and then synthesize. A good place to begin this discussion, it turns out, is the hospital's organizational chart.

Sitting at the top of the organizational chart is the board of trustees, empowered by the hospital's legal charter to direct all that goes on within the hospital. The board is self-replicating (members elect their own successors, including themselves) and typically serves without pay. Board members own no stock in the hospital because there is none. Indeed, more likely than not, they are expected to donate money to the hospital at some time, as well as provide overall direction while serving on the board. They choose who manages the hospital and provide overall strategic policy and advice to those managers.

The primary administrative officers of the hospital serve in much the same role as their counterparts in other firms, at least nominally. For purposes of this discussion, we call the most senior of such persons the hospital's president.[1] Reporting to the president is a series of vice presidents,[2] dividing the management responsibility of the hospital. A prototype of such division of responsibility might include vice presidents for finance, planning and marketing, nursing, professional departments (emergency room, laboratories, social service, physical therapy, etc.), and support departments (such as food service, laundry, supplies, housekeeping), although every hospital's organizational chart is unique. To each of these, in turn, report middle managers in various areas.

Much of the hospital's activity focuses around subunits serving particular types of patients, commonly described by the physical location of the unit or its function, such as 2-West (second floor, west wing), OB (where obstetric patients stay), Delivery (where babies are born), Newborn Intensive Care (where babies go if they are very ill or premature), the Emergency Room (ER). A physically based designation (such as 2-West) usually implies that

---

[1]The titles for such persons are quite diverse, ranging from "president" to "executive director" to "hospital administrator." Quite commonly, such a person (and his or her immediate subordinates) have received a master's degree in business, public health, or hospital administration. On rare occasion, the person is a medical doctor. In smaller hospitals, the person may have no graduate training.

[2]Titles will match that of the most senior officer. For example, hospital administrators will have assistant administrators, and presidents will have vice presidents.

this unit serves "basic" adult medical and surgical patients. These units commonly have 20 to 40 beds and operate under the immediate supervision of a head nurse, around whom all of the other activity revolves. These charge nurses (the ones in charge during their shift) direct all of the nursing care and coordinate almost all other patient care given on their units.

If the patient receives medications, the pharmacy delivers them to the floor, where a medication nurse administers them. If the patient receives physical therapy (PT), either the therapist comes to the patient's room or the patient is delivered (walking or by wheelchair) to the PT unit. If an X-ray is to be taken, a similar process occurs. If a laboratory test is needed, the phlebotomist comes to the patient's room to draw a blood sample. Meals are brought from the kitchen to the floor and given to the patient there.

All of the specialists performing these activities (pharmacist, therapist, phlebotomist, X-ray technician, food service delivery) report organizationally to the supervisor in their own department (pharmacy, X-ray, etc.), who reports up the line eventually to the relevant vice president. The activity of all of these hospital departments interacts on the floor unit, focusing around the patients. In addition to directly supervising the nurses in such units, the charge nurse also acts in a way that is similar to a traffic cop managing the flow of all of these diverse actors as they interact with the patients.

Remarkably, this complicated interaction and organizational description omit the one person who initiates all of this activity: the doctor who admitted the patient to the hospital. The doctor is typically not an employee of the hospital. The doctor has no "boss" up the line. The one person upon whom this entire activity depends has only a weak and ambiguous organizational tie to the hospital—the medical staff.

The hospital medical staff has its own organizational chart and bylaws of operation. The staff is divided by medical specialty: medicine, pediatrics, obstetrics and gynecology, and so on. If the hospital is sufficiently large, these departments may have subdivisions as well, reflecting subspecialization of the doctors: orthopedic surgery, neurosurgery, cardiac surgery, and general surgery, for example, within a department of surgery. Figure 8.2 shows a typical organization of the medical staff.

Doctors receive admission to this medical staff by application to the hospital, nominally to the board of trustees, who are responsible for the hospital's overall activity. The board invariably delegates the responsibility for this decision de facto to the existing medical staff, which commonly has a "credentials committee" established to review the applications of potential new staff members. Their report, voted on by the full staff, provides the basis for the board's decision. Thus, at least de facto, if not de jure, the medical staff, as with the board, is self-replicating.

FIGURE 8.2 Organization of the medical staff.

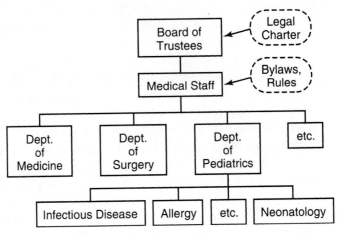

An important difference emerges between the "line management" and employees of the hospital, and the medical staff. Those within the "management" organization all have a contract with the hospital; the hospital reviews their performance, pays their wages or salary, and can fire them. By contrast, doctors admitted to the medical staff have no similar relationship with the hospital. In general, they receive no income directly from the hospital; their performance is subject to a very different and weaker review process; and, with few exceptions, they cannot be "fired."[3] Once a doctor gains admission to a medical staff, removing that privilege turns out to be exceedingly difficult.[4]

More recently, as hospitals have expanded to become "integrated delivery systems" (see later discussions of managed care in Chapter 11), some hospitals have purchased physician practices and converted the physicians involved into salaried employees rather than fee-for-service independent agents.

---

[3]Some of the line managers are doctors in some hospitals, such as the director of the laboratory, the X-ray division, or the emergency room. In other hospitals, these functions are handled by a separate firm (composed of relevant doctors), with whom the hospital has a contract to perform the management functions. Thus, for example, a radiologist may be a member of the medical staff of the hospital as well as an employee or may be a member of the medical staff as well as president of a separate corporation that contracts with the hospital to manage the radiology functions. Typically, doctors performing such a management function retain a separate relationship with their patients, sending them separate bills (e.g., for the interpretation of an X-ray).

[4]The doctor may have privileges revoked for serious medical mistakes or misbehavior, but even this has proven exceedingly difficult in the past. See Chapter 13, which describes the medical-legal system, for further discussion.

(Chapter 6 discusses some of the incentives for working that these changes create—physician productivity often falls when the pay is guaranteed by salary rather than coming through fee-for-service exchanges.) To the extent that hospitals actually own physician practices, it is of course the case that the physician can be "fired," and the hospital has the ability to set the physician's salary directly. However, the trend toward hospital acquisition of physician practices seems to have been halted, if not reversed, perhaps because of the adverse incentives for productivity that come with a full-salaried compensation (Gaynor and Gertler, 1995).

By law, most of the activities carried out with, on, and for patients within the hospital must be done either by or under the direction of a licensed physician. Thus, the doctor "writes orders" in the patients' charts that direct virtually the entire flow of activities for each patient. These orders create "demands" for activities within the hospital, which the hospital organization "supplies." If those orders require a blood test, the phlebotomist appears on the unit, draws blood, and takes it to the laboratory, where it will be analyzed by equipment purchased with the knowledge that such orders will be written. If the patient goes to surgery, the surgeon performing the surgery will literally give direct orders to the nurses and technicians (employees of the hospital) who assist in the operation, even though the surgeon is not their "boss" organizationally. The drugs the patient receives come only after the doctor writes a prescription, and similarly with any therapy, X-rays, and even the diet that the hospital offers to the patient. The doctor captains the ship, ordering when to start the engines, which direction to go, and how fast to move, and the hospital can do little but respond, no matter what orders the doctor gives. The doctor, independent of the hospital for income and supervision, nevertheless directs virtually all of the activity and, hence, the use of resources within the hospital. Figure 8.3 shows these relationships (albeit vaguely).

The hospital is really two separate organizations—the line management and the medical staff—which serve the roles of supply and demand in the "market" of hospital care.[5] The hospital is really a "job shop," in which each product is unique (although often similar to others), and the hospital is set up to provide inputs to the craftspersons (the doctors on the medical staff) who direct the output of this job shop. The patient agrees to two distinct contracts before this can all happen,[6] one with the hospital and the other with the doctor. In the contract with the hospital, the patient promises to pay for

---

[5]This viewpoint, which forms the basis for a very useful analysis of the hospital organization, appears in two articles by Jeffrey E. Harris, M.D., Ph.D. (J. Harris, 1977; J. E. Harris, 1979). As mentioned earlier, Dr. Harris is trained in internal medicine and economics.

[6]Here, we use the word *contract* to include both written documents and oral agreements.

FIGURE 8.3 The doctor directs the activity.

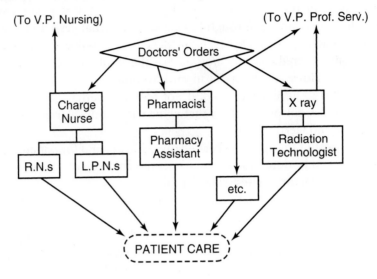

care, and the hospital promises to provide necessary medical care under the direction of the patient's physician. In the contract with the doctor, the patient promises to pay for care, and the doctor promises to provide care as needed and to supervise the activities of the hospital.

This type of arrangement has apparent disadvantages, notably that cost control may be difficult if not impossible to achieve in this type of organization. However, apparent advantages also emerge. Most notably, in the unpredictable environment of treating illness, the patient's health may be better served by having a doctor who is independent of the hospital in control of resources. In addition, the patient may be able to monitor the physician's activity better than the hospital because the patient possesses unique knowledge about the doctor's success (i.e., how well does the patient feel?).

WHO IS THE RESIDUAL CLAIMANT?

The hospital just described can and often does "make a profit" in the sense that its revenues exceed its costs. What becomes of that profit, and who makes the decisions about its allocation? This question has haunted analysts of the hospital industry for decades. Some models say that the doctors have seized control of the hospital and operate it to enhance their own profits.[7] Others say that the hospital administrator (or hospital board) operates the hospital

---

[7]This view is most carefully developed by Pauly and Redisch (1973) and by Pauly (1980).

to increase its own happiness, shifting the use of the hospital's resources accordingly.[8] Some say that the hospital uses its profits to raise wages of employees above normal levels, in effect being captured by "the nurses."[9] The legal charter of the hospital as a not-for-profit entity at least hints that "profits" will be returned to patients in the form of lower prices, although no serious analyst has adopted this view in writing.

Most likely, none of the proposed answers to this problem are wholly correct or wholly wrong. *Everybody* associated with the hospital has a finger in the pie. Who gets the bigger slice varies from place to place and time to time, and the study of such questions is probably better suited to modern political science than to economics. Let's look at each of the relevant actors and their roles in control of the hospital resources.

The Doctors as Residual Claimants

In its simplest form, the doctors-win-it-all (Pauly-Redisch) model of the hospital simply says that the doctors on the medical staff "milk" all of the hospital's profits into their own bucket by having the hospital perform (and pay for) activities that promote the profitability of the doctors' own firms.[10] This model has obvious face appeal, given the central role of doctors in directing the use of hospital resources.

The difficulties in fully accepting this model arise from two directions. First, why don't the doctors just directly own the hospital and thus eliminate the ambiguity arising from the existing situation? Indeed, in past years, doctors *did* own a majority of all the hospitals in the United States.[11] One answer to the question might be that the not-for-profit law confers tax advantages on the hospital that can be passed on to the doctors, enhancing their profits.

One study (Sloan and Vraciu, 1983) estimated that for-profit hospitals at that time paid about $15 per bed-day in income taxes, avoided by their nonprofit competitors. In addition, because of regulatory distinctions drawn, the payments from Medicare and Medicaid to nonprofit hospitals were sufficiently higher on a per-bed-day basis to add another $15–$20 per day in profitability to the nonprofit hospital. For a 300-bed hospital operating at average

---

[8]This view of the hospital administrator as "owner" first appeared in Newhouse (1970b).

[9]Martin S. Feldstein's (1971) study of hospital costs developed this theme.

[10]Chapter 6 discussed the physician-firm as an economic entity and how this differs from physicians as individual "workers" in those firms.

[11]Steinwald and Neuhauser (1970). The number of for-profit hospitals peaked in the first quarter of the 20th century at about 2,500, representing more than half of all hospitals in the United States during the early part of that century.

utilization rates, these differences could add more than $2 million per year to the hospital's profits. By the Pauly-Redisch model, the $2 million is available for the doctors as added profits.

The difficulty with this view, and the second major problem with the Pauly-Redisch model, is that on the whole, it treats the medical staff as essentially homogeneous, operating with unified goals as a single entity. It assumes that the doctors divide up the hospital's profits in even proportion to their own amount of work.

The reality differs considerably from this simple view, which proponents of the "doctor-gets-it-all" school readily recognize. Specialists of one area— for example, infectious disease—have very different ways to enhance their own profitability than, for example, pediatricians or heart surgeons. Although all of the heart surgeons may have a single voice recommending how the hospital should, for example, build a laminar air-flow surgical suite to cut down on infection during long operations, the pediatricians will likely have a different viewpoint, such as providing a clinical psychologist for testing children's developmental skills. The Pauly-Redisch model does not tell us how the hospital resolves such conflicting claims. The central difficulty is that, to a considerable degree, the model does not confront the question of choice between conflicting objectives of various medical staff members.

This conflict also circles back to the first question, the alleged financial superiority of the tax-free model. Lower taxes (and higher profits for the hospital) create higher profits for the doctors only if the hospital decides to spend those profits in particular ways. The battle of control within the hospital may itself be costly, so that the hospital dissipates some or all of the gain. For example, the choices made to appease both the pediatricians and the heart surgeons may end up costing so much that neither group gains anything from the nonprofit structure. Pauly and Redisch discuss this problem to some degree, but they leave unresolved the question of just how the doctors cooperate, if at all.

The Administrator as Residual Claimant (Organizational Utility Function)

Another view of the hospital proposes a "decision maker" within the hospital, whom we can either dub "the administrator" or "the board." This person is said to control the hospital in such a way as to maximize its own utility, much in the fashion of a consumer (see Chapter 4). The prototype model (Newhouse, 1970b) describes the decision maker as gaining utility from quantity and quality of output. Rather than having a budget constraint (as would a consumer), the hospital faces a market constraint (the demand curve for its services) and a production constraint (the technical ability to combine inputs into producing output). In the usual fashion of a maximizing decision maker facing constraints, the hospital decision maker trades off quality and quantity in such a way as to maximize utility.[12]

This model suffers from a problem similar to the second problem described for the Pauly-Redisch model: Where does "the utility function" come from? If we accept the existence of such a central decision maker with a stable utility function, then this model is very helpful.

This approach has considerable appeal and can help illuminate the types of decision making that must occur in a not-for-profit hospital, as we shall see later in this chapter.

Employees or Patients as Residual Claimants (Higher Wages or Lower Prices)

Other views of the hospital have suggested that the hospital deliberately pays its employees more than market wages, either because it wants to or because the employees have forced it to. The hospital might do this either because of a powerful employees' union (or other strong bargaining position) or because the administrator "wants to."

A corresponding view is that the hospital returns any profits to patients in the form of lower prices, simply by not collecting economic profits that it might have achieved. If one takes the legal form of *not for profit* at its face value, this might be interpreted as the "desired" choice of the legislators who establish the not-for-profit structure, but this belief holds water only if one does not consider the other possible "residual claimants," such as the medical staff or the administrator. It also is silent on the question of quality choice and thus does not really help much in understanding hospital behavior. Of course, if the decision maker's utility function includes quantity of output (as Newhouse, 1970b, modeled it), then lower prices offer one way to achieve this. Because patients respond to lower prices by demanding more care, lower prices might also directly improve "administrator" well-being.

The For-Profit Hospital: Shareholders as Residual Claimants

The for-profit hospital has different claimants to the profits of the hospital—namely, the owners. Legally, of course, they are entitled to all of the profits. However, in a market populated with nonprofit hospitals, they may have to make concessions—for example, to the medical staff—to induce them to bring patients into the hospital. These concessions may make the for-profit hospital appear similar to the not-for-profit hospital in structure, organization, equipment, and even management style. [See Becker and Sloan (1985) and Box 8.1.]

---

[12]In Chapter 9, this model is more fully developed. If you want, you may look ahead to get a flavor of how this decision-making process works.

BOX 8.1 THE PERFORMANCE OF FOR-PROFIT VERSUS NOT-FOR-PROFIT HOSPITALS

One study of the effects of for-profit ownership compared 80 "matched pairs" of investor-owned ("chain") hospitals and matching not-for-profit hospitals (Watt et al., 1986) using 1980 data. The cost data showed

	Investor-Owned Hospitals	Not-for-Profit Hospitals
Per admission	$1,529	$1,453
Per day	233	218

These differences are not statistically significant. However, the data did show significant differences in the costs of drugs and supplies (the for-profit hospitals used more).

The for-profit hospitals "marked up" their costs more than the not-for-profit hospitals, yielding higher revenue and higher net revenue (profits). After adjusting for differences in income and property taxes paid by the investor-owned hospitals ($14 per day), the study found the charges per day as

	Investor-Owned Hospitals	Not-for-Profit Hospitals
Charges per day	$257	$234
"Profit margin"	9%	4%

Another study (Sloan and Vraciu, 1983, p. 34) of hospitals in Florida found no differences between the two types of hospitals on a wide variety of dimensions. Using 1980 data, the researchers compared nonteaching hospitals with less than 400 beds in Florida. In that state, a third of all the hospital beds are owned by for-profit hospitals, strikingly higher than in most other states. The study used 52 not-for-profit hospitals and 60 for-profit hospitals, matched by size category and location. The findings on "profitability" show

Investor-Owned Hospitals
Chain—4.8%
Independent—5.4%
Not for profit—5.6%

One substantial difference between the two studies is the amount of taxes they detected. Sloan and Vraciu also calculated direct income taxes at about $14 per patient per day, just as did Watt et al. However, they found that for-profit hospitals paid $20 per day in "hidden taxes" because of the way Medicare and Medicaid pay for care differently to each type of hospital. These rules paid only "allowable costs," which are less than patient charges for both types of hospitals. However, the greater discount Medicare and Medicaid imposed on the for-profit hospitals ($20 per total patient day more) almost exactly accounts for the discrepancy in charges per day found in the Watt et al. study. The distinction is this: The for-profit hospitals list higher prices than the not-for-profit hospitals, but Medicare and Medicaid don't pay as much. On balance, the two types of hospitals seem indistinguishable.

Sloan and Vraciu also compared the list of facilities and services the hospitals indicated that they offered. They concluded that "the not-for-profits are more likely to offer such 'profitable' services as open-heart surgery, cardiac catheterization, and CT scanning, but are also more likely to offer an 'unprofitable' one like premature nursery." On other dimensions, it seemed difficult to distinguish between the hospitals.

WHERE DOES THE UTILITY FUNCTION COME FROM? A POLITICAL THEORY MODEL[13]

Modern political science theory gives some insight into how the utility function of a not-for-profit hospital can be understood. The model presented here is an *extremely* simplified version of the types of models used to understand legislative behavior, and should be taken as an introduction into a very complex and fascinating literature. This approach looks at the key aspect of the not-for-profit hospital—the board of trustees—and shows how a stable utility function can emerge from such an organization.

To keep this model very simple, let's posit that the only two things that a hospital trustee might worry about are the volume of patients treated (N, for number of patients treated) and S (for the quality of service). Chapter 9 will extend this model to a market equilibrium context. Here we seek to understand only how the utility function emerges. Also to keep things simple, we can assume that the board of trustees has only three members, and that they resolve any issues before them by majority rule vote.[14]

Each trustee has a preference function that can be shown as indifference curves, just as we used to understand consumer demand theory in Chapter 4. Figure 8.4 shows the basic idea. Trustees A, B, and C are arrayed in this diagram as having different preferences about the trade-offs between quality and quantity. We also need something akin to a budget for the hospital, such as the "income" line in consumer demand theory. The way such a "budget" emerges is described more fully in Chapter 9, but for now, we can take it as a given that the hospital confronts a "budgetlike" constraint such as the line BB in Figure 8.4.

---

[13]This section relies considerably on a model developed in Phelps and Sened (1990) and elaborated further in Phelps (2001).

[14]If there are more than three members of the board, the fundamental model doesn't change. If there is an even number, then the model must be expanded to include tie-breaking procedures, a complication that hinders our ability to understand the basic issue at hand. Thus, we use a three-person board in our discussion.

FIGURE 8.4 Preferences of three trustees of not-for-profit hospital.

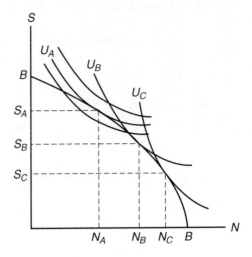

The budget line is curved rather than straight because of various market forces; it may help to recall the concept of a "production possibility curve" from the intermediate microeconomics discussions of theory of the firm. This curve has many similarities to such a curve. One can also think of it as a consumer budget line where the consumer pays increasing amounts to buy more and more of a single commodity, so that as consumption concentrates on a single commodity, the relative prices change in a way that diminishes buying power compared with the usual "fixed-price" budget line analysis.

Given the line BB as the maximum available budget, Trustees A, B, and C all know how to achieve their highest possible personal utility—they find the tangency between their own set of indifference curves and the budget line BB confronted by the hospital. Each one of them might propose that their preferred combination of quality and quantity be chosen as the hospital's operating policy. However, in a majority-rule voting scheme, Trustee B will normally win because the combination (N_B, S_B) gives higher utility to A than does C's preferred set, and similarly C prefers B's choices to A's. Thus B can form a coalition with either A or C to achieve a winning majority that dominates any other. B does not need to compromise with either A or C in general because either one of them should be willing to pick B's preferences over other alternatives. So B—the "median voter"—wins any vote on hospital policy. Hence, B's utility function becomes the hospital's utility function.

Now we come to the key point about "stability" of the preferences. Eventually the terms of office of A, B, and C will expire (or they will die in office). Not-for-profit organizations, including hospitals, invariably have succession rules built into the hospital charter that determine how retiring board members are replaced. These rules nearly always specify a simple process: The board selects new members to replace retiring (or deceased) members.

Consider now what happens if either A or C is scheduled to retire from the board. All three have a vote here, so if A is retiring, then A can best ensure that the hospital's behavior follows A's own preferences by electing a successor (say, A') who has preferences very similar to A's.

A and B will naturally form a voting coalition to replace A with somebody with A-like preferences because A does not wish to put somebody more C-like onto the board (horrors!). Also, B most of all does not want to put somebody onto the board who is more C-like than is B because if that happened, B would no longer have the median vote (mega-horrors!).

Thus A' will have preferences a lot like A, and similarly C' will have preferences a lot like C.

What happens if B is scheduled to leave the board? The same ideas apply: B obviously would like to be replaced with a very like-minded B'. A and C would like to replace B with a person with preferences more closely aligned to their own than B currently is, but they are in no position to "insist." B's best outcome is to find a very close substitute B', and neither A nor C can shift that choice. Hence, B is replaced with a very like-minded B'.

In every case, the preferences of the board remain stable even when the composition changes. It should be easy to see that this basic idea carries on when the board is expanded in size, and something similar would emerge even if different voting rules were in place.[15]

It should be clear that this basic approach can accommodate all of the models discussed earlier (physician-capture, administrator-capture, etc.) if the things that make the trustees happy are expanded from N and S to include as well physician income, employee income, administrator's salary, and so on. The only question is whether any of these groups or persons can muster enough votes in a real-world setting to get a member of the board elected who shares their concerns. Of these, as we will see in Chapter 9, the most likely group to succeed are physicians because they can (through their choices of where to hospitalize their patients) alter the budget constraint (BB) facing the hospital. Chapter 9 explores these issues more fully.

We should *expect* hospitals to appear different from each other in the nonprofit world, precisely because we should expect that the preferences of

---

[15]The political theory literature from which this idea flows looks at legislatures in general, and focuses on the roles of committees and their ability to determine the voting agenda of the main body (the legislature in one case, the board of trustees here). These issues complicate the overall picture a lot, but do not in general degrade the idea that we can find a stable preference function (utility function) on a not-for-profit board of trustees that comes from the preferences of the individual board members.

the winning (median voter) trustee will differ in different hospitals. For example, hospitals owned by the Roman Catholic church will surely include an obstetric service, but never an abortion service. Hospitals with a particularly "savvy" cardiac surgeon will emphasize capabilities and services to benefit that doctor's patients and profits. The broad message from this view of hospital control is that there is no common message. We should not expect any single group to "capture" the organization consistently because the rules of the game and the capabilities of the players differ from setting to setting.

In this environment, the hospital's legal not-for-profit status (and hence, its exemption from paying taxes and its ability to receive charitable donations) creates a further set of "interested parties" who can control the direction taken by the hospital in important ways: donors. Hospitals rely on donors considerably, both for routine activity and, more importantly, for large investment projects. Donors reap the benefits of public adulation from these acts, as well as any private pleasure they might receive. Their charitable generosity is in part, of course, supported by the income tax laws of this country: Donations are deductible to offset taxable income, so the marginal cost of \$1 of gifts (for an itemizing taxpayer) is $(1 - t)$ dollars, where t is the marginal tax rate.

Donors almost invariably specify a particular activity or facility to which their donation should be put. These donations often follow the personal health patterns of the donors or their families. For example, people who have had relatives die of cancer often give toward cancer research or a cancer treatment facility in the hospital. People who have had a premature newborn infant restored to health often contribute toward the newborn intensive care unit of the hospital (or research associated with diseases of very premature infants). In these ways, donations at any particular hospital might appear idiosyncratic, but they can and do shape the direction of the hospital's investments and the set of therapeutic interventions it has to offer.

A visit to almost any not-for-profit hospital in the United States will find not only a wall filled with names commemorating donors but also plaques scattered throughout the hospital signifying the specialized gifts of donors for particular activities or regions of the hospital. These donor's wishes, and the finances to support them, can make such donors, at least to some extent, a part of the decision-making structure of the hospital, and their "wishes" become embedded in the de facto utility function of the hospital. Thus, the "interested parties" helping to shape the preference function of a hospital include not only the doctors, staff, administrators, and perhaps its patients but also its donors.

The ideas captured in Figure 8.5 can also show how a "targeted" donation can alter the behavior of a hospital. Suppose a generous donor offers to give the hospital enough money to shift the budget line from BB to B'B' but *only if the number of patients treated is at least as large as N**. The gift shown in

.5 A restricted gift improves Trustee B's utility.

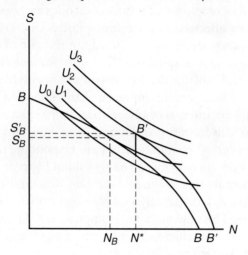

Figure 8.5 is large enough that Trustee B (and C for sure) will vote to accept the gift. Figure 8.5 shows only the preferences of Trustee B because those of A and C really don't matter; if B is made better off (i.e., reaches a higher level of utility) then B willingly accepts the gift, and because Trustee C prefers a larger N even more than does Trustee B, C will join B in accepting the gift. (Trustee A may also actually vote to accept the gift, but A's vote is irrelevant here because B and C have a voting majority.) The gift will cause the hospital to shift to a higher level of output at N^*, even if the quality of care actually were to fall slightly from S_B to S^*; B would be happier nevertheless, so the gift is accepted. It should be obvious (this is left as an exercise at the end of the chapter) that the donor could propose a gift sufficiently small that Trustee B would not be made better off by accepting the gift (coupled with the restriction that the volume of treatment at least reach N^*). In such cases, either the gift would be turned down or (more likely) the hospital leadership (and perhaps even Trustee B or C) would negotiate with the donor either for a larger gift or a less restrictive requirement about the size of N^*.

In some important cases, this approach significantly deviates from a "decision maker's utility function" approach to modeling the hospital. The approach outlined here raises an alert about changes in the legal and regulatory structure that will alter the rules of the "game" within the hospital, and thus the resulting outcomes. Each time this happens, the apparent "utility function" of the hospital shifts. For example, a labor-relations board ruling decertifying a nurses' union will shift the balance away from them. A legal ruling strengthening the hospital's ability to dismiss a doctor from the medical staff shifts the balance away from doctors. A statewide regulatory system decision to limit wage increases to 3 percent next year will clearly reduce the bargaining power of employees. Each time such an event occurs, the "utility function" of every affected hospital shifts, potentially creating systematic changes in its economic behavior. Obviously, in the case of donors, a change in the taxable status of a hospital (and hence its ability to receive charitable gifts) would markedly change the standing of donors in this environment.

Within a stable legal system, however, changes that occur from hospital to hospital should be more sporadic, rather than systematic, as individual leaders of various factions retire, die, move, or emerge. While individual hospitals change their behavior from time to time, responding to such changes in the balance of power, no systematic changes should appear. In such an environment, it is probably safe to think about hospitals (at least collectively) as behaving according to a model relying on a single decision maker with a stable utility function. This approach, for example, assists in understanding how hospitals respond to some changes in cost control regulation (but not others!), as we will see in Chapter 15.

HOSPITAL COSTS

The mix of particular activities selected by a hospital to undertake, the mix of inputs it chooses to produce that mix of outputs, and the cost of those inputs all come together to form "the costs" of the hospital. Given all of these choices, one can think about expanding the scale of the hospital, holding constant its output mix (newborn deliveries, cancer therapy, psychological counseling, substance abuse, open-heart surgery, etc.) and the cost of its inputs (wages for nurses, interest on loans, the cost of electricity, etc.). As the scale of this hospital/job shop increases, we can expect its costs per unit to change as well. How this happens forms the basis for studies of economies of scale in the hospital industry.

Such studies try to determine whether costs per unit of "output" rise or fall as the scale of the organization expands. A long series of analyses of hospitals in the United States (and elsewhere) have sought to study this. The resulting set of studies allows you to select almost any answer you wish. Some show costs rising with output (diseconomies of scale), others show costs falling with output (economies of scale), and some show approximately constant average costs over a broad range of outputs.[16] In each case, the "output"

---

[16]The earliest studies of hospital costs included Lave and Lave (1970). A more recent review of this literature (Cowing, Holtman, and Powers) appeared in 1983. Except for a few subsequent studies, this review is relatively comprehensive and provides a good starting point for the person wishing further detail on the various approaches and statistical problems associated with estimating hospital cost functions.

of the hospital is measured by the number of patients treated or the number of patient-days produced.

To undertake such studies appropriately, one must in concept compare the costs of two hospitals that are "identical" except for size, or else control for their differences in scope and complexity somehow. This may prove to be an impossible task.

As hospitals expand in size, they invariably expand in the scope of their activities as well. This may take place in subtle ways. For example, a larger hospital may be able to justify a larger diagnostic laboratory that not only does more blood tests but also automatically tests for a greater variety of items within each blood sample. Doubling the size of the surgical service may make it feasible to build and staff a postsurgical intensive care unit. A larger obstetric service may make possible the construction of a newborn intensive care unit for critically ill babies. Some of such differences appear in the "list" of capabilities of the hospital, but others do not.

We should remember that the hospital is really a highly specialized job shop, in which each case treated is unique, at least in some ways. There are similarities in types of cases, but even the most finely tuned classification systems available show large variation in the costs of treating patients within a single hospital for a single type of illness or injury; Box 8.2 shows one city's experience.

Another important distinction between hospitals concerns the types of patients they serve. Some "community" hospitals specialize in providing routine care to people living in the nearby vicinity. Others specialize in complex care, with referral patterns spanning a wide area, often with patients from more than one state. These referral hospitals invariably end up with patients who are, on average, sicker than those in community hospitals, even after holding the patients' primary diagnoses constant. For example, patients

---

BOX 8.2   VARIABILITY IN LENGTH OF STAY WITHIN DRGS

Some data from hospital admissions in Rochester, New York, show how variable the resource use can be within a single diagnostic group. The following table shows the average length of stay in days and the standard deviation (SD) for each of several common illnesses or treatments. These were selected not because they show a lot of variability, but rather because they seem fairly routine and predictable, compared with other diagnoses. These deviations are partly predictable (see Chapter 3), but in a considerable part they represent the effects of different problems of different patients, emphasizing the "job shop" nature of the hospital.

(continued)

BOX 8.2 VARIABILITY IN LENGTH OF STAY WITHIN DRGS (continued)

Diagnosis-Related Group (DRG)	Average (Days)	SD (Days)	Range (Days)
Otitis media and upper respiratory infections	2.7	1.7	1–10
Inguinal hernia, ages 18–69 without complications	2.0	1.2	1–19
Appendectomy without complications, age <70	3.6	1.6	1–15
Fracture of femur	15.4	12.9	2–54
Prostate removal, transurethral, age <70 without complications	5.3	1.7	3–14
Normal delivery without complications	2.5	0.9	1–24
Caesarean section delivery without complications	4.5	1.9	1–19

Source: Calculations by author from claims data from Blue Cross-Blue Shield of Greater Rochester.

hospitalized for "chronic obstructive pulmonary disease" in a local hospital are probably "routine" cases; those who are transferred to or deliberately travel to specialty care in "referral" hospitals probably have other complications that make their treatment more difficult.

Statistical methods to "hold constant" the case mix of hospitals when cost functions are calculated invariably cannot measure these types of differences, yet they clearly exist and are important. One study, for example, found that for a given set of diagnoses, it cost about 10 percent more per patient to treat Medicaid patients than comparable patients with private insurance (Epstein, Stern, and Weissman, 1990), probably because Medicaid patients have more advanced states of illness when they reach the hospital. All of these factors make accurate estimation of hospital cost functions quite difficult, at best.

Hospitals also differ on how well they are equipped to handle unusual events, further hindering comparison of their costs. Some of this "standby capacity" is easy to observe. For example, how many beds are usually available in case of a large disaster such as an airplane crash or office building fire? Other differences, such as the ability to conduct a complicated and rare laboratory test, are not so apparent in a study of hospitals' costs. Sometimes the same "ability" means very different things. A very powerful magnetic resonance imaging (MRI) machine can cost two or three times what a small one costs, but both appear as "MRI" in a list of the hospital's abilities.

With these caveats, we can turn to the evidence on economies of scale. Although a number of studies that have estimated the behavior of costs as scale changes exist, few have solved the knotty methodological problems well.

One attempt (Grannemann, Brown, and Pauly, 1986) has data and analysis methods that deal with many of the problems and has the added advantage that it jointly estimated the costs of both inpatient and hospital outpatient department activity (including emergency rooms). But even these researchers were not fully successful in controlling for output mix, the problem discussed earlier.

Their findings show that marginal costs of inpatient care rise both with the number of discharges and the number of patient-days the hospital produces. They estimated the marginal cost of a *discharge* at $533 (in 1981 dollars) for low-volume hospitals, $880 for medium-volume hospitals, and $1,084 for larger volume hospitals. Similarly, the marginal cost of a *day* increased from $168 to $237 and then fell slightly to $231 for the hospitals of these respective size groups. The differences in the cost of a "discharge" seem too large for the authors to believe that the differences represent efficiency of operation. As Grannemann, Brown, and Pauly concluded, "The variables included in this cost function do not fully capture the differences ... [and] unmeasured differences in case mix and service content differences may be responsible." Another way to say this is that bigger hospitals are more complex and offer a different "quality" of care than smaller hospitals, in ways that are too difficult to control for using existing data.

This study also found that in the operation of emergency departments, persistent economies of scale exist. The obvious question is why we don't see ever-larger (and fewer) versions of such departments, particularly in cities large enough to support multiple hospitals. The answer—and the key policy issue—is that such mergers (to produce costs savings) are not feasible because of uncounted costs.

Hospitals (including emergency rooms) produce services that require the presence of the patient (and often, the patient's family). Taking travel costs of patients into account, hospitals always have naturally limited markets, and the question of economies of scale do not matter much. Put another way, if we counted the cost of transporting the patient to the hospital, every hospital would have eventual diseconomies of scale. In the relevant time frame for transportation of serious emergencies, where sometimes a few minutes can make a considerable difference in outcomes, these diseconomies of scale could rapidly appear.

Cost of patient care is not the only thing that changes with hospital size. The "quality" of a hospital can also change importantly. One obvious way that quality changes reflect the usual effect of specialization is that larger hospitals can afford to employ specialists to do more jobs, and this, at least to some degree, can improve quality. To paraphrase Adam Smith, division of labor is limited by the size of the hospital. Larger hospitals can also afford to have more "standby" equipment that gets used only rarely; as the scale of the hospital increases, the effective demand for such equipment also increases, eventually making the purchase and operation of such equipment economically desirable. Thus, for people with rare diseases, their chances of getting treated by the most sophisticated (if not the best) methods increase if they enter a large hospital.

Just as hospital cost can decline with increasing size and then finally increase (the classic U-shaped average cost curve), so can specialization lead to increasing and finally decreasing quality of care. Most people have heard of some "horror story" in hospitals in which the care had become so fragmented, with numerous specialists each caring for some part of a patient's problem but nobody worrying about the "whole" patient, that major medical mishaps occur. Just as too many workers in the vineyard can trample the grapes and too many cooks can spoil the broth, too much specialization in the delivery of health care can produce a poor quality of care.

LONG-RUN VERSUS SHORT-RUN COSTS

A much more interesting question about hospital costs is how much those costs vary as the patient load varies. If a hospital's costs and patient load change together closely, then most of the costs are *variable costs*. If a hospital's costs remain pretty much the same whether it is 50 percent full or 90 percent occupied, then much of its cost structure is *fixed*.

In the very shortest of short runs (for example, an hour or a day), almost all of a hospital's costs are fixed, possibly with the exception of a few supplies (food, medicines, etc.). In the very longest of long runs, all of a hospital's costs are variable because the entire cost structure, including the decision about rebuilding the hospital, is open to question. However, as Lord John Maynard Keynes once said, "In the long run, we're all dead."[17] How much do a hospital's costs fluctuate as its patient load goes up and down? This question matters considerably right now because (for a variety of reasons that we discuss in later chapters), hospital use has fallen considerably over the past several years. Should we expect hospital costs to fall in parallel? That depends on the short-run and long-run cost structure.

One study of this question suggests that in a meaningful "short run," defined as one in which the capital stock of the hospital does not vary, about 70 percent of the hospital's costs are fixed (Friedman and Pauly, 1981). To see why this occurs, one need only look at the typical hospital's operations.

---

[17]Economist Rodney T. Smith adds this rejoinder: "Yes, but the short run determines our standard of living."

Hospitals have "wings," or units, dedicated to various types of patient care, commonly with 20 to 40 patient beds. This "unit" must be staffed with nurses, janitors, aides, and so on, 24 hours a day, 7 days a week, 52 weeks a year. In the course of normal day-to-day and even month-to-month fluctuations, whether the unit is 50 percent full (for example, 20 patients with 40 beds available) or 90 percent full (36 patients), the same levels of staff will probably be on duty. It is difficult to adjust the staffing levels even to accommodate monthly swings in hospital use because of costs of laying off staff and then retraining or rehiring them. If the unit becomes *systematically* half full, the administrator may feel comfortable reducing the staffing level some, but probably not in direct proportion to the changes in patient load.

If a hospital's occupancy rate falls considerably, it can eventually reduce its labor costs by closing down one or more units and moving the patients into another wing of the hospital (which also presumably had lost some patients). This makes the labor costs variable, but the building and beds continue to sit there, and their costs to the hospital don't change. Only by eventually eliminating new-bed construction (what would otherwise occur) can the long-run costs of hospitals be reduced completely in parallel with the reduced hospital use.

The importance of the fixed-cost versus variable-cost question appears in many policy questions. States with regulations covering hospital prices need to decide how to change the allowed price if a hospital's occupancy changes. Some regulatory programs pay for hospital care based on historical costs of the hospital. If patient loads in hospitals systematically decline through time, then the average costs of the hospital will rise and a fixed level of payment based on historical costs will place the hospital in a serious financial squeeze.

THE HOSPITAL'S "COST CURVE"

We are now in a position to consider what "the cost curve" of a hospital looks like. We begin with the variable costs, those that change as the rate of output of the hospital changes. Usually, economists draw a cost curve that resembles the one shown in Figure 8.6, in which the quantity of output appears on the horizontal axis and the vertical axis has cost/output as its scale. (This can represent price, average cost, or marginal cost.) In most productive activities (and we should not expect the hospital to differ), average variable costs will initially fall as output rises, so the average variable cost curve in such a diagram, labeled *AVC* here, has a standard J shape. The logic behind this stems from the common finding that inputs in the productive process eventually have diminishing marginal productivity (see the appendix in Chapter 3). The same phenomena produce an average variable cost curve that at first falls and then rises.

FIGURE 8.6 A hospital's variable, fixed, and total average costs.

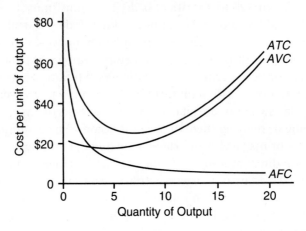

We also need to consider the role of fixed costs. For costs that are truly independent of the rate of output, *average fixed costs* appear as a curve such as AFC in Figure 8.6.[18] The average total costs, which must equal average revenue for the not-for-profit hospital, are the sum of the average variable cost and average fixed cost. Figure 8.6 shows this as the curve labeled ATC. At each level of output, ATC has a height equal to AFC + AVC.

This figure is drawn to reflect the empirical finding that much of a hospital's costs are fixed in the short run.

Quality of Care, Size, and Ownership

Many things change as a hospital's size increases. The scope of services performed expands, so more types of different illnesses can be treated with more specific and sophisticated equipment and staff. Perhaps the most important of these differences is the systematic relationship between quality of care and size—or in some cases, the patient volume for a particular type of treatment.

Several studies have investigated the relationship between hospitals' experience in performing surgery and their outcomes (as expressed by surgical mortality). These results show a strong relationship between experience and better outcomes (lower mortality). Practice, although not necessarily making things "perfect," seems to move outcomes in that direction.

---

[18]The equation producing this curve is of the form $AFC \times Q = K$, which is called a *rectangular hyperbola*.

The most prominent of these studies have been undertaken by economist Harold Luft and a series of colleagues. The first study (Luft, Bunker, and Enthoven, 1979) used outcomes for 12 operations in nearly 1,500 hospitals. For complex procedures such as coronary artery bypass grafts (CABG), open-heart surgery, vascular surgery, and even simpler procedures such as transurethral resection of the prostate (TURP), hospitals doing 200 or more of any of these procedures had mortality rates that were 25 to 40 percent lower than low-volume hospitals. Some procedures such as hip replacement showed a flattening of the mortality curve at about 100 procedures, and other procedures (e.g., cholecystectomy) showed no apparent gains in outcomes with the frequency of operations.

Critics of this first study suggested alternative explanations for the relationship, including the possibility that hospitals of superior quality attracted more patients, so that the relationship was not the one originally proposed (experience in a procedure improves outcomes) but rather what one would expect from a market that contained good information. Luft (1980) called this the "referral effect." There are also questions of "spillover effects," for instance, whether broader surgical experience improves outcomes on similar procedures. A second study by Luft (1980) identified the importance of spillover effects in some areas (various types of vascular surgery, for example) but continued to find only "own-procedure" effects for some activities such as CABG. Luft was not able to identify clearly the causal relationships involved, but the data suggest that for some of the procedures, the referral effect explained an important part of the observed association.

In the most recent of the series, Hughes, Hunt, and Luft (1987) examined the outcomes for more than 0.5 million patients from 757 hospitals, all of whom had received one of 10 specific surgical procedures. As with most of the other studies (Luft's and others cited in Hughes, Hunt, and Luft), the now-familiar relationship between surgical volume and improved mortality appeared again. In this study, however, a "low-volume doctor" effect also appeared, in somewhat of a contrast to the previous studies. The researchers found that a hospital was more likely to have poor outcomes, other things being equal, when low-volume doctors did a higher proportion of a hospital's surgery.

The literature is now clouded on the issue of doctor-specific effects but fairly consistent on hospital-specific effects. Hospitals doing more CABG, vascular surgery, and so forth, seem to experience better outcomes. Still incompletely resolved is whether this is a "referral effect" or a "practice-makes-perfect" effect.

In a more recent analysis of the risk-adjusted 90-day mortality rate for patients hospitalized after an acute myocardial infarction (AMI)—a major heart attack—McClellan and Staiger (2000) analyzed Medicare data for U.S.

hospitals in 1985, 1991, and 1994.[19] They found (in all 3 years analyzed) that higher levels of annual admissions of Medicare AMI patients improved the 90-day mortality outcomes significantly. Each 100 admissions (annually) reduced the mortality by about 1 to 1.5 percentage points (depending on the year). Because a large hospital can have hundreds, if not thousands more AMI patients than a small one, these differences mean that the quality of care differs very importantly between large and small hospitals for these types of patients. Whether this result generalizes to other medical events has yet to be demonstrated, but the results from McClellan and Staiger strongly suggest that at least for very complicated medical treatment problems, quality improves with size.

In carrying out this study, McClellan and Staiger also could estimate the differential effects of hospital ownership (holding size constant). They found that government-run hospitals had 90-day AMI mortality rates of about 1.0 to 1.8 percent higher than not-for-profit hospitals, and that for-profit hospitals had mortality rates in between the government and not-for-profit hospitals. In addition, they found that teaching status (independent of size) conferred a separate improvement in AMI mortality of about 0.2 to 1.1 percent (depending on year).

In a separate but related study, Halbrook et al. (1992) studied the "learning curve" for heart transplant surgery, seeking to determine whether the costs of treatment changed as the experience level of the transplant team increased. As the transplant team in a single hospital increased its experience, the costs fell from about $82,000 for the first case to under $50,000 for the tenth case, and further down to $35,000 for the fiftieth case and finally to $25,000 (less than a third of the original cost) for the last case in the series (seventy-first).

ANOTHER COMPLICATION: OUTPATIENT SURGERY

Hospitals not only produce many different types of treatments (the so-called job shop), but they also produce them in different ways and settings. The most obvious (and recognized) distinction is that between inpatient and outpatient surgery. The former involves the traditional case in which the patient is in the hospital for more than one day (a stay overnight is the key distinction);

---

[19]Researchers commonly look at 90-day mortality (i.e., 90 days after the heart attack) to avoid the risk that hospitals often differ considerably in their use of (for example) nursing homes or hospices as the final stop in the patient's life journey. Looking at 90-day mortality rates puts every hospital on an even basis of comparison.

TABLE 8.1 THE CHANGING FACE OF HOSPITAL TREATMENT

	1975	1980	1990	1995	2000	2005
Admissions	36157	38892	33774	33282	34991	37005
Average Length of Stay (ALOS)	11.4	9.9	9.1	7.8	6.8	6.5
Inpatient Days	412133	385031	307343	259600	237938	240539
Outpatient Visits	254814	262951	369184	483195	592673	673689
Outpatient Surgery as Percent of Total	—	16.3	50.5	58.1	62.3	63.3

Source: Health 2007, Table 103.

the latter case involves a situation in which the patient comes in, has surgery, and is discharged to home on the same day.[20]

The nature of activity at the typical U.S. hospital (and assuredly similarly worldwide) has shifted dramatically through the past few decades. Table 8.1 sets forth the key data. First, despite a significant increase in both the size and average age of the population, inpatient admissions remained essentially flat between 1975 and 2005, dipping slightly around 1990 and then recovering to previous levels. But admissions tell only part of the story—the average length of stay (ALOS) fell dramatically during this period, so that the total days of service created (the product of admissions and ALOS) plummeted, as shown in the third row of Table 8.1. Total inpatient days in 2005 were only 57 percent of what they had been a "mere" three decades ago.

Where did all the patients go? Partly into the "ambulatory" parts of the hospitals (outpatient clinics, emergency rooms, diagnostic testing and outpatient surgery)—instead of the traditional "inpatient admission" treatment path. Row 4 of Table 8.1 shows the rapid rise in outpatient visits to hospitals, from about 250,000 in 1975 to almost 675,000 in 2005—about a 165% increase over 30 years.

The final row of Table 8.1 shows the other remarkable phenomenon— the proportion of all surgical procedures done on an "outpatient" (one day) basis. Such surgery was almost non-existent in 1975. By 1990, half of all surgery was done on an outpatient basis, a fraction that has leveled off at about 63 percent in recent years. This shift of surgery out of the hospital came mostly through technological innovation—"minimally invasive" surgery primarily (see further discussions in Chapter 15), and greatly benefitted patients through faster recovery, minimal time away from home, shorter times of lost work, and of course lower health care costs than would have been the case had they been admitted for "traditional" inpatient surgery. But the loss of inpatient revenue created a major problem for hospital

---

[20]One might call this "dry cleaner" surgery: "in by 9 A.M., out by 5 P.M."

managers who confronted a collapse of historic proportions in their "bread and butter" revenue stream—inpatient days that could be billed to insurers and patients.

THE DEMAND CURVE FACING A SINGLE HOSPITAL

Each hospital faces its own demand curve. When there is only a single hospital within a geographic area, the hospital's demand curve and the market demand curve (the added-up demand curves of all of the individuals within the market) are identical. The same idea holds true in a multihospital market, with an important complication: When we "add up" the patients' demands to create the demand curve for St. Elsewhere Hospital, General Hospital, or their other competitors, we need to have a way to determine which patients in the market will choose which hospital.

We explore in Chapter 9 the mechanisms by which this process takes place, but the process is somewhat similar to that discussed for physicians in Chapter 7. For now, we need note only that the demand curve confronting a single hospital will slope downward (as does the market demand curve) and that it will almost certainly be more elastic (that is, the quantity demanded will be more sensitive to price) than the market demand curve. In a market with classic competition, the hospital's demand curve becomes infinitely elastic, but this characterization of hospital markets seems extremely unlikely.

Because hospitals are really multiservice job shops, one can meaningfully think about demand curves for each of the various things that a hospital does. These may differ importantly from "service" to "service." For example, in a town with two hospitals, only one of which has an obstetric suite, the demand curve for that hospital's obstetric services will coincide with the market demand curve. However, for other services (such as general medical and surgical cases), the demand curve for a single hospital is part of the market demand curve and is at least as price sensitive as the market demand curve, probably more so. Chapter 9 discusses these distinctions in more detail. This also raises the question of how to determine "the market" for a single hospital. This issue has been central not only to hospital planners (including those with the authority to control hospital bed capacity through "certificate of need" laws—see Chapter 15) but also in antitrust considerations that emerge more commonly now as hospital mergers become commonplace.

The standard approach to measuring markets relies on patient flow data, matching the origin of patients (e.g., by ZIP code) to hospitals. Most hospitals can tell immediately the ZIP codes of origin of their own patients

(patients' records invariably include addresses), so hospitals can tell on their own the regions from which they draw patients. If one drew a "circle" around the regions from which a given hospital draws patients, that provides one (albeit incomplete) definition of its market area. This corresponds to the standard antitrust definition of finding an area in which there is "little in from outside" (LIFO), an area sufficiently large so as to encompass the entire region from which (most) patients come to the hospital.

The next question is somewhat the reverse of determining a hospital's market—finding an area in which most of the patients in that geographic area receive their hospital treatment *from within* that region, leading to the description "little out from inside" (LOFI). This states that a market, once defined, is nearly self-contained.

Drawing a region either using LIFO or LOFI criteria creates a market area.[21] Particularly in antitrust settings, economists seek to understand the nature of competition within that market. Is there only one hospital (monopoly)? Are there two, and, if they merge, will they create a monopoly? Are there many hospitals in that market so that even after a merger, the resulting entity will not have a huge market share? These are the types of questions posed in hospital antitrust cases (and where and when such laws are relevant, in certificate-of-need hearings). Such legal cases and regulatory hearings hinge, in many ways, on an understanding of how the hospital's demand curve differs from the market demand curve. The more the hospital and market demand curves are one and the same, the more market power the hospital has and the less desirable it is from an antitrust perspective to approve a further merger. (These antitrust debates also involve questions about how not-for-profit hospitals might differ from for-profit hospitals in their economic behavior, holding constant the relationship between the market and the hospital's demand curve.)

---

[21]There is no definitive relationship between the sizes of LIFO and LOFI markets. A hospital such as the Mayo Clinic, in Rochester, Minnesota, for example, draws patients not only from its region but also from around the country and the world. However, most of the patients in its immediate region seek care either at the Mayo Clinic or a near neighbor; very few people feel compelled to seek care outside the region. Thus the LOFI region would be smaller than the LIFO region.

Alternatively, a rural area with only a small, unspecialized hospital would likely send many patients out of the region to referral centers in a large city, but it would treat almost no patients from outside the immediate geographic area (except those, for example, who are involved in an automobile accident while on vacation in the region). For these hospitals, the LIFO region would be quite small (just their own immediate region), but the LOFI region would have to expand to include the referral centers to which many patients go. In this case, the LOFI region would be larger than the LIFO region.

THE UTILITY-MAXIMIZING HOSPITAL MANAGER REVISITED

With the tools of a hospital's cost and demand curve in hand, we can return to the "utility-maximizing hospital manager" problem for a useful example of how a hospital sets its priorities and makes its economic choices. A section in Chapter 9 works through these ideas more formally, including interactions among hospitals, so this discussion only introduces the ideas.

Suppose the hospital manager cares about only two things: quantity and quality of care. In this case, the hospital decision maker has a utility function of the form $U = U(N, S)$, where N = the number of patients treated and S = some measure of quality (service). The hospital can produce any level of quality it desires, but more quality costs more. Thus, the average cost curve of the hospital depends upon the quality it offers.

The not-for-profit "rules" require that the hospital's total revenue equals its total costs, or (on a per patient basis), average revenue = average cost. The hospital can achieve exactly "zero profit" by setting a price $P(N, S) = AC(N, S)$. It will exactly "clear the market" if the quantity demanded for the quality it selects just equals the quantity supplied. This occurs whenever the demand curve and the average cost curve intersect each other.

If other things "matter" in the utility function, the same sort of logic can yield an analysis of how much of such things will be produced because we can judge how much patients value them and how much they cost to produce. Indeed, "quality" in the previous discussion could stand for anything that affected the utility function of a hospital's director, including nurses' salaries, doctors' profits, or thicker carpets on the administrator's floor. Of course, patients may not place much marginal value on these dimensions of the hospital's output, in which case the demand curves of the hospital's services won't shift much (if at all) as this dimension of quality varies.

The final idea in this discussion introduces the idea of cross-subsidies, or charge shifting, in hospitals. The previous discussion acts as if the hospital had only one output (for instance, patient-days) and only a single pricing decision to make. In actuality, the hospital has multiple outputs and a large number of prices. Thus, it has the opportunity to exploit its market power in one area (e.g., surgical patients) and to support another activity creating "utility" in another area (e.g., obstetric services). Thus, the ratio of costs to charges in the typical not-for-profit hospital can differ greatly across activities, and even those ratios can differ greatly across hospitals.

SUMMARY

In this chapter, we explore the hospital as an economic entity. The typical hospital in the United States has a not-for-profit legal status, which eliminates the usual corporate shareholder as a residual claimant. As a result, the hospital's profits must necessarily go somewhere else. Researchers have offered various models to help understand the behavior of the hospital, which generally presume that one or another person (or group) within the hospital has "captured" the hospital and uses the hospital's economic profits to further its own ends. In the doctor-capture model, the hospital's profits are passed indirectly, and possibly inefficiently, to doctors. In the manager-utility function model, some central decision maker has "captured" the hospital and guides the hospital's behavior in a utility-maximizing way. Employee-capture models and patient-capture models also seem possible, although not commonly considered.

A synthesis of these models probably better serves our understanding of the hospital. With no clearly defined legal "rights" to the hospital's profits, something else must serve the same functions as property rights might have, if they existed. This becomes essentially a problem in applied politics. The hospital's bylaws and charter define the "rules of the game" for the participants, who then seek to maximize their own gains in a contest with others in the same arena. We can expect these participants to eventually reach a standstill in their struggle, and the hospital will take on the appearance of having a single decision-maker utility function. However, this "apparent utility function" can shift if anything shifts in the political structure of the hospital, including external legal changes, the death of an important participant, or a change in the methods by which the hospital is paid. Whenever any such event shifts the balance of power in the hospital, its apparent utility function changes and so does the hospital's economic behavior.

RELATED CHAPTERS IN *HANDBOOK OF HEALTH ECONOMICS*

Chapter 20, "The Industrial Organization of Health Care Markets" by David Dranove and Mark A. Satterthwaite

Chapter 21, "Not for Profit Ownership and Hospital Behavior" by Frank A. Sloan

PROBLEMS

1. What is the distinguishing feature of the nonprofit organizational form compared with a for-profit organization? (*Hint:* What happens to any profits earned by the nonprofit hospital?)
2. Who controls most of the flow of resources within the standard not-for-profit hospital, and what mechanisms of control does the hospital president have over these people?
3. Suppose Hospital A has 500 patients per day (average) and average costs of $600 per day. Hospital B has 250 patients per day (average) and average costs of $500 per day. Hospital C has 100 patients per day (average) and average costs per day

of $550. What can you say (if anything) about the most efficient size of a hospital from these data?

4. Some studies show that the average mortality from specific surgical procedures differs depending on the frequency with which those procedures are undertaken annually by the hospital. Thus, for example, a hospital doing 200 open-heart cases annually probably has lower mortality rates than one doing 20 cases a year.

   a. Based on these data, where would you rather have open-heart surgery done, other things being equal?

   b. If some hospitals achieved reputations for being "very expert" in a particular procedure, do you think that they might actually end up with worse mortality rates? If so, how could this happen, and how would you want to interpret the mortality data? What would you need to be sure you interpreted such data correctly?

5. Most hospitals in Great Britain are owned by the government (part of the British National Health Service), and the doctors who work in them are employees of the hospital. In what ways do you think their behavior would differ from comparable doctors (same specialty, training, etc.) in a not-for-profit hospital in the United States?

6. What types of hospitals would you most expect to have sophisticated special treatment units (such as a burn-treatment unit, special capabilities for open-heart surgery, etc.)?

7. Using Figure 8.5 as the basis, construct a figure showing a gift with a restriction that quantity be at least N^* but where Trustee B decides to vote against accepting the gift. Explain carefully why you drew the curves as you did.

CHAPTER 9

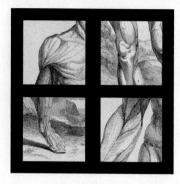

Hospitals in the Marketplace

This chapter discusses the behavior of hospitals in interaction with each other, their patients, and the doctors in their communities. Although we generally rely on the model of a not-for-profit hospital as developed in Chapter 8, nothing really differs greatly in this chapter if the hospital is a for-profit entity, and probably not much if it is operated by a local government (e.g., Cook County Hospital in Chicago). In part, this is because the "utility function" model of the hospital readily incorporates "profits" as the source of utility and because government agencies probably operate in a way that is quite similar to not-for-profit agencies in many important dimensions.

LEARNING GOALS

- Understand how hospitals simultaneously seek to attract doctors to their medical staffs and patients to their hospitals.

- Master the model of market equilibrium for a not-for-profit (NFP) hospital and discover how prices, quality, and quantity interact in these markets.

- Learn how the nature of competition has changed among hospitals as large buyers exert more power in the market.

- Digest the consequences of the large declines in demand for hospital services in recent decades and assess how industry entry and (mostly) exit occur.

Hospitals operate in a variety of markets. They must attract physicians to their staffs because physicians admit patients to the hospital. They must also attract paying patients. Many of the steps the hospital takes to do one of these also help the other, but in some ways the two types of "competition" differ, particularly under current funding arrangements. Hospitals also operate in input markets as buyers, most notably in the market for labor. Some of this labor is quite general in nature (e.g., janitorial staff), and some quite specific to the hospital (laboratory technicians). This chapter explores how each of these markets relates to the hospital and to its eventual survival and growth.

HOSPITALS AND THE MARKET FOR MEDICAL STAFF

A primary problem for a hospital is how to attract a medical staff because by law, only doctors may prescribe much of the treatment for patients that hospitals provide and only doctors can provide some of that treatment (e.g., surgery). Without doctors, a hospital cannot function. In the U.S. health care system, however, doctors typically function as independent economic entities. Thus, the hospital does not "hire" doctors, but rather "attracts" them.

This system of organizing doctors and hospitals does not occur in all other countries. In Great Britain and Germany, for example, "community" doctors typically have no ability to admit patients to hospitals. Patients who need to be admitted are referred to separate doctors on the hospital staff for treatment. They are then returned to their community doctors once they are discharged. In this kind of a setting, the hospital hires the staff doctors directly.

In the type of market organization found in the United States, the problem of attracting doctors creates a type of competition separate from what one would normally find in an industry because the doctor is somewhat like an employee and somewhat like a customer. Much economic research has made clear that doctors are an important "input" in the production of medical care in the hospital and can be analyzed in the same way as other types of labor (R.N.s, technicians, janitors, etc.) even though they are not "on payroll." However, because the hospital and doctor do not directly exchange money (payroll), the hospital must do something else to attract doctors. The solution has typically been for the hospital to compete, when necessary, by providing the doctor with facilities and services that make the doctor's practice more profitable.

As should be apparent, the question of how a hospital attracts doctors to its staff is closely tied to the problem discussed in Chapter 8 of "dividing up the profits" of the hospital. The model of the hospital developed by Pauly and Redisch (1973) focuses on this problem of attracting doctors quite intensively and ends up characterizing the hospital as if the doctors "owned" it. Of course, the hospital has other things it must or wants to do as well as attract doctors, so we would not expect a complete "capture" of the hospital by doctors, but to the extent that attracting doctors matters (as it must), the hospital does behave at least partly in ways characterized by the Pauly-Redisch model.

Some types of doctors are intrinsically more attractive to a hospital than others, depending on the hospital's goals. For example, some doctors are systematic moneymakers, creating a cash cow that helps finance other hospital activities. Other doctors provide prestige, glamour, and headlines for the hospital; they may actually create financial losses for the hospital with their activities. The mix that the hospital tries to attract depends in part on the goals of the hospital's leaders.

A primary way by which hospitals attract doctors to their staffs is to provide the doctors with the ability to do things that they cannot do elsewhere. For cardiologists, for example, the provision of a hospital with a cardiac intensive care unit (CICU) makes the hospital more attractive because it provides a high-tech environment in which to care for seriously sick patients. For heart surgeons, provision of excellent nursing staff for postsurgical patients is important, and, in some cases, provision of special operating rooms and equipment is the key attraction. For obstetricians, a good "delivery room" is available in almost any hospital, but having a newborn intensive care unit (NICU) available in case an infant is born prematurely or with a complex illness makes the hospital more attractive.

Some features of the hospital that provide general attractiveness include prompt laboratory work, the provision of good assistance to help the doctor complete the medical record, and the availability of standby emergency equipment (the so-called crash cart for cardiac arrest provides a good example) increase the general attractiveness of the hospital for doctors.

Of course, the doctor and the hospital stand in somewhat symmetrical positions in many ways. Not only does the hospital need doctors but also most doctors need access to at least one hospital to conduct their medical practice. Denying some doctors access to hospital medical staffs is tantamount to denying them the ability to earn a living, at least in some specialties. (For some specialties, such as psychiatry and dermatology, hospital privileges are not as important as they are for others, such as surgery.) Thus, in towns in which only one or two hospitals exist, the hospital may be in a stronger bargaining position with the doctor than it would be in a town with many hospitals. Similarly, hospitals in regions that are intrinsically attractive to doctors need not provide as many "goodies" to the doctors as hospitals in less desirable regions.

In every hospital, the "bargain" struck between doctors and hospitals differs, depending on the strengths of each in the marketplace and their uniqueness as a medical resource. Some hospitals, for example, require every doctor on their medical staff to provide some time in the emergency room as a quid pro quo for membership to the medical staff. In other hospitals, by contrast, the hospital not only does not exact such a "payment" but also actually provides office space for the doctor (sometimes at a very low or no charge) to see patients within the hospital.

Depending on how hospital care is paid for, it is easy to see how competition for doctors can become quite costly. Particularly in an environment in which health insurance pays for most if not all of the costs of most hospitalizations, it may well be that competition among hospitals mostly manifests itself in a technology-intensive war to attract physicians. As discussed later in this chapter, this appears to be what happened in the United States until quite recently.

HOSPITALS AND PATIENTS

A hospital must also attract patients, because they bring with them the revenue the hospital needs to pay its costs. Some of the same things that attract doctors to a hospital also attract patients, but sometimes different things matter, and sometimes the problem of attracting patients conflicts with the problem of attracting doctors. For patients, of course, a reputation of providing quality medical care is important, but other things sometimes loom large in patients' perceptions of a hospital. The quality of food; the friendliness of the nursing staff; and even, to some degree, the price of the hospital, its proximity to patients and family, and its general neatness and cleanliness can all affect the desirability of a hospital to patients.

Price matters only a little, if at all, to many patients because their health insurance pays for any costs the hospital bills. From the patient's point of view with such an insurance policy in hand, the price of care is zero in many ways, as discussed in Chapter 4.[1] For patients such as this, the hospital will mostly compete on the basis of the quality of nursing care, the food, and so on. With these types of patients, doing things that attract doctors to the medical staff and things that attract patients to the hospital often work in tandem. Moreover, because "the insurance pays for it," decisions to raise treatment quality have no apparent cost to the patient.

Some patients have insurance that pays only a specific amount per day of hospitalization, and others (about 18 percent of the U.S. population under the age of 65) have no insurance at all. For these people, price does matter in the choice of hospital. (In addition, some new forms of health insurance create something akin to price competition for hospitals. We discuss this momentarily.) For these types of patients, the things a hospital might do to attract doctors (e.g., more elaborate standby equipment in case of cardiac arrest, more numerous and more specialized intensive care units) may also prove attractive to patients, but they also raise the hospital's cost (and hence,

---

[1]It should be noted that most insurance policies pay only for "semiprivate" rooms (i.e., rooms shared by two patients). Therefore, if the patient selects a private room, often at a considerably higher price, the insurance policy usually pays only the amount it would pay for a semiprivate room. On this dimension of "quality," the patient bears the full incremental cost.

the price). For patients who pay for quality "on the margin" (for example, those who have an insurance policy that pays a fixed dollar amount per day of hospitalization, no matter what the cost of the hospital), an inherent conflict arises between attracting doctors and attracting patients.

In "the good old days" for U.S. hospitals, Medicare essentially paid dollar for dollar any costs incurred by the hospital, most Blue Cross insurance plans paid nearly full dollar, and much commercial insurance also paid billed charges.[2] For this reason, most hospitals apparently adopted a strategy of competing on quality, both for doctors and patients. One direct piece of evidence to support this claim comes from a study by Pauly (1978), comparing the costs of various hospitals with the makeup of their medical staffs. As the above discussion suggests, hospitals with "fancy" doctors (i.e., highly specialized doctors requiring specialized, rather than general-purpose, equipment and staff) also have "fancy" costs. Pauly's study shows a strong connection between the composition of the medical staff and a hospital's costs. Such a study cannot determine for sure which causes which, but logic dictates that the hospital cannot permanently attract a highly specialized surgeon to its staff (for example) without providing the equipment and support staff necessary for the surgeon's work.

Returning to the question of the modes of competition between hospitals, even with this extensive insurance coverage, it is clear that price matters, at least to some degree. Remember that a number of people (about one in every six persons who enters the hospital) have no insurance; for them, hospital care is very expensive on average. Others have insurance that pays only a lump sum per day, thus making these persons "price conscious" as well. One study attempted to estimate the demand curve confronting individual hospitals to determine just how much price mattered. This study (Feldman and Dowd, 1986) used data from a single metropolitan area (Minneapolis-St. Paul) in 1984 and estimated the demand curves facing 31 hospitals in that area, using techniques that depended upon a standard economic idea—namely, that a firm's optimum "markup" to set its price above cost to maximize profits is inversely related to the demand elasticity confronting the firm.[3] With estimates of cost and price, Feldman and Dowd inferred the demand elasticity, which stands as a proxy for the degree of competitiveness. (See also the appendix to this chapter for a more detailed discussion.)

Under one commonly invoked model of market pricing, the price elasticity confronting a noncolluding firm in the market is approximately the market

---

[2]This was not literally true, but a reasonable approximation that serves our discussion here.

[3]This is the so-called Lerner Index. Lerner (1934) first showed that the optimum markup for a monopolist is found by setting price such that the relative markup $\lambda = (P - MC)/P = -1/\eta$, where η is the demand elasticity and λ is the Lerner Index.

demand elasticity divided by the share of the market held by the firm. For example, if the market demand elasticity is -1 and the firm has 10 percent of the market, then its demand curve should have an elasticity of -10. This arises under a model of oligopoly pricing set forth by the French economist Cournot; it presumes that firm i sets its price under the belief that no other firm in the market will change its output if firm i changes its output. Although this "story" may seem unrealistic, it has some desirable properties.[4] Because the Minneapolis-St. Paul area had 34 total hospitals (with no cost data for 3, leading to the estimates for 31) and the demand for hospital care at the market level in that city should be about the same as that found in the RAND HIS ($\eta = -0.15$ for hospital care), the demand elasticity confronting any single hospital should be about $-0.15/(1/34) \approx -5.1$ if the hospitals were all in the same market and if they behaved in a simple Cournotlike way.

In fact, the estimates found by Feldman and Dowd using this approach did not differ considerably from that target. The price elasticity they inferred for private-pay patients was approximately -4; for Blue Cross patients (who have better coverage), approximately -2.3. However, using another completely different approach (directly estimating the demand facing each hospital as a function of its own price), they found price elasticities near -1, suggesting more monopoly power. These estimates represent a large share of the total literature on this topic,[5] so the matter cannot be considered conclusively settled. Nevertheless, these estimates do suggest that hospitals have some market power, confirming the desirability of using something other than a pure competitive model for analyzing the behavior of hospitals. In the next section, we can turn to what amounts to the beginnings of a model that describes how hospitals determine their price and quality jointly, an important problem in the U.S. hospital setting, with considerable implications for public policy.

A MODEL OF EQUILIBRIUM QUALITY AND PRICE

A model of how the choice to pick quality and cost of a hospital is made emerges (at least in part) from Newhouse's discussion (1970b) of the decision making of a hospital.[6] That model characterizes the hospital as having a single utility function, describing how much the hospital balances its various

---

[4]The Cournot model has the advantage that as the number of firms rises toward infinity, each firm's pricing rules approach those of perfect competition. More precisely, as $n \rightarrow \infty$, each firm's share approaches zero and the markup (Lerner Index) becomes very small.

[5]One hundred percent of that known to the author of this textbook.

[6]This discussion follows directly from this study, and some of the figures that follow are quite similar to those of Newhouse (1970b).

goals. In his simple model, the hospital desires only two things—size and quality—but the ideas generalize to other dimensions of hospital choice. We begin with this model and then discuss how various forces in the market, notably competition and insurance, alter the outcomes. The appendix to this chapter derives the solution to this problem formally.

We assume that the hospital utility function includes two characteristics—"quantity" (denoted N for number of days) and quality per day of care (denoted S for service). The hospital attempts to maximize the utility function $U(N, S)$. The patients' willingness to pay for the hospital service is represented by the inverse demand curve facing the hospital $P(N, S)$, where the willingness to pay P decreases with total quantity N (as is customary with demand curves) and increases with the quality of care S.[7] The not-for-profit hospital also faces a break-even constraint specifying that revenue equals cost $[P(N,S) \times N = C(N,S)]$. We presume that patients respond to quality and price in the normal fashion. We can assume that costs increase both with more quality S and more quantity N.[8]

If we were to draw the demand curves for different qualities, as shown in Figure 9.1a, each demand curve would slope downward, but the demand curves (willingness to pay) would be higher at higher qualities. *Remember that in this diagram, everything else is held constant except quantity (N), quality (S), and price-cost. Specifically, the insurance coverage of the patients and the quality and output of other hospitals are held constant.* In this way, the demand curve facing a single hospital is stable.

FIGURE 9.1 (a) Demand curves. (b) Average cost curves of the hospital for different levels of quality.

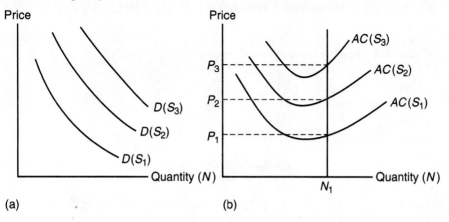

---

[7]In formal terms used in calculus, $\partial P/\partial N < 0$ and $\partial P/\partial S > 0$.

[8]Again, this means formally that $\partial C/\partial N > 0$ and $\partial C/\partial S > 0$.

Similarly, if we were to draw the average cost curves of the hospital for different levels of quality, the cost curves would stack up, each with the characteristic U shape of average cost curves (see discussion in Chapter 6 on physician-firms), so that higher quality costs more at any given level of output. These curves are shown in Figure 9.1b as approximately parallel, but nothing requires this in general.

Now combine these two sides of the market, as in Figure 9.2. Indicators for the level of quality (e.g., S_1, S_2, S_3) are omitted to avoid clutter, but we can take D_1 to mean $D(S_1)$ and so forth. In general, the demand curve for a specific quality (such as S_1) must intersect the corresponding average cost curve at either two points, one point (just tangent), or never. Points at which the demand and cost curves intersect are important because they show the combinations of price, cost, quality, and quantity that keep the hospital in equilibrium. The hospital can charge a price equal to its average cost for that output and quality, and at that price quantity demanded will just equal quantity supplied. In other words, these points of intersection are equilibrium points. If no intersections occur, that choice of quality is not feasible because it would always cost the hospital more to produce that level of quality than patients would be willing to pay, no matter what the level of output.

The next thing to note is that when two intersections occur, the one to the lower right is the best one for the hospital because it has more output, and, by assumption, hospitals would prefer to produce more hospital care, so long as quality doesn't suffer. Thus, the upper left of any intersections of a quality-specific demand curve and average cost curve doesn't matter.

We can find the set of all possible equilibrium combinations of quality and quantity using these tools. First, pick any level of quality, for example, S_1, and draw the corresponding average cost AC_1 and demand curve D_1. The

FIGURE 9.2 Equilibrium combinations of quality and quantity.

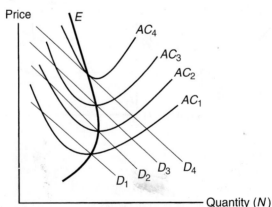

lower right of the two intersections is one possible equilibrium choice for the hospital. Now repeat that process for some other quality level, for example, S_2, and again for S_3, and all other possible combinations. Figure 9.2 shows all such possible combinations of cost and demand curves, tracing out the entire set of quantity-quality points that jointly satisfy both the demand conditions facing the hospital and its zero profit constraint. This collection of points is the line EE, a continuous line so long as quality can vary continuously. In general, this collection of points can slope either downward or upward, but only the downward-sloping portion should matter because on the upward-sloping portion of that set of points, the hospital could increase both N and S, which (by our assumption) are both "goods" to the hospital decision maker. In other words, if the hospital inadvertently found itself at some quality level on the upward-sloping portion of the EE curve, it could increase both quantity and quality and still be in equilibrium.

We can pick the "best" of all possible equilibrium points for the hospital by using the concept of an "indifference curve" (an idea set forth in Chapter 4 on the demand for medical care). Because we have assumed that the hospital decision maker has a utility function that increases with two "goods" (N and S), we can draw a set of indifference curves for such a decision maker. The discussion in Chapter 8 shows why this set of indifference curves (those of the median-voter board member) should remain stable through time. Figure 9.3 shows such indifference curves. The problem of finding the best possible combination of N and S is found by taking information from the EE curve in Figure 9.2 and

FIGURE 9.3 Indifference curves for quality and quantity.

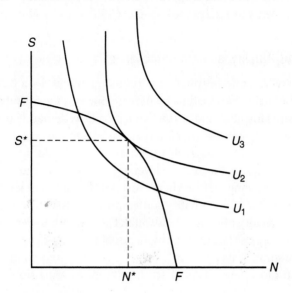

redrawing it into Figure 9.3. We can do this because each point on the *EE* curve describes a unique combination of quality (*S*) and quantity (*N*). Thus, the points on the *EE* curve can map into an opportunity-possibilities frontier *FF* for the hospital, with the optimum mix of *N* and *S* defined by the familiar tangency to an indifference curve of the hospital decision maker at N^* and S^*. This indicates at which single point on the *EE* curve the hospital will choose to operate.

INSURANCE AND COMPETITION IN THE HOSPITAL'S DECISION

The next step in understanding hospital decision making is to ask what various market (economic) events would do to the location and slope of the hospital's demand curve because for all of the discussion surrounding Figures 9.1, 9.2, and 9.3 "everything else" was held constant, including the quality and quantity of other hospitals and the scope and style of the insurance plans of the patients using the hospital. If we can learn what happens to demand curves in response to various stimuli, we can at least begin to infer what happens to the hospital's best choices for output and quality, and hence for the cost per hospital-day.

All of the previous discussion presumes that the hospital is a monopolist, or more specifically, that the family of demand curves facing the hospital (one for each level of quality) does not change as the pricing, quality, or output of any other hospital changes. In some small towns with only one hospital, this accurately describes the world. In many cities, however, the relevant market is shared by a few hospitals—more than one, but not so many that we can safely presume a purely competitive market. A more complete analysis of this problem appears in Phelps and Sened (1990).

Other Hospitals' Quality and Output Changes

What happens when one hospital changes its quality and no other hospitals respond? We can begin the analysis by picking one specific hospital (for example, St. Elsewhere Hospital) and asking what affects its demand curve's location and slope (elasticity). Suppose that another hospital in the region (for example, General Hospital) increases its quality—for example, by adding a new intensive care unit or by increasing the average level of training of its nursing staff. All of the demand curves facing St. Elsewhere Hospital (for different levels of quality) will shift. Demand for higher quality confronting St. Elsewhere will fall because of the increased quality of General Hospital. Demand for lower quality service at St. Elsewhere may rise because the higher quality (and price) at General Hospital may drive some of its patients elsewhere. On net, this will tip the *EE* curve confronting St. Elsewhere Hospital so that the downward-sloping portion is flatter in Figure 9.2, by rotating the *EE* curve counterclockwise. In Figure 9.3, the opportunity-possibilities frontier *FF* will also flatten out, making the most desired point one of higher output (more *N*) and lower quality (smaller *S*). This suggests that hospitals tend to specialize in different styles of output (different qualities) depending on their tastes and preferences, but that the market will not generally behave explosively.[9]

Entry by a new hospital does the same thing to St. Elsewhere's demand curves, with the shift being greater for those qualities for which the new entrant specializes. Thus, if a lower quality hospital enters, St. Elsewhere's demand curves will shift most for low quality and not much for high quality. If the new entrant has precisely the same quality as St. Elsewhere, then all demand curves would shift similarly, and the entire *EE* curve (Figure 9.2) and corresponding *FF* curve (Figure 9.3) would just shift inward.

The ultimate equilibrium appears as a variant on the standard monopolistic competition analysis. As noted, entry by other hospitals will cause some of St. Elsewhere's patients to shift to the new entrant. How long can this continue? If the demand curve shifts so far for a given level of quality that it no longer touches the *AC* curve for that quality level, then St. Elsewhere can no longer produce at that quality. If the same thing happens for all possible qualities that St. Elsewhere might produce, it will not be able to cover its costs of production at any quality level and would be forced out of business.

In general, for hospitals with access to the same technology, any entering hospital would face the same problem as St. Elsewhere faces—that is, attracting enough customers to have demand curves crossing *AC* curves for at least one point. The new entrant could not in fact enter unless it had some tangencies or intersections of demand and *AC* curves at one or more qualities. The limiting case occurs when each hospital in the market has its demand curves *at all levels of quality* just touching their *AC* curves at one point—that is, just tangent to the *AC* curves. This obviously will occur on the left side of the *AC* curve, where *AC* is declining and the hospital's capacity is underutilized. This is the classic excess-capacity story of Chamberlin's (1962) monopolistic competition. Figure 9.4 shows St. Elsewhere's opportunity set in this equilibrium, with the *EE* curve just a collection of tangencies of demand curves to *AC* curves for various levels of quality. Any further entry will cause St. Elsewhere's market opportunities to collapse. If every hospital in the community has similar *EE* curves, then the market is stable, with no incentives for any hospital to enter or exit.

---

[9]An explosive market would have the following characteristic: If hospital A increased its quality (perhaps by mistake), then Hospital B's optimal response would also be to increase quality. This would in turn cause Hospital A to increase quality more. . . . Soon all of the resources in the universe would be sucked into the abyss of hospital quality.

FIGURE 9.4 Excess capacity.

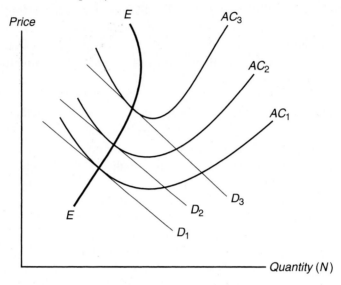

Changes to Patients' Insurance Coverage

We can also think about what would happen if hospital insurance coverage changed for the patients in the market. As a thought experiment, consider what would happen if more patients suddenly became insured with standard "coinsurance"-type insurance. We know from Chapter 4 that such insurance rotates demand curves clockwise around the point at which the demand curve intersects the quantity axis. In other words, the demand curves become steeper, and, in general, are further to the right than previously. This causes the *EE* curve to shift outward to the right in Figure 9.2, causes the opportunity possibilities frontier *FF* to expand outward in Figure 9.3, and leads to a higher equilibrium quality and quantity for the hospital. This would happen for *all* hospitals in the market because the expansion of insurance causes the demand curves for all hospitals to rotate outward, rather than cause an increase on one hospital's demand to come at the expense of another (as happens when one hospital increases its quality unilaterally). Thus (and this should really come as no surprise), better insurance not only increases the quantity of care demanded but also increases average quality, and hence average cost.

The world of managed care has altered the way hospitals are paid to a considerable degree, as also has the way Medicare pays hospitals. Analysis of these issues appears in subsequent chapters (Chapter 11 for private managed care and Chapter 12 for Medicare).

INTERACTION OF DOCTORS AND HOSPITALS: "GOODIES" FOR THE DOCTOR

This same type of model can help us understand how hospitals and doctors interact and how hospitals "compete" with each other for medical staff. For example, consider a doctor in a monopolistically competitive market with n physician-firms total, each initially with "typical" demand curves such as D_n and cost curves such as AC_1 in Figure 9.5. (This figure shows the same situation as Figure 7.1, where the idea of monopolistic competition among doctors was developed, but this one is more complex; AC_1 and D_n represent the situation shown in Figure 7.1.) Now suppose that the hospital used some of its surplus in a way that reduced doctors' AC curves. (The hospital has numerous ways it could do this, such as providing specialized surgical equipment that the doctor can use at no charge, renting in-hospital office space at reduced or no charge, making available interns and residents to "cover" the doctor's patients on nights and weekends, etc.) This would shift the AC curve downward, to something such as AC_2 or AC_3. If the costs for each doctor shift as low as AC_3 because of the hospital's largesse, then the existing doctors are no better off because the costs will have shifted so low that entry into the market will occur. (This takes place when the AC curve is just tangent to the demand curve D_{n+1} that each doctor would have with $n + 1$ doctors in town, shown as AC_3; indeed, AC_3 was chosen so that it is just tangent to D_{n+1}.) However, if the hospital picks some intermediate amount of largesse

FIGURE 9.5 Monopolistically competitive physician markets with differing degrees of hospital investment to reduce physician-firm costs.

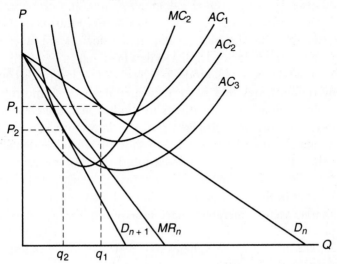

to bestow on its doctors, it will lower their costs to AC_2, which will not support another doctor in town and hence will not induce entry. At this point, the doctors can begin to price monopolistically (see Box 7.2 on monopolistic pricing), setting $MR_n = MC_2$, the marginal cost curve corresponding to AC_2, and the price will be P_1. (If entry occurred, the price would fall to P_2 in the monopolistically competitive environment.) This is drawn in Figure 9.5 as the same price that had prevailed before (at the tangency of D_n and AC_1), but this just represents another deliberate choice in drawing Figure 9.5. The price could rise or fall from P_1 depending on whether the AC shift was above or below AC_2. The key point is that the doctor receives a direct benefit because costs fall for the physician-firm and the optimal pricing response *must* make the physician-firm more profitable. Of course, it's also important that the hospital not "overdo it" (i.e., reduce costs at or below AC_3) to the point at which entry is provoked.

INTERACTION OF DOCTORS AND HOSPITALS: PATIENTS FOR THE HOSPITAL

The story is not yet complete, for we must reach an understanding of why the hospital would agree to do something to cut the physician-firm's costs as just described and as shown in Figure 9.5. One can ask why the doctor becomes a "stakeholder" in the hospital, or, in the model of the not-for-profit hospital developed in Chapter 8, why the physician-firm's profits enter the utility function of the hospital "director." One obvious answer is that the doctor can provide something the hospital badly needs: patients. Patients cannot "admit" themselves into a hospital; a doctor who has "admitting privileges" in the hospital must admit each patient. Thus, the very location of the demand curve for each hospital depends on how many doctors are on its staff and how many patients the doctor admits to that hospital.

We can now see how this model reaches closure. Hospitals compete for doctors by doing things that make their physician-firms more profitable; doctors respond by admitting patients to the hospital, thereby shifting out the demand curve (or, more properly, demand curves for all levels of quality) for the hospital. As the earlier discussion showed, when the demand curves shift out, the EE curve expands outward and the hospital can accomplish more of its desired goals. The doctors who bring the patients to the hospital share somewhat in the fruits of this expanded EE curve, but not completely.

This market seems generally to have a stable equilibrium, in which hospitals compete for doctors (and hence patients) by providing cost-reducing "benefits" to its medical staff (Phelps and Sened, 1990). Doctors in return bring patients to the hospital. In a market in which doctors can move freely from one community to another and in which hospital staffs are "open" to new doctors, the equilibrium has the characteristics described here, with doctors getting some but not all of the possible economic returns that their patients provide for the hospital.

In recent years, hospitals have begun to integrate their own services with those of physicians, commonly by hiring physician groups as hospital employees. This brings the doctors into more direct control of the hospital, and seeks to channel the patients of those doctors into the hospital when hospitalization occurs. Most commonly, the physician practices purchased by the hospital involve primary-care doctors (internal medicine, family practice, and general pediatrics) because a wide network of such practices can provide a strong referral base for the specialists in the hospital's practice. However, the trend for hospitals to acquire physician practices has abated, possibly because the incentive effects for physician effort under a flat salary (lower work effort) counteract the potential benefits of the affiliation. (Recall the work of Gaynor and Gertler, 1995, discussed in Chapter 6.)

COMPETITION—"OLD STYLE" VERSUS "NEW STYLE"

This discussion of hospital and doctor behavior leads naturally to a more extended discussion of how hospitals compete. Of course, in addition to competing for doctors, they must also compete for patients because patients' preferences have at least some effect on where they are hospitalized.[10] This section explores how this competition takes place and how it has changed over the most recent decade.

We might (loosely) characterize the "old-style" hospital market in the United States as one in which most of the people going to the hospital had insurance that covered most of their expenses, so that demand curves were quite inelastic. (Some of Feldman and Dowd's estimates confirm this assertion.) In general, we could even draw the following tentative conclusion: With "old-style" insurance, the hospital's problem of attracting patients was solved mostly in concert with its problem of attracting doctors—namely, by increasing the quality of the hospital.

In this type of market, increasing the number of hospitals could have an unusual effect on costs and prices. Because more hospitals would relatively increase the doctors' bargaining power, we might expect that areas with more

---

[10]Some doctors have admitting privileges at several hospitals and admit their patients to the one the patient most prefers. Of course, some patients also choose doctors on the basis of where they have admitting privileges, which makes the attractiveness of the hospital the key issue to doctors.

hospitals (more competition) would have to compete more intensively for doctors. In this case, competition would be cost increasing by driving every hospital to a higher quality level to attract doctors (and patients).

An alternative type of insurance (and market equilibrium that would result) a "new-style" insurance occurs if a large fraction of the insured population has incentives or administrative mechanisms that induce a high degree of cost consciousness on the part of patients.

We have seen something of a natural experiment in hospital insurance over the past several years that provides some insight into hospital behavior, which is important for understanding how hospital–doctor–patient markets work. The first step came when Medicare (which pays for about one-quarter of all hospital admissions) switched from a pay-dollar-for-dollar system to a very different system called the *prospective payment system* (PPS), which pays a flat amount to each hospital for a given category of admission.[11] For now, all we need to know is that it suddenly put into the decision-making process a cost consciousness that had been notably absent previously.

During the same period, particularly in a few states, cost-conscious insurance spread through other sectors of the health care market as well. Some private insurance plans adopted very aggressive shopping-for-deals strategies, and even some state Medicaid programs for low-income people began to seek competitive bids for hospital care. The insurers began to negotiate with hospitals and doctors, offering to send them all of the patients enrolled in their insurance plans in exchange for a "good price." The insurers enforced this with their subscribers by paying 100 percent of the hospital bill for "approved" providers, but a lower amount for others.[12]

The results of this change, which began in the early 1980s, create the possibility that the economic environment might have shifted between the "old style" and this new cost-conscious style. In particular, whereas competition might have been cost enhancing in the old style (due to the pursuit of doctors and competition for patients with increasing quality), competition under the "new style" is much more likely to create cost reductions.

A perfect "test bed" for this type of analysis appeared in California during the mid-1980s because the change in Medicare pricing coincided with a large increase in the market share of cost-conscious private health insurance as well as a shift to competitive bidding for the state's Medicaid hospital business. Under the "old style," competition indeed was cost increasing for California hospitals; in the new-style era, the opposite appears to be happening more and

---

[11]This change in Medicare pricing is discussed in much more detail in Chapter 12.

[12]These insurance plans, called *preferred provider organizations* (PPOs), are discussed in more detail in Chapter 11.

more. In one analysis (Melnick and Zwanziger, 1988), the role of competition appeared quite dramatically. In markets characterized by low competition,[13] hospital costs (adjusted for general inflation) increased by only 1 percent in the 1983–1985 period, historically a very low rate. In markets characterized by high competition, inflation-adjusted hospital costs *decreased* by more than 11 percent during this same period. This decrease represents a very unusual event in the history of U.S. hospital costs and suggests (as Melnick and Zwanziger describe it, p. 2669) that "pro-competition policies are having dramatic and potentially far-reaching effects on the nature of hospital competition, leading to increased competition based on price."

An outpouring of studies in the same vein occurred during the 1990s. This body of work analyzes the relationship between market concentration and price and cost behavior, and in particular, looks for changes in the relationships as managed care spread across the land. This work has now acquired the tag-line of the role of competition in the Medical Arms Race (MAR), and the basic idea says that in "old style" insurance that reimbursed hospitals generously for any expenses incurred, a MAR would be the natural outcome, but that when managed care emerged as a potent market force, competition would eliminate the ability of hospitals to engage in this behavior. Thus, one expects to find a direct link between the lack of competition and higher prices and costs (i.e., continuing MAR behavior) in the 1980s and 1990s. For example, Conner, Feldman, and Dowd (1998) used U.S. hospital data to show that costs rose much more rapidly between 1986 and 1994 in more heavily concentrated markets. Dranove, Shanley, and White (1993) looked at the "list" prices and the actual transactions prices for a set of very standardized services (radiology, laboratory, basic "hotel" services, etc.). They found that in 1983, market concentration (their measure of the lack of competition) was unrelated to price-cost margins, but by 1988, when competition had spread widely, they found a significant relationship between concentration and margins (i.e., those communities with little competition had higher markups in 1988, while those with lots of competition had prices close to costs). Prices were *negatively* related to concentration in 1983 and *positively* related in 1988. This also is consistent with the idea that competition had switched from attracting doctors (MAR) to competing on price (in the face of large pressure from managed care insurance plans).

---

[13]The measure of competition was the Hirshman-Hirfindahl Index (Hirshman, 1945; Herfindahl, 1950), HHI $= \sum_{i=1}^{n} s_i^2$ (where s_i is the market share of each hospital). If each seller is of the same size, the HHI equals the number of sellers, which is of course 1 in a monopoly. The U.S. Department of Justice uses the HHI as a test of whether monopoly power is present, particularly when deciding whether to contest mergers.

ENTRY AND EXIT: THE PIVOTAL ROLE OF FOR-PROFIT HOSPITALS

One of the characteristics of a market economy widely admired by economists, if not others, is the ability of market forces to generate investment in a hurry when new demand emerges. Unusually high economic returns create incentives to enter an industry. Not-for-profit hospitals, by contrast, may not respond as swiftly to changes in demand. For example, if a community grows very rapidly or, more particularly, if demand grows for a service in some community, one might expect that the first line of response could well be a for-profit hospital.

The same characteristic of rapid entry in the face of rising profits may cause for-profit firms to exit an industry faster than nonprofit firms when profitability (i.e., demand) falls.

It is difficult to characterize market responses to changes in demand fully in the hospital industry because (1) some states forbid or severely curtail the presence of for-profit hospitals and (2) governments sometimes subsidize or create hospitals where they would not otherwise exist. However, the growth of for-profit hospitals in regions of the country that grew rapidly over the past several decades lends credence to the idea that the for-profit response is faster than not-for-profits are capable of producing. The casual observation that for-profit hospitals have grown most rapidly in California, Florida, and Texas supports this idea because these areas have had rapidly growing populations and even more rapidly growing demand for hospital care. This is because they are popular retirement states, and elderly people systematically use much more than the average amount of hospital care. In one early study of the role of for-profit hospitals, Steinwald and Neuhauser (1970) indeed found that growth of for-profit hospitals was correlated positively with population growth more than was true for the not-for-profit hospitals.

Demand for hospital services is now shrinking, particularly in California and other areas where "competitive" health strategies have been prominent and where there has been the growth of substitutes, particularly ambulatory surgery. Box 9.1 shows trends in U.S. hospital use from 1981 to current times.

THE HOSPITAL IN LABOR MARKETS

We now turn to a different problem confronting the hospital—its market environment for buying its inputs, such as equipment, supplies, and labor. The demand for the services of a hospital in turn creates a derived demand for the inputs that a hospital uses, including those of capital (for example, buildings and equipment) and various types of labor. These derived demand curves slope downward, just as do the demand curves for the final product. Sometimes, these demand curves are called *factor* demand curves, with reference to the phrase *factors of production*. Demands for input factors depend in part on the quality of the hospital's service and the mix of complexity of patients' problems. Because larger hospitals seem to specialize in more complex patients, it would seem natural that they demand both more total staff per patient and a more highly trained staff.

Hospitals compete for these inputs, just as firms in any other industry do. In some cases, they compete only against other hospitals, for instance, for very specialized forms of labor. In other cases, they compete against a very broad spectrum of the economy, for instance, for secretaries, janitors, food service workers, and so on. In the former case, the industry itself in part determines the wages paid within the industry. In the latter case, worker's wages are almost certainly determined in broader markets in which the hospital has no pivotal role at all.

To see how and why this works, think about two generic types of labor, one specialized to the hospital sector and the other used broadly across all industries.[14] As a shorthand notation, we might call these types of labor "nurses" and "janitors," understanding that the labels connote nothing about skill level but the extent to which the occupation crosses the bounds of many industries. Thus, "nurse" represents nurses, various types of technicians, therapists, medical records librarians, and so on, and "janitor" represents janitors, food service workers, accountants, computer programmers, lawyers, and so on. These prototypes form extreme cases, whereas much of the labor working in hospitals fits "in between" these cases. For example, nurses work not only in hospitals but also in doctors' offices, in public health settings, and as private-practice nurse practitioners. The fundamental difference between these two types of labor is whether the supply curve confronting the hospital industry in a particular community is likely to be upward sloping or flat. The distinction has the following importance. When the supply curve is upward sloping, if the hospital attempts to expand its output or quality (by hiring more "nurse" labor), it will have to pay an increasingly higher wage, and if it contracts its demands for "nurses," then the equilibrium wage will fall. However, in the market for "janitors," changes in the hospital's demands will have no effect on the market wage because "janitors" can find ready employment elsewhere. Thus, if the hospital tries to expand its output or quality by hiring more "janitors," it can do so without driving up the wage rate. The reason is that the pool of people available for hiring includes not only those janitors

---

[14]The same discussion applies to other types of inputs for the hospital, such as equipment and supplies, which might be quite special for the hospital or wholly generic.

BOX 9.1 THE DEMISE OF DEMAND FOR THE AMERICAN HOSPITAL

Aggregate hospital statistics reveal a striking decline in the use of hospitals in the United States, beginning in the mid-1970s. One can compute the average daily census (the number of actual patients occupying beds in U.S. hospitals) as the product of the number of beds times the occupancy rate. In these data, we see a steady decline over 30 years from a bit more than 1 million patients per day to about 600,000 per day. Much of the decline occurred in the 15-year period between 1981 and 1996 (see Figure A).

FIGURE A Total Hospital Inpatient Days, U.S. Community Hospitals, 1981–2006

Source: AHA Trendwatch Chartbook, 2008, Chicago: American Hospital Association, 2008.

The causes of this drop in demand are numerous, but two things stand out in particular: the advent of "pay by the case" (prospective payment) that created large incentives for hospitals to reduce length of stay (initiated by Medicare's PPS in 1983 and rapidly mimicked by private insurance plans thereafter) and the technological shift of surgery from inpatient (and long stays) to "ambulatory" (same-day) surgery. Although hospitals captured most of the same-day surgery, the long and low-cost hospital days following up on the surgery (as the patients recovered) vanished from the revenue stream.

Figure B shows the shift through time from 1981 to 2006 for the percentage share of all surgeries conducted as inpatient versus outpatient. In 1981, about 80 percent of the surgery occurred on an inpatient basis. By 2006, the share was under 40 percent. Most of this shift came with the advent of minimally invasive surgical techniques: "laparoscopic surgery" for abdominal and other soft-tissue operations and "arthroscopic surgery" for bone and joint surgery.

FIGURE B

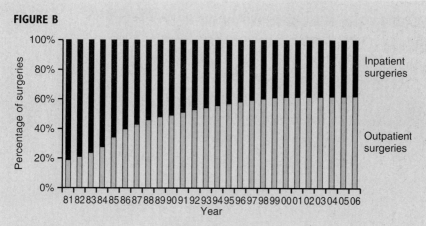

Source: AHA Trendwatch Chartbook 2008, Chart 3.14.

"Hospital-days" is the product of hospital admissions (Figure C) and average length of stay (Figure D). We can see two very different trends in these component parts. Hospital admissions plummeted from 1981 to (again) about 1995 and then began to grow again through various forces (population aging, changes in insurance coverage, and technological change that created new ways to cure people but still required hospitalization). Had this been the only thing happening, the U.S. hospital industry would have survived more easily.

FIGURE C

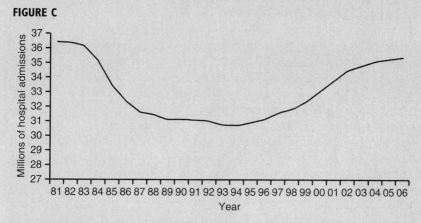

Source: AHA Trendwatch Chartbook 2008, Chart 3.2

(continued)

BOX 9.1 THE DEMISE OF DEMAND FOR THE AMERICAN HOSPITAL (continued)

FIGURE D

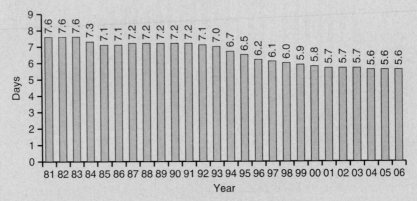

Source: *AHA Trendwatch Chartbook 2008,* Chart 3.5

However, beginning at about 1983 (and likely showing the effects of the Medicare PPS's introduction), average length of stay (ALOS) began to creep down, flattened out briefly, and then continued in a headlong dive downward, with 2005 levels of 5.6 days compared with 1981 levels of 7.6 (a reduction of more than 25 percent).

The decline in ALOS is all the more remarkable because so many "easy" surgical patients (who would mostly have had short lengths of stay) shifted to ambulatory surgery (Figure B).

All of this decline in demand came in the same period in spite of a population growth from 215 million to 296 million people (about 38 percent total growth) and an increase in the average age (revisit the discussion relating to the tables in Chapter 1) that would also increase demand if nothing else was happening.

How did the U.S. hospital industry accommodate this drop in demand? Partly it did so by closing some hospitals. The number of hospitals had fallen by 2005 to about 82 percent of the 1975 peak level. Furthermore, the industry took beds out of service, usually a "wing" at a time, to reduce staffing most efficiently. By 2005, the total number of U.S. hospital beds had fallen to two-thirds of the 1975 peak.* But the hospitals were not able (or willing) to close beds fast enough to remain at the peak efficiency occupancy rates of 75–80 percent. The average occupancy rate fell to 65 percent (in 1995) and has slowly crept back up as more beds are taken out of service.†

*This also took place with differential closure rates for hospitals of different sizes. The largest drop occurred in hospitals in the 50–100 bed size; almost a third of them closed during this period.

†A close analog occurred in 2008 during the rapid increase in the cost of petroleum products, including jet fuel. This cost increase—passed in part but not completely to

passengers in initial phases—caused overall demand for air travel to shrink. Airlines responded in part by raising prices and in part by reducing capacity. In this case, they systematically removed from service those older aircraft that had the worst fuel efficiency ratings. This is akin to taking a "wing" out of service in a hospital (pardon the expression). Also some airlines went out of business or merged with others (just as some hospitals closed in the face of reduced demand). Even as airlines removed aircraft from service, the "load factor" (exactly akin to the average occupancy rate in hospitals) declined because demand fell faster than the airlines removed aircraft from service.

currently unemployed but also all those working in all other industries. By the same token, if the hospital reduces its demand for janitors, those laid off can find ready work elsewhere, so the wage rate will not fall.

Figure 9.6 portrays these two cases, with the wage rates for nurses shown in Figure 9.6a at two levels of demand and the (unvarying) wage rate for janitors Figure 9.6b.

What might cause the demand for labor to shift outward in this way? The most obvious answer is that anything causing a shift in the demand for hospital care will also shift the demand for labor used in the hospital. A key example is provided by the introduction of Medicare in 1965, which created a large increase in the amount of medical care (including hospital care) demanded by the elderly. That shift in demand for hospital care also created a shift in the *derived* demand for labor of all sorts. The shift in the demand for nurses would create an upward pressure on the wages of nurses because the

FIGURE 9.6 (a) Wage rates for specialized hospital workers. (b) Wage rates for unspecialized hospital workers.

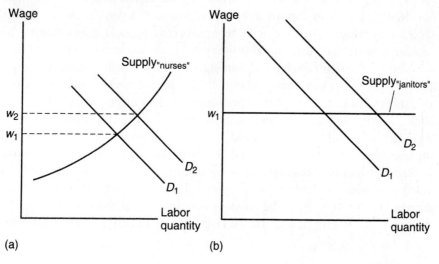

supply of nurses (at least in the short run) is upward sloping, or "inelastic." This in turn would cause the costs of the hospital to rise. As a first-order approximation, the change in the costs of a hospital (or any other firm) behaves according to the following rule: The percentage of change in costs equals the percentage of change in the factor price multiplied by the cost share (%ΔCost = %Δwage × cost share). Thus, for example, if nurses constitute half of the cost structure of a hospital and nurses' wages rise by 10 percent, then hospital costs will rise by 5 percent. The increase is less if the hospital has the ability to substitute other forms of labor (or equipment, capital, or any other productive input) for nurses as the wage of nurses rises, but the first-order effect is as stated.

NURSING "SHORTAGES"

Hospital markets frequently have the appearance of a shortage of some types of labor, most commonly, registered nurses (R.N.s), as distinct from the generic "nurses" we discussed earlier. This phenomenon has appeared repeatedly in the U.S. health care literature, most recently during the early 2000s. A true "shortage" in an economic sense means that something is constricting the wage rate or the supply beyond normal market forces because we would expect that whenever the quantity demanded exceeded the quantity supplied, the normal market response would cause the wage rate to rise, thereby eliciting a larger supply while causing the quantity demanded to fall at the same time. In equilibrium, of course, the quantity supplied and demanded are the same, at the equilibrium wage rate.

From the perspective of competitive markets, therefore, a "nursing shortage" suggests that something is constricting either the supply or the wage rate. Neither situation appears to exist in the United States. People can decide to enter nursing freely, and a large number of schools offer training to become a nurse. The traditional training program for much of this century was a hospital-oriented school of nursing, offering a 3-year training program leading to a degree in nursing. Many of these schools were operated in close affiliation with large hospitals. More recently, community colleges began to offer a 2-year program leading to an associates of arts (A.A.) degree in nursing, after which the student could take state licensure examinations and become a legally registered nurse (R.N.). Some colleges offer a 4-year course of study leading to a bachelor of science in nursing, and graduate study in nursing is now available at some universities, providing M.S. and Ph.D. degrees. At the M.S. level, the training is often specialized (for example, in intensive care nursing), and the Ph.D. programs mostly prepare nurses for teaching and research or high-level administrative positions. Nevertheless, the widespread availability of these programs suggests strongly that there is no artificial constriction on the supply of nurses. In light of this, we would anticipate a competitive labor market from the supply side, at least on the decision to enter nursing.

Monopsonistic Markets

One alternative explanation that has appeared cyclically along with nursing "shortages" is that hospitals have market power in the labor markets for nurses and are responding in an appropriate way to that market power. Note that the presence of market power is not illegal; colluding to obtain that power is. However, by the very nature of the hospital, whereby it has market power on the product side (i.e., faces a downward-sloping demand curve for its final product), we could well expect also that it has market power on the supply side, at least for types of labor that are specialized to the health care industry. It is precisely this type of labor that we called "nurses" generically earlier in this chapter.

To see what happens when a hospital confronts an upward-sloping supply curve for labor, look at Figure 9.7. This curve shows the supply of labor (adding up all of the hours of supply from individual participants) and the hospital's derived demand for labor, sloping downward in the usual fashion. The third curve in Figure 9.7 is the marginal factor cost (identified as *MFC*) curve, so called because it shows the hospital how much its factor payments (total wages to "nurses") rise as it tries to expand its use of "nurses." The *MFC*

FIGURE 9.7   Hospital confronting an upward-sloping supply curve for labor.

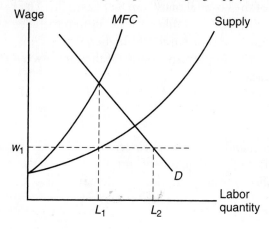

FIGURE 9.8 Monopolization of the market for labor by a union.

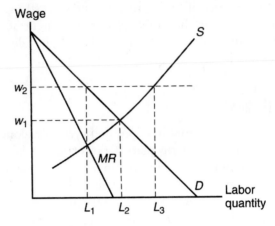

curve rises faster than the supply curve because of the market power of the hospital in the labor market; it has *monopsony* power.[15]

A hospital in this setting will choose the "right" amount of labor by finding the point at which the *MFC* curve crosses its demand curve, at the point labeled L_1 in Figure 9.7. The "going wage" for the market will then be set at the point at which the market supply curve and the vertical line L_1 intersect, at the wage rate w_1. Of course, at that wage rate, the hospital would gladly hire L_2 amount of labor, but at that wage rate, a competitive labor market will supply only L_1. The gap between L_1 and L_2 represents the "shortages" of R.N.s confronting U.S. hospitals.

One study of the market for nurses in Utah found an apparently considerable degree of potential monopsony power in it (Booton and Lane, 1985). Three firms controlled 26 of the state's hospitals, and one firm controlled more than half of the hospital market in Salt Lake City. Their study estimated that a 10 percent increase in unfilled vacancies in nursing by hospitals would lead to more than 4 percent *lower*, not higher, wages. This is precisely what would happen in a monopsonistic market if the gap between L_1 and L_2 represents "unfilled vacancies."

SUMMARY

Hospitals face demand curves for their services that shift inward or outward, depending on the price and quality of competing hospitals. Only if the hospital is a monopolist (one hospital) does the demand curve for a hospital match

---

[15]Again, we should emphasize that nothing is illegal or immoral about this. It's just a fact of life, like gravity, or sticky fingers after eating a jelly doughnut.

the demand curve for the market. Any hospital also can choose its quality, and the demand it confronts (think of it as willingness to pay for the hospital's services) will shift upward as the quality increases. In general, we can state that demand curves for a hospital shift upward (outward) whenever

- A competing hospital's price increases.
- A competing hospital's quality falls.
- The extent of hospital insurance held by patients increases.

Hospitals also must decide about their scope of services. In part, the interaction between doctors and hospitals hinges on these types of decisions. When hospitals want to attract more patients, they need doctors to do this; to attract more doctors, they need to provide special facilities that assist the doctors' practices. Thus, the "scope of services" decisions importantly determine much of the overall success of a hospital.

We can think of hospitals as confronting a family of demand curves, with a different curve for each quality of care that the hospital might produce. Each level of quality also has associated with it a different cost curve, so there is a family of average cost curves just as there is a family of demand curves. The not-for-profit rules of the hospital require that it set a price so that revenue just covers costs, which means that it must operate where demand curves intersect average cost curves. The set of all such intersections, called the *EE* curve in the text, provides the set of all feasible choices of quality, quantity, and price. The hospital can select which of these feasible choices is best by comparing the preferences of the hospital's fictitious "director" (using a utility function) with the available choices. One choice will provide the highest utility, and this becomes the point actually chosen by the hospital.

Hospitals use resources to produce their services, leading to derived demand curves for inputs. The technology of production available (the production function) and the costs of inputs determine the choice of inputs. One particularly interesting part of the hospital's decision is that it may have monopsony power in some labor markets, such that the hospital can alter the price paid for labor (such as nurses) as they change the amount of labor they demand. In these cases, hospitals may set their wage offers to some staff (e.g., nurses) in a way that creates the appearance of a permanent shortage.

RELATED CHAPTERS IN *HANDBOOK OF HEALTH ECONOMICS*

Chapter 27, "Antitrust and Competition in Health Care Markets" by Martin Gaynor and William B. Vogt

Chapter 28, "Regulation of Prices and Investment in Hospitals in the U.S." by David S. Salkever

PROBLEMS

1. Using graphs such as those shown in Figures 9.2 and 9.3, carefully explain how a hospital decides what level of quality to produce.
2. Using graphs such as Figures 9.2 and 9.3, show what happens to the quantity and quality of a not-for-profit hospital that has been a monopolist and suddenly has a new competitor in town.
3. What necessarily happens to average quality in a hospital market when the generosity of insurance coverage increases? How does this relate, if at all, to the data appearing in Chapter 1 on increases in spending through time in the hospital sector?
4. If you looked in the want ads section of your local newspaper, would you expect to find more advertisements run by hospitals in your town seeking nurses or janitors? Similarly, among ads for nurses, would you expect the ads to focus more on "general" nurses or specialized nurses, such as those with training to work in intensive care units? Why?
5. What factors do you think most contribute to the declining occupancy rates of U.S. hospitals over the past decade? (You should think both of technological change and financial incentives.) Data show that occupancy rates have begun to stabilize in recent years, despite the continuing forces for declining use of the inpatient hospital facility. To what do you attribute this phenomenon?
6. Does the not-for-profit status of most U.S. hospitals make them more or less likely that any single hospital will close its doors in the face of falling demand? Why?
7. If hospitals began to affiliate within regions, would you expect that "unnecessary duplication of facilities" would increase, decrease, or stay the same? Why?

APPENDIX TO CHAPTER 9

The Hospital's Quality and Quantity Decision

One way to determine the best choice of quality and quantity is to use a calculus technique called *Lagrange multipliers*. This technique finds the best choice to maximize utility subject to the constraint that revenue does not exceed cost (the limitation of the not-for-profit form of organization). The Lagrangian formulation of this problem says to maximize the function L, which is the sum of the objective function and λ times the constraint (written to equal zero). Then the technique takes the partial derivatives of L with respect to each variable, including the new variable λ, and sets each equal to zero. The resulting equations define the best mix of output and quality:

$$L = U(N, S) + \lambda[P(N, S) \times N - C(N, S)] \qquad (9A.1a)$$

Define the derivatives by subscripts, so (for example) $\partial U/\partial N = U_N$, and similarly for U_S, and C_N and C_S. The conditions to maximize the hospital's utility require that:

$$U_N + \lambda[P(N, S) \times (1 + I/\eta) - C_N] = 0 \qquad (9A.2a)$$

$$U_S + \lambda(P_S N - C_S) = 0 \qquad (9A.2b)$$

$$P = C/N = AC \qquad (9A.2c)$$

where η is the own-price elasticity of demand confronting the hospital (holding service quality constant). Reorganizing equations 9A.2a and 9A.2b to solve each for λ gives

$$U_N/[C_N - P(1 + 1/\eta)] = \lambda \qquad (9A.3a)$$

$$U_S/(C_S - P_S N) = \lambda \qquad (9A.3b)$$

In this familiar form, the decision rules emerging from the maximization say to set the ratio of marginal utility to marginal cost equal for both of the choices N and S. In equation 9A.3a, the net cost of N is marginal cost minus marginal revenue. In equilibrium, MC exceeds MR, which in turn requires expanding production past the monopoly level (where $MR = MC$). The hospital "spends" potential profit on the expansion of sales. In one corner solution where $U_N = 0$, the firm simply picks the monopoly price, using its market power as a cash cow to augment quality.[16] So long as C is nondecreasing in N and normal demand conditions prevail (so marginal revenue falls as N rises), the net cost of N increases with larger N.

A corresponding condition holds for service intensity ("quality"); the marginal cost to the hospital is $C_S - P_S N$, the logical equivalent of the difference between marginal cost and marginal revenue; again, the hospital "spends" potential profits on more quality. So long as cost is nondecreasing in S and demand is increasing in S, the "net cost" of S to the hospital also increases with S.

---

[16]This might correspond closely to Pauly and Redisch's (1973) model, in which "service" was selected to create more profits for doctors. Conversely, a Baumol-like "sales maximization" model would have $U_S = 0$ and would milk the quality dimension to expand sales.

Because the "costs" of both N and S increase as their own scale increases (at least in the relevant range of behavior), the hospital faces decreasing returns to scale in production of utility in both N and S. Thus, the opportunity-possibility curve is concave to the origin for the relevant choice set, as shown in the figures in the body of the chapter.

Policy Applications of the Model

The model here has some interesting policy applications as well. We can solve equation 9A.2a for the equilibrium price and then use that result in further discussion:

$$P = \left(C_N - \frac{U_N}{\lambda} \right) \frac{\eta}{(1 + \eta)} \qquad (9A.3c)$$

This is similar to the standard "markup pricing" of a monopolist, except for the term U_N/λ, which represents (scaled to dollars by λ) the utility benefits to the hospital director from additional output.

This characterization of the optimal price helps explain two particularly interesting questions in the economics of hospital behavior. The first returns to the analysis by Feldman and Dowd (1986) described in the text. They used an equation similar to 9A.3c to estimate the demand elasticity facing a hospital. To do that, they solved their version of equation 9A.3c for η, which is

$$\eta = \frac{-P}{[(P - MC) - U_N/\lambda]}$$

The only difference between their work and the approach defined in the immediately preceding formula is that they assumed the hospital sought to maximize profits alone, so that $U_N = 0$. Thus, they calculated $\eta = -P/(P - MC)$, as one would for a profit-maximizing monopolist. The estimates they derived are the larger valued elasticities reported in the text. The direct estimates of demand curves gave values of η near -1, which Feldman and Dowd appeared not to believe. In part, their disbelief arises from the well-known monopolist's rule that one never willingly operates in the region where demand is inelastic (i.e., $|\eta| < 1$) because marginal revenue is negative. The monopolist can always make more money by raising price and reducing output if demand is inelastic. However, as equation 9A.3c shows clearly, if the hospital's utility function sufficiently emphasizes quantity of output, then the hospital will willingly operate in the realm of inelastic demand. Indeed, it might even willingly charge a negative price (bribe people to use the service) under some situations.

The second issue arising from this analysis concerns the oft-studied question of "cost shifting" in hospitals. All hospitals have prices that they use when sending bills to every patient. However, many customers (usually big insurance organizations or government insurance plans) do not pay "charges," but rather something less, often an approximation to the actual average costs of the hospital. Groups that continue to pay billed charges often complain about the arrangement and are particularly worried that when, for example, Medicare or Medicaid reduces its payment to hospitals, the hospital merely shifts its costs to the charge-paying customers by billing at higher prices. (The hospital keeps sending the bills with higher charges to the government plans as well, but the government plans ignore them and send back their own calculations of "costs.")

The model of behavior developed here extends directly to the question of cost shifting. Suppose there are J groups of patients, each with demand elasticity $\eta_1, \ldots \eta_j, \ldots \eta_J$. Suppose also that the hospital doesn't really care more about providing service to one group than another and that each costs the same to serve. Thus, overall costs

$$C\left(\sum_{j=1}^{J} N_j\right)$$

are just the cost of providing the total amount of care, and total revenue is

$$\sum_{j=1}^{I} P_j N_j$$

The optimal strategy for the hospital sets a different price for each group, using the rule

$$P_j\left(\frac{\partial C}{\partial N} - \frac{U_N}{\lambda}\right)\frac{\eta_j}{(1 + \eta_j)}$$

Thus, although producing care for each group costs the same, the groups can end up paying different prices. The smaller the demand elasticity, the higher the price.

Dranove (1988b) has used this type of model to show what should happen in a hospital that faces an arbitrary reduction in payments by a government program. We can think about a government program with a fixed price per day (or stay) as one in which the demand elasticity is very high, indeed, infinitely high. Dranove shows what happens to the price paid by "charge-paying" patients with smaller demand elasticities. The worst fears of the charge-paying customers are "confirmed" in his model: Lower Medicare or Medicaid payments lead to higher prices for everybody else. Furthermore, he actually estimated the response of hospitals in Illinois to a substantial reduction in that state's Medicaid payments and found that for each $1 reduction in Medicaid income, $0.5 was recouped from charge-paying customers.

CHAPTER 10

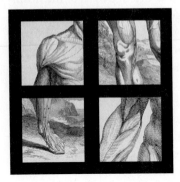

The Demand for Health Insurance

The world around us generates risks of innumerable variety. Fire can damage or destroy homes. Thieves can steal automobiles, and careless drivers can crash them. Vandals can smash plate glass windows. Any person or business can purchase insurance against the financial consequences of these risks. Similarly, illness can make it impossible for people to go to work, and they will lose income. Disability insurance offsets the financial loss. People can even insure against the financial consequences of death for their families.

Many persons purchase insurance against these and other risks. Almost every homeowner carries fire insurance, and most automobile owners carry collision insurance. Life insurance is commonplace. Perhaps the most pervasive of all insurance is that which insures against the costs of medical care. About 80 percent of the US population under 65 (before Medicare becomes mandatory) have health insurance through

LEARNING GOALS

- Discover the basic principles of people's dislike for financial risk and how they deal with it.

- Grapple with the complex "risk-aversion" model, hopefully winning at least two falls out of three.

- Master the difference between the premium and the price for an insurance policy, and learn the basics of insurance policy pricing.

- Integrate information on demand for medical care into the model of demand for health insurance and understand how "moral hazard" losses affect the demand for insurance.

- Learn how health insurance markets run the risk of "market failure" due to asymmetric information and ways to avoid the problem.

- Understand the role of employer-based insurance in the United States and the major effects of the U.S. tax laws on the demand for health insurance.

either private or governmental programs. Table 10.1 outlines the current coverage levels:

TABLE 10.1

Age	Employer	Other Private	Total Private	Government	Total
All ages	61.0	5.1	66.1	14.0	80.1
Under 18	55.2	4.2	59.4	29.9	89.3
18–44	60.1	4.9	65.0	8.6	73.6
45–64	68.3	6.9	75.2	6.3	81.5

Source: Health 2007, National Center for Health Statistics, Health, United States, 2007, Hyattsville, MD: 2007. Tables 136–138.

Government coverage includes both Medicaid (the state-federal partnership for low income families) and Supplemental Children's Health Insurance Program (SCHIP). The high coverage rates for children under 18 are mostly due to SCHIP, which Chapter 12 discusses in more detail.

In this chapter, we explore key issues related to health insurance purchases. We begin with a discussion of the demand for health insurance, blending together traditional economic models of demand for insurance with the specific characteristics of the nature of health insurance and how it alters the demand for medical care. This is followed by a discussion of the supply of health insurance and a brief excursion into the for-profit versus not-for-profit organizational form that also is prominent in the health insurance market. Next we study key issues of market equilibrium in health insurance, and the prospect of a "market failure." Finally, we look at the role of the U.S. income tax system in subsidizing demand for health insurance and the resulting increase in the scale and scope of the health insurance coverage of U.S. citizens and the concomitant increase in the size and scope of the U.S. health care system.

THE DEMAND FOR HEALTH INSURANCE

We must think about the demand for health insurance and the demand for medical care together; the two cannot be separated meaningfully. Of course, this raises the obvious question of whether it is easier to think first about the demand for health insurance or the demand for medical care. We have solved that problem by thinking (in Chapters 4 and 5) about the effects of insurance on medical care, without any particular concern for why a person might have a particular insurance plan. We can now return to the question of how a consumer selects that insurance, taking into account how the insurance (whatever it might be) will affect the demand for medical care.

The Source of Uncertainty

The fundamental uncertainty driving the demand for health insurance arises not because of any financial events but because of the random nature of health and illness. The rational response of a consumer who becomes sick (to seek a cure for the illness with appropriate medical care) creates a financial risk. Health insurance protects against this *derived* risk.

In a hypothetical world in which no medical care exists, people still might buy insurance against the risks of poor health, but it would differ considerably from the type of health insurance we see now. Without medical care, each person's stock of health would be a unique and irreplaceable object, similar to an original painting by Picasso or the original copy of the United States Constitution. The loss could be tragic, and no amount of money could replace these unique items. Money, however, might help in a different way. With sufficient money, a person might purchase a near substitute that would create almost as much utility as the original object. Of course, that money might be used to buy another Picasso, or it might be used to buy a new car. Because substitutes exist for almost everything, money will surely help offset the loss of even unique objects for which no markets exist. Life insurance cannot replace the loss of a person, but the money can substitute, for example, for the earning power of the working person who dies.[1]

With health insurance, we typically seek something else. We know from Chapters 4 and 5 that people use more medical care as the severity of their illness increases. Although nothing *compels* a sick person to seek medical care, it is a rational act, so long as the care has some positive benefit in improving health and doesn't cost too much. Some people complain sardonically that "health insurance" is nothing of the sort because it doesn't insure our health. Of course, this is correct, but meaningless. Our society simply does not possess the technology to insure health. We must accept the second-best alternative of insuring against the financial risks associated with buying medical care.

REASONS PEOPLE WANT INSURANCE

A Simple Indifference Curve Approach

Before we move to a more complex (yet more useful) approach to understanding the demand for insurance, let's consider the simplest possible problem—a world with only two random states—using the familiar tool of indifference curves.[2] In this simple world, the outcome is either state 0 (the

---

[1]Cook and Graham (1977) discuss the insurance of irreplaceable objects.

[2]This figure comes from Ehrlich and Becker (1972) hereafter EB, with some notation changes.

economic loss happens), which occurs with probability p, or state 1 (no loss), which occurs with probability $(1 - p)$. The consumer can shift income between these two states using an insurance that charges a market-determined rate $\gamma = -dI_1/dI_0$. Think of γ as the relative price of income between the good and bad states of the world.

Figure 10.1 shows the initial "endowment point"(E) at which the consumer would be without insurance (i.e., with "endowed incomes" I^e_1 and I^e_0, where $I^e_1 - I^e_0$ is the loss that occurs in the bad state. The "budget line" AB (which necessarily runs through the initial endowment point E) allows shifting income from state 1 to state 0 at the rate γ (which is shown as the slope of AB). The slopes of the indifference curves $(U_1, U_2, \ldots$ etc.) are such that income is more highly valued in state 0 (or more precisely, the marginal utility of income is higher when income is lower).[3]

The consumer is not in equilibrium at point E (with utility $= U_1$) because by shifting income along the AB line, it is possible to reach a higher level of utility at point P on U_2. No higher point than E^* can be reached because any higher point would be beyond the resources allowed by the budget constraint AB.

This optimum at E^* has some interesting properties. Because the underlying "risk" of the bad event has underlying odds of $p/(1 - p)$, it's useful to normalize the price of insurance γ relative to those odds. We can write $\gamma = [p/(1 - p)]\gamma^*$, where γ^* is the "real" price of insurance and $p/(1 - p)$ is the actuarially fair odds of the risk. One way to think about γ^* is that it's the "markup" the insurance company charges above the rate that actuarially fair odds would suggest. If $\gamma^* = 1$, the insurance is called "actuarially fair" and if $\gamma^* > 1$, insurance has a positive real price. In the equilibrium (EB

FIGURE 10.1

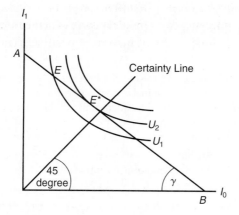

[3]This condition is required for the decision to maximize utility.

prove this in their 1972 paper), the ratio of marginal utilities of income in the two states equate with γ^*, which is a very familiar outcome—the ratio of the marginal utilities of two goods in diagrams such as this always equals the relative prices of the same two goods, as implied by the tangency of the budget line to an indifference curve.

The basic point is that people with preferences such as these will want to shift income from good times to bad times. Insurance provides the mechanism to do that, and utility can rise by using insurance in this way.[4] They do so more if the marginal utility of income changes rapidly with income (we would see this in Figure 10.1 as steeper indifference curves) and more so as the price of insurance falls (a flatter budget line AB in Figure 10.1). Thus, insurance "acts like" any normal good, with more of it demanded when the price falls—so long as we define the price appropriately as γ^*.

This sets the stage for a more complicated (but eventually more useful) approach to understanding the problem of why consumers desire insurance in financially uncertain environments, an approach using a graph that plots utility vs. income, a task to which we turn next.

A More Detailed Approach

People seem to dislike risk. The pervasive purchase of insurance of many types offers concrete evidence of this dislike. People willingly (and often) pay insurance companies far more than the *average* loss they confront in order to eliminate the chance of really risky (large) losses. We describe people who behave this way as *risk averse.*[5]

Risk aversion arises quite naturally from a simple assumption about people's utility functions. Recall earlier that we described a utility function $U(X, H)$ for individuals, and we said that more X or more H created more utility. In other words, the *marginal utility* of either X or H is positive.[6] Because income (I) can be used to purchase X or medical care, which can increase H, we can also say that the marginal utility of income is positive.[7] The basic idea is that

---

[4] The reader can play with Figure 10.1 to see what happens as the price of insurance changes. Rotate the budget line AB around the initial endowment point E; as the relative price of insurance falls (the line becomes flatter), the new equilibrium will shift more income into state 0, and visa versa. Once the price of insurance becomes sufficiently high—when the budget line is tangent to the original endowment point E—insurance no longer has any value to the consumer.

[5] Some people simultaneously buy insurance and gamble. This sort of behavior creates a real puzzle. At this point, we will simply ignore such contradictory behavior.

[6] In the language of calculus, $U_x = \partial U/\partial X > 0$ and $U_H = \partial U/\partial H > 0$.

[7] This link between income and utility allows us to redefine $U = U(X, H)$ into a comparable "indirect" utility function $V = V(I, p_x, p_m)$. Utility increases with income (holding prices constant), so $\partial V/\partial I > 0$. Utility also falls as prices rise, holding nominal income constant, so $\partial V/\partial p_m < 0$, for example.

a person has a fixed and stable set of preferences, so that once we know how much X and H the person has, we know his level of utility. A process of rational decision making also tells us that once we know a person's income and the prices for X and m, we can also determine the person's utility.[8]

Risk aversion arises from a simple additional assumption—namely, that the marginal utility of income, while positive, gets smaller and smaller as a person's income gets larger. In other words, if we were to plot a person's utility against her total income (which, recall, corresponds to increasing ability to buy X and m), the diagram would look like the one shown in Figure 10.2. The person's utility would always increase as income increased (because "more" is "better"), but the graph of utility versus income would always flatten out more and more. In Figure 10.2, this is shown by the two tangent lines at incomes I_1 and I_2. The slope of the tangent line shows the marginal utility of that income level. At I_2, the slope is flatter, which is the equivalent to saying that the marginal utility of income is smaller.

A person with a utility function shaped in this way is *risk averse* and will always prefer a less risky situation to a more risky situation, other things equal. This is called *diminishing marginal utility,* and the idea is central to the question of why people buy insurance. At this point, this is really the same consumer decision problem—how to select insurance in a financially uncertain environment—as we saw in Figure 10.1, with two possible outcomes (a good and a bad state of the world).

FIGURE 10.2   Marginal utility at two income levels.

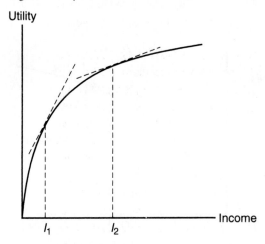

---

[8]For a detailed description of this process, including the direct measurement of consumer welfare from quantities, prices, and income, see McKenzie (1983) or McKenzie and Pearce (1976).

The Risk-Averse Decision Maker

We explore briefly the nature of risk aversion by considering a very simple gamble. (*Problem 8 at the end of this chapter works through this case in more detail; be sure to complete it.*) Suppose the person with the utility function shown in Figure 10.2 starts out with an income I_2 but knows that some externally generated risk (over which the person has no control) may reduce this year's income to I_1. If this risky event occurs with probability f, then the statistical expected income of this person is $E(I) = fI_1 + (1 - f)I_2 = I^*$. Now look at Figure 10.3, where, to make things simple, we can select a particular value for f, for example, $f = 0.4$. If $I_2 = \$20,000$ and $I_1 = \$10,000$, then $E(I) = (0.4 \times 10,000) + (0.6 \times \$20,000) = \$16,000$.

What is the expected *utility* of a person confronting this risky gamble on income? Using the utility function in Figure 10.3 tells us the correct answer. If the income level I_2 occurs, then the utility associated with that, $U(I_2)$, measures the person's level of happiness. If I_1 occurs, then similarly $U(I_1)$ is the right measure. The *expected utility* for the person with this risky income is $fU(I_1) + (1 - f)U(I_2)$. In the specific case we have used, $E(U) = [0.4 \times U(10,000)] + [0.6 \times U(20,000)] = E(U)$.

Because of diminishing marginal utility, $U(20,000)$ is not simply twice $U(10,000)$ but is smaller. The *expected utility* $E(U)$ of this risky income lies 60 percent of the way between $U(10,000)$ and $U(20,000)$ on the vertical axis of Figure 10.3 (the 60 percent figure coming from the probability $f = 0.6$ that I_2 will occur).[9]

FIGURE 10.3 Expected utility when probability of $I_1 = 0.4$ and probability of $I_2 = 0.6$.

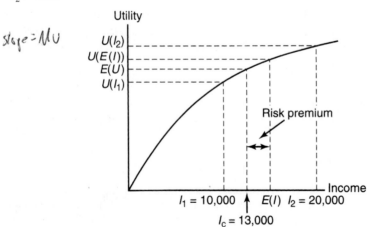

slope = MU

[9]Note that in Figure 10.3, $E(U)$ is actually shown below the proper level. Otherwise, the lines for $E(U)$ and $U[E(I)]$ would bunch together too much.

Because this gamble has an average income (expected income) of $16,000, we could also find the utility associated with that expected income of $16,000, U(E(I)) in the figure. *Note that U(E(I)) exceeds the expected utility (E(U)) of the risky gamble.*

We could find certain income I_c that would create utility of $E(U)$ by reading the utility-income graph the other way—that is, moving across the graph at $U = E(U)$ until coming to the utility–income curve and then dropping down to the income axis to find the corresponding income. This "certainty equivalent" income I_c is less than $16,000, shown as $13,000 in Figure 10.3. The difference between the certainty equivalent and the average income is called the *risk premium*. It represents the maximum that a risk-averse person is willing to pay to avoid this risk, *if he made decisions in such a way as to maximize expected utility.*

This model of consumer behavior when confronting uncertain (risky) financial events stands at the heart of the economist's way of thinking about such decisions. Economists presume that people act to maximize expected utility. When they do so, they buy insurance against risky events.[10]

To restate things slightly, if the Solid-as-a-Rock Insurance Company came up to this risk-averse person and offered the following deal, this risk-averse person would say yes:

Each year, you give me your paycheck, whether it is $10,000 or $20,000. In turn, every year, we will give you a certain income that is larger than I_c.

How far can I_c got below $E(I)$ (here, $16,000)? That depends on how fast the person's marginal utility of income diminishes as income rises. Intuitively, the more tightly bent the graph of utility versus income (as in Figures 10.2 or 10.3), the more the person dislikes risk. The straighter this graph is, the more neutral the person is about risk. A perfectly risk-neutral person has a utility function plotted versus income that is a straight line.

The more the person dislikes risk, the bigger the gap between I_c and $E(I)$. It can be shown that the risk premium $[(E(I) - I_c)]$ a person will willingly pay to avoid a risky gamble is directly proportional to the variability of the

---

[10]Caveat emptor! Some important work, mostly arising out of the field of psychology but some out of economics, shows that people don't behave according to this model in all settings. However, no clearly competing alternative has yet emerged that can fully explain all of the anomalies either, and the expected utility model does predict much of the key behavior we see in the purchase of health insurance. See Hershey, et al. (1984).

gamble (the variance, in statistical terms) and to a specific measure of how rapidly marginal utility declines as income increases.[11]

The welfare gain that people receive from an insurance policy is simply any difference between the risk premium they would willingly pay and the amount the insurance company charges them for risk bearing. In discussing this, we need to be very careful about definitions of terms. The *risk-bearing amount* charged by the insurance company is any amount above and beyond the amount of benefits that the insurance company can expect to pay. We define these terms more precisely in the following section.

Of course, events involving illness are much more complicated than this simple risk, but the idea of risk aversion remains the same. If a person's utility function is defined in terms of X and H and is "stable" in the sense that the *function* itself doesn't change as health changes, then the ideas of this simple risk-aversion example carry through to the complicated world of health insurance. We can now proceed to consider the particular problem of selecting a health insurance policy.

CHOICE OF THE INSURANCE POLICY

In Chapter 4, we defined the simplest of all health insurance policies, one with a consumer coinsurance rate C that paid $(1 - C)$ percent of all the consumer's medical bills, leaving the consumer to pay C percent. Although many insurance policies are more complicated than this, this simple insurance plan captures the essence of many real-world plans and allows us to explore the issues associated with selecting the insurance. In this simple world, the consumer is confronted with the problem of finding the value of C that maximizes expected utility.

To think about this problem clearly, we need to begin with some common statistical definitions. Box 3.2 provides the most basic definitions of mean and variance that we need. (If this material seems unfamiliar after review, any beginning text in statistics can probably provide additional help.) If an insurance company intends to stay in business, it must charge the consumer an insurance *premium* that at least covers the *expected benefits* it will

---

[11]For the calculus freak: Define the second derivative of the utility function as $d^2U(I)/dI^2 = U''$ and the first derivative as $dU(I)/dI = U'$. Now define $r(I) = -U''/U'$. John Pratt (1964) has proven that the risk premium a person will pay when confronting a risky gamble is approximately $0.5 \times r(I) \times \sigma^2$, where σ^2 is the variance of the risky income distribution.

A related measure is the *relative risk-aversion measure* $r^*(I) = Ir(I)$. This is simply the income elasticity of the marginal utility of income, that is, the percentage of change in marginal utility associated with 1 percent change in income.

pay out plus any administrative expenses. Suppose the insurer knows precisely the *distribution* of medical expenses that a person confronts for the coming year, although neither the insurer nor the consumer knows actual expenses that will arise.

The insurance contract says that the insurer will pay $(1 - C)p_m m$ if the consumer buys m units of medical care at a price p_m each. We have assumed so far only one type of medical care for simplicity in discussion. The idea readily generalizes to many types of care. Suppose that the consumer *might* buy N different amounts of medical care during the year (for example, each corresponding to one of N different illnesses the consumer might acquire) and that each one of these would occur with probability $f_i(i = 1, \ldots N)$. Then the *expected benefit payment* from the insurance company to the consumer is

$$E(B) = \sum_{i=1}^{N} f_i(1 - C)p_m m_i$$

or, more simply, $(1 - C)p_m m^*$, where m^* is the expected (average) quantity of care.

Herein lies the most complicated part of the problem. As we learned in Chapters 4 and 5, the amount of m that people select depends upon the coinsurance of their health insurance plan. Thus, the insurance company cannot blithely assume that m^* is the same, no matter which insurance plan (which coinsurance) the consumer chooses. The insurance plan is chosen in advance (at the beginning of the year, for example), but that choice affects all subsequent choices of medical care. When the consumer actually gets sick or injured, the medical care demanded depends upon the coinsurance C previously chosen.

The dependence of m on C has sometimes been described as "moral hazard," but (as Pauly, 1968, has pointed out) this behavior has nothing to do with morals and it isn't even hazardous, in the sense that it is predictable. (The RAND HIS results provide the type of information one needs to make the right calculations.) "Moral hazard" is really just a predictable response of a rational consumer to the reduction of a price. In this case, the insurance plan causes the out-of-pocket price to fall when medical care is purchased. This price response by consumers is somewhat of an unwanted side effect of insuring against the risks of health loss by paying for part or all of the medical care people buy when they become sick.

The effects of the insurance coverage on demand for care feed back on the demand for insurance itself. Recall the discussion of the demand curve for medical care, or more particularly, the "value curve"—called the "inverse demand curve." The demand curve (and the inverse demand curve) slopes downward, so the marginal value of a particular amount of m consumed falls as the total amount of m rises.

Because health insurance reduces the price of medical care, it induces people to buy some care that creates less marginal value (as measured by the inverse demand curve) than it actually costs to provide the care.[12] The induced demand due to the health insurance coverage creates a *welfare loss* in the market for medical care. The insurance policy breaks the link between the costs of care and the price charged for it because the health insurance is paid for no matter which illness the person actually gets and no matter what amount of medical care the person buys.

This welfare loss from buying more medical care offsets the welfare gains that consumers get by reducing the financial risks. The choice of the best coinsurance rate C balances these two ideas—reduction of financial risk versus the effects of increasing demand for care (Zeckhauser, 1970).

A Specific Example[13]

We can explore these ideas better by thinking of a *very* simple world in which only two illnesses might occur (with probability f_1 and f_2). Because probabilities must add to 1, "not getting sick" has probability $(1 - f_1 - f_2)$ in this simple world. Think now about a specific insurance policy that the consumer might select, for example, with $C = 0.2$. Then (as in Chapter 4) the demand curves for medical care depend on the particular illness that actually occurs. If illness 1 occurs, the demand curve is D_1, and similarly it is D_2 for illness 2. For illness 1, the insurance plan induces the consumer to buy m_2 of care, but an uninsured consumer would buy m_1. The welfare loss generated by this purchase is indicated by triangle A in Figure 10.4. Similarly, if illness 2 occurs, demand is m_4 (versus m_3 for a consumer without insurance), and the welfare loss is shown as triangle B.

The medical spending associated with the risk of illness is a distribution that (in this example) has outcomes m_2 (with probability f_1) and m_4 (with probability f_2). Thus, the expected insurance benefit is $p_m (f_1 m_2 + f_2 m_4) (1 - C)$. To place things in very concrete terms, if $C = 0.2$, $p_m = \$500$ per hospital-day, $m_2 = 4$ days in the hospital, $m_4 = 9$ days in the hospital, $f_1 = 0.3$, and $f_2 = 0.1$, then the expected benefit to be paid by the insurance company is $\$500[(0.3 \times 4) + (0.1 \times 9)] \times (0.8) = \$840$.

The total insurance premium is the expected benefit (the $\$840$) plus any "loading fee" for risk bearing. Insurance companies commonly compute a loading fee as a percent of the expected benefit (as a subsequent section discusses). For example, if the loading fee is 10 percent, then the actual premium

---

[12]This is the same type of welfare loss discussed in the section on variations in medical care in Chapter 5.

[13]Appendix A at the end of this chapter provides more detail for this problem.

FIGURE 10.4 Medical spending associated with two levels of illness.

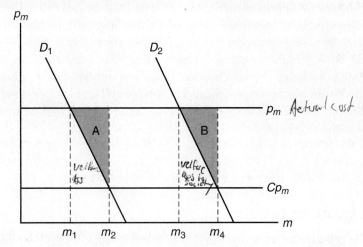

charged will be $924, of which $840 is expected benefit, and $84 is the insurer's fee for risk bearing, profits, and administrative costs.

The net welfare gain to the consumer depends on two things: the amount of the risk premium (willingness to pay for risk reduction) and the size of the triangles A and B. Appendix A (see the end of the chapter) works out a specific computation for this problem, but for now, we can just assume the results. If triangles A and B have areas equivalent to $200 each, then the *expected* welfare loss in purchasing medical care is $(0.3 \times \$200) + (0.1 \times \$200) = \$80$. (Recall that illness 1 and hence welfare loss A happens with probability $f_1 = 0.3$ and illness 2 with welfare loss B happens with probability $f_2 = 0.1$ in our simple world.)

We would have to know the consumer's utility function to derive the maximum risk premium for this risk. (See the discussion regarding Figure 10.3 about risk premiums to remind yourself of what this term means.) Suppose this risk premium were $220.[14] This means, of course, that the consumer would be willing to pay $220 (risk premium) *plus* $840 (expected benefits) = $1,060 for the insurance policy, minus the $80 in "moral hazard" welfare losses, for a net of $980. If the insurance company actually charges $924, then the consumer gains $980 − $924 = $56 in welfare from the risk reduction.

---

[14]In the simple problem presented here, the variance of the uninsured risk equals $1,552,500. For a risk-aversion parameter of −0.0003, a "moderately high" level of risk aversion, the risk premium is approximately $233. See footnote 11 for the formula.

The consumer who wishes to maximize expected utility will (in concept) think about all possible coinsurance rates that the insurance company might sell and will pick the one value for C that gives the highest net gain. Each value of C selected requires the same balancing: Lower C reduces risk more but creates higher welfare losses such as illustrated by triangles A and B. Higher values of C create less risk reduction but don't generate as much welfare loss in purchasing medical care. We revisit this example shortly to discuss the effect of income taxes on this decision and the net well-being from having an insurance policy.

Effects of the Medical Care Demand Elasticity on the Demand for Insurance

A key idea in the health insurance problem is that the expected "moral hazard" loss ($80 in the example) depends directly on the elasticity of demand for medical care. If the demand curve were very inelastic (such as $\eta = -0.05$), then there would be very little change in demand due to the insurance coverage, and the expected welfare loss would be much smaller, for example, $20. Conversely, if the demand elasticity were much larger, the welfare loss would also be much larger.[15]

The welfare loss arising from the purchase of insurance tells us something particular about the link between medical care demand and health insurance demand: *The more price responsive (price elastic) the demand for medical care is, the less desirable it is to insure against that risk with "normal" types of health insurance.*

The reason for this is that large price responsiveness (elastic demand) creates higher welfare losses in the demand for care for any given level of insurance coverage. Figure 10.5 shows this for two demand curves with different price responsiveness. Demand curve D_2 is not very price responsive (very steep demand curve), so if an insurance policy is acquired with copayment rate C, the increase in demand on demand curve D_2 is only to quantify m_4 from m_3 without insurance. The welfare loss is the small triangle B. However, if the demand curve is much more elastic (price responsive), as shown by D_1, then the consumption with the insurance policy rises to m_2 from m_1

---

[15]Specifically, the welfare loss for any illness is measured by the size of the triangle $(1/2)\Delta p \Delta m$, where Δp is the change in effective price due to insurance and Δm is the change in demand due to that change in price. For a simple insurance policy paying $(1 - C)p$ for each unit of m purchased, $\Delta p = (1 - C)p$. We can find Δm from the demand elasticity; $(\Delta m/m) = \eta(\Delta p/p)$. Thus, the percentage change in m is $(1 - C)\eta$. A little algebra makes it easy to prove (see problems at the end of the chapter) that the welfare loss for any illness i is approximately $-\eta(1 - C)^2 pm_i/2$.

FIGURE 10.5 Two demand curves with different price responsiveness.

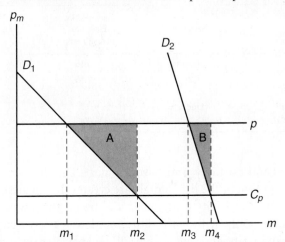

and the welfare loss is the triangle A, obviously much larger than B. Indeed, if demand for medical care were perfectly price insensitive, more complete insurance would be a better idea.

The formal model of risk aversion can be brought to bear on this issue in more detail, but the problems delve into calculus that this textbook generally eschews. For the advanced reader, Appendix B shows this approach in more detail.

Patterns of Insurance Coverage

This relatively complicated model of consumer behavior (the model that consumers act to maximize expected utility when confronting risky events) contains several clear predictions about empirical regularities that we should observe in the demand for insurance. It says that (1) demand for insurance should be higher the more that financial risk (variance) confronts the consumer; and (2) demand for insurance should be lower the more price elastic is the demand for the type of medical care being insured. How well do these ideas stand up in practice?

One simple test asks what portion of the population carries health insurance against specific risks such as hospital care, surgical procedures, dental care, psychiatric care, and so on. It turns out that the patterns of coverage conform well to the expected utility model as it applies to health insurance.

As shown in Table 10.2, the type of coverage most commonly held is for hospital care, which is the type of care creating the greatest financial risk (highest variance) and which has the smallest elasticity of demand. In-hospital surgical and doctor expenses rank next in risk, and share with hospital costs

TABLE 10.2 PATTERNS OF INSURANCE COVERAGE

Type of Health Care	Variance of Risk	Demand Elasticity (RAND HIS)	Percent of People Under 65 Insured
Hospital	Highest	−0.15	80
Surgical and in-hospital medical	High	−0.15	78
Outpatient doctor	Medium	−0.3	40–50
Dental	Low	−0.4	40

the lowest demand elasticity, and have the next-highest extent of coverage. Finally, at the bottom of the list, dental care creates the smallest financial risk and has the largest elasticity of demand and by far the lowest frequency of coverage. Indeed, only within the last few decades has dental insurance enjoyed any popularity, and that (as we will see in a later section) is probably only because of favorable tax treatment for health insurance.

The Price of Insurance

We normally expect that demand for a good or service falls as its price increases. With an insurance policy, we must be careful to define the price appropriately. The price is not simply the premium paid because that premium includes the average expense of something that the consumer would have to pay anyway. The price of insurance is just any markup above those expected benefits that the insurance company adds. To return to the previous discussion, suppose the expected benefits are $E(B) = (1 - C)p_m m^*$. The insurance premium (the amount actually paid by the consumer each year) can be defined as

$$R = (1 + L)(1 - C)p_m m^*$$

The price of insurance is L, the "loading fee" of the insurance company above expected benefits. If $L = 0$, the insurance is "free" in the sense that there is no charge for risk bearing or administration of the insurance plan.[16] Demand for health insurance behaves in response to this "price" just as other goods and services do to their own price—the higher the price, the less insurance will be demanded. In the case of our simple insurance policy with a coinsurance rate

---

[16]Insurance that is priced so that $R = E(B)$ is called "actuarially fair" insurance. In this notation, $(1 + L)$ is the same as γ in the discussion of Figure 10.1. Of course, no insurance company can afford to sell "actuarially fair insurance" because insurance companies use real resources to conduct their operations.

C, this simply means that at higher loading fees (higher L), the consumer will select a higher coinsurance rate (C) and the portion paid by the insurance company $(1 - C)$ will be smaller.

If the health insurance policy has a deductible in it (see Chapter 4), the same idea holds: Higher loading fees cause the consumer to select higher deductibles.

The "price of insurance" comes—as is true in the market for any good or service—from the meeting of demand and supply for the service. Chapter 11 takes a brief excursion into the world of the supply of insurance to understand how insurance companies operate and how their "side of the market" affects the price of health insurance—the "loading fee."

Prevention Added to the Picture

If we were to consider preventive medical care—vaccinations, regular check-ups, routine diagnostic tests such as Pap smear and mammography for women or tests for prostate-specific antigen (PSA, an indicator of possible prostate cancer)—as a "medical risk," we would never seriously consider insuring such expenses. These events are by definition highly predictable—more like grocery bills than medical expenses, in some sense. Nevertheless, it makes good sense to insure (i.e., subsidize) preventive medical care because it can reduce financial risk and at the same time reduce the expected "welfare losses" from excess demand created by standard medical insurance.

Figure 10.6 shows how this works. In Figure 10.6a, we see the situation in which the individual has no insurance. Remember that demand curves are all "conditional" on an particular medical event. Let's use the risk of influenza

FIGURE 10.6

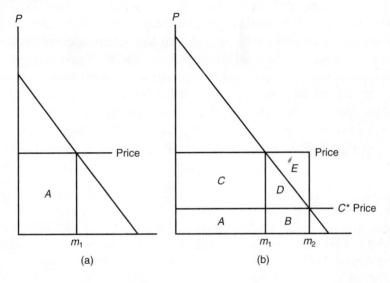

(a)   (b)

("the flu") as a specific example. For a person getting the flu, the rational response is to purchase m_1 of medical care, incurring a financial expense pm_1, represented by the rectangle A in the figure. If a preventive activity (e.g., a flu shot) reduces the probability of this event, then both the expected financial outlay and the financial risk of the individual have declined.

Suppose that without a vaccination, the flu occurs with probability $\pi = 0.3$. The expected medical expense (in the statistical sense) is πpm_1, and the financial risk (the variance) is $\pi(1 - \pi)[pm_1]^2$. If (at the extreme end of the success spectrum) the vaccination eliminates the risk entirely, then the financial gain from risk reduction is the risk premium attached to that risk—approximately the variance $\pi(1 - \pi)[pm_1]^2 \times r$, where r is the Pratt-Arrow risk aversion measure.

In Figure 10.6a, the area of the rectangle A represents pm_1, so for this situation, elimination of the risk creates a gain of $\pi(1 - \pi)A^2$. To continue with specific dollar figures, suppose the flu treatment cost \$500, and with $\pi = 0.3$ (without the vaccination), the variance is $500 \times 500 \times 0.3 \times 0.7 = 52,500$. For a risk-aversion parameter of $r = 0.0002$, the dollar value of removing that risk is \$10.50.

The individual is also better off in an expected value sense by eliminating a potential \$500 outlay, the expected value of which is $\$500 \times 0.3 = \$150$. The individual will "save" \$150 in expected medical expenses and will gain \$10.50 in the value of risk reduction for a total expected financial gain of \$160.50, and, of course, avoid the annoyance of having to put up with the flu. That gain must be offset against the money and time cost of getting the flu shot. Of course, if the flu shot is less than 100 percent effective, all of these change proportionately.

Now consider Figure 10.6b where the individual has health insurance that pays 80 percent of the cost of medical care. Demand increases from m_1 to m_2 because the health insurance reduces the price paid for treatment. Suppose demand increased by 20 percent,[17] so total medical expenditure rises from \$500 to \$600 and the out-of-pocket expense is 20 percent of that, or \$120, represented by areas A+B in Figure 10.6b. The individual's risk reduction from getting the vaccination has shrunk because the individual's health insurance pays for 80 percent of the care. By assumption for this example, $m_2 = 1.2m_1$, so the financial risk is now $\pi(1 - \pi)(0.2pm_2)^2 = 0.04$ times the original risk and the risk premium, using the same value of r, falls to \$0.60.[18]

---

[17]To tie this back to Chapter 4, the arc-elasticity of demand would thus be -0.136. Verify this with your own calculation.

[18]If there were no change in demand, the risk would fall proportionally to C^2 (i.e., $0.2 \times 0.2 = 0.04$). But medical use increased by 20 percent (by assumption), so we must multiply the original m by $1.2 \times 1.2 = 1.44$. The product of $1.44 \times 0.04 = 0.0576$.

The individual also will capture 20 percent of the reduction in expected medical expense if the risk is eliminated, which in this example is $0.2 \times 600 = \$120$ if the person actually gets the flu. If the original risk was $\pi = 0.3$ and that risk falls to zero, the expected gain in financial outlay is $0.3 \times \$120 = \$36$. Thus, the total direct financial gain to the individual from getting the vaccination is $\$36 + \$0.60 = \$36.60$. Contrast this with the expected $\$160.50$ gain for the person without insurance.

How does all of this affect the individual's decisions about vaccination? The answer depends on the mechanisms by which the insurance is priced, which adds still another dimension to the problem. The insurance company "sees" a person at risk for the flu with a potential $\$480$ outlay (80 percent of $\$600$) if that person gets the flu (which will occur with probability $\pi = 0.3$ if the person does not get the vaccination). This area is shown as $C + D + E$ in Figure 10.6b. If the individual decides to get the vaccination (and hence remove the risk), the insurance company saves an expected outlay of $\$144$.[19]

If the insurance plan does not consider the person's behavior, then the "private" incentive for getting the flu shot is blunted (pardon the expression). Insurers have several ways to induce consumers to get appropriate preventive care. First, they can, of course, include preventive medical care as an insured service, reducing the consumer's financial outlay for the cost of the preventive service (e.g., the flu shot). Prevention can be covered even more generously than "acute" services if the insurer so desired.

Second, the insurer can alter the insurance premiums based on the consumer's behavior. This happens commonly in life insurance (prices for life insurance contracts depend directly on such things as smoking behavior, so one can commonly find contracts priced much higher for smokers than non-smokers) and automobile insurance (when its cost takes into account both actual driving record and so statistical propensities for people to have auto accidents[20]). This practice is known as "experience rating" for the insurance. It happens seldom in health insurance, and really almost not at all in group health insurance, the most common mechanism for providing health insurance in the United States.

Insurers' incentives to subsidize prevention also differ greatly depending on the particular nature of the preventive activity. Flu shots have an immediate (within the year) payoff because the flu virus mutates annually and each year's flu shot is specialized to the "strain" moving around the world. Smoking cessation and obesity reduction often have payoffs far into the future, and

---

[19]The astute reader will note that some of the "moral hazard" loss also goes away, but it's embedded in the insurance company's share of the expenditure.

[20]Thus, for example, male teenagers pay more for auto insurance coverage than females of the same age, and males age 35 pay less than males age 20.

insurers investing in such activities can capture only a fraction of the potential gains as their current year customers move to new jobs or change insurance carriers. Many preventive activities have most of the "payoff" into the future, which means that neither the insurer nor the insured individual really has strong incentives relating to preventive medical care. This is another example of an "externality" issue in health care, a topic explored further in Chapter 14.

Finally, particularly when insurance is offered through employment groups that are experience rated to the group or self-insured by the employer, we often now find that employers include "wellness plans" in their human-relations portfolio. Employers in such situations can reduce the time and financial cost of their employees seeking preventive care (e.g., by having on-site flu vaccination programs) and share in the gains through not only reduced health care costs but also reduced absenteeism or reduced work performance due to sickness. Workplace programs are now increasingly common for such illnesses and injuries as low-back injury prevention, smoking cessation, weight loss, and (less commonly) depression. Employers have a more concrete "tie" to their employees than does the insurer (even through the same group) because the insurer has two ways to "lose" the customer (new job or changing insurer) while the employer has the risk only that the person will change jobs. Thus, employers would seem to have stronger incentives to promote prevention than do insurers.

INSURANCE MARKET STABILITY: THE QUESTION OF SELF-SELECTION

Despite the widespread presence and persistence of health insurance, a lingering question persists, at least in theory, about the intrinsic stability of the health insurance market. The problem hinges on the difference in information held by buyers of insurance (consumers) and sellers of insurance (insurance companies). The buyers know more about their own health than the sellers. Thus, the risk exists that insurance companies will put an insurance plan into the market that uses one set of actuarial projections about the costs of insured people but ends up attracting a special subset of the population with unusually high health care costs. Obviously, the insurance company would go broke if this happened repeatedly. This is called the problem of "self-selection," or "adverse selection." It represents another way in which uncertainty and incomplete information intrude considerably into the economic analysis of health care.

Self-selection could manifest itself in many ways. People who believe, for example, that they might have cancer because of unusual weight loss, couples

who plan to have a baby, or people who think it is time to get their hemorrhoids or hernia repaired all have special reasons to buy high-coverage health
insurance. They will try to subscribe to an insurance plan with excellent coverage. People with better health risks obviously do not want such people in their
insurance pool because the average costs and hence the premiums will be
driven up. We might characterize this process as "bad risks chasing good risks."
This phrase creates the vision of people racing from group to group in a frenzy
of sickly people seeking coverage and healthy people trying to evade sickly people. Of course, this doesn't literally happen, but it is useful to think about the
idea to understand how and why the insurance market does remain stable.

A Simple Model of Selection and Self-Identification

The process of "sick people chasing healthy people" has a potential solution,
but it comes at a cost in economic well-being to the healthier group: Insurance companies may find it in their interest to market sets of plans causing
people to self-identify their "type" (sickly versus healthy) through their selection of insurance. If such plans can be found, then insurance companies can
avoid the problem of adverse selection. In their efforts to do so, however, the
insurance companies deny the healthier group the chance to buy insurance
they really would prefer.

Figures 10.7 and 10.8 show how this process works, but it takes a bit of
discussion to really understand it. Begin in Figure 10.7 with a "budget line"

FIGURE 10.7 The (curved) budget line for other goods (X) and insurance coverage
($1 - C$) and optimal purchase decision.

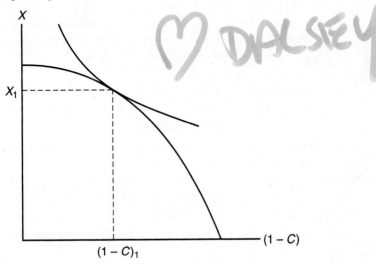

FIGURE 10.8 Optimal purchase decision for sickly and healthy persons (experience rating).

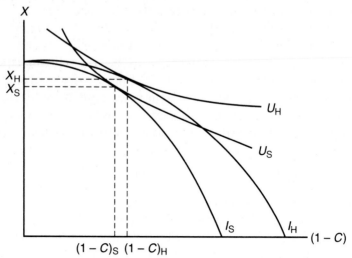

showing the market-available trade-offs between buying other goods (X) and insurance coverage $(1 - C)$, both standard "goods" in the usual sense. The budget line is curved because as C falls (coverage increases), the insurance premium increases more than proportionately because not only is the insurer "picking up" more of the health care bill, but also the total bill increases in size due to the effects of insurance on demand for care. (Chapters 4 and 5 discuss these phenomena in detail.) Thus, expanding coverage $(1 - C)$ causes the ability to purchase X to diminish at an increasing rate; hence, the curved (rather than straight) budget line in Figure 10.7. The optimal insurance coverage occurs at the usual tangency of a consumer's indifference curve with the budget line, with X_1 and $(1 - C)_1$ chosen as the optimal amounts of other goods and insurance coverage.

Figure 10.8 complicates this by allowing two types of people, "sickly" and "healthy," into the world. The former has higher (from the insurance company's point of view) expected costs than the latter. It is important to note that the indifference curves of these two types have different slopes. The sickly person's preferences are tipped more toward insurance coverage, and the healthy person's more toward other goods. Thus, although none of the indifference curves for each person can cross (in the usual fashion), when we draw the indifference curves for these two individuals on the same picture, their *sets* of curves can (and do) cross. In particular, the healthy person's indifference curves are all flatter in this diagram, tipping preferences more toward X.[21]

If the insurer could identify healthy and sickly people accurately, it would offer insurance plans that charged a higher premium to the sickly people; hence, the "budget line" for sickly people (I_S) would be lower than the budget line for healthy people (I_H). (Put another way, given equilibrium market prices, at every coverage level one might think about, the healthy person would be charged a lower premium than the sickly person, and hence would have more to spend on other goods X.) Figure 10.8 shows the optimal choices for two otherwise-equal people, one of whom is sickly (and identified as such by the insurer) and the other healthy (and similarly identified). Because the healthy person doesn't have to pay as much for the insurance coverage as the sickly person, the healthy person can consume more of everything, being, in effect, the person with the higher effective income.

Now consider what happens if the insurer can't tell one of these people from the other. The sickly people would try to buy insurance along the budget line that was intended (by the insurer) only for healthy people, and the insurer would end up selling insurance policies at a loss to sickly people.[22] To prevent this, the insurer limits the set of policies it sells at "healthy-person" prices to the set from the point E^* back to the left on the budget line I_H, shown in Figure 10.9 as a boldface line. In other words, the insurer will only offer "low-coverage" (high-C) plans at rates based on "healthy" (low-risk) spending experiences. Put a slightly different way, the set of plans offered along the I_H budget line are only those creating less utility to sickly people than the "optimal" plan for the sickly person along the I_S budget line. The insurer can't afford to offer any plans with more generous coverage along the I_H budget line, because they would attract undetectable sickly people, and hence the insurer would lose money on each such sale.

Once that constraint is placed on the policies available at low-risk prices, the sickly person will prefer to purchase the plan where the indifference curve U_S is tangent to the budget line I_S—as before, at point E_S, since that choice creates higher utility than the lower-coverage plan at E^* would create. In

---

[21]For the mathematically addicted reader, recall that the slope of the indifference curves at any point is the ratio of the marginal utility of insurance coverage to the marginal utility of other goods, that is, $-U_{(1-C)}/U_X$. Thus, as preferences of healthy people tip more toward X, the marginal utility of X rises, and the indifference curves are flatter than those of the sickly person.

[22]Since the actual spending by both sickly and healthy people within a single year is highly variable, the insurer has no way to determine whether the person was sickly or healthy (that is, had relatively high or low propensity to use care) based on a single year's experience.

FIGURE 10.9 Separating equilibrium outcome with utility loss to healthy consumers.

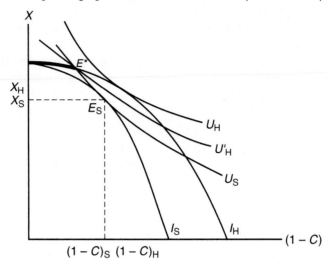

other words, the high-risk persons will self-identify themselves and pay the "experience-rated" insurance premium appropriate to their risk class along budget line I_S. The low-risk persons will buy the plan that provides the maximum possible utility, given the constrained choice set, namely at the point E^*, providing utility U'_H.

Note that the low-risk (healthy) person has been made worse off by the incomplete information because this person can now achieve only U'_H, lower than the amount achievable (U_H) if the insurer could accurately determine which type of buyer was which. In this type of "incomplete-information" or "asymmetric-information" market, the insurers' natural competitive action makes healthy people worse off while leaving the utility of sickly people unchanged. This "separating-equilibrium" approach is widely believed to be the standard outcome in a competitive market because no competitive insurer could afford to do anything except limit the types of insurance plans offered to "low-risk" types in a way similar to that shown in Figure 10.9 (Rothschild and Stiglitz, 1976).

One alternative solution adopted by some governments (including the state of New York) is to require "community rating" for insurance. Figure 10.10 shows a budget line that has a range of insurance plans offered (different values of C) but—by law—is offered at the same price to all individuals within a given community. This is called "community rating," which is different from the "experience rating" that a market such as the one in Figure 10.8 implies and from an outcome such as the separating equilibrium shown in Figure 10.9. We can call this budget line I_{CR} (CR for community rated). The optimal insurance plan for the healthy people now comes at a tangency of the U''_H

FIGURE 10.10 Mandatory community rating outcome, with possible improvement for healthy and sick consumers.

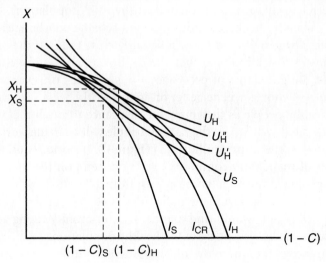

indifference curve and the I_{CR} budget line. Because I_{CR} (in this example) lies close to I_H, U_H'' offers more utility than U', and the healthy people have been made better off by mandatory community rating. Sickly people have also been made better off, shifting to more coverage (at a lower cost) than they would choose when facing the I_S budget line, and their utility rises from a similar tangency (not shown to avoid overcluttering the diagram) in the family of U_S curves to the new budget constraint I_{CR}. (Only the U_S curve tangent to I_S is shown.) Remember here that the U_S curves are for a "sickly" individual and the set of U_H curves are for a healthy individual, so while none of the U_S indifference curves can cross one another, they do cross the U_H curves because the H and S people have different preferences for insurance coverage $(1 - C)$ and other goods X. Indeed, as the figure shows, the U_S curves are tilted so that tangencies always occur with more coverage than for the U_H curves. In this world, mandatory community rating is Pareto superior, in the sense that every person has been made better off.[23]

---

[23]Italian economist Vilfredo Pareto (1848–1923) defined a set of *economic equilibria* in which nobody could be made better off without at the same time making somebody else worse off. These are called *Pareto equilibria*. (This set implies that all possible gains from mutually desirable trade have been accomplished.) Pareto's life's work is steeped in irony. His most durable work was the proof that a purely competitive economy achieves this Pareto goal, yet he spent much of his time working toward planned economies, and he held democracy in high contempt. Italian fascism was largely based on his work.

The relative location of I_{CR} between I_S and I_H depends, of course, upon the relative mix of sickly and healthy types in the community. If the sickly people are relatively rare (as a fraction of the total population), the prices charged by insurers in the community-rated scheme will be fairly close to those for healthy people, and I_{CR} will lie fairly close to I_H. If the population consists mostly of sickly people, then the I_{CR} budget line will lie closer to the I_S line, and the guarantee of everybody's being better off evaporates. The sickly people, of course, will be better off in this world because of the subsidy from the healthy people as they purchase insurance through the mandatory community-rated system, but the healthy people will be made worse off than they were in the separating equilibrium (Figure 10.9) world. Thus, the potential benefits of mandatory community rating depend on the mix of healthy and sickly people in the population, at least from a Pareto-improvement perspective. Of course, government policy designed to transfer wealth from healthy to sick people would find mandatory community rating acceptable, even if it reduced the well-being of the healthy population.

In summary, the presence of unobservable differences in people's propensity to become sick leads to a variety of outcomes in either a competitive or regulated market that makes the healthy people worse off than they would be with full (and "free") identification of their "type." In a freely competitive market, insurers restrict the offerings to healthy types to contracts with limited coverage (high C), thereby reducing their utility. One solution adopted in some areas requires mandatory "community rating"—offering insurance contracts to everybody in the community at the same rate. This has the potential for improving the well-being of the healthy types compared with the separating-equilibrium solution (as shown in Figure 10.9) by expanding the range of insurance policies available to them, albeit at a "surcharge" to help pay for the insurance policies of the sickly types. It also has the possibility of making the healthy types even worse off than in the separating-equilibrium case, depending on the mix of healthy and sick people in the community.

Transactions Costs as a Basis for Stability

Sometimes the "community-rating" solution emerges, at least in part, without any government regulation. Within any single employer group (the predominant form of providing insurance in the United States), the costs of buying insurance outside of the group greatly exceed those of plans within the group, making switching very unlikely. (There is a separate problem arising from employer-provided insurance known as job lock; see Box 10.1.) Interestingly, virtually all employers have a "community-rating" scheme within their firms, at least nominally, providing the same health insurance

BOX 10.1 JOB LOCK FROM HEALTH INSURANCE

Two previous discussions converge to an interesting problem for many Americans: Because U.S. workers primarily receive their insurance through employment groups, becoming unemployed (either quitting, being laid off, or being fired) implies losing one's main source of insurance, at least until another job is found. Does the fear of becoming uninsured inhibit people from quitting their jobs when they otherwise might? This phenomenon, known as *job lock,* turns out to be an important economic phenomenon. Using 1987 data, Madrian (1994) estimated that health insurance-related job lock reduced the annual voluntary turnover rate from 16 percent of workers to 12 percent. The concern is greatest among people with ongoing medical problems because many insurers (and employment-related groups) have exclusions that eliminate payment for "preexisting medical conditions" for a period of time (e.g., 6 months after beginning work at the new firm).

In response to concerns about this problem, the Congress passed and President Clinton signed into law in August 1996 the Health Insurance Portability and Accountability Act (HIPAA) of 1996. This law requires group insurance plans to include any new members, regardless of any preexisting conditions, and at the same price as the insurance is available to other group members. It does not affect the terms and conditions of nongroup insurance. The same legislation increased the tax deductability of health insurance for self-employed persons and built in some tax breaks for both long-term care insurance and the provision of long-term care itself.

coverage for everybody working in the firm at the same price. Because the employment group is brought together for some purpose other than buying insurance (e.g., building cars or selling groceries), insurers usually need not worry about the problem of bad risks chasing good risks. It is difficult for "bad risks" to attach themselves to a particularly desirable insurance plan because they must be healthy enough to work and possess skills desired by the employer through which the insurance plan is offered.

Avoiding self-selection in insurance plans seems to be an important function of the work group arrangement for selling insurance. A key to making this system work is that the work group must all use the same insurance plan, so the preferences of the "median" worker dominate the choice of plan. Probably for this reason, a minority of employer groups offer a choice of more than one insurance plan to their employees.[24]

---

[24]An exception involves the option of a health maintenance organization (HMO), which federal law requires employers to offer as an option to employees in any area where a federally certified HMO exists.

Finally, we should note that the issue of self-selection and market stability may matter considerably more in such areas as long-term care insurance than in more traditional hospital insurance. Long-term care insurance is mostly viewed as pertaining to the elderly. If the demand for such insurance mostly arises from retired people, then the mechanism of the work group is not available to stabilize the market. How much this matters remains to be seen because these markets are only just beginning to form. However, the very fact that such markets have formed slowly and incompletely may address the question.

INCOME TAX SUBSIDIZATION OF HEALTH INSURANCE

The other important part of the "price of insurance" for most health insurance purchases in the United States is the income tax system. We noted earlier that employers pay for a significant fraction of all workers' health insurance premiums in the United States. Over the past several decades, payments by the employer toward the health insurance premium have increased from about two-thirds of the total premium to more than four-fifths (Phelps, 1986b) and have since declined to slightly less than 80 percent.[25]

Because modern economic analysis tells us that the worker really ends up paying for this premium anyway in terms of lower wages, why go through the extra step of having the employer pay for it? The answer lies hidden in the bowels of the Internal Revenue Code. Employer payments for health insurance are not taxed as income to the employee but remain a legitimate deduction for the employer. Thus, these employer premiums escape the tax system. As a result, they make health insurance cheaper than any other good or service the employee might buy because the employer purchases the health insurance with before-tax dollars.

Relative to everything the employee might purchase with after-tax dollars, health insurance costs only $(1 - t)$ as much, where t is the employee's marginal tax rate. Rather than paying $R = (1 + L)(1 - C)p_m m^*$ for an insurance policy (with after-tax dollars), the employee (and the group, when thinking about the best policy to choose) can buy health insurance for an effective premium of $(1 - t)R = (1 - t)(1 + L)(1 - C)p_m m$. Thus, the *effective* price of insurance is not L but $L - t(1 + L)$. In other words, the rate L is still paid, but the tax effect provides a subsidy of $t(1 + L)$. This makes the cost of insurance very

---

[25]Using data from Employee Benefits Research Institute (1992), the employer's share of total premiums was 73 percent in 1970, had increased to 83 percent by 1980, and stabilized at 84 percent by 1990. As of 2005, the employers' share had declined to 78 percent according to most recently available estimates.

low indeed! Because the marginal tax rate (t) for the median worker in many firms is about 0.25 to 0.35 over recent years (Barro, 1993, Congressional Budget Office, 2005) and because actual loading fees (L) from insurance companies are about 0.1 to 0.3 for large groups, many people find themselves in a position in which the net price of insurance is negative! For example, if $t = 0.25$ and $L = 0.2$, then $L - t(1 + L) = 0.2 - 0.25 \times 1.2 = 0.2 - 0.3 = -0.1$.

Calculating marginal tax rates has become increasingly complicated, even more so with recent tax reforms and the growing applicability of the Alternative Minimum Tax (AMT).[26] As of the most recent tax brackets available (2008) at this writing, the marginal tax rate ranges in steps through 0, 10, 15, 20, 25, 28, 33 and a top rate of 35 percent. Box 10.2 shows the exact steps for a person to file individually. For a very detailed analysis of marginal tax rates, the truly eager reader can digest the data in Congressional Budget Office (CBO) (2005).

On top of that, Social Security wage taxes (which appears as the Federal Insurance Corporation of America, or FICA, on paycheck stubs) add an additional 6.2 percent tax on earned wages up to an annual maximum that is indexed by inflation. For example, in 1995, that cap was $61,200 and by 2001 the cap had increased to $80,400. In addition, on *all* wage income, there is an additional tax of 1.45 percent to support the Medicare system. *Both* the employer and the employee pay both of these wage taxes.

Most economists also presume that the employer's share is passed along to the employee in terms of wages lower than would otherwise be received. (The logic for this comes from a branch of economics knows as general equilibrium theory.)

Finally, state income taxes (and city income taxes in cases such as New York City) add to the marginal income tax rate. State income taxes are also normally graduated, ranging from lows of 0 percent (Alaska, Florida, Nevada, New Hampshire, South Dakota, Tennessee, Texas, Washington, and Wyoming have no state income taxes) to other states with top marginal tax rates in the vicinity of 10 percent or higher.

---

[26]The AMT was designed to catch a few (fewer than 200) wealthy individuals who avoided income taxes with large deductions, but the Congressional Budget Office (2004) now says "In 2010, if nothing is changed, one in five taxpayers will have AMT liability and nearly every married taxpayer with income between $100,000 and $500,000 will owe the alternative tax." (Congressional Budget Office, "Revenue and Tax Policy Brief: The Alternative Minimum Tax" April 15, 2004, page 8.) The AMT phases out (through incomes of $150,000 to $415,000) the taxpayer's ability to take many otherwise legal deductions, preserving only a few (charitable donations, happily for colleges and universities, and homeowner interest are the key deductions remaining.). For persons with incomes of more than $415,000, the top marginal tax bracket is 28 percent, but for those in the range of phaseout of deductions, the effective rate can reach 35 percent. The Wikipedia encyclopedia entry on AMT is quite useful to help the reader understand the nuances of the AMT.

Box 10.2 provides even more detail (and some example problems) of the issues that arise in calculating marginal tax rates.

BOX 10.2 MARGINAL TAX RATES IN THE UNITED STATES

Calculating marginal tax rates (which determine the extent of the subsidy to employer-paid health insurance premiums) sounds like a simple matter, but the truth becomes far more complicated. Let's begin with a simple reading of the U.S. Tax Rate schedules from 2008. In general, we will consider a single person; similar issues arise if you look at married persons filing jointly or separately.

If Taxable Income is Over ($)	But Not Over ($)	Then the MTR Is (%)	The Tax Due Is ($)
0	8,025	10	0.1 × (Income)
8,025	32,550	15	803 + 0.15 × (Income − 8,025)
32,550	78,850	25	4881 + 0.25 × (Income − 32,550)
78,850	164,550	28	16,456 + 0.28 × (Income − 78,850)
164,550	357,700	33	40,452 + 0.33 × (Income − 164,550)
357,700	∞	35	104,192 + 0.35 × (Income − 357,700)

Every year (under current federal tax law) the incomes that define the brackets (those in the left-hand column of the preceding table) are adjusted to account for the past year's inflation.

However (as the TV ads for a set of kitchen implements often say, "But wait! That's not all!"), we have many more complications. The first of these is Social Security tax (known as FICA, the Federal Insurance Corporation of America, the federal agency that actually collects Social Security payments and pays out income to retirees). That tax is a constant amount paid by the employer and the employee *up to a specified income amount* after which the tax goes to zero. Again using tax rates for 2000, the FICA tax was 6.2 percent on the first $76,200 of wage earnings, matched by the employer. Self-employed persons must pay both the employer and employee share, so their rates are double those for employed workers.

For a number of reasons, most economists believe that the equilibrium in the labor market will lead employers to pass along their share of the Social Security tax to employees in the form of lower wages because employers will consider the costs of hiring workers overall in their decisions about how much to pay and how productive the workers are. (One simple point to help understand this: The market must maintain some sort of equilibrium between self-employed and regularly employed workers, and the law requires self-employed workers to pay both the employer and employee share. That makes "official" what most economists believe happens in all employment settings.)

Are we through yet? No way! There's also a federal tax to support Medicare, currently at 1.45 percent of all earnings with no wage cap. And employers must match this share, too.

But wait! That's not all! There are still state income taxes, some of which have income brackets much like the federal tax structure. (Some states have no state income tax, including Nevada, which taxes people who cannot understand probability theory by collecting a small portion of all the gambling revenues in the state. That income suffices to operate the entire state government, mostly paid by "outsiders" who have come to gamble and gambol in Nevada, and they have no state income tax. Other states with no income tax rely on other mechanisms such as sales taxes, property taxes, and the like to finance the costs of state government.)

New York state is a higher-than-average tax state, but the schedules look fairly standard. Again for single persons, the tax table looks like this:

If Taxable Income Is ($)	But Not Over ($)	The Marginal Tax Rate Is
0	11,000	4.00% of taxable income
11,000	15,000	4.5% of all income over $11,000
15,000	17,000	5.25% of all income over $15,000
17,000	30,000	5.90% of all income over $17,000
30,000	—	6.85% of all income over $30,000

This is a somewhat odd, bumpy tax schedule (the one narrow bracket of $2,000 in the middle is quite unusual), but the important thing to note is that the marginal rate of 6.85 percent occurs at a fairly low income—an income easily achievable for a college graduate with a few years of experience in the market for sure.

Are we through yet? No, not quite. First, if you live in New York *City*, there's an additional income tax that has marginal tax rates of 3.0495 percent up to 3.8276 percent (leaving all of us to wonder where they got *those* numbers!).

And finally (yes, really finally), we must note that if the taxpayer itemizes deductions (but only if so), then the income taxes paid to the state are deductible from income before calculating the federal income tax due. This deductibility makes it impossible to know exactly the marginal tax rate of any individual unless you also know whether they itemize deductions when filing federal taxes.

Let's try this all out now. Do each of these calculations and then check against the answer that follows. [No cheating now!]

Problem 1: What's the marginal tax rate for a single person living in New York State (but not New York City) who has $25,000 taxable income?

(continued)

BOX 10.2 MARGINAL TAX RATES IN THE UNITED STATES (continued)

Answer: The federal income tax marginal rate is 15 percent, the New York State marginal rate is 5.9 percent, the FICA tax is 6.2 percent each for the worker and employer, and the Medicare tax is 1.45 percent each for the worker and employer. If the taxpayer does not itemize, then the marginal tax rate is 15% + 5.9% + 2 × 6.2% + 2 × 1.45% = 15% + 5.9% + 12.4% + 2.9% = 36.2%.

Problem 2: What happens if the same person itemizes? *Answer:* The implied state tax becomes 85 percent of the 5.9 percent, because the deduction of state income taxes on the federal tax schedule removes 15 percent of the 5.9 percent. So the marginal tax rate falls by 15 percent of 5.9 percent or by just under 0.9 percent. So the marginal tax rate is just slightly more than 35.3 percent.

Problem 3: Suppose that the same person as in Problem 1 had earned $29,000 rather than $25,000. *Answer:* The federal marginal tax rate goes up to 28 percent at an income of $26,250, so the marginal rate would go up from 15 percent to 28 percent, and the overall rate would rise from 36.2 percent to 49.2 percent.

Problem 4: Now suppose instead that the income had increased to $31,000 instead of $29,000. *Answer:* The federal rate is still 28 percent, but the New York State rate now climbs to 6.85 percent from 5.9 percent. If the person is not itemizing, the marginal tax rate is now another 0.95 percent higher and now exceeds 50 percent, or to be precise, 50.15 percent.

Problem 5: Suppose the same person as in Problem 4 had lived in New York City. *Answer:* Add another 3.7706 percent for the New York City income tax.

Problem 6: Suppose the same person gets married and the spouse does not work. *Answer:* You need to know the marginal tax rate for married couples filing jointly. Let's just look at the marginal tax rate for somebody earning $29,000 (as in Problem 3) but Married, Filing Jointly. The federal rate falls back to 15 percent. The New York State rate is 5.90 percent for a married couple with that income. So instead of paying a marginal tax rate of 49.2 percent (as in Problem 2), the same person will pay the same rate as found in Problem 1 at the lower income. Marriage saves you income taxes by widening out the brackets before the marginal tax rate increases.

Problem 7: Suppose the same individual as in Problem 1 had an MBA before entering the labor force and had an annual taxable income of $80,000 instead of $25,000. *Answer:* The federal marginal tax rate becomes 31 percent and the New York State marginal tax rate is 6.85 percent. But the individual is now over the FICA limit for the year, so the 6.2 percent share for the employee and employer drops away as marginal taxes. The Medicare tax remains as long as the Chicago Cubs never win a World Series (that is to say, forever), so it still applies as a marginal tax. So the marginal tax rate is 31% + 6.85% + 2.9% = 40.75%. Of course, somebody with an MBA is probably savvy enough to itemize deductions, which means that she pay only 69 percent of the state tax out of pocket (because the federal marginal tax rate is 31 percent), and the tax becomes $31\% + 6.85\% \times 69\% + 2.9\% = 31\% + 4.7265\% + 2.9\% \approx 38.6\%$. Remarkably, once a person's income gets above the FICA cutoff income ($76,200 in 2000), the person's marginal tax rate actually falls below that paid by persons with much lower incomes.

What constitutes the "marginal" tax for a household? If each worker's wages are under the FICA limit (which is the case for a very large fraction of U.S. workers), the marginal tax is the sum of the household members' federal income tax marginal rate plus the 6.2 percent FICA tax *twice* (employee's and employer's share), plus the 1.45 percent Medicare FICA tax *twice*, plus (an almost-final complication) either part or all of their state income marginal tax rate. Because state income taxes are deductible when calculating federal income tax liability, for people who itemize their federal income tax calculation (rather than using the simplified short form), the appropriate marginal state tax is $(1 - t_f)t_s$, where t_f and t_s are (respectively) the appropriate federal and state marginal tax rates as shown in the tax code.[27] The last wrinkle, relevant only for high-income families, is a formula that reduces the value of some deductions as income rises, thereby effectively increasing the marginal tax rate for those families by another few percentage points.

The magnitude of this tax subsidy has become truly staggering, even for those accustomed to multiple-billion-dollar federal budget numbers. Projections of recently available growth rates to 2010 show an estimate of employer payments exceeding $500 billion annually. (See Table 10.5.) Because the marginal tax rate that would be applied to these premiums averages about 35 percent (see CBO, 2005), this implies forgone tax revenues of about $175–$200 billion annually. The employer contributions have grown at a compound rate

TABLE 10.5 EMPLOYER AND EMPLOYEE INSURANCE CONTRIBUTIONS (BILLIONS OF $)

	Year							
	1987	1993	1997	1999	2001	2003	2005	2010(est.)
Employer premium payments	84.2	158.3	191.5	229.2	272.4	319.3	366.9	520.0
Employee contributions and nongroup premiums	43.9	89.9	112.4	124.3	147.1	182.7	202.1	315.0
Total	128.1	248.2	303.9	353.5	419.5	502.0	569.0	835.0
Percent by employers	65.7	63.8	63.0	64.8	64.9	63.6	64.4	62.3

---

[27]The last portion of Box 10.2 has some specific examples.

of about 7.5 percent in recent years. The share of total private health insurance premiums paid by employers has remained quite stable since the mid-1980s in the 63 to 65 percent range (including individuals' payments for nongroup insurance as part of the individuals' payments).

What puts any limit at all on the demand for insurance in this setting? One limit, of course, is the group insurance choice. The group plan is a compromise over the interests of many workers, some of whom surely have different preferences than others. The heterogeneous nature of the group (for example) with respect to age also puts an eventual lid on the demand. Because every worker in the group pays the average premium (over all workers) regardless of age or health habits, younger workers will find an extremely generous health insurance plan too expensive for their preferences, even with the tax subsidy. Because they "vote" on the plan, they help constrain the choice.

The other natural limit for health insurance, of course, is the welfare loss generated by extending coverage too far. As C approaches zero (full coverage), the welfare loss caused by overpurchases of medical care increases further and further. Even with a tax subsidy for insurance, it is probably preferable to quit before full coverage is reached for most people.

Revisiting the Fictitious Insurance Purchase Example

Earlier in the chapter, we had a simple example of a consumer deciding whether or not to purchase an insurance policy against the simple risk that a 4-day hospitalization might occur (with probability 0.3) and that a 9-day hospitalization might occur (with probability 0.1). For a moderately risk-averse consumer, we found that the net gain from purchasing the insurance policy was $56 after all was taken into account. (Go back and review that example, in the section called "A Specific Example" including Figure 10.4 earlier in this chapter. We use it again here.)

Now consider what happens if the same insurance policy is acquired through a group insurance plan and the consumer's marginal tax rate is 0.3 ($t = 0.3$). Not only does the consumer gain all of the benefit previously stated, but also the tax liability confronting this consumer drops by 0.3 times the insurance premium—that is, $0.3 \times \$924 = \$277.20$. This "tax benefit" swamps the overall gain from the insurance policy alone ($56 net). Indeed, it could readily tip the decision about whether or not to purchase the insurance.

To see how this could happen, suppose that an otherwise identical consumer was not as risk averse as the first consumer we described and had a risk premium (willingness to pay to avoid risks) of only $70, rather than the $220 in the original example. Then *without the tax subsidy,* the net benefit of buying the insurance would be negative because the costs ($924 premium and the welfare loss triangles A and B, with expected value of $80) exceed the willingness to pay for the insurance ($840 expected benefit plus $70 risk premium = $910). In a world with no tax subsidy, this person would not buy this insurance policy. (He or she might well buy one with larger coinsurance.) However, adding in the "tax benefit" of $277, we can see that this insurance policy is now attractive, and the smart consumer will choose it. This expands the amount of insurance in force and will increase the overall demand for medical care.

Note that the same thing can happen as the marginal tax rate changes. Even our second "mildly risk-averse consumer" would not take this insurance policy if the marginal tax rate were smaller. For example, if this consumer were in a 10 percent tax bracket rather than a 30 percent bracket, the "tax benefit" from buying the insurance policy would be only $92, not $277, and this would not be enough to offset the other costs of insurance.[28]

EMPIRICAL ESTIMATES OF DEMAND FOR INSURANCE

Studies of demand for insurance have taken two approaches. The first studies the choices actually made by individuals or groups (Phelps, 1973, 1976; Goldstein and Pauly, 1976; Holmer, 1984; Marquis and Holmer, 1986; Marquis and Phelps, 1987). In such studies, the differences in income (for example) allow estimating how demand varies by income. Differences in the group size generate variation in effective price, allowing estimates of price responsiveness. The other approach uses aggregate data over time, estimating how total insurance premiums (for the entire economy) change in response to changes in income, loading fees, tax subsidies, and so forth.

Income Effects

In most studies using individual data, estimated income elasticities are generally positive, but less than 1 for almost any measure of insurance chosen. Measuring the "correct" income is difficult for insurance chosen in a group setting because the median worker's income presumably is more important than any other worker's income. Aggregate data (such as Phelps, 1986b; Long and Scott, 1982; Woodbury, 1983) avoid this problem. Generally, the income elasticity of demand for insurance (as measured by premiums) in such studies is more than 1, and it may be closer to 2.

---

[28]The policy costs the consumer $924 for the premium plus $80 in welfare loss, for a total cost of $1,004. The willingness to pay is the expected benefit of $840 plus the risk premium of $70 plus the tax benefit of $92, for a total of $1,002.

Price Effects

The effects of the price of insurance on demand constitute an important question for public policy because of the way the income tax system subsidizes health insurance purchases. Unfortunately, the range of estimates from the literature is disquietingly large. Again, the source of data seems to determine the magnitude of the estimate. Aggregate data usually provide price elasticity estimates (using variation in the marginal tax rate through time as a price change) in the neighborhood of −1.5 to −2 (Phelps, 1986b; Long and Scott, 1982, Woodbury, 1983). Studies using data on individual households have varied somewhat in their findings. When the size of the work group is used to generate price variation, the estimates are also typically large, in the range of −1 (Phelps, 1973, 1976; Goldstein and Pauly, 1976; Ginsberg, 1981). Other studies use differences in the marginal tax across households to determine the effect of price on insurance demand (Taylor and Wilensky, 1983) and get smaller estimates (about −0.2).

Certainly there is clear evidence that the price of insurance matters considerably in demand for it. The question of just how much is not as well settled as the question of demand for medical care itself because nothing comparable to the RAND HIS exists for studies of demand for insurance. One other piece of evidence arises from the tax cuts initiated by the Reagan administration. Those tax cuts reduced the desirability of extensive insurance because they reduced the tax subsidy for almost all working persons. (The top marginal tax bracket fell in several steps from 50 percent to 28 percent.) In response, the number of persons with hospital insurance began to fall in the United States in 1983, the first year after the tax cut took place. The peak enrollment occurred in 1982 (188.4 million), fell to 181 million by 1985, and dropped further to an estimated 165 million to 170 million by 1995. This represents the first time since World War II that a systematic decline in the number of insured persons occurred, and this decline took place in a period of rising population, employment, and income. Looking at this picture another way, in the early 1980s, 90 percent of the under 65 population had private health insurance coverage, and by the early 1990s, the figure had fallen to 72 percent.[29] The consequences for the total number of people without insurance (and their characteristics) is a subject discussed in Chapter 16.

---

[29]Using data from the Health Insurance Association of America, in 1984 there were 175.6 million Americans under the age of 65, 158.1 million of whom (90 percent) were covered by private health insurance (Health Insurance Association of America, 1989, Table 1.1). By 1991, the comparable numbers were 219 million citizens under the age of 65, 158 million of whom (72 percent) had private health insurance, nearly 90 percent of which came through employer groups (Health Insurance Association of America, 1993, Figure 2.1). Thus, there was an absolute loss of 17.5 million persons with insurance during a time when the under 65 population increased by 44 million people.

THE OVERALL EFFECT OF THE TAX SUBSIDY ON THE HEALTH SECTOR

The cumulative effects of the federal income tax subsidy of health insurance could be very large indeed (Vogel, 1980). The health insurance subsidy produces a secondary effect in the market for medical care because the increases in insurance coverage in turn increase the demand for medical care. The leverage that this interaction can generate has the potential for substantially altering the shape and size of the health care system.

One study (Phelps, 1986b) estimated that employer-group health insurance premiums would be only about 55 percent as large today if the tax subsidy were not in effect. Cutting the premiums in half is not as radical a restructuring of insurance coverage as it might seem. Recall (for a simple insurance policy) that $R = (1 + L)(1 - C)p_m m$ and that m falls as C rises. Based on estimates of how m varies with C, an increase in C of about 25 to 30 percentage points (e.g., from 0 to 0.25 or 0.25 to 0.5) would cause premiums to fall by the required amount. In turn, this change in insurance coverage would cause the demand for medical care to fall among those insured persons. Again, the RAND HIS results tell us that demand is about 20 percent lower for $C = 0.25$ than for $C = 0$, and about 10 percent lower for $C = 0.05$ than for $C = 0.25$. Thus, total medical care could decline by some 10 to 20 percent among the persons under the age of 65 who are insured by this mechanism.

In addition, if private health insurance had (from the beginning) contained higher coinsurance or deductibles (without the tax subsidy), the structure of Medicare would probably reflect that difference as well. Medicare was clearly patterned after private health insurance when it was instituted in 1965, with essentially full coverage for hospital care and a "major medical" type of insurance for doctor services, with a $50 deductible and a 20 percent coinsurance. Thus, private insurance with greater cost sharing probably would have led to public insurance with more cost sharing as well. In the aggregate, it seems possible that the health sector would be at least 10 to 20 percent smaller without the tax subsidy for health insurance. Lest this seem "small," we can translate that difference into something that represents 1.5 to 3.0 percent of the gross national product.

"OPTIMAL" INSURANCE

The model used by economists to study demand for insurance (the expected utility model) offers one further insight into the question of how insurance contracts might look without the tax subsidy in place. According to that model (Arrow, 1963), a consumer seeking to maximize expected utility will select a policy with full coverage above a deductible, when the losses are fully independent of the insurance coverage (truly random losses). The size of the deductible increases as the loading fee increases. Arrow also showed that the optimal policy has a coinsurance feature included when the insurance company, as well as the consumer, is risk averse. Taking into account the effect of coinsurance on demand for medical care, Keeler et al. (1988) estimated the expected utility among a variety of insurance policies, based on the RAND HIS results. The "best" plans all contain a coinsurance rate of about 25 percent and an initial deductible of $100 to $300, comparable to deductibles of $200 to $600 in 2010 dollars.

Most current health insurance plans that pay for doctor services out of the hospital have about this structure. In a survey of employers, only 5 percent of covered employees had plans with no deductibles, and more than half had deductibles in excess of $150 by 1990 (Employee Benefits Research Institute, 1992). The theory of demand for insurance, coupled with the empirical results from the HIS, suggests that consumers would be better off with less complete coverage. Elimination of the income tax subsidy would certainly move people in that direction, and (based on the estimates in Phelps, 1986b) the magnitude of change from the full coverage to a major-medical type of plan would correspond with the premium changes predicted to occur. Indeed, the shift toward higher deductibles followed closely on the heels of the decline in the marginal tax rates in the early 1980s. In a comparable 1980 study, only 10 percent of all covered employees had deductibles in excess of $150, compared with the 55 percent number found in 1990 (Employee Benefits Research Institute, 1992).

OTHER MODELS OF DEMAND FOR INSURANCE

The model of expected utility maximization has enjoyed wide popularity among those studying demand for insurance. Nevertheless, the model has some particular defects in terms of precise predictions about how people behave in settings containing uncertainty. The strongest challenges have come from the discipline of psychology, most notably from Kahnemann and Tversky (1979) and Tversky and Kahneman (1981). Their prospect theory model sets aside the idea of a stable utility function (one that does not change, for example, as income or health changes). Instead, they offer a model in which deviations from "today's" world affect behavior. Everything is viewed in terms of "where you are." The model goes on to suggest that people prefer risk (are willing to accept gambles) for degradations in their well-being but are risk averse with regard to improvements. A key part of these authors' approach is that the basis from which one views the problem (the perspective) alters the decision and the apparent attitudes toward risk. For example, with regard to the widely popular lotteries found in many states, standard expected utility theory predicts that people will not participate because the expected value is negative (the state keeps some of the money paid in) and the gamble involves risk. In prospect theory, however, the consumer's response to a financial gamble depends on the weights and the frame of reference. Because (in this approach) people overweight low-probability events, Lotto-like gambles will seem more attractive.

SUMMARY

Health insurance offers a way to protect against financial risk. Economists' models of expected utility maximization predict certain patterns of insurance purchases, including the presence of deductibles, copayments, and insurance against the riskiest (large, uncommon) events, rather than lower-risk events (common, relatively low cost). These models predict the actual patterns of insurance purchases well, but not perfectly.

Most insurance is sold through groups, most commonly by employer work groups. This insurance provides to consumers the added benefit of reducing income taxes. In some cases, the tax benefit is large enough to tip the balance between buying and not buying insurance.

Health insurance creates a subsidy for medical care, so a "welfare loss" emerges each time medical care is purchased because consumers are induced (by the lower price of care generated by the insurance policy) to buy more medical care than they otherwise would. Indeed, they are "tricked" into buying care that costs them (through the insurance premium) more than it is worth in restoring health. This is an added "cost" of health insurance that doesn't show up on anybody's accounting books, but it is a real cost in any economic sense.

Health insurance provides a way to diversify financial risks associated with illness, but the markets for such insurance plans have grown increasingly complex. Firms selling such insurance have important distinctions. Some sell group insurance; others sell to individuals. Nongroup plans run the risk of considerable adverse selection, which group plans (especially those organized around the work group) avoid.

Market failure looms as a risk in health insurance markets because of the asymmetric information between individual buyers of health insurance (who may be unusually sickly) and health insurers. Various mechanisms to solve this potential problem exist, the most notable of which is the use of large groups (e.g., those assembled in the workforce) as the basis for insurance contracts. Another way to solve the problem for the society as a whole (including those not working in the labor force) is for the government to require "community-rated" insurance. Under some circumstances, both the relatively sickly and the relatively healthy segments of a society might gain by such a regulation, but it is also possible for the regulation to help the relatively sickly only at the expense of the relatively healthy.

Group insurance, coupled with favorable tax treatment for employer-paid premiums, has made health insurance a popular but not universal fringe benefit. A growing pool of persons remains uninsured through either conventional insurance or various government programs. Many of these people are employed with wages at or near the minimum wage. Various proposals to create universal insurance in the United States typically rely on mandated coverage for workers and their families as a cornerstone of these universal insurance plans. A more extended discussion of these issues appears in Chapter 16 in the context of comparison with the health care systems in other nations.

RELATED CHAPTERS IN *HANDBOOK OF HEALTH ECONOMICS*

Chapter 11, "The Anatomy of Health Insurance" by David M. Cutler and Richard J. Zeckhauser

Chapter 12, "Health Insurance and the Labor Markets" by Jonathan Gruber

PROBLEMS

1. "People most commonly buy insurance against hospital costs because it is that type of medical care that has the biggest average expense for individuals year in and year out." Comment.

2. "The single most important health policy choice in the United States over the past four decades has nothing to do with the Department of Health and Human Services, but rather with the Internal Revenue Service." Comment.

3. Prove that the welfare loss triangle described in footnote 15 has a value of approximately $-0.5\eta(1 - C)^2 p_m m_i$ for medical event i.

4.
   a. Obtain tax tables for the current year (you can easily get them from the Internet) appropriate for your state. (If you live in one of those select states with no state income tax, this problem is a little easier for you. However, if you live or work in New York City or many other cities you also have city income taxes to worry about.) Calculate the effective marginal tax rate for a single-person household with the following combinations of wage and total income:

Wage Income ($)	Total Adjusted Gross Income ($)
20,000	22,000 (high school graduate)
50,000	55,000 (engineer)
70,000	80,000 (MBA)
150,000	200,000 (lawyer)

Don't forget FICA taxes, FICA Medicare taxes, and state income taxes. (Presume that the person does not itemize deductions, so that state income taxes are not deductible federally.) To do this properly, you also need to learn this year's cut-off for FICA payroll taxes, a number you can get either from your professor in this class or one of his or her colleagues in public finance. If your school's economics department heavily emphasizes theory and doesn't pay much attention to such issues, a quick search of the internet using phrases such as "FICA tax rate" will readily provide current data.

    b. Calculate the incremental cost to this person from changing employer-paid plans from one with a $1000 premium to one with an $1100 premium.

5. How are "adverse selection" (in insurance markets) and "demand inducement" (in physician-service markets) related, if at all?

6. (This question relates to appendix C and is intended for more advanced students.) Think of two otherwise identical hypothetical countries, one of which has widely eliminated contagious disease and the other for which contagious disease remains a major cause of death. Where would an active market for health insurance be less likely to emerge, and why?

7. Not-for-profit health insurers have several market advantages over for-profit insurers, including the ability to avoid premium taxes (taxes that function as a sales tax does, e.g., 3 percent of a premium paid). Would you expect that this would automatically result in a lower premium paid by people buying insurance? (*Hint:* What else might the insurance plan do with the money? Think of the model of hospital control in Chapter 8, and extrapolate to a firm providing health insurance.)

8. This problem uses a utility function of the form $U = 1 - \exp(-0.0001 \times \text{Income})$ where $\exp(z)$ means "e^z." (Remember that $e = 2.718281828459045\ldots$ and is the basis of natural logarithms.) For this particular function, utility takes on a value of 0 for an income equal to zero and rises steadily (but at a diminishing rate) so that as income becomes very large, utility approaches 1.0. A more general form says $U = 1 - \exp(-r \times \text{Income})$, which has an equivalent form, $U = (e^{r \times \text{Income}} - 1)/e^{r \times \text{Income}}$, where r is the risk-aversion parameter (0.0001 in our specific case). At income $= 0$, $U = (e^0 - 1)/e^0 = (1 - 1)/1 = 0$, and at very large incomes, $U \to e^{r \times \text{Income}}/e^{r \times \text{Income}} = 1$.

    The problem analyzes a gamble in which Income $= 10,000$ with probability 0.4 and Income $= 20,000$ with probability of 0.6, so $E(\text{Income}) = 16,000$. Figure A (page 340) graphs $U = 1 - \exp(-0.0001 \times \text{Income})$ for incomes between 0 and 25,000 with values of 10,000, 16,000, and 20,000 indicated by vertical lines.

    Figure B (page 340) zooms in on the relevant portion of this diagram. It shows the incomes of 10,000 and 20,000, along with their comparable levels of utility, as calculated next:

$$U(10,000) = 1 - \exp(-0.0001 \times 10,000) = 1 - \exp(-1) = 0.63212$$
$$U(20,000) = 1 - \exp(-0.0001 \times 20,000) = 1 - \exp(-2) = 0.86466$$

Thus *expected utility* $= 0.4 \times 0.63212 + 0.6 \times 0.86466 = 0.77165$.

FIGURE A

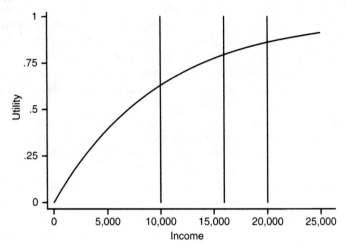

FIGURE B

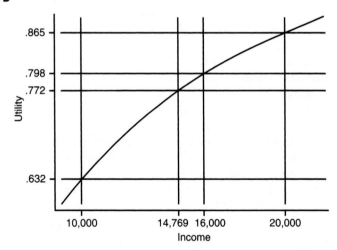

Figure B also shows $E(\text{Income}) = 0.4 \times 10,000 + 0.6 \times 20,000 = 16,000$, and the utility associated with that income, 0.798. That is, $U = 1 - \exp(-0.0001 \times 16,000) = 0.798$.

Now work *the other way* from the expected utility of 0.77165, and ask what specific income, if available with certainty, would produce the same level of utility as does the gamble. That turns out to be an income of 14,769. Thus, 14,769 is the *certainty equivalent income*, I_C, for the simple gamble we are using in this problem.[33]

---

[33]To find this, solve the equation $0.772 = 1 - \exp(-0.0001 \times I_C)$ for I_C, where I_C is the certainty equivalent income. The answer is 14,769. To do this, remember that $\ln(e^z) = z$.

The *risk premium* is the difference between $E(I)$ (16,000) and I_C (14,769). Thus, the risk premium is $16,000 - 14,769 = 1231$.

PROBLEM (to test your understanding of these concepts):

What would the risk premium be in this problem if the gamble had an income of 20,000 with probability 0.9 and an income of 10,000 with probability 0.1? The correct answer is that the risk premium is 586 in this case. Show your work.

Here are the proper steps. (a) Calculate expected income, $E(I)$. (b) Calculate expected utility, $E(U)$. (c) Calculate the income associated with that expected utility—the certainty equivalent I_C. (d) Take the difference between $E(I)$ and I_C. That's the correct answer.

Why is the risk premium lower in this case? The primary reason is that the risk's variance is lower. This type of gamble is a binary event (two outcomes), and binary events have their largest variance when the probability is nearest 0.5. In the gamble at hand, the variance in the first case is $[0.4 \times (16,000 - 10,000)^2]$ $+ [0.6 \times (16,000 - 20,000)^2] = (0.4 \times 6,000^2) + (0.6 \times 4,000^2) = (0.4 \times 36)$ $\times (10^6 + 0.6) \times (16 \times 10^6) = (14.4 \times 10^6) + (9.6 \times 10^6) = 24 \times 10^6$.

In the second case, the variance (similarly) is $[0.1 \times (19,000 - 10,000)^2]$ $+ [0.9 \times (20,000 - 19,000)^2] = (0.1 \times 9,000^2) + (0.9 \times 1,000^2) = (8.1 \times 10^6)$ $+ (0.9 \times 10^6) = 9.0 \times 10^6$, only three-eighths as large as in the first case.

APPENDIXES TO CHAPTER 10

Appendix A: A Detailed Calculation of Welfare Loss

The problem in the text has the following characteristics: Suppose the person confronts an illness risk such as the following:

Probability	Uninsured Demand	Insured Demand
0.3	3	4
0.1	8	9

Each day of hospital care costs $500. The uninsured risk has an expected value of $500[(0.3 \times 3) + (0.1 \times 8)] = \$500 \times 1.7 = \$850$. The variance of that uninsured risk is $(0.3 \times \$1,500^2) + (0.1 \times \$4,000^2)$ $- \$850^2 = \$1,552,500$.

With the insurance policy, the patient buys more medical care but pays for only 20 percent of it. The insured risk has an expected value to the patient (the patient's share) of $(0.2 \times \$500)[(0.3 \times 4) + (0.1 \times 9)] = \$100 \times 2.1$ $= \$210$. The variance of this risk is $(0.3 \times \$400^2) + (0.1 \times 900^2)$ $- \$210^2 = \$84,900$. Thus, the *change* in risk to the consumer by purchasing this $C = 0.2$ insurance policy is $\$1,552,500 - \$84,900 = \$1,467,600$.

According to Pratt (1964), the risk premium a person would be willing to pay for this reduction in risk is approximately $0.5 \times r \times$ (change in variance). If the risk-aversion parameter $r = -0.0003$, then the risk premium the consumer would be willing to pay for this reduction in risk is approximated by $0.0003 \times 0.5 \times \$1,467,600 = \$220$. This approximation works best when the risk is normally distributed and begins to fail most rapidly when the distribution of the risk is highly skewed.

Now consider the welfare loss from the extra demand for medical care, the triangles A and B in Figure 10.4. Consider first what happens for illness 1. The change in quantity is 1 day. The change in marginal value is $0.8 \times \$500 = \$400$. The welfare loss triangle for that event is $0.5 \times \$400 \times 1 = \$200$. Similarly, if illness 2 occurs, the change in demand is also 1 day (although there is no reason why it has to be the same), the change in marginal value is again $400, and the welfare loss from that event is also $200. Thus, the expected welfare loss from "moral hazard" is $(0.3 \times \$200) + (0.1 \times \$200) = \$80$.

These data are sufficient to allow calculation of the net welfare gain from purchasing an insurance plan with $C = 0.2$ as described in the text. The risk premium is $220, and the loading fee charged by the insurance company is 10 percent of $840, or $84. Then the net gain from risk reduction is $220 - \$84 = \$136$. The welfare loss from the "moral hazard" is $80, as computed in the previous paragraph. Thus, the net gain from purchasing the insurance is $136 - \$80 = \$56$.

A useful approximation to the welfare loss triangles (see Problem 5) has the following computations: The arc-elasticity of demand for the first illness is -0.2143. The change in price is $400. The approximate welfare change is $0.5 \times \$400 \times 4 \text{ days} \times (-0.2143) = \$171$. This occurs with probability 0.3, for an expected loss of $51.43. The "exact" calculation shows a welfare loss of $200 rather than $171.

Appendix B: The Calculus of the Risk/Moral Hazard Trade-off

One approach to understanding how risk avoidance and moral hazard balance off for a rational consumer comes from specifying the welfare losses associated with risk bearing and those associated with "moral hazard" activity, considering that each of those changes as the degree of insurance coverage changes, and finding the insurance coverage (copayment rate) that minimizes the total expected welfare loss from risk bearing plus moral hazard.

Phelps (2002) approaches this problem by using second-order Taylor Series expansions to describe the welfare loss from risk bearing (following the approach used by Pratt, 1964) and the welfare loss from the changes in consumption (following the approach specified by McKenzie and Pearce, 1976). In this problem, it turns out that both of these welfare losses are quadratic expressions involving the coinsurance rate C, so that these Taylor Series approximations can be summed, and then the minimum-loss value of C readily derived. Phelps (2002) shows that the optimal value of C is found by the equation

$$C^* = -E(pm_i\eta_i)/[r\sigma^2 - E(pm_i\eta_i)]$$

where p = price, m = quantity of medical care, η is the demand elasticity, r is the risk aversion parameter, and σ^2 is the uninsured variance of the risk facing the individual.

From our understanding of the meaning of each of these components, a nice intuitive meaning comes out of this equation:

$$C^* = (\text{Moral Hazard Loss})/(\text{Moral Hazard Loss} + \text{Risk Premium})$$

which can be simplified even further by the simple assumption of a constant elasticity of demand across all illness events (perhaps an heroic assumption!), in which case

$$C^* \approx -\eta/(-\eta + \omega COV^2 r^*)$$

where COV = coefficient of variation = σ/μ, $r^* = rI$ = relative risk aversion, I = income, and $\omega = E(pm)/I$.

This last equation highlights ideas expressed in the main text of this chapter: The optimal coinsurance rate is higher the larger is the demand elasticity, and is smaller the larger the financial risk (variance) facing the consumer is. This also shows that the budget share in medical spending matters—the larger the share of the budget at risk, the more it makes sense to acquire better health insurance.

Phelps (2002) uses data from the RAND Health Insurance experiment to calculate the optimal values of C for various types of medical risks, using the HIS data to estimate the variance (and higher-order moments of the Taylor Series expansion), and then solve for the optimal value of C.

Not surprisingly, hospital care—the highest risk and the lowest demand elasticity—had the most complete coverage, and preventive care (lowest risk, highest demand elasticity) had the highest demand. The optimal coinsurance rates found in Phelps (2002) are as follows:

Type of Risk	Optimal C
Hospital care	0.05
Physicians services	0.50
Dental services	0.60
Preventive services	0.95

Appendix C: The Statistics of an Insurance Pool

An insurance pool reduces an individual's risks by trading in that person's risky gamble for an insurance premium with a much lower variance. To understand this, consider a very simple insurance policy against a random risk X_i for individuals $i = 1 \ldots N$, each with mean μ and variance σ^2. (The conditions are similar when means and variances differ by person.) The total premium that must be collected is

$$P = \sum_{i=1}^{N} \mu = N\mu \qquad (10C.1)$$

and the per person premium is

$$\frac{P}{N} = \sum_{i=1}^{N} \frac{1}{N} \mu = \mu \qquad (10C.2)$$

The average per person premium P/N is a weighted sum of the means (μ), where the weights are $w_i = 1/N$ for each variable. The variance of the average premium is

$$\sigma_T^2 = \sum_{i=1}^{N} w_i^2 \sigma_i^2 \qquad (10C.3)$$

if the risks are uncorrelated. When each σ_i is the same σ and each w_i equals $1/N$, this becomes

$$\sigma_T^2 = \sigma^2/N \qquad (10C.4)$$

because the summation occurs N times and each has a weight of $(1/N)^2$. Thus, the variance confronting the "average" person in the pool falls proportionately as N rises.

If the risks are correlated, the average variance is $\sigma^2[1 + (N - 1)\rho]/N$, where ρ is the typical correlation between any two people's risks. If $\rho = 0$ (uncorrelated), then the average variance collapses to σ^2/N. If illness were perfectly correlated across individuals, so that when one person got sick, everybody got sick, then $\rho = 1$ and the ability to spread risks is completely nullified. In that extreme case, the average variance is $\sigma^2[1 + (N - 1)]/N = \sigma^2$. In real data, risks are correlated across persons for only a very small amount for medical expenses, so pooling in insurance plans works well.

CHAPTER 11

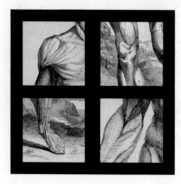

Health Insurance Supply and Managed Care

This chapter analyzes two aspects of insurance markets beyond those covered in Chapter 10 (Demand for Health Insurance). First, we will learn about the supply side of health insurance. Second, we will see how insurance markets have evolved to deal with the fundamental dilemma created by health insurance as discussed in Chapter 10, i.e., the increase in medical care use created by traditional health insurance and the costs associated with that increase in medical care utilization. These new forms of insurance, dubbed "managed care," provide ways to control medical care utilization, but only at a cost of inconvenience and annoyance to insured individuals.

LEARNING GOALS

- Discover how "managed care" can help resolve the tension between risk reduction and control of health care costs.

- Acquire a working understanding of the alphabet-soup menagerie of managed care plan types.

- Learn what mechanisms managed care plans have to control health care costs and the extent to which these do (or do not) work well.

- Digest the effects of managed care market penetration on health care providers, and consider the long-run market equilibrium consequences of these changes.

THE SUPPLY OF INSURANCE

Insurance companies perform two primary tasks, the first of which is more obvious to the consumer, and the second is more fundamental. The obvious activity is the processing of claims. When a patient incurs an expense for medical care, either the doctor's office bills the insurance company directly or else the patient pays the doctor and then submits the bill to the insurance

345

company for reimbursement. The insurance company compares the medical expense with the person's insurance coverage and then issues a check to the doctor or patient, as appropriate.

The risk-bearing activity, the second task performed by insurance companies, is less obvious but more important. Insurance companies are in the business of bearing and spreading risk. Because consumers dislike risk, if they are able to shed that risk, somebody must acquire it. Insurance companies perform this task.

The simple exchange of risk from one person to another does little to reduce risk in our society; it merely transfers it from one person to another. However, by pooling risks, insurance companies can actually reduce average risk. If the risks are completely independent, the average risk (the risk per person in the group) of an insured group with N members is $1/N$ times the variance that each individual confronts.[1] If the risks are correlated across persons, then the risk can't be reduced as much. Thus, for example, a group of people all living in southern California can't gain much by pooling their risks against earthquake losses because if one home is destroyed by earthquake, probably others will be as well.

In health care, the presence of contagious diseases such as colds and influenza contribute to the correlation of risks, but overall, the correlations across people are very small, and risk spreading can work quite well.

The Production Function of Health Insurers

Health insurance companies exist to spread risk. They do so, of course, by paying for part or all of the medical expenses associated with illnesses of the people insured by the company. The operating costs of insurance companies include the tasks of processing insurance claims and making appropriate payments. Thus, the observable products of insurers are claims payments, and we can talk meaningfully about the production function for these products. These tasks primarily involve people and computers, which are the main inputs, along with buildings, in the production of health insurance claims. These costs are paid for by the loading fee charged by the insurance company described previously in this chapter.

The loading fee for the insurance company rises and falls as its costs rise (wages of workers, for example) and fall (computing costs, for example). The structure of an insurance policy itself also affects the loading fee. If the insurance plan has complicated provisions that require many human decisions before a payment can be made, the loading fee will of necessity be higher. If the insurance is a "standard" plan that can be administered mainly by computers, loading fees will be smaller. The number and complexity of

---

[1]Appendix C to Chapter 10 provides the proof and discussion.

claims filed by insured people similarly affect loading fees. Insurance plans with large deductibles, for example, generate fewer claims because people don't bother filing small claims on the policy. Plans with many small claims, such as dental insurance, probably generate higher loading fees than plans with a smaller number of large claims, such as a surgical insurance plan.

The other relevant cost of insurance companies is a negative cost—the "cost" of money. Because insurance companies collect the insurance premium at the beginning of a year (or whenever the insurance contract begins) and pay claims throughout the year as patients send them in, the companies get to hold the money in the interim, earning a return on their investment. Competitive forces generally lead to the pricing of the insurance contract to account for any earnings from the insurance company's investment portfolio. For a typical health insurance contract with a one-year duration, the average time between payment of the premium and payment of the "typical" benefit is 6 months. Thus, the higher the "real" return on capital for the insurance company, the lower its loading fee.[2] Over the past several decades, the real return (net of inflation) for insurance companies has fluctuated between 0 and 10 percent, averaging about 5 percent.[3] Thus, with an average holding period of half a year, the insurance company can earn about 2 to 3 percent of premiums as investment income. Although it is conceptually possible for the premiums collected by the insurance company to be *less* than the average benefit paid out, portfolio earnings commonly do not suffice to offset the entire operating costs of the insurer, and loading fees are positive.

Flavors of Insurance Companies

As in the case of hospitals, many health insurers in the United States operate as not-for-profit organizations. The companies, most commonly "Blue" plans (Blue Cross or Blue Shield), were organized under special enabling legislation passed during the first half of the century. These Blue plans operate with several advantages over their for-profit competitors.

---

[2]The "real" rate of earnings is approximately the actual rate of interest earned minus the rate of inflation. For example, if the insurance company can earn 10 percent on its investment portfolio and there is 6 percent inflation in the economy, then the real rate of return is 4 percent.

Health insurance companies pay out most of the premium in terms of health care costs. Only a small part (the administrative costs of the insurer) depends on the overall price level in the economy. Because health care prices have increased faster than overall prices for almost all of the past 40 years, health insurance companies really need to concern themselves with the rate of price increase for the bundle of goods and services they pay for in benefits, such as hospital care and physician services, versus the interest rate they receive.

[3]The Department of Commerce gathers data on insurance companies' return on investment.

First, by virtue of their not-for-profit organizational form, they are exempt from taxation. Many states levy a special "premium tax" (such as a sales tax applied to health insurance premiums) on all insurance sales, including those for-profit health insurance organizations (such as Aetna, Travelers, New York Life, Prudential, and similar large national insurers). The Blues escape such taxes by being tax exempt, which gives them an automatic price advantage in the market of several percent in many states. They also avoid other taxes, including federal and state corporate income taxes, property taxes, and the like.

Second, Blue plans do not face the extent of regulation in many states that other insurers do, including regulations about minimum cash reserves that are imposed upon other insurers.

One might appropriately ask why these plans have not swept the market, given these legally supported advantages. One answer is that the Blue plans, being organized on a state (or substate regional) basis, miss some opportunity for economies of scale that larger insurers can capture. Second, as a philosophical matter, the Blue plans for a long time adhered to a style of insurance that differed from that offered by commercial insurers. Although the commercial insurers evolved a "major medical" insurance policy (a plan covering a wide scope of services, typically with a deductible such as $100 and a coinsurance rate of 20 percent), the Blue plans opted for first-dollar coverage for hospital care (Blue Cross), but with common limitations on the number of hospital days covered (Anderson, 1975). Early Blue Cross plans covered only 30 days of care (later 60 and then 120), but this clearly placed considerable risk on individuals who might be hospitalized for a long time because they faced having their insurance coverage run out. This type of coverage is "upside down" from the point of view of a risk-averse consumer; it insures low-risk events (first hospital day) but not high-risk events (very long hospitalizations). Similar constraints on payments for physicians' services in Blue Shield plans may also have made the plans less attractive to consumers. Thus, although the Blue plans operated with cost (and hence price) advantages, other features of their insurance offerings made it less likely that they would capture the entire market.

Group Insurance

Most health insurance in the United States (and in many other nations as well) is sold not to individuals or families but to large groups. Group insurance offers two advantages over individual insurance: It provides economies of scale and a way to avoid adverse selection.

Economies of Scale

Many of the costs of developing and selling an insurance policy are nearly the same whether 10 or 10,000 people are enrolled in the plan. Group insurance sales take advantage of this economy of scale. Group insurance purchases also eliminate some of the activities often involved in the sale of nongroup insurance, such as gathering and analyzing information about the health history of persons buying the insurance. Insurance companies can do this because of the role of groups in eliminating adverse selection.

The economies of scale associated with group insurance are considerable, and the loading fees that result reflect these gains. At the most basic level, we can see the importance of group insurance in reducing the price of insurance by looking at the aggregate data for recent years. Table 11.1 shows the premiums paid by consumers, the benefits paid by the insurance company, and the ratio of these two, which equals $(1 + L)$. Although the numbers vary from year to year (depending on how well the actuaries forecast the benefit payments), the group policies always have a much lower loading fee (averaging about 15 to 20 percent in most years), compared with nongroup policies that have an average loading fee of 50 to 100 percent or more. As a consequence, one of the key factors affecting demand for health insurance in this country is access to group insurance. When a person belongs to some group (as people do when they work for a firm that provides insurance as a benefit), the chances are much greater that the person will have insurance coverage.

Large groups have bigger economies of scale than small groups, so the price of insurance should be even lower in big groups than in small groups. Table 11.2 shows typical loading fee by group size.

TABLE 11.1 PREMIUMS, BENEFITS, AND LOADING RATIOS FOR GROUP AND NONGROUP INSURANCE OF COMMERCIAL INSURANCE COMPANIES FOR HOSPITALS AND MEDICAL/SURGICAL INSURANCE

Year	Group Insurance			Nongroup Insurance		
	Premium[a]	Benefit[a]	Ratio[b]	Premium[a]	Benefit[a]	Ratio[b]
1970	6.2	6.0	1.02	2.3	1.1	2.10
1975	13.1	11.6	1.13	3.1	1.6	1.97
1980	31.5	25.9	1.22	4.9	3.0	1.65
1985	59.5	44.3	1.34	7.9	4.7	1.68
1990	93.7	79.4	1.18	8.9	5.8	1.53
1995	117.0	102.0	1.15	12.9	8.4	1.50
2000[c]	125.0	105.0	1.19	20.0	13.3	1.50

[a]In billions of dollars.
[b]Calculated as premiums/benefits.
[c]Estimated.

TABLE 11.2   TYPICAL LOADING FEES BY GROUP SIZE

Number of Employees	Loading Fee[a] (As Percent of Benefits)
Individual policies	60–80
Small groups (1–10)	30–40
Moderate groups (11–100)	20–30
Medium groups (100–200)	15–20
Large groups (201–1,000)	8–15
Very large groups (more than 1,000)	5–8
Overall for all plans (weighted average)	15–25

[a]Varies annually.

Several studies of demand for insurance have shown that the insurance coverage selected in large groups is systematically greater than in small groups (Phelps, 1973, 1976; Goldstein and Pauly, 1976). In fact, the size of a work group appears to be one of the best predictors of the amount of insurance any family in the United States will have.

Group insurance solves the adverse selection problem detailed in the previous section by selling insurance to a group of people assembled for some purpose other than buying insurance. For example, an employment group (all of the people working for a particular company) probably has its share of good and bad health risks, but on balance, the risks should be pretty average. Thus, the insurance company can sell insurance without having to go through the trouble of examining people, taking histories, and so on, which is common with individual insurance policies.

MANAGED CARE: A RESPONSE TO THE INCENTIVES OF TRADITIONAL INSURANCE

Health care has evolved in recent years into an economic form that defies comparison with other sectors of the economy—the "managed care" sector. One cannot contemplate the modern U.S. health care system adequately without understanding the nature of managed care organizations (MCOs), what they attempt to do, what management tools they have at their disposal, and why consumers would bother to join them (instead of staying with a traditional insurance plan such as discussed in Chapters 4, 5, and 10). Managed care spans a wide variety of organizations, but the key idea is that MCOs are actively involved both in the delivery of health care and in the provision of health insurance. Sometimes they originate as health care delivery organizations but more often as insurance companies. However, as they evolve into the "middle ground," they can begin to look quite similar, no matter what their origins or history. They come in many flavors; Box 11.1 provides definitions of the most common types.

BOX 11.1 THE ALPHABET SOUP OF MANAGED CARE

The world of managed care organizations (MCOs) has evolved into a series of loose classifications that, it turns out, are almost invariably examples of TLAs.*

HMO: The "classic" and most widespread phrase for these organizations is the health maintenance organization, a phrase coined in the 1970s meant to describe a fairly specific organization in which the insurance plan, the doctors, and the hospital either were all the same organization or were closely affiliated. The doctors usually worked in the same (large) medical office building, often adjacent to or part of the hospital itself. The original Kaiser Permanente plans on the west coast were perhaps the prototypes. In such plans, the doctors are on salary, the plan owns the hospitals used by patients, and patients (except in emergency) must use the plan-affiliated providers for their care.

The essential feature of the pure "staff model" HMO is that the plan is paid on a "capitation" basis ("per head"), which means that the HMO receives a fixed sum of money each year to provide all of the medical care the enrollee needs, no matter what. This offers the greatest incentive for cost control and cautious use of medical interventions (and to some observers, an incentive so strong that it might harm patients' health).

The term has evolved in common use to imply almost any kind of managed care organization and in some settings has almost the same meaning as MCO.

FFS: Fee-for-service, the antithesis of MCOs. Traditional insurance (including Medicare at its inception) offered defined coverage for billed charges for any service provided for the patient. FFS creates the least constraints on both provider and consumer behavior, and has higher costs for a given degree of its financial protection to consumers because of its unconstrained environment.

IPA: Independent practice association, a step away from the "pure" HMO. In an IPA, the doctors work as independent doctors in their own offices, and normally have a mix of patients enrolled in traditional FFS plans as well as capitated or "managed" patients.

PPO: Preferred provider organization. A PPO is a cousin of the IPA, but relies more on selecting a subset of all available providers and making contractual agreements with them that mostly focus on price. The "preferred providers" have patients steered to them by the PPO insurance plan in exchange for a lower price. The lower price allows the PPO to offer a lower total insurance premium, which attracts enrollees, which in turn creates a larger patient base that the PPO can use to negotiate with providers. Doctors are paid on a fee-for-service system, usually with a set of negotiated fees for each service offered.

*Three-letter acronyms.

(continued)

BOX II.I THE ALPHABET SOUP OF MANAGED CARE (continued)

POS: Point of service plans. Often called HMOs without walls, POS plans often have a capitation arrangement with providers for their enrollees, but the doctors are spread around in their own offices as in an IPA or PPO. The key difference is that in a POS plan, the compensation to the provider is per patient per year rather than FFS. Patients have strong financial incentives to use the POS plan doctors because their insurance either covers nothing if they use out-of-plan doctors (the extreme form) or has a very high copayment rate, but they can make the choice at the "point of services" (the time when they seek care.) rather than annually.

CDP: Consumer-directed plan. This primarily is a plan with very large front-end deductibles, typically with a health savings account (**HSA**) attached over which the consumer has direct control for medical care spending.

The federal government allows individuals to make contributions of up to $900 (at this writing) annually to an HSA account and not pay income taxes on that amount, but the law also has minimum deductibles for plans that are eligible—$1,100 per person per year in current law.

We begin this chapter with a discussion of the consumer's decision—why would a consumer enroll in an MCO?—and then turn to the incentives available to MCOs (both provider and consumer interventions) to accomplish their goals?

WHY MANAGED CARE?

Managed care organizations evolved as a response to a problem created by a solution to another problem. Health insurance (as we saw in Chapter 10) exists fundamentally to reduce individuals' financial risks. Variability in health outcomes provides the fundamental source of risk, and intelligent responses to those illnesses and injuries (buying appropriate medical care) create the derivative financial risk. In response to these risks created by illness, individuals chose to purchase health insurance. But the traditional forms of that insurance, including classic Blue Cross and Blue Shield "first-dollar" coverage and then "major medical" insurance (first sold by commercial insurance companies) created another problem in return as they sought to reduce the financial risk—they altered people's behavior in choosing medical care in an ultimately undesirable way. Managed care evolved to help deal with that problem.

As we learned in Chapters 4 and 5, traditional health insurance creates a welfare loss by reducing the price of medical care at the time consumers (with their doctors) choose how much medical care (including the types of treatment, training of specialist, etc.). With an artificially low price, consumers are led to consume too much care, but (as we can infer through the voluntary purchase of the insurance) they gain more through the reduction in financial risk than they lose through excessive consumption of medical care. The discussion in the preceding chapter shows how a rational consumer balances off those gains and losses, and how the "optimal" insurance differs greatly, depending on the risks arising from the illness (and treatments thereof) and the elasticity of demand for the medical services themselves.

Managed care seeks to improve upon the problems created by traditional insurance by interfering in some way with the decisions about the amounts and types of health care chosen. Contracts between the consumer and the MCO limit the consumer's access to medical care in some ways in order to offset the incentives for overuse of medical care. The consumer who enrolls in an MCO in effect says "stop me before I kill again" (although perhaps with less extreme wording). The MCO inserts various incentives and constraints into the system to reduce the quantity of care and to shift to lower cost alternatives when more than one treatment choice is available.[4]

Managed care organizations are still evolving in their understanding of which interventions actually work, which seem to be acceptable to consumers, and how to price the insurance contract when including various combinations of "management." The mechanisms used to constrain health care consumers' choices affect both provider and consumer behavior. Because of the important "principal-agent" relationship between doctors and patients (whether involving demand inducement or not), influencing provider behavior has proven important in these arrangements. However (as we shall see below), those mechanisms that rely upon altering provider behavior are subject to potential legal attack because they inevitably alter the principal-agent relationship between the patient and the doctor. Subsequent sections in this chapter explore the main types of these "management" tools and analyze their consequences.

At this point, it is worth noting that MCOs have not succeeded in the market "merely" because they have created insurance plans that cost less than

---

[4]Various alternatives exist, particularly in single-provider or single-insurer systems of countries such as Great Britain and Canada, to achieve the same goals. In those (and similar) countries, access to care is deliberately limited by availability of various services, and commonly rationed by waiting lists. (For an elegant discussion of the operation of the British National Health Service, see Aaron and Schwartz, 1984.) Various regulatory controls in the United States have attempted to deal with the same issue at the governmental level, as Chapter 15 will discuss in detail.

standard fee-for-service (FFS) plans, although to the casual observer this may seem to be the primary reason for their success. However, lower premium costs *alone* would not necessarily attract rational consumers to MCOs. One can always achieve a lower insurance premium, of course, by accepting insurance with reduced coverage (higher copayments and deductibles, for example) or reduced scope of benefits (no coverage for prescription drugs, dental care, etc.). But that simply moves the consumer along a trade-off of lower cost premiums in exchange for greater financial risk. The essential value of the MCO comes in its ability to reduce insurance premiums to the consumer while retaining the elimination of financial risk that a comprehensive FFS insurance plan offers.

When consumers decide to enroll in an MCO (instead of a traditional FFS plan), they in effect precommit to a plan that they know in advance will constrain their choices because such precommitment can actually improve their overall expected utility. Analysis of economic "games" commonly shows the value of precommitment to rational economic agents, both on the consumer and supplier side of the market.[5] Box 11.2 discusses an ancient and famous legend involving precommitment as well.

Enrollment Patterns

The most recent information available about enrollment trends shows a rapid switch to managed care of some sort. In the early 1980s, most people had some sort of FFS plan. By the early 1990s, one out of seven of the population had some form of HMO, while the remaining insured people has FFS plans. Of those, IPAs, PPOs, and POS-like plans had by far the largest share, and "pure" HMOs (in the traditional sense) were down to 3.2 million enrollees, barely above 1 percent of the U.S. market.

---

[5]For example, on the provider side, precommitment can help organize an implicit collusion between sellers by which a "dominant firm" precommits to match the price of any lower price. This precommitment dissuades other firms in the market from cutting their prices, thus creating a tacit collusion to keep prices high. On the consumer side, a common form of precommitment can be seen in the purchase of U.S. Savings Bonds. The consumer makes a small investment in the bond up front, and its value grows through time, but the owner cannot "cash out" the bond until a specified number of years has passed. This precommits the bond owner to a plan of savings that could be achieved through smaller annual deposits into a savings account, but without the precommitment, the consumer runs a risk of failing to meet the annual savings goals, and hence not having as much money saved at the end.

BOX 11.2 A CLASSIC MYTH INVOLVING PRECOMMITMENT

An early Greek myth helps us understand the concept of precommitment—
that concerning Ulysses (or Odysseus), the hero in Homer's *Odyssey*. Ulysses
deliberately constrained his own behavior in advance to accomplish something else he greatly desired. His precommitment prevents him from taking an
irrational (and in his case, fatal) course while still allowing him to achieve
other goals. In most economic models involving precommitment, the same
issues arise.

   Ulysses, returning home from his travels, must sail by an island populated
by some apparently irresistible women called Sirens, the songs of whom
attracted sailors to hear them, but, alas, always fatally, as they crashed their
ship upon the rocks.* Ulysses wished to hear the famous song, but obviously
did not wish to crash his ship, so he filled the ears of all his crew with wax so
they could not hear, and then had himself carefully tied to the mast of his ship
so he could not alter its course. The crew sailed by safely, and Ulysses was able
to hear the famous Sirens' Song, but only by having arranged in advance that
his own actions would be constrained. Thus, he was able to accomplish his
immediate goal of hearing the Sirens and to accomplish his long-run goal of
maintaining a safe passage homeward. Ulysses' idea of "tying himself to the
mast" has become symbolic of somebody who takes actions in advance to
constrain his own later actions. Managed care has many of these same elements for consumers of medical care.

*Homer, never made clear the motives for the Sirens to do this but perhaps they prof-
ited by scavenging the remains of the ships. Homer does allude to the scattered ruins
of the victims' ships on the rocks.

   By 1996, the best data summarize plans obtained through employment
groups, but because that represents the vast majority of all private health
insurance, we can take these data as being representative of the market as a
whole. By 1996, only 27 percent of these enrollees persisted in an FFS plan,
and by 1999, only 8 percent remained.

   Thus, it seems fair to say that at this point in the evolution of health
insurance, traditional FFS insurance has almost evolved out of existence.
During the evolution to managed care, the most rapid growth has come in
PPOs, which increased from almost no market share in the early 1980s to
28 percent in 1996 and 41 percent by 1999. POS plans, a relatively new
entrant, moved from 14 percent in 1996 to 22 percent in 1999. Classic

HMOs (combining pure HMOs and IPAs) remained about static between 1996 and 1999 at about 30 percent. (All 1996 and 1999 data are from Dudley and Luft, 2001.)

A View from the Physician Side of the Market

Another view of the managed care market looks at physician participation. In a recent survey of physicians (2000), the American Medical Association (AMA, 2003) asked respondents about their reliance on managed care patients, both in terms of the proportion of doctors who have managed care contracts (they are almost ubiquitous!) and the percent of their practice revenue derived form managed care contracts. Table 11.3 summarizes the responses for various types of medical practices. Overall, 88 percent of doctors has *some* managed care contracts and derived 41 percent of their income from managed care patients. Of the total revenue overall, only 7.3 percent came from "capitation" contracts that pay the doctor an annual amount to treat patients rather than on an FFS basis. (This latter number varied from 3.9 percent for surgeons to 15.3 percent for pediatricians.)

The 41 percent of revenues deserves special attention. This actually represents a much higher fraction of the private health market than one might immediately imagine. While some states that have managed care Medicaid and a fraction of Medicare patients choose a managed care option, most of the managed care revenue comes from private patients under age 65. Government programs (mostly Medicare and Medicaid) pay for about 45 percent of the total costs of health care, leaving 55 percent for private payment. It is against this 55 percent that the 41 percent revenue share should be judged. On this simple basis, it would appear that about three-quarters of all

TABLE 11.3 MANAGED CARE PENETRATION FROM THE PHYSICIAN PERSPECTIVE

Specialty	Percent with Managed Care Contracts	Percent of Revenue from Managed Care Contracts	Percent of Revenue from Capitated Contracts
All physicians	88.1	40.8	7.3
General/Family	91.6	42.5	11.4
Internal medicine	91.2	38.0	9.6
Surgery	89.6	38.3	3.9
Pediatrics	94.1	54.9	15.3
OB/Gyn	93.9	56.4	4.1
Radiology	91.8	42.0	7.0
Other	78.9	31.8	2.4

Source: AMA (2003), Tables 36, 37, and 38.

physicians' medical practice revenue from nongovernmental patients came from managed care contracts.

TYPES OF INTERVENTIONS

To deliver on its promise to lower costs of health insurance while controlling risk to the consumer, MCOs must find acceptable ways of limiting access to medical care. They do so through altering the incentives and "rules of the game" for both consumers and providers of health care. In this next section, we will learn about the mechanisms MCOs commonly employ to achieve their goals.

CONSUMER SIDE

A number of interventions in managed care deal directly with consumers' behavior; the interventions seek to modify consumers' choice in seeking care and their decisions about what care to receive once their doctor has made a recommendation.

Copayments The most common and readily understood intervention used by almost every managed care plan is the simple imposition of copayments at the time medical care is used. Most plans now use a system in which patients pay a fixed amount on each occasion (for example) that they see a doctor. This amount typically ranges from $5 to $20. The consequences of such a copayment approach were explored in Chapter 4, and will not be discussed further here, except to note the issue about search incentives. As we learned in Chapter 4, a copayment model with this type of structure obliterates the incentives for consumers to search for a lower price because (once having paid the fixed amount per physician visit, prescription, etc.) the consumer has no financial advantage from seeking a lower priced provider, and hence presumably has minimal if any incentive to carry out any search. However, almost every managed care plan in operation already has negotiated prices with providers who are eligible for treating patients in the plan, in effect having done the searching for the consumer. Thus, they really don't care if the consumer searches or not, and are quite willing to have a copayment system that does not encourage search. The advantages to the insurance plan from using something like a $10 copayment appear to center mostly on administrative costs—the doctor's office collects the copayment at the time of the visit, and the insurance company has already agreed how much it will pay the doctor for each procedure or visit delivered to the patient.

Second Opinion Programs Another approach in some managed care plans offers (and in a few occasions, requires) "second opinions" before they will pay for surgery. In a second-opinion arrangement, the insurance plan will pay for a second doctor's opinion, but it is made clear to the second doctor that they will not provide the treatment. They are asked only whether they concur with the original recommendation.

The second opinion process focuses on the intrinsic financial incentive problem embedded in the doctor–patient relationship in a fee-for-service arrangement. The "agent" (the doctor) has financial incentives to recommend treatment more aggressively than the "principal" (the patient) might prefer (Dranove, 1988a); because of asymmetric information, the patient cannot always tell when the advice has been altered in an important way. By offering to pay for a second opinion, the insurance plan not only signals to the patient the possibility of receiving "tilted" advice from the doctor but also creates a way for the patient to get advice from a doctor who has no possible financial stake in the outcome.

Despite the intrinsic appeal of second opinion programs, they have not worked very well in altering patients' choices, and relatively few managed care plans at least in widespread use now require them. Several things work against the second opinion program: First, patients are often reluctant to use the second opinion when it seems as if they are challenging their doctor. Next, the second opinion almost invariably comes from another doctor in the same region (because for it to be otherwise, the patient would have to travel some distance for the second opinion). This means that the "styles" of doctors are likely to have some within-region similarity, as we learned in the analysis of regional variations in Chapter 3. Thus, an initial recommendation for surgery will likely find a concurring second opinion even if the doctor giving the second opinion gives a completely honest opinion about the case because we know that doctors within the same region have related styles of decision making.

Gatekeeper Models Another approach, widely used in managed care programs, is called a "gatekeeper" model. In these managed care programs, the patient *must* see a primary care doctor (family practice, internal medicine, pediatrics, or in the case of pregnancy, obstetrics) before seeing any specialist, and a specific referral from the primary care provider (PCP) is necessary before the insurance plan will pay for specialist treatment. The PCP visit obviously costs the insurance plan something, so it must expect some reduction in treatment to occur to justify that expense.

The belief that overall treatment costs will fall in a gatekeeper model comes from several sources. The key situation is one in which either the PCP or a specialist might treat the patient (and many illnesses and injuries fall into this category). The specialist normally receives a higher fee than the generalist (the PCP), and at least on some occasions, we know that specialists tend to use other medical resources (laboratory tests, hospitalization, etc.) more intensively than generalists.[6] Thus, the insurance plan can rely on the normal economic incentives for the generalist to "hold onto" the patient rather than referring the patient to a specialist, and can anticipate that the total costs of treatment will be lower than if the patient were treated by a specialist. The basis of the gatekeeper model, then, is to prevent the patient from bypassing the PCP and going directly for specialty treatment, a specific example of "tying oneself to the mast."

Data supporting the efficacy (or not) of gatekeeper models are extremely sparse. One early study of the first gatekeeper model in Seattle, Washington (Moore, Martin, and Richardson, 1983), provides a case study of a failed plan (which offered incentives to providers that did not support the gatekeeper concept).

Provider Side

Traditional health insurance sought to control health care costs exclusively through the use of consumer-side incentives (copayments and deductibles). Modern managed care plans use such strategies, but also deal with the incentives faced by providers. This section discusses the major utilization and cost-control strategies that focus on providers.

Payment Strategies for Doctors

Perhaps the most traditional and widely studied method of altering provider behavior in managed care involves compensation of the doctor, who (by training and law) sits in the position of prescribing and managing all of the patient's care. The key issues in this matter have already been discussed in Chapter 7.[7]

---

[6]One classic study of this looked at doctors' recommendations for terminal cancer patients. General internists recommended within-home and hospice care more often, whereas cancer specialists (oncologists) recommended hospitalization and intensive care more often (Kissick et al., 1984).

[7]The assiduous student should here reread the summary of the very important study by Hickson, Altmeier, and Perrin (1987) discussed in the final section of Chapter 7. Or better, find the original article from *Pediatrics* in a medical library and read it directly.

Salary Versus Fee-for-Service The idea of paying doctors a fixed annual salary (instead of paying on a FFS basis) arose most prominently in the "classic" HMOs (such as Kaiser Permanente), for which all of the medical treatment for enrolled patients is provided by a closed panel of physicians who all receive fixed salaries. This HMO literature provides a good source of information about the effects of physician compensation, although we cannot treat it as definitive because the HMOs do other things besides change physician compensation. For example, HMOs often tout their use of preventive services as a way of reducing health care costs, and emphasize the value of continuity of care provided through a single integrated organization. That having been said, we can turn to the HMO versus FFS literature for guidance about the effects of salary-based compensation.

The concept originated with the Kaiser Permanente Corporation in the 1940s in Portland, Honolulu, and Los Angeles, as a way to provide health care benefits to corporation employees. The insurance plan hires the doctors (in the pure form, on a straight salary) or contracts with a specific group of doctors to provide care, and either builds its own hospital or contracts for the services of a hospital within the community. The original Kaiser Permanente group plans also all had their own associated hospitals. The key feature of such programs is that the providers of care (doctors, hospitals, etc.) have no financial incentive to provide extra care to the patients enrolled with the insurance plan because the insurance plan, the hospital, and the doctors all share common financial interests.

This payment form is often called "capitation payment" because the payment for caring for patients comes on a "per person" or "per head" basis (hence the name "capitation"). Capitation payment is really the essential part of a pure HMO because of the financial incentives contained therein. In standard FFS insurance plans, providers always do better financially by providing more care to patients. The insurance company is "at risk" in a large way, the providers are not "at risk" at all, and the patients are "at risk" only to the extent of their deductibles, coinsurance, and so on. In this type of world, the two parties closest to the decisions about using medical care—providers (notably, doctors) and patients—have no financial interest in conserving scarce resources. The "third party"—the insurance company—has the financial risk but the weakest ability to do anything about expenditure control. In fact, the only interest the insurance company has in controlling costs is the extent to which mechanisms can be devised to control costs that help make the insurer's premium costs to insurance buyers more attractive, and the tax subsidy to health insurance blunts the value of accomplishing that.

By contrast, in the pure capitation model, doctors and hospitals are paid either on a flat salary (in the case of doctors) or on the basis of agreements about how many "covered lives" they will take care of. The providers agree to provide all "necessary" care for the patients in exchange for a specific amount of payment per patient per year.

This arrangement greatly changes the incentives for doctors and hospitals. They no longer make money on volume business. They make money by finding ways to prevent the use of care, and they have strong financial incentives to do just that. They have legal and market incentives to provide "adequate" amounts of care, which can help ensure that patients are not undertreated, but they most certainly do have incentives to conserve on resources.

In many of the "pure HMO" plans, the doctors operate as a separate legal entity (commonly, a large multispecialty group practice) that enters a contract with the HMO-insurance company to provide care for the enrolled patients, agreeing to use the HMO's hospital exclusively. The patients pay a fixed premium for the year, for which all care is provided (sometimes, with small copayments for physician visits). The physician group shares in any extra money remaining at the end of the year. Thus, the group has strong financial incentives to avoid expending resources unnecessarily. The HMO can avoid some of the coordination problems of large groups (see Chapter 6) through rules and supervision, and—importantly—by being able to fire doctors who do not cooperate.

These plans create a supply-side incentive to restrict the amount of medical care rendered. Not surprisingly, the major cost savings generated by this form of care come from reduced hospitalization of enrolled patients, the one very costly activity over which physicians have almost exclusive control. Extensive studies of HMOs (see Luft, 1981, for a summary) have repeatedly shown their reduced propensity to use the hospital, compared with FFS arrangements with extensive insurance coverage. (Note that the relevant comparison is the rate at which medical resources are used in a full-coverage insurance plan because HMO patients have no financial risk and an out-of-pocket price at or very near zero.)

These nonexperimental findings were confirmed in the RAND Health Insurance Study (HIS), which enrolled some (randomly assigned) patients into an HMO in Seattle. These HMO patients were compared with other HIS enrollees with full-coverage insurance and with a set of patients previously enrolled within the HMO. The first comparison (with full-coverage FFS patients) tests the effect of the HMO-incentive system, holding constant the coverage from the patient's point of view (row 1 versus row 3 of Table 11.4). The second comparison (with previously enrolled HMO patients) tests a separate issue: namely, whether the HMOs have been getting an unusually favorable or unfavorable set of patients in their usual enrollment (row 1 versus row 2). This is the "self-selection" problem previously discussed. It has loomed important in the long debate about HMOs because the previous comparison studies,

11.4 HMO HOSPITAL USE AND TOTAL COSTS IN THE RAND HIS

	Percent Using Hospital	Percent Ambulatory Any Care	Total Cost ($)
HMO experiment group	7.1	87	439
HMO controls[a]	6.4	91	469
Fee for service with $C = 0$	11.1	85	609

[a]Previously enrolled in HMO, not as part of RAND HIS.

such as those undertaken by Luft and others, always contained the risk that the results achieved by the HMO were due to a favorable patient mix.

Two important results emerge from this study. First (in parallel with the previous nonexperimental results of Luft and others), the HMO plan used considerably fewer resources than the comparable $C = 0$ FFS plan in the same city (Seattle). (The importance of using the same city as a comparison is heightened by the cross-regional variations in hospitalization shown in the work of Wennberg and others; see Chapter 3.)

Second, the RAND HIS studied the health outcomes of people enrolled in the experimental HMO and compared those with people on the full-coverage FFS plan. As Sloss et al. (1987) reported, at least on a battery of 20 physiological measures of health status that encompass every major organ system (vision, musculoskeletal, digestive, etc.), the HMO enrollees fared at least as well as the corresponding FFS enrollees with full coverage ($C = 0$). Thus, at least in this HMO, the reduced use of resources did not lead to reduced health outcomes for the enrollees.

The Proper Balance of Incentives Economists always worry about incentives, and when one looks at the problems associated with FFS payment (incentives to overprescribe treatment) and those of a flat salary-based compensation (shirking and incentives to withhold treatment if doctor share the savings), then it comes as no surprise that people have begun to think about a blend of payment schemes that provides the best possible outcome. Ma and McGuire (1997) did just this, modeling the physician's behavior with a compensation system that provided both a flat salary (of smaller size, of course, than if the total compensation were salary) and a FFS (again, smaller in size than if the FFS were the only payment). The best blend between the two depends on the strength of the adverse effects generated by each payment system (all of which can, in concept, be measured). If demand inducement effects are relatively large, then the salary component rises and the FFS component shrinks. If shirking and withholding matter more, then the reverse holds (Ma and McGuire, 1997).

The proper balancing between salary and FFS depends in part on how hard doctors work under different compensation arrangements. As reviewed in Chapter 6 (see discussion in the section entitled "The Size of the Firm— Group Practice of Medicine") an important analysis of physician productivity under various compensation arrangements (Gaynor and Gertler, 1995) showed that as physicians are paid more and more on salary (versus by the treatment), their work effort shrinks, and the effect gets worse in larger firms as the ability of managers to monitor the work effort of the physicians deteriorates. In small groups, salary-paid physicians worked about two-thirds as much as doctors paid in an FFS model. In the largest groups, the work effort by salaried doctors dropped to 40 percent of that found in comparably sized FFS groups. This effect is precisely captured in the Ma and McGuire approach.

Implementing the Ma and McGuire approach in a real-world setting involves conjectures (data to support a carefully designed plan simply do not exist) on the part of insurance plan managers about the strength of the effects of demand inducement and shirking. Gaynor and Gertler's work provides reasonably strong evidence on the relationship to work effort and compensation. However, detailed understanding of the importance of demand inducement is missing. Most likely, the extent of demand inducement will vary considerably from setting to setting, perhaps by treatment, perhaps by the educational level of the consumer, perhaps by the degree of competition and information in the market. Such a level of detail about demand inducement simply does not exist now, so the balancing act implied by Ma and McGuire must rest more on conjecture than on firm analysis at this point.

Holdbacks A separate but common method for controlling costs in MCOs occurs when the insurance plan "holds back" a part of the payments due to physicians (say, 15 percent) until the end of the year, to see whether total treatment costs within the plan have come within targets. If the plan comes in at or under target costs, the holdback is dispersed to all of the doctors (in proportion to the payments that they have already received). If the MCO has unusually large costs, then the holdback is kept to help the MCO cover total costs. The logic is that because the doctors control the use of medical care, they should have an incentive to control the costs by sharing in any losses that the MCO might encounter.

This approach certainly helps the MCO deal with cost overruns when they occur, but its ability to actually lower costs remains in doubt. The central problem from an analytic point of view is that the doctors within the MCO have little economic incentive to engage in lower cost medical treatments because of the holdback, and indeed, if they do "cooperate" with the MCO, they are likely to suffer relative to their peers. The concept of a global holdback is best analyzed using noncooperative game theory, and this fits into the class of games known as a Prisoner's Dilemma. In such games, cooperation (here, to save money) almost always falls apart, and hence can have no effects on total medical care use. The problem is directly analogous to the global spending cap problem analyzed in Box 12.1 which discusses a similar feature in Medicare; you may wish to jump ahead and read that material now.

Payment Strategies for Hospitals and Related Organizations

Hospitals have distinct characteristics about their services that make them eligible for a particular form of payment that lies in between FFS and capitation—the so-called payment by "the case." Because a hospital "event" has clearly defined boundaries—the admission and discharge of the patient—insurance plans can pay hospitals for single hospitalization events in a lump sum. This is not the same as FFS payment (in which the hospital bills and is paid for each distinctive event that happens to each patient) nor capitation (in which the hospital is at risk not only for the cost of each hospitalization but also for the number of such events during the year).

The quintessential case-based payment system emerged from the federal government's desires to control hospital costs under the Medicare program, creating a "prospective payment system" (PPS) involving nearly 500 "diagnostically related groups" (DRGs).[8] A number of private insurance plans has adopted this payment system as well. Chapter 12 (Medicare) discusses the details of the DRG system and where the system arose, and thus will not be discussed further here.

Provider Selection

Many MCOs rely on careful selection of providers to control costs of care. The benefit comes from two sources. First, if intrinsic differences between the costs of various providers actually exist, then finding the low-cost providers makes good sense for an MCO. Second, whatever the actual cost structure of providers, if they have been pricing (in the "old" market structure) above their actual costs of treatment, then negotiating the price downward has salutary effects for the MCO.

Perhaps the most important evidence on the efficacy of PPO plans is their rapid growth in the market (from 28 to 41 percent of the market in the short span between 1996 and 1999, for example). Price-conscious employers and employees choosing lower cost health insurance would find PPOs increasingly attractive (as these data show) if they developed a relatively low

---

[8]Another pair of TLAs for the student of MCOs to learn!

premium structure through their primary cost-containment activity: bargaining with providers. Glied (2000) surveys the literature on managed care and finds no unambiguous result with respect to PPOs compared with alternative (FFS) plans.

One reason why PPOs might not achieve their full possible benefit is that they seldom actually use available information to select among providers carefully. One study of the primary care physicians in Rochester, New York (encompassing almost all doctors in the region), shows large and systematic differences in the total costs of treating patients among doctors in a very "open" IPA panel of physicians. The top 10 percent of doctors had charges per patient per year that were twice those of the lowest 10 percent. Furthermore, these differences controlled carefully for the underlying illness conditions of patients, and they replicated well from year to year. Thus, the authors concluded that doctors in this study have identifiable and reproducible practice styles that allow their grouping into relatively lower and relatively higher cost providers (Phelps et al., 1994). Yet neither of the competing IPA insurance plans in the community opted to limit their panel of physicians to the relatively lower cost providers. Their choices invariably embraced the philosophy of bringing into the "panel" of allowed providers all those who wished to participate, apparently on the hypothesis that more doctors meant more patients and hence a larger market share. (Both plans are not for profit, and may prefer market share as a goal rather than net plan profits.)

Do MCOs select doctors on the basis of quality of care as well as cost of treatment? One study on this issue uses New York State's periodic report on the quality of care (measured by risk-adjusted mortality rates, or RAMR) of surgeons and hospitals for coronary bypass artery grafts (CABG). Mukamel and Mushlin (1998) studied the probability that an MCO would contract with a cardiac surgeon, and found that MCOs preferred to contract with doctors with better RAMR and also tended to avoid low-volume providers (holding RAMR constant). The preference for high-quality "outliers" was higher in the New York City metropolitan area where (presumably) more choices were available to the MCOs. This one study, at least, suggests that quality of care also affects provider choice (when it can be measured) in addition to cost of treatment.

In this light, a rather remarkable change occurred in a large insurance carrier in California in 2001; Blue Cross of California, first among its peers, abandoned rewards linked to cost control in its HMO MCO plans and structured a new set of bonus payments to physicians directly tied to patient satisfaction with the plan.[9] The new system, applying to the 1.5 million HMO enrollees among the 5.5 million overall enrollees of Blue Cross in California, offered

---

[9]Reported on the AP wire service, July 10, 2001.

incentive payments of up to 10 percent bonuses for the highest satisfaction scores, as measured by random surveys of patients enrolled in the plan.

MCOs also select hospitals as well as individual doctors. In a study utilizing California data from 1983 to 1997, Zwanziger, Melnick, and Bamezai (2000) studied the consequences of California's introduction of selective contracting both through the state's Medicaid program ("MediCal") and by introducing legislation allowing selective contracting in private insurance markets. They developed measures of competition among hospitals and measured the rate of cost growth and how it changed due to selective contracting entering the market. They found a strong negative relationship between the degree of competition (the market concentration) and the rate of cost growth after selective contracting emerged—more competitive markets had less cost growth.

Still another form of "selection" occurs when MCOs limit the choices of consumers (and their doctors) regarding prescription drugs. Many MCOs now have a "formulary" of drugs that receive the highest coverage (typically generic drugs when available) and one or two more expensive (to the patient) tiers of drugs where the patient's out-of-pocket costs can be considerably higher. Chapter 15 discusses insurance coverage of prescription drugs in more detail.

Prices and Fee Schedules

The essential feature of PPOs (as noted in Box 11.1) is to bargain with providers about price. The circularity of success in such programs is compelling, particularly in markets in which providers have had the opportunity to price above marginal production costs. The cycle looks like this: A PPO enrolls a group of people with the promise of a low premium (based on the expectation of low prices from providers). It negotiates with providers (doctors, hospitals, nursing homes, etc.) by promising to bring them a high volume of patients (those they have enrolled) in exchange for a favorable price.

To the extent that a PPO is successful in recruiting more patients, it enhances its ability to convince more providers to join the organization, which gives it more leverage in bargaining for a better price. Similarly, as the PPO adds more providers to its panel, it becomes more attractive to more consumers (particularly those who do not wish to change providers as they change insurance plans). Hence, successful growth in either the patient or provider market can enhance the ability of a PPO to grow in the other market. The only limiting factor eventually may be the proportion of patients who object to managed care and are willing to pay more for more generous alternatives. (Recall that PPOs usually come with other restrictions on utilization as well in the traditional managed care environment.)

If setting prices did not affect providers' behavior, then the only "achievement" coming from price negotiations between MCOs and providers would be to lower the overall premium because the plan would pay less for each unit of service provided, and hence have lower benefit payments and thus can charge lower premiums for the insurance coverage. But price negotiations do more than that—they affect the quality of services that doctors and hospitals will provide and such negotiations can also alter the mix of services provided by altering relative prices of different procedures.

On the question of quality of service, we can understand readily the relationship between quality and price in many standard consumer purchases, ranging from restaurant meals to guitars to automobiles and homes. We should expect nothing different in health care. Chapter 9 details mechanisms by which not-for-profit hospitals will select output, price, and quality when facing consumers with standard insurance plans. MCOs alter that arrangement by bargaining on price with the hospital but leaving the hospital able to alter quality and quantity within the constraints provided by the price bargaining. A review of Figures 9.1 through 9.3 (with the altered perspective of a hospital negotiating with an MCO) would be a good idea at this point.

The same effect of price negotiations on quality will hold also for physician firms and other similar providers; for example, if the PPO bargains for a lower price, one ready response for the physician firm would be to shorten the time of each patient visit. Other characteristics of quality will also change in response to a lower fee from the insurance plan, including (in the longer run) upgrading the medical equipment in the office, the inventory of available supplies, the quality of furniture in the waiting room, and, indeed, even the number of magazines (and the degree to which they are current) in the waiting room.

PPOs must also attend to the question of *relative* prices among services (unless they are a POS model that pays providers on a capitation basis). Rogerson (1994) develops a formal mathematical model of the problem in a structure almost identical to that posed in the discussion of quality, quantity, and hospital preferences in Chapter 9. He concludes that when a payer with significant market power (a large PPO or Medicare, as the next chapter discusses) sets prices for individual services, the not-for-profit hospital will respond by adjusting quality in a specific way: For those goods for which demand is not quality sensitive (one might think perhaps of urgent care where the consumer had little time to contemplate alternative choices), the hospital will lower quality and hence cost (relative to the price offered by the PPO or Medicare) and capture a higher "margin" to help support other hospital goals. In those services for which demand is very sensitive to quality (one might think of highly predictable events such as childbirth), the hospital will maintain high quality.

Intervention in Specific Treatment Choices

Another class of interventions occurs at the time specific medical decisions are made. In general, the interventions discussed previously for patients (copayments, gatekeeper, etc.) and providers (selection of providers through profiling, holdbacks, price setting) all take place "in the large." Many MCOs also use two types of interventions for decisions "in the small" to help control medical costs.

Prior Authorization Particularly for expensive interventions (surgery, hospitalization, major diagnostic tests), many MCOs require that the physician receive prior authorization from the insurance plan. Often approval is routinely granted, but sometimes with limits attached. For example, a hospitalization may be authorized for a length of stay of X days, at which point if the doctor wishes to extend the stay, further authorization is required. Although often granted by the MCO, the demand for the authorization sometimes tips the balance in the doctor's decision making about discharging the patient to home or not. The "hassle" of getting the authorization offsets the gains from extending the stay, hence sometimes leading to reduced length of stay. These protocols can also help MCOs establish "norms" for treatment that help control costs.

Denial of Payment Another powerful device for MCOs to control costs is denial of payment, probably the most controversial of the various cost-control devices. Unlike prior authorization mechanisms (about which the patient and provider know in advance of treatment), denial of payment takes place *after* treatment has been rendered. In that case, either the doctor (and hospital) or the patient (or some mix of them) has to "eat" the costs of treatment. The spectre of denial of payment leads physicians to be very cautious about venturing into treatment protocols for which the risk of denial of payment looms as a possibility. Because they materialize after treatment has already been rendered, the conflicts they cause between MCOs and the provider and patient can be considerable.

There exists, of course, a fuzzy boundary between denial of payment and denial of treatment through prior authorization. In many cases, refusal of an MCO to authorize a treatment is described as a denial of payment. Sometimes even the process of making a decision about whether to deny authorization or not can lead to major disputes. One of the landmark cases in the area of patients suing MCOs over denial of treatment centered on the time lapse between a request for treatment and the actual decision (see the discussion of MCO liability in Chapter 13 for details).

WHICH INTERVENTIONS WORK BEST FOR MANAGED CARE?

Among this extensive array of interventions ("tools") that managed care can use to control costs, which matter most in terms of expenditure control? In an in-depth study of a particular medical condition (acute heart attacks), Cutler,

McClellan, and Newhouse (2000) (CMN) found a provocative and potentially important conclusion (if the result generalizes to other illness conditions). Using claims data from a set of Massachusetts health insurers (staff model HMO, PPO, and indemnity plans), they studied the rates of use of various types of treatment for acute myocardial infarction (AMI) and ischemic heart disease (IHD, a milder form of heart disease) and the prices paid for those services.

Selecting a specific and generally unpredictable medical event (AMI) prevents a problem bedeviling other comparisons of managed care versus indemnity insurance: "self-selection." As discussed in Chapter 10, sickly individuals tend to seek better insurance. (Insurance companies also will want to find ways to identify sickly people and either charge them more or induce them to enroll elsewhere.) Thus, it is widely understood that the average managed care patient is healthier than the average indemnity patient. By studying what happens when these patients actually have a heart attack, Cutler et al. could bypass most of these "self-selection" issues.

What they found will surprise some people. Basically, the AMI patients received about the same types of treatment in all types of health plans studied, in this case including hospitalization rates, average lengths of stay, cardiac catheterization (a specific study of blood flow to arteries supplying the heart), bypass surgery, and angioplasty (various procedures to open clogged arteries without surgery). The cost savings from the managed care approach came almost entirely from the price per unit of service negotiated.

Overall, the average payment from traditional indemnity plans for AMI patients was $38,500. For PPO plans (which basically have only the price tool at their disposal), the average was $26,500 (about 70 percent of the indemnity plan level). For HMO (more aggressively managed) plans, the average was $23,600 (about 60 percent of the indemnity plan level). This occurred despite the HMOs actual use of invasive procedures (bypass surgery and angioplasty) slightly more often than the indemnity plans (in contrast to the typical stereotype of managed care "stinginess" about treatments).

CMN found similar patterns for treatment of patients with IHD; the average reimbursement for IHD patients was about $7,000 for indemnity insurance, $5,000 for PPOs, and $4,000 for HMOs. The patterns and proportions are quite similar to the AMI results: The PPO paid about 70 percent of the costs paid by indemnity plans, and the HMOs about 60 percent.

Two facts from these studies stand out. First, given the already widespread growth of managed care plans in the market, it would appear that managed care has already squeezed out a considerable level of "fat" in the prices for health care. Second, about three-quarters of the possible gains from "managing" care come from simple price negotiation and the remaining quarter from actual "management." It is dangerous, of course, to draw broad generalizations from the study of only two disease conditions in one region, but these results at least begin to shine some light on the overall question asked by CMN: "How do managed care plans do it?"

LONG-RUN ISSUES

As one might expect, when a major change such as managed care sweeps across a market, a number of subsequent changes will reverberate through the market, particularly in "input markets" that may require longer time periods for adjustment. Hospitals experience lower demand for their services, and either convert to other uses such as long-term care or actually close (see Chapter 9). The new insurance organizations will also experience growing pains as they experiment with different cost-control strategies to find out which are more effective, which annoy providers and/or patients too much, and which cost more to implement than they return in value.

As MCOs grow and solidify their hold on the insurance market, we can look ahead to various long-run consequences in health care markets. These include effects on physician location and retirement and the behavior of insurance markets themselves.

Physician Incomes, Geographic Distribution, Mobility, and Retirement

The market for physician services has been particularly stressed by the arrival of managed care. In part because of general incentives and in part because of the specific choices of MCOs to emphasize primary care (versus specialty care), the relative financial status of primary and specialty providers has been turned somewhat topsy turvey, particularly in markets with large MCO penetration. This in turn should ultimately affect specialty choice for physicians in training, retirement decisions, and the like. We can observe some of this happening already.

One way to look at the long-run outcomes is to compare the staffing patterns of traditional group-practice (salary, staff model) HMOs with the U.S. health care system as a whole. Although the pure staff model HMO is far from the favorite of consumers in the U.S. market, it sets a benchmark of personnel utilization that is worth understanding. Table 11.5 shows the staffing patterns of various HMOs and compares it with the U.S. physician supply in a similar year (1992). (The U.S. mix is quite similar now because the stock of active physicians changes relatively slowly even if the flow of new graduates were to change abruptly in its mix, which has not occurred.)

The data shown in Table 11.5 approximate the equilibrium demand for physician services in a strongly managed care environment. They show an important decline in the utilization of specialists of all types. If we extrapolate

TABLE 11.5 COMPARISON OF HMO STAFFING PATTERNS WITH NATIONAL PHYSICIAN SUPPLY

	HMO Staffing[a]				
	Seven Kaiser Plans[b]	Kaiser Portland[c]	GHC Seattle[d]	1992 U.S. Supply[e]	U.S./HMO Ratio[f]
Total	111.2	136.8	121.7	180.1	1.5
Primary care	53.6	56.3	57.1	65.7	1.2
Medical subspecialties	11.8	14.7	11.5	17.8	1.4
Surgical subspecialties	27.8	33.0	34.3	43.8	1.4
Hospital based	9.7	16.5	—	22.0	1.7
Other	10.2	12.3	—	20.3	1.8

[a]All figures represent full-time equivalent physicians per 100,000 population. Totals and subtotals may include some subspecialties not listed.
[b]1983 data from four to seven Kaiser Permanente sites (depending on specialty).
[c]1992 data from Kaiser Permanente Portland HMO, staff model HMO with 378,000 members. Primary care includes "urgent care" physicians.
[d]1992 data from Group Health Cooperative of Puget Sound, staff model HMO with 475,000 members.
[e]Nonfederal patient care M.D. and D.O. physicians, excluding residents and fellows in training.
[f]Ratio of the fourth column to unweighted average of HMO data from the first three (or two) columns.
Source: Weiner (1994, P. 224).

these data to the United States (a risky enterprise because these are staff model HMO data, not more popular PPO and IPA staffing arrangements), as the demand for specialists declined, those with multiple $100,000 earnings would find their annual incomes plummeting and perhaps even reach the stage of unemployment. We must view these data with some caution because the staffing mixes reported in Table 11.5 are more than two decades old, but the general conclusion about physician supply probably stands, even if future patterns of physician demand do not perfectly match those appearing in this table.

Medicare's payment schemes instituted in 1992 will enhance these trends because they lower the earnings of specialists emphasizing procedures (surgery, etc.) and increase the earnings of doctors emphasizing cognitive skills (internists, family practice doctors, etc.). Chapter 12 discusses the Medicare payment reform known as Resource-Based Relative Value System. However, here we can study separately the effect of managed care growth on physician earnings.

In one study, for example, Simon, Dranove, and White (1998) used sophisticated statistical models to assess the changes in physician earnings using data collected by the American Medical Association (AMA) on physician practices (a 1 percent sample using telephone interviews with a 60–70 percent response rate annually). They conclude that managed care penetration into a market enhances *primary care* physicians' earnings significantly and in parallel significantly cuts into the earnings of a group of hospital-based specialists (radiologists, anesthesiologists, and pathologists, or RAPs) by comparable amounts. Specifically, each 1 percentage point increase in MCO market share in the insurance market added $2,263 to the annual earnings of primary care doctors in their study. Because the markets saw MCO market share rise by more than 15 percentage points in the time period they studied (1985–1993), they estimate that these primary care doctors experienced an average increase of about $34,000 per year due to MCO growth, a 50 percent growth from their base income average of $69,000. By contrast, RAPs experienced a $1,993 decline per percentage point increase in MCO market share, for an overall "hit" of about $30,000 a year.

Economic theory (and the evidence we saw in Chapter 7 in the discussion regarding Table 7.2) tells us that physicians tend to locate in ways that equalize earning opportunities across regions. Greater MCO penetration into markets did affect the mobility of some physicians, but not all: Younger physicians were more likely to move in the face of an influx of MCOs than older doctors. This is as we would expect; they have more time to "amortize" the costs of the move than older physicians (Escarce et al., 1998). Specialists were more likely to move than generalists (in accord with the notion that generalists, if anything, experience positive income outcomes from MCO growth). Other types of physicians seemed unaffected in location decisions by MCO growth in the market (Polsky et al., 2000). As one might expect, those physicians who moved generally headed toward markets with the same or lower MCO penetration, with few moving to a market more intensively populated by MCOs.

The same set of authors report that large MCO penetration into a market caused many physicians to retire early, with results varying by specialty (Kletke et al., 2000). Not unexpectedly, older physicians were most likely to move to retirement, and among that group, both generalists and medical/surgical specialists opted for earlier retirement. As an example of the magnitude of this effect, they compared the retirement probabilities of generalists in a high-HMO penetration market (45 percent) with a low penetration market (5 percent) and found that retirement probabilities were 13 percent higher in the high-penetration market than in the low-penetration market. Medical/surgical specialists' retirements differed by 17 percent in the same comparison.

Market Segmentation

In Chapter 10, we explored the issues originally posed by Rothschild and Stiglitz (1976) regarding the possibility that health insurance markets might "separate" into submarkets for low- and high-risk consumers. The restrictions on access to care that are the cornerstone of cost management in MCOs may do exactly that.

To begin this discussion, return to Chapter 10 and the discussion surrounding Figures 10.7 and 10.8. The key idea there (reworked slightly from Rothschild and Stiglitz' original presentation) is that insurance companies have difficulty in identifying relatively healthy and relatively sick individuals. One mechanism insurance companies have to accomplish this (and hence regain the ability to charge a premium to the sickly individuals that will reflect their higher health care use) is to limit the degree of insurance coverage to the point at which sickly people find the more-generous plan desirable, even at a higher premium. The cost of this arrangement (in social welfare terms) is that the relatively healthy people in the population find their coverage opportunities limited (at prices reflecting their generally lower cost health outcomes).

Could the restrictions on managed care plans serve the same role? The essential feature of all MCOs is to restrict (or deny) access to care in myriad ways (second opinions, gatekeeper arrangements, denial of payment to providers in ambiguous cases, etc.). These are precisely the sorts of restrictions that a very sick person would find particularly undesirable, and a relatively healthy person would find relatively less obnoxious (because they are sick less often). Does the selection of health plans by people follow this sort of model?

Glied (2000) reviewed two dozen published studies on the issue of selection in MCOs. The primary method of identifying "sickly" and "healthy" individuals in these studies was to look at prior year medical spending as a measure of the propensity to get sick. Her summary of this literature states that "overall, the results of selection studies suggest that managed care plans in the private sector tend to enjoy a 20–30% prior utilization advantage over conventional indemnity plans while Medicare plans enjoy a similar advantage over traditional Medicare", p. 745.

These results suggest that the primary outcome of MCOs may not be to control medical cost so much as to create a viable mechanism by which insurance carriers can identify relatively healthy people and attract them into an insurance plan that sickly people will find relatively unappealing. If so, then the MCOs provide a crisp mechanism for achieving the sort of market segmentation that was discussed in Chapter 10 using the example of "copayment" as the selection device.

To date, we have no strong randomized controlled trial data to show the effects of various MCO strategies on utilization and cost control, and, indeed, it seems unlikely that such studies will appear in the near future. The problems in conducting a "definitive" study, either using a prospective randomized controlled trial (RCT) format or careful econometric analysis, seem formidable because the array of possible "management tools" is so large, and the combinations of them employed by MCOs will make it almost impossible to define the effects of any one of these strategies cleanly.

SUMMARY

Managed care organizations in their various flavors have emerged as a potent force in the U.S. health care market. The evolution should not come as unexpected. Traditional insurance plans help protect consumers from the financial risk imposed by illness but in turn create incentives for overconsumption of medical care that ultimately drive up medical spending (both quantity and quality) beyond a desirable point. Nor should it come as a surprise that in a market-driven economy such as that in the United States, inventive entrepreneurs create alternative organizations that deal with the risk and at the same time provide mechanisms to control the spending.

Numerous types of MCOs have emerged during the past two decades to compete with traditional insurance and with the "pure" staff-model HMO that was the only viable alternative to FFS insurance for decades. We now have an alphabet soup of IPAs, PPOs, and POS plans, and now IDS as various models. All seek to accomplish the same goals: protect the consumer against financial risk while controlling the incentives for overuse of medical care. The tools available to accomplish this include incentives placed on the patient (copayment, gatekeeper requirements, second opinion programs), on the provider (holdback mechanisms, provider selection), and on individual medical events (prior authorization, denial of payment).

Each of these mechanisms to control cost comes with some inconvenience to patients, providers, or both. How much inconvenience U.S. consumers of health care are willing to tolerate has yet to be determined and will certainly change through time. (Avoidance of inconvenience is likely a luxury good and will increase as U.S. per capita income grows.)

RELATED CHAPTERS IN *HANDBOOK OF HEALTH ECONOMICS*

Chapter 13, "Managed Care" by Sherry Glied

Chapter 27, "Antitrust and Competition in Health Care Markets" by Martin Gaynor and William B. Vogt

PROBLEMS

1. Identify the key distinctions between a staff-model HMO and an IPA model HMO. Which of these models do you think will have more ability to reduce utilization, and by what mechanism(s) do you think this will occur?

2. Suppose you were advising a PPO about selecting doctors to join the "panel" of approved doctors. What characteristics of physicians might you seek out? (*Hint:* Think of the physician-specific variations from Chapter 3; think of malpractice

propensities of some doctors; think of patient satisfaction with their care and how the doctors' behavior could affect that.)

3. Would you expect enrollment in managed care to increase or decrease in the future, presuming that future trends include (a) increasing technology available to treat illnesses, which would of course bring with it (b) increasing cost of medical care, which would be accentuated by (c) increasing per capita income over time (as a general trend)?

4. Discuss the potential value of second-opinion programs in light of what you know (see Chapter 3 for a refresher) about the variability of physician practice patterns across regions. If a second-opinion "consultation" comes from a doctor in the same geographic region as the original opinion, is it more or less likely to agree with the first doctor, compared to having the second opinion drawn from a wholly separate region?

5. Gatekeeper models of MCOs require patients to see a primary care doctor before going to see a specialist. What two key economic principles would be involved in a successful gatekeeper program? (*Hint:* One of these involves "technical" matters, and the other involves incentives to providers.)

6. If MCOs continue to grow in market share (compared with traditional FFS insurance), what do you think the consequences will be for physician incomes (in general)?

7. If MCOs contine to grow in market share, what do you think the consequences will be for the specialty mix of physicians?

CHAPTER 12

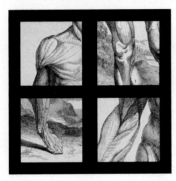

Government Provision of Health Insurance

In 1965, capping decades of political and legislative turmoil, the U.S. Congress passed and President Lyndon Johnson signed a law adding Titles XVIII and XIX to the Social Security Act. Title XVIII created a universal and mandatory health insurance program for the elderly called *Medicare,* subsequently expanded to include persons permanently disabled for at least two years and persons with otherwise fatal kidney disease (so-called end-stage renal disease, or ESRD) who need kidney dialysis treatments or transplants to remain alive. Title XIX created federal-state partnerships for states to establish health insurance plans for low-income people, broadly called *Medicaid.* These amendments to the Social Security Act created several important changes in our society, both politically and economically. As a political step, they changed the role of the U.S. government in the provision and control of health care, increasing its scope and presence considerably.

LEARNING GOALS

- Learn the basic features of federal insurance programs (Medicare, Medicaid, and SCHIP) and how, when, and why they emerged in their particular forms.

- Understand the economic implications of these program design features in terms of demand, risk management for individuals, and cost.

- Follow modifications to Medicare payment mechanisms to hospitals (DRG, diagnosis-related group, or program) and physicians (RBRVS program) and understand the economic and health impacts of these programs.

- Learn how capitation programs (HMO, PPO, etc.) work in Medicare and Medicaid, and understand how risk-adjustment mechanisms can affect the viability and value of such programs.

The economic consequences of Medicare and Medicaid were only poorly understood initially, in part because no clear picture existed about the effects of insurance on demand for medical care at the time the law was under discussion (1964 and 1965). Thus, when Medicare and Medicaid actually took effect in July 1966, nobody had the really clear ability to predict what would happen. In retrospect, almost nobody understood the effects on demand in the short run or the long-run effects on demand for technology.

As time passed, the increase of costs in Medicare and Medicaid became *the* dominant issue in federal health policy discussions. Before Medicare and Medicaid had reached their twentieth birthdays, their structures had changed importantly to limit dollar outflows from the federal treasury. These changes have, in turn, spawned changes in the structure of private insurance.

The first changes (instituted during the Nixon administration's price controls) attempted to control costs by limiting the fees doctors and hospitals received for each procedure. Later changes were more radical, shifting the payment base for hospital care from the smallest of procedures the hospital billed for to a single payment for each admission. As we shall see, this shift in payment precipitated large structural changes in the health care delivery system in the United States. Some states even shifted their Medicaid systems to a capitation system, in which providers received a single payment for a year's worth of care for a Medicaid recipient.

More recent changes have not merely altered the way basic Medicare programs are administered but also have added major new programs. The original program included the mandatory Part A for hospitalization insurance and voluntary Part B for physician services. In 1997, as part of the Balanced Budget Act (BBA), a new Part C, Medicare + Choice, was added, expanding the ways in which Medicare enrollees could use private sector insurance in lieu of Medicare's basic plan. The same legislation also created the new program Supplemental Children's Health Insurance Program (SCHIP). Finally, in 2006, a new Part D added prescription drug insurance.

The Centers for Medicare and Medicaid Services (CMS), successor to the Health Care Finance Administration (HCFA), administer all of these programs.[1]

To understand the effects of Medicare and Medicaid and the importance of some of the changes in their structures, we first need to develop a clear

---

[1]Although for many years notoriously slow in creating reports on the health care system it administered, CMS now has an active and lively statistical reporting system on line, located (as of this publication date) at www.cms.hhs.gov/home/rsds.asp, which can produce enough data to bury even the most sophisticated analyst. Many useful summary data, generally up-to-date within approximately two years, are available through this site. For example, in 2008, most of the data tables were current to 2005.

picture of how these plans were originally structured. Then we can portray the changes in their structures through time.

It is also important sometimes to delve into the detail of program structure and administration to thoroughly understand the economic implications of these programs. Thus, the discussion that follows will be a blend of history, description, and economic analysis.

THE MEDICARE PROGRAM

Initial Structure

When Medicare was originally put in place, its designers had two options to which they could turn for comparison—the private U.S. health insurance market and foreign health care systems. Most foreign systems involve a degree of nationalization (e.g., government ownership of hospitals) that probably would have proven politically unacceptable in the United States.[2] Instead, Medicare's designers turned unabashedly to the private health insurance in force during that period for a design template.

The template had a fairly standard appearance for the time: Hospital care would receive highest priority, with coverage beginning from the moment a person entered the hospital ("first dollar" coverage). Physician care would be paid under a "major medical" concept, with an initial deductible to accrue annually, a coinsurance provision to help control costs, and a "usual, customary, and reasonable" fee schedule to set provider fees.

The Medicare program had two parts: Part A paid for services provided by hospitals. Enrollment in Part A was mandatory for every person receiving Social Security benefits (including those over the age of 65, plus people who are "permanently disabled"). The entire cost of Part A is paid by the Medicare Trust Fund, a separate government account funded by additions to each worker's current-year Social Security tax.

Part B (covering physician services), called *Supplemental Medical Insurance,* was made voluntary, although the premiums paid by enrollees were so low that enrollment has been very nearly 100 percent from the beginning of

---

[2]Since the administration of Franklin Roosevelt in the 1930s, some people have actively sought a comprehensive national health insurance (NHI) plan. The closest the United States has come to this probably occurred during the Truman administration in 1948–1952, but NHI proponents were unsuccessful then, and their political advantage waned during the postwar years of prosperity during the Eisenhower administration (1953–1960). Subsequent attempts to achieve NHI came during the administrations of Presidents Nixon, Carter, and Clinton, all without success. The issue was also a focal point in the 2008 presidential election.

the program. At the outset, the program's planners had little idea how much the program would actually cost, but they intended the Part B premium charged to enrollees to cover about half of the Part B program costs, in order to get the largest possible enrollment. (The monthly premium at that point was a now-incredible $3 per month.) At present, the premium to enroll in Part B is set at approximately one-quarter of the anticipated cost and had risen to $96.40 per month as of 2009. Had the individual's share of Part B costs remained at 50 percent, this would now be almost $200 per month, 70 times higher than the initial level in 1965, representing a 13 percent compound annual growth rate for every year since the program's inception.

Hospital Coverage At the time of Medicare's design, the predominant insurance for hospital care was through Blue Cross, which had historically offered 30, 60, or 90 days of coverage for hospital care, and nothing thereafter. Insurance sold by for-profit commercial insurance companies had also grown considerably, so by 1965, the group insurance market was nearly evenly split between the Blues and commercial insurance. The model set by the Blues still held considerable sway, and Medicare adopted the Blue approach directly.

In its initial design, Medicare Part A paid for hospital care in the following way *for each episode of illness* of the patient:[3]

Day 1: Patient pays U.S. average cost of hospital care.

Days 2–60: Medicare pays 100 percent of hospital charges.

Days 61–90: Patient pays 25 percent of average U.S. cost per day; Medicare pays the remainder.

Days 91–150: Patient pays 50 percent of average U.S. cost per day, drawing down a "lifetime reserve" of 60 days.

Day 151 and beyond: Medicare pays nothing.

The first-day "deductible" cost for hospitalization tracked directly with average hospital costs until 1987, at which point Congress set it at $520 and established a different formula for its update. Since the 1987 formula was put into place, changes in the Part A deductible have closely tracked overall changes in the Consumer Price Index, so (for example) by 2009, the Part A deductible had reached $1,068, double the original value, while the CPI index had increased by 90 percent in the same period.

---

[3]Episodes of illness begin when the patient enters the hospital and end when the patient is discharged. If the patient is readmitted within a week of discharge, Medicare rules consider it the same episode of illness. This prevents doctors and patients from "gaming" the Medicare system to eliminate copayments, for example, by discharging a patient after 59 days and readmitting him or her the next day.

From the viewpoint of standard economic models of insurance demand, this structure of hospital insurance is completely "upside down" because it provides nearly "first-dollar" coverage but offers no serious protection against "catastrophic" (very large but rare) financial risks. (Review the discussions on risk aversion Chapter 10 if the logic behind this statement is not apparent to you.) We discuss the two responses to this risk—private supplemental insurance and (later in this chapter) the provision of catastrophic coverage by Medicare.

Physician Care

The Part B coverage of Medicare actually includes a much broader range of services than physician care, but the great majority of Part B benefit payments occur for physician services. Medicare planners had two prototypes available within the private health in insurance market in the United States after which they could model Part B. One model would have used the traditional Blue Shield approach, providing nearly full coverage for physician services, but only for hospitalized patients. The alternative model came from the "major medical" insurance sold mostly by commercial carriers. Under this approach, essentially all physician services would be covered (both in and out of the hospital), but the participants would have an annual deductible to meet before coverage began and a coinsurance rate for all services. The Medicare Part B program closely followed the "major medical" model.

Under the structure of the initial Part B plan, Medicare paid for doctor services (as well as some prescription drugs, medical appliances such as wheelchairs and crutches, etc.) with a very traditional insurance model, encompassing a $50 annual deductible, a 20 percent coinsurance rate, and a fee schedule by which providers would be paid. Congress increased the annual deductible to $60 in 1973, to $75 in 1982, and then to $100 in 1991, where it has remained until a recent change to $135.

The inflation-adjusted deductible that would equate to the original 1965 level of $50 per year would now be near $350 because the CPI increased by almost a factor of seven between 1965 and 2008. Thus, the "real" deductible has fallen substantially through time and is now less than 20 percent as large (in buying power) as it was in 1965. Put differently, the equivalent deductible in 1965 would be about $10, rather than the $50 chosen by the Congress. This can have important effects on the use of medical services under Part B by Medicare enrollees.[4]

---

[4]Review the RAND HIS results concerning the effects of a deductible on health care use from Chapter 5.

Program Additions Through Time

Since the original legislation in 1965, several major additions to Medicare have been made; most important are the two major changes in 1997 and again in 2006. We will explore these new programs next.

MEDICARE HMOs (MEDICARE ADVANTAGE)
How They Work

In 1997, as part of the BBA (the same legislation creating the SCHIP program), Medicare extended the ways people could enroll in various HMO plans.[5] Medicare Advantage allows eligible members to enroll in various private insurance plans in lieu of using standard Medicare coverage. These plans must cover at least the same services that Medicare covers, but they need not cover them in exactly the same way. The most prominent of these choices is the Medicare HMO, a "classic" capitation insurance plan as described in Chapter 11. Medicare (PPOs) and even Medicare Fee for Service plans also emerged under Medicare Advantage, but the most common enrollment choices are the classic HMO plans.

When a Medicare-eligible person enrolls in a Medicare HMO (or PPO or—FFS—plan), Medicare pays a fixed monthly amount per capita (varying by region) to the plan for each enrolled person (per capita payment), and the plan in turn provides all medical care for the enrolled individuals. The capitation payment varies by region (and is of course adjusted over time), but—importantly—it also contains higher payments known as *risk adjustments* for people with known expensive medical conditions. Without this provision, the plans would, of course, actively discourage enrollment of all but the healthiest people.

Risk Adjustment

When Medicare Part C was created in 1997, the payment to Medicare HMOs used an average adjusted cost per case, but the adjustments employed only two factors: regional differences in costs and demographic mix of the enrollees (age and gender). The BBA of 1997 required that a more refined risk-adjustment measure be phased in beginning in 2000.

---

[5]The 1997 BBA legislation named the program *Medicare + Choice* (commonly M + C), and it officially became Part C of Medicare (beyond the Part A hospital coverage and Part B physician coverage plans). The name changed again in 2003 legislation to Medicare Advantage, the current moniker.

At the time of the phase in, it was clear that enrollees in Medicare HMOs were healthier on many dimensions (e.g., self-reported health status, numbers of chronic conditions, functional mobility) than the average Medicare population (Aber and McCormick, 2000). Before risk adjustment began, patients enrolling in Medicare HMOs actually increased total program expenditure (opposite from the desired effect) because the HMOs were paid essentially an average cost per enrollee while treating patients with better than average health.

When the initial risk adjustment began in 2000, Medicare capitation payments to the plans fell by significant amounts. Some Medicare HMOs left the industry; enrollment in them fell (see Figure 12.1) as these new payment rules were implemented—in part because providers withdrew and in part because changes in offering services probably caused some enrollees to switch back to standard Medicare coverage. But as Medicare realigned the risk-adjustment methods in 2004, particularly with a more refined risk-adjustment system based on clinical diagnoses (Pope et al., 2004), enrollment in the Medicare Advantage plans again began to increase and now has more than 8 million participants (of 44 million Medicare enrollees).

These results show just how much risk-adjustment systems matter. Figure 12.1 has three distinct time periods that exemplify different aspects of risk-adjustment methodologies. In the first period (1998–2000) without risk adjustment, Medicare overpaid the HMOs (which happily competed for enrollment among Medicare beneficiaries). During the second time period (2000–2004) during which the initial risk adjustment system was operational, payment to Medicare HMOs fell, some plans withdrew (the number of plans offering Medicare HMO services fell from more than 400 to less than 250), and enrollment plummeted from about 7 million to about 5.3 million in 2003.

FIGURE 12.1 Total Medicare Private Health Plan Enrollment, 1999–2007.

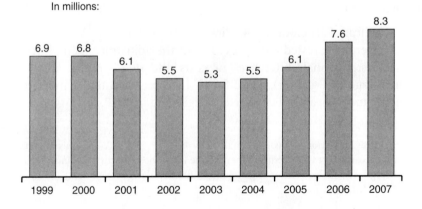

In millions:

1999	2000	2001	2002	2003	2004	2005	2006	2007
6.9	6.8	6.1	5.5	5.3	5.5	6.1	7.6	8.3

In 2004, the beginning of the third period, Medicare shifted to a more refined adjustment system that HMO plans viewed as more reasonable, and rapid entry into the field occurred (the number of Medicare contracts with private firms rose from 240 to more than 600 in just five years), and enrollment increased from 5.3 to 8.3 million people.

According to recent reports (Kaiser Family Foundation, 2007), although the large share of Part C enrollees chose a classic HMO or a PPO plan, the most rapid growth has occurred in the Medicare Fee for Service (MFFS) plans, which had 1.3 million enrollees of the 8.3 million in all Medicare Advantage programs at the time of the report (2007). In any event, about 20 percent of all Medicare enrollees in 2008 used a plan authorized by Part C rather than traditional Medicare enrollment with steady increases in enrollment in recent years.

The Supplemental Children's Health Insurance Program

Save the women and children first. . . .
Old Sea Chantey

Of particular concern to federal policy makers in recent decades has been the high rate at which children in the United States go without health insurance. The presumption is that uninsured children often did not receive the benefits of early preventive care (checkups, vaccinations, etc.)—medical interventions that often have among the lowest cost per quality-adjusted life years (QALYs—see Chapter 3) of any known medical interventions. Of particular concern were children in families with incomes too high to qualify for Medicaid but nevertheless with low access to private health insurance (most notably provided through employment groups), a group often called *tweeners* in policy discussions. The Supplemental Children's Health Insurance Program (SCHIP) legislation was enacted in 1997 to help bridge this gap. SCHIP had a 10-year horizon and authorized a total of approximately $40 billion for federal contributions, after which a refinancing bill was required in 2007 (more about this later).[6]

SCHIP (like Medicaid) operates as a federal-state partnership with each state designing its plan and the federal government setting ground rules and assisting in the financing. On average, the states pay 30 percent of total program costs and the federal government pays (on average) the remaining 70 percent, but the program (like with Medicaid) requires a higher sharing rate for states with high per capita income. By law, the federal share for SCHIP varies

---

[6]SCHIP was part of the BBA of 1997.

from 65 percent (for the highest income states such as California and New York) to 85 percent for the lowest income states. (By contrast, the Medicaid share that the federal government pays span's from 50 percent to 75 percent.)

As with Medicaid, states with high per capita incomes tend to design and fund more generous SCHIP programs. Although the formula seemed as intended to funnel money to low income states, federal contributions actually are larger on a per capita basis to high income states than low income states.

Under the 1997 legislation, states have three ways to improve coverage for children in this "tweener" group. Each state can provide SCHIP through its Medicaid program, establish a wholly new SCHIP program, or use a combination of the two. Because of this three-pronged approach, a meaningful assessment of SCHIP's success or failure cannot be made on its own but by measuring the numbers and rates of uninsured children in the United States before and after the program's creation.

The results hearten supporters of SCHIP, but a review of the actual proportion of children without insurance (the "non-coverage rate") (see Figure 12.2) shows that the program has eliminated less than one-third of the uninsured children in the country. The United States has about 73 million children in the relevant age group (under 18), so the initial levels of uninsured children—about 11 million—represent about 15 percent of that population, and the steady state levels of about 8 million uninsured children represent about 11 percent of the relevant population.

FIGURE 12.2 Uninsured and Government-Insured Children

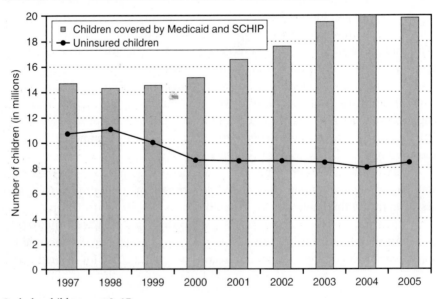

Includes children ages 0–17.
Source: U.S. Current Population Survey, 2006

The other observation from these data concerns the apparent substitution of government for private insurance. While the number of uninsured children declined by about 3 million during the program's first eight years, the number actually covered by Medicaid *and* SCHIP rose from about 14 million to about 20 million for an increase of 6 million children. The gap between the increase of 6 million enrollees and the reduction in the uninsured of 3 million children formed the crux of the 2007 reauthorization debate.

The 2007 Reauthorization Battle—Substitution and Crowding Out

The 2007 reauthorization of SCHIP proved to be a memorable political battle with important economic consequences. As has been noted (and carefully studied with regard to Medicaid, the SCHIP program's generosity expands as the per capita income in states expands. The original 1997 legislation targeted families below 200 percent of the official Federal Poverty Line (FPL) (a number that changes annually and varies by family size) but allowed exceptions in both directions. To identify eligibility, most states (26) used the 200 percent rule, some (15) have a higher limit, and a few (9) used a lower number, the lowest being 140 percent. Some states wished to expand that limit to 350 to 400 percent of the poverty line, and the legislation passed by both houses of the U.S. Congress included that expansion. However, President George W. Bush vetoed the legislation (twice), and the Congress could not muster the necessary votes for an override.[7]

The political debates in 2007 regarding inclusion centered in many ways on the extent of *crowding out,* the situation in which the availability of public insurance programs reduces the demand for private insurance. Expanding the income eligibility for SCHIP would clearly increase the extent of crowding out by SCHIP for private insurance. The debate in part centered on "how much," which in turn hinged on the nuanced difference between *substitution* and *crowding out.* By usual definitions, *substitution* means dropping private coverage immediately when public coverage is acquired.

One study of the NY SCHIP program (Shone et al., 2007) based on interviews with SCHIP enrollees found that only 7.5 percent of SCHIP enrollees had actually given up private insurance when they enrolled in SCHIP.

Crowding out encompasses a wide set of behaviors, including direct substitution as well as anything else that reduces the use of private insurance. For example, a person might change jobs from one employer who offered insurance coverage for children (higher benefits and lower wages) to another who offered higher wages but not the good benefit of insurance for children. The

---

[7]Thus, compromise legislation that extended SCHIP for three years with previous rules about eligibility was finally passed and signed in late 2007.

family then enrolls in SCHIP. This change would be classified as a crowding out event, not a substitution.

The Congressional Budget Office has estimated that "between a quarter and a half" of SCHIP enrollment in its first decade represented crowding out (CBO, 2007). A recent analysis by Gruber and Simon (2007) that assessed crowding out more broadly indicates that crowd out rates could be as high as 60 percent when entire families are considered, although their work does not apply directly to SCHIP.

As one might expect, crowding out increases as the income eligibility level increases for a program such as SCHIP. Private insurance coverage, of course, is closely linked to income through the standard mechanism of employer-group insurance; that is, people who have jobs have more income and more accessible insurance. Thus, when the 2007 reauthorization bill sought to increase the income limit for the SCHIP program from 200 percent (as originally written) to 400 percent (thereby doubling the income at which families would be eligible), the crowding out issue became central. One analysis (Winfree and DeAngelo, 2007) estimated that crowding out rates would increase from 34 to 42 percent (in the under 200 percent of poverty group) to 54 to 60 percent in families with incomes between 200 percent and 400 percent of the federal poverty level.[8]

Crowding out is a key issue in debates not only about SCHIP but also about any government program and affects the way both economists and politicians think about ways to design a universal insurance program in the United States, a topic to which we will return in Chapter 16. To politicians, the issue is often phrased in terms of "fairness" language (e.g., if wealthy people take advantage of programs designed to help the poor, is it fair?). Depending on their political persuasion, politicians may also view this as a public sector versus private sector issue.

Beyond these considerations, economists often also consider the efficiency with which public programs achieve their stated goal. Crowding out represents one form of inefficiency, but paying for things people would purchase on their own is another. The federal income tax subsidy to private health insurance provided through employment groups is another. The debate often hinges on whether the subsidy creates an incentive to change behavior on the margin or is (in contrast) inframarginal, in which case incentives do not change. These issues arise in almost any discussion of governmental programs for which a private alternative exists.

---

[8]The federal poverty level varies with family size, and the levels are set annually by the U.S. Bureau of the Census. For 2008, the level for one person was about $10,500, a number which approximately doubles as family size rises to four and then doubles again for a family of nine or more.

Part D Prescription Drug Insurance

Part D of Medicare presents several enigmas. First, why is prescription drug coverage desirable now when it was not in 1965 when the original Medicare legislation was enacted, or for that matter, in 1988, when the Medicare Catastrophic Care Act was passed (and then rescinded in 1989)? Second, why does Part D have a strange donut hole in the coverage?

Let's first look at the reasons drug insurance became part of the formal structure of Medicare. Recall that in 1965 when Medicare was enacted, out-of-hospital prescription drugs constituted a relatively small part of the total health care budget, and few high-expense drugs were the treatment of choice for disease conditions. In other words, out-of-hospital drugs really did not create much financial risk for patients. So what happened? Technical change!

New drugs evolved in the time after Medicare's introduction in 1965 that could treat medical conditions that had been untreatable or conditions for which surgical intervention had been the only choice. The array of such new drugs is almost dizzying but includes, for example, those to control cholesterol (hence avoid heart surgery), to avoid or control ulcers (also avoiding surgery and/or psychiatric treatment) and heartburn (also sometimes avoiding surgery), to prevent fertility, to enhance fertility, to avoid erectile dysfunction, to treat cancers, to avoid the side effects of cancer drugs, to treat AIDS, to treat depression and schizophrenia, and on and on. These new drugs (see Chapter 15 for further details) are expensive to develop and test, their purchase created new and significant financial risk to consumers. Remember that these risks do not necessarily appear in the average medical spending per capita. Prices for many drugs fell through time, reducing the financial risk for persons using those drugs. But new drugs also appeared on the scene that were very expensive, and for people using these drugs, the financial risk increased. The demand for insurance (and also the political pressure to cover prescription drugs within Medicare) depends on the financial risk (variance) not the average amount of spending for the entire population.

Because risk creates demand for insurance, increased financial risk should create demand for drug insurance. Indeed, not only did most private insurance for the under 65 population cover prescription drugs by the time the U.S. Congress began to consider prescription drug coverage in Medicare, but also Medigap policies had commonly included prescription drug coverage (see the following discussion about Medigap plans). Thus, both the commonality of the coverage in private insurance plans and the increasing financial risk from prescription drug use made the inclusion of prescription drugs more compelling within Medicare. While the Congress included prescriptions in the failed Medicare Catastrophic Coverage Act of 1988 (repealed in 1989), Part D really created the first broad prescription drug coverage within Medicare.

How Part D Functions Medicare Part D is voluntary; enrollees pay for premiums, and low-income individuals receive a substantial federal subsidy. The average monthly premium for basic Part D coverage began in 2007 at about $30 per month with steady increases scheduled over time. The program has large deductibles ($275 per year initially, also scheduled to increase regularly) and a 25 percent coinsurance up to an "initial coverage limit" of about 10 times the deductible ($2,510 in 2008), at which point the "donut hole" appears, and coverage goes away until the individual has spent about 15 times the original out-of-pocket deductible (about $4,050 in 2008). Using 2008 figures, to reach the initial coverage limit of $2,510, an individual will have spent $275 for the deductible and 25 percent of the remaining $2,510 ($558.75) for an out-of-pocket total of $833.75. The individual must then spend another $3,216 (approximately) before catastrophic coverage kicks in. All of these numbers increase with scheduled adjustments year by year, so the interested reader will have to search the Internet to find current values.

Part D's insurance plan is very unusual in that its design was created to balance between offering usable insurance coverage and controlling federal spending within the Medicare program. (The federal subsidies for low-income individuals create the federal budget outlay that is of concern to planners.) The program offers catastrophic protection to persons with very large annual drug expenses but not to people with intermediate to large expenses (about $2,500 to $5,700 in total drug costs). Other designs would control the spending (e.g., with even larger deductibles), but politicians who created the actual medicare Part D structure apparently sought something that would immediately affect many Medicare enrollees, so they created the "donut hole" model.

Private Supplements to Medicare: "Medigap" Insurance

Medicare Part B called *supplemental insurance* is voluntary, but because it is so highly subsidized (by law, the annual premium to enrollees is now set at 25 percent of the expected cost), almost everybody in Part A also enrolls in Part B. However, another type of supplemental insurance is less common but important to understand in assessing the economic value of Medicare: private supplemental insurance, generally called *Medigap*. About 10 million Medicare enrollees (a bit less than a quarter of the total) subscribe to these private plans to supplement their Medicare coverage.[8]

---

[8]A somewhat larger number of Medicare enrollees have supplemental private insurance as a retirement benefit from previous employment, but this has become an increasingly uncommon employment benefit, and this number is likely to shrink through time.

The word *Medigap* implies (correctly) that Medicare coverage leaves some large holes or gaps in the spectrum of coverage. The hospital coverage under Part A creates some risk by providing increasingly less coverage for long hospital stays, and eventually an individual who has a very long hospital stay can actually run out of coverage. In addition, individuals can face large daily copayments even with hospital stays as short as 61 days of a single hospitalization, higher ones after the 90th day, and even higher ones after the 120th day. Part B also creates some significant risks, most notably with the open-ended 20 percent copayments for physician and surgeon fees.

The original Medicare program did not cover any out-of-hospital prescription drug expenses, leaving another large financial risk, which was of increasing importance as expensive new pharmaceuticals became the treatment of choice for many illnesses. While the introduction of Part D resolved some of these financial risk issues, its structure (as noted previously) has the large donut hole when drugs are not covered, an issue of particular concern for individuals with chronic illnesses who need regular and expensive drug treatments.

Medigap policies "fill in the gaps" through private insurance contracts. Designed expressly to do this task, Medigap policies often have a complex array of choices. Medicare originally defined 10 standardized plans (labeled Plan A, ... Plan J), all of which "picked up" the Part A and B deductibles and copayment to some degree with plans that pick up either 100 percent, 75 percent, or 50 percent of the charges not paid by Medicare (depending on the plan chosen). With Part D Medicare now available for prescription drugs, Medigap plans do not offer drug coverage, but two new standardized plans (K and L) offer more limited coverage initially but eventually have a "stop loss" feature that limits out-of-pocket expenses for covered individuals to $2,220 for an individual or $4,440 for a family.[9] These plans are the first plans available to Medicare enrollees that have an absolute "stop-loss" feature built into them.

The annual premiums for Medigap policies vary not only according to the plan chosen but also to the region of the country because of regional differences in medical practice patterns and expenses incurred by enrollees. According to one survey of Medigap premium costs,[10] the average across the nation in 2005 ranged from about $1,150 to about $1,750 for plans without prescription drug coverage, with striking differences across regions. For

---

[9]These limits closely match spending limits (stop-loss features) in the major federal insurance initiative for under 65 persons, the health savings account or consumer-directed health plan programs.

[10]Business Wire, August 29, 2005, "Striking Differences Persist in Medigap Premiums Despite Identical Benefits."

example, in Plan C (the most generous of the plans not covering prescription drugs in 2005), the national average premium was $1,766, with an overall low premium of $698 and a high of $9,798 — a 14-fold difference. While some of this can be attributed to regional differences in medical care use (see discussion in Chapter 3), the lack of competition in some of these markets surely plays an important role as well.

The key issue involving Medigap is the underlying risk remaining within the standard Medicare program. If basic Medicare contained good stop-loss provisions, few people probably would buy Medigap insurance. And, because Medicare HMO plans (which promise, like pure HMOs in the under 65 market, to cover all needed medical care for a fixed annual fee) create the stop-loss function through other mechanisms, researchers have found that higher Medigap premiums in a region lead not surprisingly to more Medicare HMO enrollment (McClaughlin, Chernow, and Taylor, 2002).

Another feature of the Medigap plans reflects an important economic issue. Because of the risk of self-selection—that is, people with worse health status seek better insurance coverage—there is a risk that the Medigap market might unravel (see the discussion of market failure in insurance markets in Chapter 10). Medicare policy makers require that insurance plans using the term *Medigap* not only offer policies with the standard coverage definitions (as discussed earlier—plans A through L alphabetically) but also have annual periods of open enrollment when anybody can enroll for the same premium (for a given plan).[11] Albeit only in specific times, this approach mandates the same "community" rating for all individuals and represents a good example of regulation that attempts to improve market functioning when otherwise market failure risks loom large.

OPERATIONAL CHANGES IN MEDICARE

Since its inception, Medicare has undergone numerous operational changes, almost all of which have the obvious intention to reduce Medicare outlays. The changes in Medicare through time included the following (with the year these changes appeared):

- Fee limitations for doctors (1972).
- Per diem limits set on hospital reimbursements (1972).
- Required Part B enrollees' premiums to cover one-quarter of average program costs.

---

[11]This is similar to the rule for Medicare Advantage (Part C) enrollment in private Medicare HMOs, PPOs, and MFFS Plans.

- Changes in the ways doctors can charge higher than the "allowed fees" (1983).
- Shifts from per service to per admission payment for hospitals—the Prospective Payment System (October 1983).
- Shifting to a new physician compensation system (resource-based relative value system) (1992).

Limitations on Fees

Remember from Chapter 7 that physicians commonly charge different prices for the same service, so a broad dispersion of fees generally prevails in a single geographic area. This dispersion creates a problem for insurance carriers. They must decide what is the "right" price to pay for a doctor office visit under the insurance plan, for example. The problem becomes more acute when one realizes that the dispersion in prices *might* be related to quality, and it *might* be related directly to monopolistic or monopolistically competitive pricing practices (Schwartz and Wilde, 1982a).

At its inception in 1965, Medicare paid for doctor services under Part B using a technique following directly from private insurance ideas—a "usual, customary and reasonable" concept of private insurance carriers. Medicare's terminology uses the terms *customary* and *prevailing. Customary* refers to the fee at the 50th percentile of the distribution of fees each doctor charges, so half of each doctor's fees lies above and half below that doctor's customary fee for a given procedure. *Prevailing* is a concept that locates *each* doctor's fee within the overall fee distribution in the community. Medicare used the 75th percentile in the distribution of fees within the community to define *prevailing.* If the doctor's customary fee exceeded the prevailing fee for the same service, Medicare paid only the prevailing fee. This fee screen, which by definition affects 25 percent of all doctors' bills, constituted essentially the only limit imposed by Medicare on payments to physicians in its initial structure.

All of this relatively hands-off policy, as discussed in the preceding paragraph changed abruptly in 1971 when President Richard Nixon instituted some economywide price controls, beginning with a 90-day freeze on all prices and wages on August 15 of that year, followed by a series of controls that limited the rates at which prices could increase. While these controls were soon lifted for the remainder of the economy, two sectors—petroleum and health care—remained controlled, with ongoing limits on the rate at which fees could increase.

The Nixon era price controls generally allowed physicians' fees to increase from their historic level (which varied, remember, from physician to physician) at a rate determined by a "cost index" designed (if not perfectly) to reflect the costs of a physician-firm's business. More specifically, changes in the "prevailing fee" screen in each region of the country were limited beginning in 1972 to changes in the Medicare Economic Index, a weighted average of overall inflation, changes in the costs of physicians' practices, and changes in the overall earnings level of the country.

A second change occurred as a part of the Omnibus Deficit Reduction Act of 1984. Physician's fees were frozen again until the beginning of 1987, at which time a complicated series of rules allowed some doctors to increase their fees somewhat, while placing very strict limits on others. The important distinction was whether the doctor had chosen to become a "Medicare participating physician," a topic we discuss in the next section.

The fee schedule arrangements under Medicare produce additional financial risk for patients (Ruther and Helbing, 1980), but they also increase the incentives for patients to undertake comparison shopping. How much they actually do shop still remains unknown, but probably not much, given the dispersion in prices that Medicare's data reveal.

Medicare Assignment of Benefits

The economic consequences of fee limitations depend in part on another apparently arcane part of Medicare law, known as *assignment of benefits*. Medicare pays for 80 percent of the doctor's fee *up to* a schedule of "allowable" fees determined for each region of the country. If any doctor's fee is higher than that allowed fee, the effective insurance coverage can fall. For example, if the allowed fee is $80, Medicare Part B would pay $64. If the doctor's actual fee is $100, Part B would still only pay $64. If the doctor's fee is $50, Part B would pay $40.

Physicians have had the option to bill the patient for any balance above the Medicare payment (called *balance billing*). However, if they do this, they must collect the entire fee from the patient, and the patient submits the charge to Medicare for reimbursement. Alas for the doctor, some patients do not pay their bills. The physician-firm can circumvent much of this risk by taking "assignment of benefits," whereby the patient signs over the payment of the Medicare fee to the physician-firm. Thus, the doctor is virtually guaranteed the payment of the 80 percent share of the Medicare-allowed fee and must try to collect only the remaining 20 percent from the patient.

Physicians must balance two economic forces in making this choice. If they accept assignment, they may be forced to accept a lower total fee, but they collect it with higher probability. If they do not accept assignment of benefits, they can charge higher fees but may not be able to collect all of them.

Physicians should be more willing to accept assignment the closer their own fees are to the allowed fee from Medicare. Indeed, if the doctor's fee is lower than the Medicare-allowed fee, the doctor can lose nothing by accepting assignment. In addition, the doctor should be more eager to accept assignment of benefits if the chances of default by the patient are high. One study of physicians' acceptance of assignment of benefits found all of these phenomena actually occurring. Physician-firms accepted assignment of benefits less often when patients were deemed less likely to default (i.e., higher income of the patients in each firm's practice and less unemployment in the area), and they were less likely to accept assignment the higher the fee they would normally charge exceeded the Medicare allowed fee (Rodgers and Muscaccio, 1983). The proportion of claims for which doctors accepted assignment varied over time and space, but, on average, it would not be misleading to say that about half of the claims were "assignment of benefits" and half were direct billing to patients.

Beginning in late 1983, Medicare introduced the concept of "participating physician," which altered the way assignment of benefits takes place. Before this change, physicians had to decide on a case-by-case basis whether to accept assignment or not. If they designate themselves as participating physicians, however, they *automatically* accept assignment of benefits for all patients. Of course, if they don't become participating physicians, they still have the option to accept assignment on a case-by-case basis.

A substantial majority of physicians chose to become participating physicians because of the important carrot-and-stick arrangement built into the program. The government had earlier frozen the fee structure of physicians (i.e., locked into place their profile of allowed fees). For physicians who did elect to become participating physicians, Medicare increased the allowed fees at a rate faster than that for nonparticipating physicians. The incentive worked. The assignment rate (including those from participating physicians), which had hovered in the 50 to 55 percent range for years, jumped to 69 percent of all claims submitted by doctors the year the rule was changed, and the assignment rate has now reached almost 90 percent, with almost 95 percent of covered charges coming through assigned claims.

This increase in assignment of benefits flows naturally from the rates at which physicians signed participation agreements (and are thus obligated to accept assignment of benefits). At the beginning of the relevant period (1983), only 30 percent of all Medicare-active physicians had signed agreements to be participating physicians, and these doctors accounted for a mere 36 percent of claims to Medicare. However, a scant decade later, the participation rate had increased to 60 percent, and those doctors accounted for more than 85 percent of all claims to Medicare. (The remaining assigned claims came on a case-by-case basis from nonparticipating physicians.) What happened can now be seen clearly in retrospect: When Medicare put the major economic "carrot" (being the unfreezing of their fee schedules) in front of the most active physicians in the Medicare program, those who joined were those most active in treating Medicare patients.

The Prospective Payment System (PPS)

Beginning in October 1983, Medicare radically changed the way it paid hospitals for care delivered to patients.[12] The "old" system had paid hospitals on the basis of activities performed for each patient: an hour of operating room time, five physical therapy visits, 20 doses of an antibiotic, a disposable enema kit, or a day in an intensive care unit. Each had a price that appeared on the patient's bill.[13] Additional days in the hospital each received an additional charge for room and board, plus all of the associated billings from physicians for those days. While average hospital length of stay declined systematically after the inception of Medicare (from about 13 days in 1965 to less than 10 days in 1982), almost certainly due to technical progress in medical science, the change in Medicare's structure initiated in fiscal year 1984 abruptly altered the incentives for U.S. hospitals.

The new approach, phased in over a 4-year span, began to pay hospitals on a per case basis rather than a per item or per service basis.[14] For the first time, doctors and hospitals treating individual patients were confronted with a fixed budget for the care of each patient.

We can put this type of payment in perspective by returning to the models used in Chapters 8 and 9 about hospital behavior. Think for a moment about a hospital treating only Medicare patients. With the old-style insurance, Medicare patients would exhibit a demand curve that was nearly price insensitive, and hence quite "steep" in appearance, as shown, for example, by D_2 in Figure 10.5.

The PPS essentially offered a fixed price per hospital episode to the hospital, which we would draw in a figure such as Figure 9.2 as a flat line, cutting

---

[12]The federal government operates on a fiscal year (FY) that begins in October of the previous year. Thus, FY 1984 was the first year of the PPS system, although it began in the autumn of 1983. This system introduces some possibility for confusion when interpreting time-series data because some show calendar years (for which the last quarter in 1983 has PPS in effect) and some show fiscal years, which are "pure" for purposes of evaluating PPS.

[13]Medicare paid according to a formula known as "ratio of costs to charges applied to charges" (RCCAC) that formed the actual basis of payment. However, the key idea was that each item or service used led to an additional billing by the hospital.

[14]During fiscal year 1984, 25 percent of the hospital's payment was based on the national (PPS) norm, and the remaining on hospital-specific prior year cost rates, adjusted as allowed by government rules. In fiscal year 1985, the mix went to 50 percent hospital and 50 percent PPS, and in the next year, the mix shifted to 75/25. By November 1987, seven weeks into fiscal year 1988, the system was 100 percent on the PPS system.

across the price-quantity diagram just as we would normally draw a market price confronting a price-taking firm. In other words, the Medicare PPS system makes the demand curves confronting the hospital very price elastic in the sense that the hospital can get "all the business it wants" at the price offered by Medicare but no business at a higher price. The hospital, as the model in Chapter 9 describes, would pick the quality such that the demand curve was tangent to an *AC* curve, and this would define the quality of the hospital's offering. Of course, if the demand curve is completely price elastic (i.e., a flat line), then that tangency would occur only at the point of minimum average cost. By setting prices in this way, the PPS system at least potentially forces hospitals to operate efficiently (at minimum *AC*), and it determines the quality of care by the level of price offered.

The prices actually offered by Medicare come from a system known as *diagnosis-related groups* (DRGs) that assigns each patient admitted to the hospital to one of a fixed number of groups (the current list has about 500 DRGs). The payment for a patient within any DRG varies somewhat by region and hospital type (e.g., teaching or nonteaching), but from the hospital's point of view, the price per *admission* is fixed. The hospital in most cases receives the same revenue from Medicare no matter what is done to the patient during the hospital admission or how long the patient stays in the hospital.[15]

The physician who admits the patient to the hospital is now put in a quite different position than was the case under the former payment scheme. Previously, the doctor could undertake any procedure or prescribe any service or device that might benefit the patient. The hospital would be paid (by Part A), the doctor would be paid (by Part B), and the patient would feel that "everything possible" was done to effect a cure. Under the new arrangement, the hospital stands to lose money, perhaps a large amount of money, if the doctor continues treating patients in the old style because each resource used costs the hospital money, but the added revenue under the new plan is zero.

Length-of-Stay Effects Hospital medical staffs in this situation face a problem similar to that of the group practice first described by Newhouse (1973): Each doctor's attempt to save money brings only a small proportional reward. However, the medical staff of a hospital somehow *must* respond to

---

[15]The exceptions occur for patients who stay in the hospital an extremely long time relative to the average for patients within the DRG. Those patients become "outliers," and the hospital begins to be paid on a basis quite similar to the old per service system for continued care after that point. Although this outlier system is an important component of the DRG system from the hospital's point of view, it represents a complication that we need not focus on here.

the incentives generated by Medicare's new DRG system, or the hospital runs the risk of going broke, particularly if it is a relatively expensive hospital to operate.[16]

The most obvious dimension of adjustment for the hospital and its doctors is to shorten length of stay (LOS) for patients. It is easy to monitor, providing something that committees of doctors can review readily. Guidelines on LOS are easy to develop and interpret. Doctors who systematically deviate from such guidelines could come under pressure from other members of the medical staff to respond.

All such efforts would be fruitless, of course, if doctors had no discretion in length of stay. However, we know from overall hospital use data that length of stay differs substantially by region. Thus, we have good reason to believe that *if the hospital's medical staff can find a way to coordinate doctors' behavior,* LOS would fall in response to the DRG incentive.

Apparently, hospitals were successful in achieving such coordinated effort. Data from the Health Care Financing Administration (see Table 12.1) show the remarkable declines in LOS among Medicare recipients. Without doubt, the DRG system under PPS was extremely successful in its goal of reducing hospital lengths of stay, as the data in Table 12.1 demonstrate.

To put these changes in proper context, recall (from footnote 14) that the PPS system came in as a phased plan, whereby in the first year, only 25 percent of a hospital's costs were determined prospectively, and 75 percent retrospectively (i.e., based on the hospital's own historic costs). This phase-in period essentially ended at the end of fiscal year 1986, so fiscal year 1987 represents a year when the incentives no longer were becoming tighter.

One study of Medicare spending in both Part A (hospital care) and Part B (physician services) found that government spending had fallen in 1990 in Part A by $18 billion, about a 20 percent savings over what would have otherwise been anticipated, with no offset in Part B spending (Russell and Manning, 1989).

The changes in LOS are all the more remarkable when one understands that a considerable volume of medical and (particularly) surgical activity that had previously been done within hospitals shifted to the outpatient setting with a fast-rising trend in "dry-cleaner" surgery.[17] Hospital admissions fell at an annual rate of 2.5 percent for people over 65, so by 1988, a mere five years after the DRG system had been installed, overall Medicare admissions to hospitals declined by 13 percent. A large percentage (perhaps more than half) of

---

[16]Actually, even if the hospital has been "doing well" under the DRG system, it can still make more money by reducing LOS and ancillary expenses. These "profits" would allow the hospital to advance its other goals.

[17]"In by 9:00, out by 5:00."

TABLE 12.1   TRENDS IN LOS FOR MEDICARE PATIENTS IN SHORT-STAY HOSPITALS

	LOS (Days)	Percent of Change from Previous Year
Calendar years		
1967	13.8	—
1970	13.0	−3.8
1975	11.2	−2.6
1980	10.6	−0.9
Fiscal years		
1981	10.5	−0.9
1982	10.3	−1.9
1983[a]	10.0	−2.9
1984[b]	9.1	−9.0
1985	8.6	−5.5
1986	8.3	−3.5
1987[c]	8.5	2.4
1988	8.5	0
1989	8.9	4.7
1990	9.0	1.1
1991	8.7	−3.3
1992	8.5	−2.3
1993	8.1	−4.7
1994	7.6	−6.2
1995	7.1	−6.2
1996	6.6	−7.1
1997	6.4	−3.0
1998	6.2	−3.1

[a]Tax Equity and Fiscal Reform Act (TEFRA) rules in place.
[b]Phase in of prospective payment system (PPS) begins.
[c]Phase in of PPS complete.

these reduced admissions simply meant that a surgical procedure had been shifted to an ambulatory surgical center (ASC), a new technology experiencing phenomenal growth in the 1980s.[18] The ASCs obviously pull from the hospitals patients who would otherwise have had a very short length of stay. This means that the average LOS of those remaining patients has fallen considerably more than the Medicare aggregate data show.[19] In fact, this quite likely

---

[18]See Box 9.1, Figure B, for relevant time-series data.

[19]Some simple calculations suggest that the decline in LOS has been as much as 20 to 25 percent for the remaining Medicare patients. Problem 1 at the end of this chapter explores the mathematics of this problem.

accounts for the growth in LOS in fiscal years 1987 through 1990 shown in Table 12.1.

The U.S. hospital system had another push to reduce length of stay for Medicare patients beginning in FY 1993 (as Table 12.1 shows) and most dramatically occurring during FYs 1994–1997. What was happening here? As the PPS came into full force, hospitals' accommodations in LOS brought them to a position of a generally positive "margin" on Medicare patients, peaking in 1984–1985 at about 13 percent "profit rate." That margin plummeted and for all U.S. hospitals had essentially reached zero by 1989 and fell to −2.4 percent by 1991 (Guterman, 2000). Apparently in response to this major financial pressure, hospitals began to move to reduce LOS even further, leading to the burst of effort particularly in the 1994–1996 period. In response, hospitals' profit margins again moved up to 15–17 percent by 1996 and 1997. The government's response to this improved financial position, which we shall study in more detail later, was to squeeze the U.S. hospital system again through the BBA of 1997, a piece of legislation with such profound effects that it has its own section later in this chapter.

Use of Other Services One reason why doctors were able to adjust the LOS for their patients is because the process of producing "health" allows for substitution. In terms of hospital length of stay, for example, one can substitute more intense treatment within the hospital, and one can also use nonhospital facilities as an alternative site of care. This clearly mattered considerably in reduced LOS in Medicare patients. In the first 3 years of the Medicare PPS system, use of skilled nursing facilities (SNFs, pronounced "sniffs" among the cognoscenti), a standard Medicare benefit, increased by 5.2 percent, 12.8 percent, and 5 percent, respectively, for a combined increase of 23 percent. Use of home health care, another standard benefit, increased by even more during the same period.

Finally, Medicare added a temporary benefit for hospice care in 1983 and made it permanent in 1986. This provides a low-technology "caring" environment for dying patients as an alternative to dying in the intensive care unit of a hospital (at the other extreme). Hospices emphasize supportive services such as home care; pain control; and psychological, social, and spiritual services rather than attempts to cure the patient. The annual number of patients using hospices under Medicare funding has increased to almost 1 million per year and now appears to represent about two-thirds of all persons with Medicare who die.[20]

---

[20]About 1.5 million people in Medicare's population die each year. Thus, the 1 million hospice users constitute about two-thirds of dying persons. Most of these hospice sources are provided by hospitals and nursing homes.

Sicker and Quicker? An obvious issue in the PPS system is the potential effect on patients' health. Numerous opponents of the program implemented by Medicare made dire predictions about deleterious effects on patients' health outcomes. We have substantial reason to believe in advance that such concerns were not valid—the wide variations in length of stay across different regions of the country did not create any obvious differences in longevity or other measures of health, for example. Nevertheless, the government-mandated commission set up to monitor the effects of the PPS system, known as the *Prospective Payment Assessment Commission* (ProPAC), had spent considerable effort documenting what effects, if any, the shorter stays generated by PPS might have on patients' health.

One indicator of poor outcomes for patients is the rate at which they are readmitted to the hospital.[21] The rate of readmission to the hospital within 30 days, a standard indicator of "poor outcomes," is about the same under PPS as in the previous 5 years. Readmission rates had been increasing systematically through time, in part due to the increasing average age of the Medicare population. However, the rate of increase slowed during PPS years, indicating that the incentives to reduce LOS had not contributed notably to any behavior that would cause readmissions to increase.

Another indicator of poor outcomes for patients is mortality. Particularly because of the incentives to discharge patients early, a common measure of mortality is the death rate within 30 days of a hospital discharge. This comparison is not so obvious as it might seem because two conflicting forces have altered mortality rates through time. Improved technology has reduced the overall mortality among the Medicare (elderly) population from 6.6 percent per year (at the beginning of the program in the late 1960s) to 5.1 percent by the time PPS was introduced. This represents, of course, a period of time when the average age of the Medicare population was increasing, both through socio-demographic effects and because of the increases in life expectancy due to technological change. Thus, trying to predict effects of the PPS on mortality requires holding both of those things constant. The mortality outcomes during the first years of the PPS are completely consistent with the belief that no change occurred in mortality due to the PPS.

A separate analysis of mortality rates within selected disease categories shows the same general result (Kahn et al., 1992). In five high-mortality disease categories (congestive heart failure, acute myocardial infarction, fractured hip, pneumonia, and stroke), mortality rates actually declined in a

---

[21]Recall that the hospital cannot benefit financially by discharging patients and then readmitting them to collect a new DRG payment because if the readmission takes place within 7 days, it is counted as the same spell of illness, and hence the hospital receives no new DRG payment.

comparison of years just preceding and just following the introduction of PPS in three of the five disease categories, and was statistically unchanged in the other two. The ALOS in the patients in these disease categories fell by 24 percent in the comparison, making the mortality results all the more remarkable. While patients were discharged (on average) in less-stable condition, this did not result in worse mortality outcomes. It now seems that implementation of PPS did not create any systematic degradation in patients' health and safety, despite the reduction in LOS.

Consequences for Hospitals The PPS system creates a dramatic change in the financial environment of hospitals in the United States. One might expect that some of them will fare poorly and others well in such a system. The whole idea of PPS was to put a financial squeeze on "expensive" hospitals and make them become more efficient and to put a stronger sense of market control into an industry that had, in many ways, lost contact with normal economic forces.[22] What can we now say about the results, having seen PPS in place for a quarter of a century?

Without a doubt, the downward pressure on hospital use affected hospitals' financial conditions adversely. Hospitals' net revenue margins (as a percent of total costs) had climbed steadily from 1970 through 1983, with a brief 2-year dip in 1971–1972 as a result of the Nixon-era price controls. That trend reversed itself in 1984, the first year of the PPS system, and continued through 1991, when hospital margins began to recover.

Hodgkin and McGuire (1994) analyzed the source of this downward pressure on hospital margins by assessing the rate of change through time in the average Medicare payment under the PPS system and the comparable changes in hospitals' costs. Three changes affected costs: changes in costs of goods and services the hospitals buy (wages, supplies, etc.), in hospitals' productivity (a cost-reducing change), and in the mix of patients. For the decade following the introduction of PPS, Hodgkin and McGuire calculated the year-by-year changes in hospitals' "exogenous" costs (those outside the control of the hospital, by and large). They estimated these cost changes in the range of 5.6 to 9.0 percent per year, while at the same time, the Medicare payment structure

---

[22]Many observers characterize the PPS system as an intense regulation, likening it to a price control. Others view it just as any other "contract" between a large buyer and its suppliers. Obviously, the force of government makes PPS different from private contracts, but the arrangement still has much in common with a normal contractual arrangement, perhaps more than it has in common with a "regulatory" regime. Perhaps most importantly, the PPS system does not directly alter the relationships that hospitals have with other insurance carriers or patients.

to hospitals was augmented by values between 0 and 5 percent per year, averaging about 3 percent per year. The consequent "squeeze" on hospitals led to the declining margins described earlier.

One possible response of hospitals is to decrease "intensity of treatment," not only through reduced length of stay but also through other changes in treatment as well (such as the frequency of physical therapy, frequency of laboratory tests performed, etc.). Studies both by ProPAC (1989) and Hodgkin and McGuire (1994) show that intensity fell significantly for Medicare patients, and in fact began to fall at the very beginning of the phase in of PPS, apparently as a cost-reducing measure in anticipation of the full force of PPS.

The downward pressure on hospital margins (as noted) turned around in 1991, and hospitals returned to a period of considerable per case profitability from 1991 through 1997. The change came with improved operating efficiency from the U.S. hospital industry, as the responses to the PPS squeeze came into full force. Costs per Medicare case had followed a steady uptrend from the inception of the PPS program until 1991, when suddenly costs per case flattened off and actually declined slightly in the early 1990s. Medicare's formulas for reimbursement did not keep up with this shift from the previous trend and continued to climb along the previous path. The result was an improving profit margin on Medicare cases that peaked in 1997 at about a 17 percent margin.

This lush profitability, combined with a steadily degrading fiscal position of the Medicare Trust Fund (the funds set aside to fund Medicare payments in future years), led the U.S. Congress to respond with the 1997 BBA, to be discussed shortly in a separate section. At this point, it suffices to say that the BBA "recaptured" the improved profitability of U.S. hospitals for the Medicare Trust Fund, and drove operating margins of many U.S. hospitals back into the red in a few brief years.

Hospital occupancy rates fell throughout the country, from pre-PPS levels of about 72 percent (national average) down to less than 65 percent. Tables 12.2 and 12.3 show the basic data. They represent the combined effect of declining lengths of stay (both for Medicare and patients under 65) and changes in hospital admissions. Many observers had felt that hospitals would accelerate their admissions in the PPS era (or at least try to get their medical staffs to cooperate to do so), using the general concept of "induced demand" as the tool and the motivation of lost profits per case. However, as the models of hospital behavior in Chapter 9 suggest, behavior in this realm can be anything but easy to predict in the world of not-for-profit behavior. As the overall payment level from Medicare declines relative to costs (as Hodgkin and McGuire, 1994, demonstrated), some hospitals could choose to reduce admissions *and* quality in the face of these restricted payments. (Chapter 15, in the discussion surrounding Figure 15.5, addresses this issue in more detail when treating Medicare DRGs as a binding price control.) HCFA data, in fact,

TABLE 12.2 ECONOMIC CONSEQUENCES OF PPS BY YEAR

	Hospital Employment Annual Rates of Change (%)		Hospital Occupancy (%)	
	Total FTEs[a]	Inpatient FTEs[a]	Occupancy Level	Rate of Change
1980	4.7	4.5	75.9	1.9
1981	5.4	5.1	75.8	−0.1
1982	3.7	3.4	74.6	−1.6
1983[b]	1.4	0.8	72.2	−3.2
1984[c]	−2.3	3.5	66.6	−7.8
1985	−2.3	4.3	63.6	−4.5
1986[d]	0.3	1.4	63.4	−0.3
1987	0.7	−0.7	64.1	1.1
1988	1.1	0.7	64.5	0.6

[a]FTE stands for "full-time equivalent."
[b]TEFRA rules in place.
[c]PPS phase in begins.
[d]PPS phase in complete.
Source: ProPAC (1989).

show that Medicare admissions followed essentially the same pattern as Medicare LOS upon the introduction of PPS, but with a one-year lag before the response set in. Admissions fell about 6 percent in 1984 and about 10 percent in 1985, and then they stabilized at that new level.

The concurrent shift to ambulatory surgery in the population under 65 has accelerated both of these trends. Table 12.3 shows the declines in admissions by size category. The strong relationship between size and loss of patients emphasizes the nature of patients for whom this type of substitution is possible. Small hospitals typically carry out procedures that are relatively uncomplicated, and therefore these hospitals are much more susceptible to competition from ASC-like organizations. Although the Medicare PPS system may have contributed somewhat to the growth of the ASCs, it seems

TABLE 12.3 CHANGES IN ADMISSIONS, 1983–1985

Number of Beds	Percent Change
<50 beds	−22.0
50–99	−17.1
100–199	−11.4
200–299	−8.4
300–399	−5.1
400–499	−5.8
500+	−2.7

Source: Health CARE Financing Review (1989, Table 3.3).

clear that at least some of the economic hardship facing small hospitals comes from other directions than the PPS itself.

With much of the hospitals' costs fixed in the short run (see Chapter 8), these downward shifts in demand are bound to require a response from hospitals. One response hospitals have tried is to reduce costs. As Table 12.2 shows, hospital employment began to fall in 1984, the first PPS year, and has remained very stable subsequently for inpatient full-time equivalent (FTE) personnel. This is quite consistent with studies of hospitals in New York State that confronted the strongest regulatory pressure on revenues (Thorpe and Phelps, 1990).

The external financial market responded as well. Because hospitals in general cannot issue equity financing (because not-for-profit hospitals have no shareholders), bond financing remains by far the most important way of raising capital for these hospitals. Beginning in 1983, bond ratings (the capital market's measure of the financial stability of the lending hospitals) worsened dramatically. More than 300 bond issues had their ratings downgraded, compared with only 60 whose ratings have improved during this period (Pro-PAC, 1989, Figure 4.5).

The Balanced Budget Act of 1997[23]

As noted, the cycle of government action and hospital reaction has typified the course of cost control in Medicare almost from its inception. Initial hospital reimbursement mechanisms (full-cost reimbursement) led to cost increases far beyond any predictions at the time Medicare was implemented in 1965, leading to price controls in the 1970s, and finally the PPS system in the early 1980s (dramatically changing the incentive structure for hospitals). Hospitals adapted to this change through the 1980s, shortening length of stay and building into place a series of major cost-reduction programs in most hospitals throughout the land. The cumulative effect of these programs finally took hold in 1991 when the downward spiral in operating margins for Medicare patients ended. Costs per case remained flat or declined slightly for the remainder of the decade, but Medicare reimbursements continued to grow at previous rates. As a consequence, hospital margins again erupted into *very* positive territory, causing yet another Congressional reaction, this time the Balanced Budget Act (BBA) of 1997 (called the Bad, Bad Act by many hospital industry participants).

The essential feature of the BBA was a shift from planned increase in hospital reimbursement rates to significant reductions for a few years, with an intended "leveling off" after a large bite had been taken out of the system. PPS

---

[23]Recall that this legislation also created Medicare Part C and SCHIP, as discussed previously.

payments generally follow a cost-index ("market basket" of things hospitals have to buy to operate, including labor, supplies, etc.). The BBA specified that the rates of increase for 1998 through 2002 would be *below* market basket, allegedly returning to market basket levels in 2003.[24] The cumulative effect would be hospital payments under Medicare that were 5.6 percent lower than they would otherwise have been. Because many U.S. hospitals operate at general "margins" of just a few percent, it is clear that such major reductions in compensation could have significant effects on hospitals' profitability and even survival. Medicare's goal—to create $112 billion in savings over a 5-year period (and lower payments thereafter from the lower base that would remain)—of course came directly out of the revenue streams of the hospitals providing services to Medicare patients. In terms of increase, the goal was to cut the annual rate of increase in total Medicare expenditures from 8.8 percent (the baseline estimate of what to expect) to 5.6 percent. In fact, the annual growth rate from 1998 forward has been only 3.9 percent, partly due to the cuts made by HCFA in payment rates and partly due to other cost-cutting moves by hospitals.

It became clear that the payment reductions caused by the BBA greatly increased the financial problems of many hospitals in the United States. In response, the Congress amended the BBA in 1999 with the Balanced Budget Refinement Act (BBRA), adding back $11 billion in payments for the 2000–2002 period. This restored about 10 percent of the initial revenue reduction set out in the BBA. At this writing the effects of BBA and BBRA seem to have stabilized.

Physician Prospective Payment

The success of prospective payment in reducing hospital costs prompted the inevitable question: Why only hospitals? Indeed, Congress anticipated this issue when it initiated the Prospective Payment System system for Medicare hospital payment and at the same time authorized a series of studies of the potential benefits from prospective payment for other types of medical care, most notably, physician payment. It authorized the formation of the Physician Payment Review Commission (PPRC) in 1986 to provide recommendations about altering the way Medicare pays physicians.

Resource-Based Relative Values The first large study investigating ways to alter physician payment came from Harvard University's School of Public Health

---

[24]The deviations from market basket were set in the BBA as follows: 1998, 0; 1999, −1.9 percent; 2000, −1.8 percent; 2001, −1.1 percent; 2002, −1.0 percent. For subsequent years, 0.

in late 1988, which developed a series of relative values of various procedures performed by physicians and surgeons, called the *resource-based relative value system* (RBRVS).[25] We should not understate the complexity of this task; the standard coding system for physicians' activities, the Current Procedural Terminology (CPT), describes some 7,000 different activities that physicians might perform. The Harvard study actually gathered data on 372 of these procedures and extrapolated these findings to the remaining procedures.

The RBRV system has some similarities to a system originally developed by the California State Medical Association called the *California relative value system,* or *California RVS,* that had been widely used for years until banned by the Federal Trade Commission (FTC).[26] The California RVS described the relative worth of procedures within single specialties, but it deliberately avoided making cross-specialty comparisons. The RBRVS study deliberately made cross-specialty comparisons. The underlying logic of the method used by the RBRVS study was to produce what might be called "equal pay for equal work," or to pay physicians according to the time and complexity of their effort equally, whether the task at hand was neurosurgery, psychiatric consultation, or removal of warts.

The study drew the distinction between "invasive procedures" and "evaluation and management" (E/M), which corresponds (imperfectly) to the distinction between practice styles of surgeons and internists (respectively). The study's authors can apply their relative values to actual dollar charges and simulate the effects of using their payment plan, holding total Medicare outlays unchanged. *This assumes that the mix of services provided to patients in the long run remains unchanged.* The results were quite startling. Fees for many surgical procedures would fall by one-third to one-half. Fees for "cognitive" (E/M) services would rise by comparable percentages. According to their simulations, overall Medicare outlays for E/M services would rise by 56 percent and for invasive procedures would fall by 42 percent. Laboratory payments would fall by 5 percent, and fees paid for imaging (X-rays, CT scans, MRI scans, etc.) would fall by 30 percent (Hsiao, Braun, Kelly, and Becker, 1988; Hsiao, Braun, Yntema, and Becker, 1988).

---

[25]The study's result appeared in summary in the *New England Journal of Medicine* on September 29, 1988, and in considerable detail in the October 28, 1988, issue of the *Journal of the American Medical Association,* consuming the entire issue. The final report for the study at Harvard on RBRVS consumes four reams of paper per copy.

[26]The FTC banned the use of the RVS system because it thought it facilitated doctors' collusion on pricing. The argument was that doctors had to agree on only a single number—the dollar value of each RVS unit—and they then had a complete set of prices upon which they had agreed. The logic of this argument is incomplete; use of an RVS also simplifies the consumer's search problem, because it allows a complete understanding of any doctor's pricing structure simply by knowing the conversion factor from RVS units to dollars.

Now that the RBRVS system has been fully implemented (since 1996) several studies have appeared to show the actual impact of the system on physician incomes. The generalist fared about as well as predicted, with cumulative increases from 1991 (the year before RBRVS began) to 1997 (the year after it became fully implemented) of 36 percent in average Medicare payment rates compared with the Harvard study's pre-implementations estimates of 39 percent. Surgery-intensive specialists, although suffering declines, did not fare as poorly as had been originally predicted, in part due to successful lobbying for special treatment in the implementation phase of RBRVS. Cardiothoracic surgeons, for example, had a cumulative decline of 9.3 percent in average Medicare payment rates compared with a predicted decline of 35 percent. Ophthalmologists experienced an 18.4 percent decline compared with a predicted loss of 25 percent (Iglehart, 1999).

Still left unanswered are many of the most interesting and important economic questions regarding such a system, concerning (1) changes in the mix of medical interventions in the short and long run and, perhaps more importantly, (2) changes in the patterns of specialty training in the long run. In part, of course, the answers to these questions depend considerably on what private-sector insurance plans do in parallel. Their adoption of a payment scheme similar or identical to Medicare's RBRVS, would strongly reinforce the effects of Medicare's actions, particularly on long-run specialty choice.[27]

Episode-of-Illness-Based Payment Plans (Physician DRGs)

The RBRVS really does not enter the realm of "prospective" payment, because it still essentially pays on a per service basis. One could alternatively think of paying for physician services on a DRG-like system. The complexities of such a system seem considerable, however.

DRG payments "work" for hospital care because of three key things: (1) the episode is well defined, with a beginning (admission to the hospital) and an end (discharge); (2) only one economic agent (the hospital) delivers care that the DRG pays for; and (3) the DRG system is able to account for an important part of the overall variation in hospital costs. Without these factors, the PPS would be much more difficult to operate, and perhaps it would not be feasible at all. We consider the role of each of these in turn.

---

[27]Medicare graciously created a natural experiment regarding the importance of induced demand when the RBRVS system was implemented. The final section in Chapter 7 discusses some of the key studies using this natural experiment, notably those by Nguyen and Derrick (1997) and Yip (1998). Both studies found evidence of demand inducement.

Clearly Defined Episodes The clearly defined beginning and ending of the hospital episode seem crucial to operating a DRG-like system. In ambulatory care, particularly for patients with chronic illnesses, no such definition of an episode can exist. Thus, an episode-based PPS seems infeasible. It might still be possible to use such a system for inpatient care provided by physicians, but ambulatory DRGs seem completely impractical for this reason.

Multiple Economic Agents A second complexity arises when more than one physician takes care of a patient within an episode of illness, as commonly occurs both within and outside of the hospital. The only meaningful way to operate a DRG system is to have one physician payment for each illness, no matter how many doctors participate in the care. Otherwise, one has made no meaningful change from a per service payment system. This fact raises a second set of concerns, which has to do with which doctor gets the DRG payment. This matters considerably because, in effect, the doctor would become the "prime contractor" for the treatment and other doctors would become "subcontractors." This choice would likely affect, for example, whether "conservative" or surgical therapy would be recommended to the patient for some illnesses. Allowing the patient to designate who the "prime contracting" doctor is provides the greatest patient autonomy in these choices and may also be the only legally admissible choice because the Medicare benefits come to the patient initially, not to any doctor.

Potential Within-Group Cost Heterogeneity Medicare DRG payments work fairly well in the hospital inpatient setting, in part because the system of DRGs does not leave the hospital confronting major within-group variability in cost of treating patients. (The large number of DRGs and the "outlier" system described earlier deal with this problem.) Within-group reduction in patient illness variability makes the system politically palatable because it has a sense of face validity about it. Completely unknown is the ability of anybody to organize a comparable system for physician payments. In part, the complexity of defining such a system has deterred investigators from even attempting to study the problem. The first issue discussed—the absence of a clear time frame by which to define the "group" of treatments—is probably the most essential source of trouble.

Time-Based Payments (Capitation)

An alternative payment plan would use physician payments that were wholly prospective, no matter what the condition of the patient—a per year "capita-tion" system. Capitation plans are not new, of course. Prepaid group practice plans have used these arrangements for decades. A big gap still remains between those plans and a physician-based capitation system for Medicare. Although capitation provides, in many ways, the strongest incentives for controlling costs, it imposes a large financial risk on individual providers (at least in its pure form). Prepaid group practices get around this problem by enrolling large numbers of individuals and families—tens to hundreds of thousands of enrollees per plan. With enrollments per plan on that order, the law of large numbers begins to protect the plan with regard to overall variance of expenses because the variance in expense per member falls with the number of enrollees (see Appendix C to Chapter 10 for a discussion of the relevant statistics). However, with a single physician's practice, enrollees number only in the hundreds, and the financial risk that a pure capitation plan imposes on the physician is considerable. (A "pure" capitation plan would put the primary-care physician at risk for all health care expenses of the patient, or at least all nonhospital expenses.) Some sort of sharing of the risk seems inevitable, either through insurance arrangements, formation of large groups of physicians, or (most likely within Medicare) some sort of stop-loss provisions that would limit the per patient or overall risk of doctors involved in a capitation type of plan.

We should recall here that the Part A DRG plan, as it applies to hospitals, already includes a "stop-loss" provision for the hospitals for each hospital admission. If any patient's length of stay exceeds certain bounds (different for each DRG), the patient is declared an "outlier," and the hospital begins to be paid similarly to the old Medicare methods, that is, on a per unit basis. Some sort of protection such as this seems inevitable for any successful physician capitation system within medicine as well. Balancing that risk bearing with the appropriate incentives for the doctor is a step in the formulation of Medicare policy that has not yet been taken. Indeed, proposals to use capitation within Medicare for physician payments typically speak of capitation payments to insurance plans rather than to individual physicians.

Of course, all of Medicare Advantage (Medicare Part C) rests on the foundation of capitation payments to health plans to care for Medicare enrollees. The importance of having good risk-adjustment measures to avoid selection problems appeared clearly in regard to the history of Part C plans, first with no risk adjustment (and relatively healthy people enrolling in Medicare Part C), then with an initial adjustment that drove health plans out of the market, and finally (in 2004) a revised adjustment mechanism that has spurred the increase in health plans and enrollment (see Figure 12.1 and its discussion).

Global Payment Caps

A completely separate system for controlling doctors' fees has been proposed in recent years and has on occasion reached at least the level of committee approval in the U.S. House of Representatives.[28] The proposed system of global payment caps has (again) some roots in private insurance plans. Some IPAs have such overall limits on payments to their overall panel of physicians. Those IPAs' contracts with physicians, typically "hold back" a portion of fees (for example, 20 percent) that each doctor would normally receive. If overall physician spending within the IPA exceeds targeted amounts, the deficit is taken out before "hold-back" funds are returned to the physician.

As a financial device to control costs, global caps have both advantages and disadvantages. One of the advantages is that they allow the paying entity (insurance plan) a high level of guarantee about total costs for physician services. Unfortunately, the mechanisms to achieve this may almost guarantee that the overall limit is exceeded, possibly in a way that penalizes those doctors most who have made the biggest efforts to make the system "work."

To see the problem in its clearest detail requires the use of a mathematical model known as "game theory" (see Box 12.1). Nevertheless, the ideas are relatively simple and correspond closely to the standard "prisoner's dilemma." In the prisoner's dilemma, the usual story begins with two people (thieves or spies, for example) who have both promised each other in advance that if caught they won't squeal on the other. The dilemma arises when jailers take each prisoner aside and promise harsh treatment for not cooperating and lenient treatment for confessing in a way that implicates both prisoners. Because the prisoners have no ability to communicate (collude) with one another, the "best" private response for both prisoners is to defect from the original agreement—to squeal on their partner—and (a key idea) this is the best strategy regardless of whether the partner squeals or keeps quiet.

The physician payment problem differs somewhat, but not greatly. Suppose all physicians agree in advance to cooperate with the insurance carrier to keep costs down. Then each single doctor figures out her own optimal strategy, which involves charging the plan as rapidly as possible, no matter what other doctors do. If other doctors continue to "cooperate" to keep costs down, then the "fast-charging" doctor gets to keep all of the money billed, clearly coming out ahead. If all other doctors adopt the same strategy (collectively), they will trigger the holdback of the insurance carrier, and every

---

[28]The proposal was put forth in an overall deficit-reduction bill that passed the Ways and Means Committee in June 1989.

BOX 12.1 GAME THEORY REPRESENTATION OF THE GLOBAL SPENDING CAP

		Other Doctors' Behavior	
		Control costs ("save")	Intense billing ("spend")
Individual Doctor's Strategy	Save	10,000	8,000
	Spend	12,500	10,000

Suppose the insurance plan sets up a target of $10,000 in fees billed by each doctor and promises to withhold enough money so that if the total billings exceed $10,000 × N (where there are N doctors in the pool), each doctor will be paid an amount that is proportional to her total billings, with the total paid to all doctors equaling $10,000 × N.

Each doctor must select a strategy—either to "save" costs or to "spend" rapidly—that is, bill as many procedures as possible at the highest fees allowed. If, under normal behavior, each doctor bills the plan $10,000, each is paid $10,000, assuming all doctors "save" to control costs. Thus the doctor's payoff if she "saves" and all other doctors do similarly is $10,000.

Now, suppose that this single doctor "saves" costs, but all other doctors bill intensively. If all doctors bill (for example) $12,500 under such circumstances, then total billings relative to target billings are ($12,500 × N) ÷ (10,000 × N) = 5/4. According to the plan rules, each doctor will then be paid 4/5 of his billings. Thus, the doctor who "saves" gets paid $8,000, and all other doctors get paid $10,000.* Cooperation costs the doctor $2,000 if all other doctors don't cooperate.

Finally, if all doctors "spend" resources at the $12,500 rate, each is paid $10,000 in revenue. Of course, if actual resources have been used to produce care to patients that leads to the extra $2,500 in billings (in addition to the usual $10,000 in care provided), the doctors are all worse off. If the only thing that happens is that all doctors raise their fees by 25 percent, then the economic consequences of imposing the global revenue cap are nil; everybody raises prices, everybody is paid a proportional share of them, and the total spending corresponds to what would have been there without the cap.

*This isn't exactly accurate, because the total billings are really $12,500 × (N − 1) + $10,000 if one doctor "cooperates" with the cost-saving venture. This approaches $12,500 × N very rapidly as N increases, so for expositional purposes, we can use $12,500 × N as the total billings.

physician's payments will be reduced by, for example, 20 percent. Any doctor who has not "overbilled" by 20 percent will end up losing money under those circumstances. For this reason, all doctors' incentives lead them to charge fees as high as possible and to bill as many procedures as possible when such global spending caps are put in place.

The ability to use "group persuasion" to control such proclivities is quite real in closed physician groups, which is one reason why physician group practices can sometimes use "holdback" devices effectively. In large open-panel IPA plans, almost no successful persuasion is possible because the doctors are so dispersed geographically and organizationally. At the national level, any possible use of group persuasion to control total spending seems wholly doomed. Any total-fee cap within Medicare can lead only to a "race to the cash register" that will surely trigger the mechanism. Ironically, if any physician-firms "cooperate" to try to keep total spending down, they will only suffer financial losses. In such economic games as this, Leo Durocher was correct in saying that "nice guys finish last."[29]

THE MEDICAID PROGRAM

Introduction

Enacted in 1965 with the original Medicare legislation, Medicaid has an entirely different purpose and structure than Medicare. Rather than acting as a single federal program, it operates as a state–federal partnership with each state designing its own program within federal guidelines and with the federal government sharing the program costs. The sharing formula provides a larger federal share for states with low per capita income, the federal share ranging from 50 to 75 percent.

Unlike Medicare, which has universal eligibility and enrollment for the population over 65, Medicaid has income limits for eligibility[30]; it is the health insurance program for the poor. Eligibility usually hinges on the federal poverty level (FPL) multiplier as published annually by the Bureau of the Census for families of different sizes and used by each state.

Medicaid covers almost all types of health care for enrollees and—importantly—covers some that Medicare does not. The most important difference is long-term (nursing home) care, which Medicare covers only for posthospital recovery for limited periods. Medicaid covers nursing home care indefinitely for eligible citizens.

---

[29]Durocher was a combative baseball player and manager.

[30]While Medicare has no income-related eligibility, SCHIP has such limits, and Part D of Medicare provides assistance to pay for prescription drug insurance premiums based on income. Medicine has had income-related Part B premiums since 2006.

Multiple dimensions of Medicaid programs differ across states: who is eligible (as defined by the FPL income multiplier), what services are covered (although federal guidelines set minimum standards), and how providers are reimbursed. The reimbursement aspect is important because budget control efforts have caused many states to offer very low fees to providers for treating Medicaid patients, thus often limiting the range of options for Medicaid enrollees.

Who Is Covered

Medicaid legislation requires that anybody within a state who is eligible for income assistance also is eligible for Medicaid. The Medicaid program summarizes the "mandatory" eligibility for each state's program as follows:[31]

- Those who meet the requirements for the Aid to Families with Dependent Children (AFDC) program in effect on July 16, 1996.
- Fewer than six children in a family's income is more than 133 percent of the FPL.
- Obstetric services for pregnant women with family income of more than 133 percent of FPL.
- Supplemental security income (SSI) recipients in most states.
- Adoption/foster care recipients under Title IV of the Social Security Act.
- Specially protected groups (typically individuals who lose their cash assistance due to earnings from work or from increased Social Security benefits but who may keep Medicaid for a period of time).
- Children less than 19 years old born after September 30, 1983, with family income less than the FPL.

Many states have more generous definitions of poverty. A low percentage (say, 133 percent of the FPL) leads to fewer eligible people within a state than would a high percentage (say, 250 percent of the FPL). States can choose different percentage numbers for different groups (infants, young children, older children). The highest rates currently are 300 percent in Maryland, Vermont, and the District of Columbia, and around 250 to 275 percent for Minnesota, Wisconsin, and Rhode Island. The lowest rates hover around 133 percent to 150 percent for infants and 100 percent for older children in many states, more prominently in the west.[32]

---

[31]http://www.cms.hhs.gov/MedicaidGenInfo/03_TechnicalSummary.asp

[32]http://www.statehealthfacts.org/comparemaptable.jsp?ind=203&cat=4 provides current data on every state.

The percentage of the population in any given state enrolled in Medicaid will obviously increase (other things equal) for lower PCI, but these states also tend to have less generous enrollment rules, pushing things in the opposite direction. Nationally, 20 percent of the population is typically enrolled on Medicaid at any point in time, with state-by-state enrollment ranging from lows of 11 to 12 percent to highs of 27 to 29 percent.[33]

What Is Covered and How?

Federal rules require that Medicaid cover standard health care services, both inpatient and outpatient, including a wide array of preventive activities (both vaccinations and screening examinations, prenatal care, laboratory and diagnostic imaging, and nursing home services for adults, and specified others). Most of the state plans cover more than the minimum services, commonly adding prescription drugs, prosthetic devices, optometrist services, rehabilitation services, nursing home services for children, and a wide array of diagnostic services.

Some Medicaid services can require cost sharing.[34] Programs that cannot have any cost sharing for pregnant women, children under age 18, patients in a hospital or nursing home who are expected to contribute most of their income to institutional care, and individuals using emergency and family planning services.

How Is It Financed?

The Federal Medical Assistance Percentage (FMAP) primarily finances Medicaid. The program compares each state's average per capita income (PCI) with the national average, which is determined annually by using a predetermined formula. By law, the rate cannot go below 50 percent of PCI or higher than 83 percent. In recent years, 12 states received only 50 percent, the average was about 60 percent, and the highest was about 77 percent.[35] As noted

---

[33]California is the highest with 29 percent of the population enrolled in Medicaid (called *MediCal* there), followed closely by the District of Columbia, New Mexico, and Mississippi. The comparison of California (a relatively high-income state) and Mississippi (a very low-income state) shows the balancing of "need" and "resources" in choosing program coverage.

[34]New York's cost-sharing program, for example, charges $3.00 per clinic visit, nothing for a private physician visit, $3.00 for an emergency room visit, $1.00 for X-rays, $.50 for lab tests, $3 for top-tier drugs, $1.00 for generic drugs, and $25.00 for the last day of hospitalization.

[35]The 1997 BBA created a permanent rate of 70 percent for the District of Columbia and Alaska gets special consideration because of the unusually high cost of living in that state, which distorts the PCI number.

previously, the federal share of costs is higher for children enrolled in SCHIP and averages about 70 percent nationally.

States' decisions about program generosity (enrollment eligibility rules, breadth of services covered, and provider reimbursement) are based on both income and price effects, such as individual consumer budget decisions. States with more PCI tend to have more generous programs but also face higher prices for their medicaid programs because the rules creating the FMAP cause the federal share to be lower. Previous analyses of Medicaid state plan rules show that the income effect dominates the price effect in general, so states with higher PCI tend to have more generous enrollment rules and a higher percentage of the population eligible for Medicaid (Granneman, 1980).

How Are Providers Compensated and What Are the Effects on Access?

Medicaid pays most health care providers poorly. The American Hospital Association published an analysis that shows the ratio of reimbursement rate to hospital costs. See Figure 12.3. These data show that Medicare reimbursement has varied above and below 100 percent payment over the years but on average is only slightly below 100 percent. Private payers (mostly those with private insurance, of course) pay well above 100 percent and average about 125 percent during the years on this chart. According to these American Hospital Association calculations, Medicaid, in stark contrast to Medicare and private insurance, pays between 80 to 95 percent of costs, averaging about 90 percent through the years.

FIGURE 12.3 Hospital Payment as Percent of Hospital Costs by Payer Type.

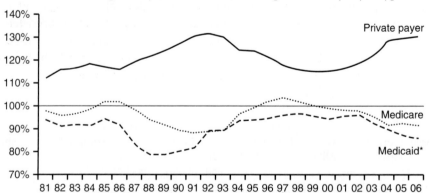

*Medicaid includes disproportionate share payments for hospitals treating large proportions of Medicaid patients.
Source: American Hospital Association Trendwatch Chartbook 2008, Chart 4.6.

Physician compensation appears to be even lower (relative to Medicaid) than hospital compensation. In a recent analysis, Decker (2006) compared Medicaid physician compensation rates across the nation with comparable Medicare rates. She shows that on average, Medicaid rates are only about 65 percent of the Medicare rate for comparable activities (ranging from 55 percent to 75 percent through the years of her sample).

Decker also showed how these rates affect the provision of health care. On average, only about 40 percent of all doctors accepted Medicaid patients in their practices, and the rates at which they did this varied directly with the generosity of fee schedules.[36] These findings support earlier studies of the same issue (Sloan, Mitchell and Cromwell, 1978; Cohen, 1993; Showalter, 1997).

Furthermore, Decker found that Medicaid patients had shorter visits with doctors (about 4 minutes, or 20 percent less time per visit on average) than patients with other insurance. Finally, she showed that Medicaid's compensation generosity affected the visit length in the directions we would expect: The nearer Medicaid came to Medicare compensation, the longer the visit for Medicaid patients.

These and similar results support the widely shared beliefs among providers that Medicaid compensation for providers is uncommonly low, and that, in turn, affects access of low-income persons with Medicaid coverage to health care, both in terms of finding physicians who will treat them and the amount of time they spend in patient visits.

The limited-access issue is so prevalent in hospitals that Medicaid has built in an extra payment—the *disproportionate Share* (DSH) payments—to those treating an unusually large number of Medicaid patients for their region. DSH payments typically are channeled either to public (county) hospitals or to hospitals treating Medicaid patients at a specified rate above the state average (e.g., one standard deviation). The data in Figure 12.3 include DSH payments for hospitals; without these funds (which average about $16 billion annually nationally), the compensation rate from Medicaid would be even lower for hospitals.

---

[36]In areas where medical schools and their affiliates operate, medical school "clinics" often become the major provider of care. Medical school faculty constitute a nontrivial proportion of the physicians who actually will accept Medicaid patients. Furthermore, particularly because of laws forbidding emergency rooms from denying treatment to patients, Medicaid patients in areas without medical schools nearby may turn to emergency rooms for "regular" care.

How Does Medicaid Pay for Long-Term Care

Medicaid is unique among government insurance programs in that it pays for long-term care (LTC) in nursing homes. In recent years, Medicaid has paid for approximately half of all long-term care expenses in the United States, about twice the national average of LTC enrollment. In fact, LTC accounts for more than one-third of total Medicaid spending.

When one reviews survival data in the United States, it should come as no surprise that that most of the recipients of Medicaid LTC support are women. Women outlive men by about 5 years, on average, and our society tends to have women marry men several years older than they are, creating an expected "widowhood" period of 5 to 7 years. Because living alone is one of the key reasons why people eventually choose LTC, and surviving widows often have diminished assets through time, the combination of these factors leads to the following observed patterns: Three-quarters of all nursing home residents are female, and in the oldest age group (85+ years), more than 80 percent are female.[37]

As with all other aspects of Medicaid, the LTC program has both income and asset tests for eligibility. Almost all persons using this program are elderly and live on retirement incomes, (generally at low levels), but they often have significant assets, most commonly home equity and other personal property. Because this program has income and asset restrictions, this feature has created a complicated cat-and-mouse game in which individuals (often with the consultation from financial planners and lawyers) seek to dispose of assets (to children, typically) to make themselves eligible for Medicaid.[38] Medicaid programs respond by creating "look-back" rules that consider assets transferred within a specific time of the Medicaid application as still being owned by the individual applicant. The Deficit Reduction Act of 2005 expanded the "look-back" period from 3 to 5 years.

SUMMARY

Medicare's structure has evolved through a series of important changes since it began in 1966. Most of the changes have sought to control outlays by CMS (for Medicare) and by both CMS and state governments (for Medicaid).

---

[37]Data from Health, 2007, Table 104.

[38]State Medicaid programs do not include homes in this asset calculation, so one standard mechanism is to shift assets into home value (e.g., by paying down home mortgages). For the curious reader, try conducting an Internet search on the terms (Medicaid asset protection attorney), and you can sample the offerings from the legal profession. A search using Google found 2.3 million responses for these terms.

In 1983, hospitals became the target of Medicare cost controls, with the introduction of the prospective payment system (PPS) using flat-rate payments based on diagnosis-related groups (DRGs). This system of payments dramatically reduced hospital length of stay (predictably, given the financial incentives). Admission rates also plummeted, possibly because of the parallel growth of new technology (leading to more ambulatory surgery) throughout the country. Declines in admissions most affected small hospitals that tend to undertake relatively simple operations, those that ambulatory surgery centers could most easily undertake.

A more recent change in Medicare again centered on physician payments. Implemented in January 1992, Medicare moved to a new fee-schedule payment system based on a study of "work effort," formally called the *resource-based relative value system.* Under this system, the remuneration for so-called cognitive services (thinking and talking with patients) would increase markedly, while fees for procedures (operations and specific diagnostic tests) would fall markedly. This system of paying physicians, especially if followed by private insurance carriers, could greatly alter the appearance of the U.S. health care system.

Other recent changes in Medicare altered the program structure again on the consumer (benefit) side. Reforms in 1997 greatly expanded the ways in which Medicare enrollees can use private provider plans (HMOs, PPOs, etc.) as alternatives to Medicare's FFS system. Under this revised system, Medicare pays the plans a monthly capitation fee and the plans provide enrollees' health care. That reform also created SCHIP, another federal-state partnership to increase insurance coverage for the children.

In 2006, the most recent Medicare reform added Part D to the benefit structure, allowing enrollees to purchase prescription drug insurance plans under federal guidelines. The program offers premium subsidies to families with low income to enhance their enrollment into Medicare.

This chapter also briefly explores the intricacies of the Medicaid program, the federal-state partnership to provide health insurance for families and individuals with low incomes. Federal rules severely limit states' ability to charge copayments to enrollees, adding utilization pressure because medical care is essentially free. States commonly respond in attempts to control budgets by paying providers at rates significantly below either those offered by private insurance or Medicare, which inhibits provider participation in treating Medicaid patients, thereby in effect substituting provider rationing (through lack of participation by providers) for price rationing.

We also see how the federal financing rule interacts with state income levels, so higher-income states tend to have more generous programs even though Federal share of program costs declines formulaically as state PCI rises.

RELATED CHAPTERS IN *HANDBOOK OF HEALTH ECONOMICS*

Chapter 14, "Risk Adjustment in Competitive Health Plan Markets" by Wynand P.M.M. Van de Ven and Randall P. Ellis

Chapter 15, "Government Purchasing of Health Services" by Martin Chalkley and James M. Malcomson

Chapter 17, "Long-Term Care" by Edward C. Norton

PROBLEMS

1. This problem considers the meaning of a decline in average long-term stay (LOS) for Medicare patients when some short-stay patients have shifted out of the hospital at the same time the DRG system came into being.

   Suppose in 1982 that for two groups of Medicare patients of equal size, the average LOS was 10 days overall. The short-stay group (cataracts, etc.) had an average LOS of 2 days.

   a. What was the average LOS of the long-stay group?

   Now suppose that the overall Medicare average fell to 8.5 days 5 years later and that all of the short-stay patients from previous years now received their surgery in ambulatory surgical centers (ASCs).

   b. What is the relative decline in LOS for the long-stay group? To find this, compare your answer to part (a) of this question with the 8.5-day LOS.

   c. How would your answer change if only half of the short-stay group got their surgery in ASCs in the later year?

2. What effects on hospital use would you most expect from the prospective payment system (PPS) as developed using diagnosis-related groups (DRGs) as the method of hospital payment? What effects might this have on patients' health outcomes? (*Hint:* The relevant catchphrase is "sicker and quicker.")

3. What single feature of the original Medicare program is most likely to cause an economist to say that "Medicare stinks as insurance"? (*Hint:* Think about aspects of the Medicare coverage that create high financial risk.)

4. The private insurance that people buy to supplement Medicare insurance, it most commonly covers up-front deductibles and least commonly covers "high-end" risks (see Table 12.2). Does this pattern of coverage accord well or poorly with the model of demand for insurance set forth in Chapter 10? What should we conclude from this?

5. Describe "balance billing" in the Medicare program, and discuss how it affects the financial risk confronting Medicare enrollees.

6. The new method of paying for doctor services under the Medicare program will increase payments for "cognitive services" (thinking and counseling) and decrease the payments for "procedures" (surgery and invasive diagnostic tests).
   a. What do you think will happen to the demand for residency training in orthopedic surgery, geriatric medicine, and pediatrics?
   b. What effect, if any, would you expect for hospital use?

7. U.S. hospitals saw plummeting "margins" following the introduction of Prospective Payment and again in 1997 following the programmatic reductions in hospital payments from the Balanced Budget Act. Because U.S. hospitals are (in general) not-for-profit organizations, what do you think the primary response will be to deal with the reduced funding stream from Medicare patients? Discuss in your answer the possibilities of changing the scope of services offered by the hospital, changing the general quality of care, and changing the efficiency of the hospital's operation. Why do you expect that any (or all) of these might be areas of change?

CHAPTER 13

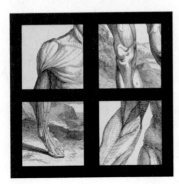

Medical Malpractice

Earlier sections of this book have alluded to the important role of the medical malpractice system. In this chapter, we explore the structure of this system and learn what is known about the ways in which malpractice law affects providers and patients. These roles and effects are not clearly known at present, and the subject generates considerable controversy in many circles. No discussion, including this one, can avoid offending some parties involved in malpractice law and/or the delivery of health care because most participants in the health care system and the medical-legal system hold strong views on the subject, often in conflict. Perhaps only the issues of reforming medical malpractice law stand as importantly in the public eye as

LEARNING GOALS

- Learn the basic concepts of liability and tort law in the U.S. legal system.
- Know the basic goals of a liability system: deterrence and compensation.
- Discover the basic concepts of the Learned Hand Rule for liability.
- Assess the importance of defensive medicine in response to liability rules.
- Find out how malpractice insurance alters incentives for deterrence.
- Learn the extent to which the current system actually deters injuries.
- Discuss large-scale reform to the medical legal system and its advantages and disadvantages.

those of cost control that pervade much of the U.S. health policy debate. As we shall see, even these issues are not wholly separate because many people blame the increasing costs of our health care system on the increases in medical-legal risk and expenses associated with the legal system.

BACKGROUND OF THE LEGAL SYSTEM IN THE UNITED STATES

Medical malpractice is a legal concept, related not so much to the practice of medicine as to the law of personal injury, the law of contracts, and, in a very few cases, criminal law. Thus, before we can study medical malpractice events, malpractice insurance, and the consequences of both, we must review the legal system in the United States.

The first issue of legal importance arises from the U.S. Constitution, which does not withhold for the federal government that part of the law relevant to medical malpractice. Therefore, by default, this area of the law becomes the domain of each state. This means that we do not have *a* malpractice law to consider but 50 of them. Each state specifies its own laws regarding everything about medical malpractice. The states also control the way doctors, nurses, hospitals, and all other providers of care are licensed.[1] Although the laws have evolved in similar ways across most states, important differences remain, and these differences allow some analysis of the effects of these laws on the rates at which malpractice occurs, the costs of defensive medicine, and the premiums paid for medical malpractice insurance, all issues we discuss in detail in this chapter.

Figure 13.1 shows the important parts of the legal system in every state that affect medical malpractice. This figure looks something like the standard biological classifications, but the "kingdoms" represent "criminal" and "civil"

FIGURE 13.1   The legal system as it affects medical malpractice.

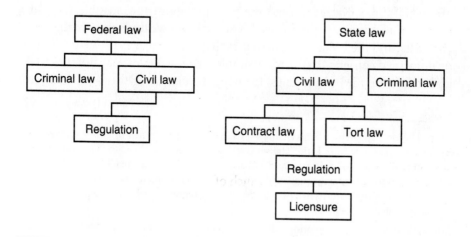

---

[1]The federal government directly licenses the use only of drugs controlled by federal narcotic laws.

law, not "plant" and "animal." With very few exceptions, the relevant law for medical malpractice is part of the civil law. Within the civil law, three major branches pertain to medical malpractice: tort law, contract law, and the laws regulating the insurance industry.

Tort law provides the basic apparatus to define medical malpractice.[2] This law provides the basis by which one person may bring a lawsuit against another to recover damages for personal injury, one of the many forms of a tort.[3] In tort law, the *plaintiff* makes a claim with the court that the *defendant* has harmed him. The lawsuit specifies the defendant's acts and the damage those acts imposed on the plaintiff and asks for *relief.* In medical malpractice suits, the relief most commonly means the payment of financial damages, an amount that the lawsuit commonly specifies. Sometimes the relief includes an order from the court to the defendant—for example, that the defendant stop doing the thing that caused the damage (a "cease and desist" order).

The key issue in medical malpractice cases is one of *negligence.*[4] Many medical events have bad outcomes—for example, the patient does not improve, gets worse, or dies. The law recognizes that many of these events would occur no matter what the doctors, hospitals, nurses, and other medical professionals might have done. In the most simple terms, on which we will elaborate shortly, the law says that a plaintiff has been negligently harmed by the defendant if and only if the injury to the plaintiff was preventable and that it was "reasonable" to undertake the activity that would have prevented the injury.

Some medical malpractice lawsuits stem not so much from whether an injury occurred (or was preventable) but from whether the doctor (or other provider) appropriately warned the plaintiff about the possible risks of a treatment that the plaintiff received. These cases have their roots in the law of contracts, and the broad set of activities that these encompass includes issues of "informed consent." In the most simple terms, a doctor may not undertake a procedure on the patient unless the patient consents. (Otherwise, the doctor

---

[2] As will become apparent, whereas many words in medicine have their origins from the Greek, most legal terms arise from Latin. The word *tort* comes from the Latin word *tortum,* meaning "twisted or distorted." The context here probably better translates as "made wrong." We get the word *tortuous* from the same origin, and those who have encountered the legal system may feel that this sense of the word, as in a twisted maze, better represents what happens in a legal context such as medical malpractice.

[3] The verb *to litigate* means to bring a dispute to a court of law. This also comes from the Latin word *litigare,* which means "to dispute, quarrel."

[4] This comes from the Latin word *negligere,* meaning "to neglect." We get the word *negligee* from the same base, via the French, although in the latter example, it is the amount of fabric that seems to have been neglected.

would, in the eyes of the law, be attacking the patient, a form of assault and battery.) For the consent to have legal meaning, the law requires that the patient have reasonably full information about the possible risks involved. Failure to provide or to document that a doctor did provide information sufficient for an informed consent has led to many a lawsuit. For this reason, doctors, particularly those who undertake specific "procedures" (such as surgical operations), spend considerable time documenting how they have described the risks to the patient and (almost invariably) have patients sign a statement that describes the risks involved.[5] Box 13.1 describes an apocryphal legal event involving informed consent that contains other legal lessons as well.

Lawsuits brought by patients suing for alleged medical malpractice may or may not end up in a trial, which may or may not include a jury. Either the defendant or the plaintiff may insist on a jury trial, but if both agree to waive that right, the trial can proceed with only a judge hearing the case and rendering the entire verdict. Both sides hire attorneys-at-law (lawyers) to present their cases to the court and to provide legal counsel. Both sides may hire experts to testify about the case, including, in medical malpractice cases, issues of negligence, medical causality, and the extent of damages incurred by the plaintiff.[6] Other "witnesses of fact" may testify about events that transpired, but only experts may render opinions about those events. As we will see, this process consumes large amounts of resources, so that even plaintiffs who win their litigation often recover far less than half of the total resources devoted to the case.

Most lawsuits in this country, including medical malpractice cases, do not culminate with a trial. Rather, the case is settled in advance of trial, quite often with no payment from the defendant to the plaintiff. (In these cases, we usually say that the plaintiff just drops the case.) One study of claims closed by medical malpractice insurers found that more than half the cases were settled with no payment at all to plaintiffs (Danzon and Lillard, 1982).

Gould (1973) first explored the logic for early settlements. He showed that, because of the costs of carrying out a trial, settlement is very likely to occur in tort cases whenever the parties agree on the probability that the plaintiff would win the case. If they agree that the plaintiff's case is very strong, the defendant will settle for an amount quite near the amount requested in the lawsuit. If both believe that the plaintiff's case is weak but has some chance of success, they may well settle for a much smaller amount,

---

[5]Some doctors record the session during which they describe the risks to the patient. Later they keep the recording in the patient's record.

[6]A cynic once said that the world consisted of three kinds of persons: liars, damned liars, and expert witnesses, presumably ranked in order of their tendencies toward mendacious behavior.

BOX 13.1 AN APOCRYPHAL STORY ABOUT INFORMED CONSENT

Issues of informed consent loom large in some medical malpractice litigation, and, as noted in the main body of the text, some doctors take considerable effort to document the information they give to patients to "inform" them before receiving their consent to operate. One case reveals how the issue of informed consent can affect the strategy involved in a specific trial. This case involved a doctor, Dr. X, who did repeated back surgery on patients with apparently unfavorable outcomes being quite common. Dr. X had been successfully sued by numerous patients, and, indeed, one plaintiff's attorney in town apparently made a substantial living from his fees in lawsuits involving this doctor.

Each medical malpractice case stands on its own merits, so even if a doctor has lost 20 malpractice cases in recent years for the same procedure, information from those previous cases cannot be admitted as evidence into the 21st case. In one of Dr. X's cases, his own testimony opened up the floodgates that allowed his past history of lost litigation (and poor outcomes for the patients) into evidence. This specific case involved the question of informed consent. The dialogue in the trial apparently went something along these lines (this is not from the trial transcript):

> PLAINTIFF'S ATTORNEY: Now, Dr. X, did you advise the plaintiff of the risks associated with having this type of surgery?
>
> DR. X: Yes, just as I always do.

This response contains five too many words from the point of view of legal strategy. (It also demonstrates why lawyers advise their clients to answer unfriendly questions as briefly as possible and not to volunteer anything beyond that.) The last phrase opens up the question about Dr. X's common practices. It admits into evidence other patients who have had the same procedure.

The case proceeded next by having a long series of Dr. X's former patients appear on the witness stand giving testimony for the plaintiff. All were in various stages of pain; had permanent injury; and, in some cases, could not walk. The questions from the plaintiff's attorney proceeded along the following lines:

> PLAINTIFF'S ATTORNEY: Did Dr. X operate on your back?
>
> WITNESS: Yes.
>
> PLAINTIFF'S ATTORNEY: Before that operation, did Dr. X inform you of the possible risks of that surgery?

The answer, of course, was immaterial. The plaintiff's attorney had succeeded in parading a long sequence of Dr. X's former patients into the courtroom. Their mere presence demonstrated that Dr. X had commonly achieved very poor outcomes with this operation. Without the issue of informed consent arising, the attorney would never have been able to bring those former patients into this case. Of course, that option also required an overly wordy answer on the part of Dr. X to a key question.

making the plaintiff happy to get something out of a "thin" case and the defendant happy to get out from under a potentially expensive risk. The logic for settling such cases closely resembles the logic for purchasing insurance that we discussed in Chapter 10. (A further discussion about the incentives for early settlement appears in the next two sections regarding the economics of settling and the value of establishing a reputation in the legal arena.)

Danzon and Lillard's study (1982, p. 53) found that settlements average three-quarters of the size of their best prediction of what a trial award would have been had the case proceeded to trial. They also found that settled cases tend to have much smaller awards than those going through trial; the larger stakes in cases with most severe injuries incline both plaintiffs and defendants to show a reluctance to settle. Danzon (1983) has concluded that "self-serving rationalism [i.e., pure economic incentives] largely explains the outcome of malpractice claims on average." Of course, this still leaves considerable latitude for court error, different motives (including revenge, malice, and spite), and suboptimal strategy pursued by plaintiffs and/or defendants in individual cases.

Each state's tort law defines the general terms by which plaintiffs may file medical malpractice suits against providers of medical care. These laws specify the nature of what constitutes negligent behavior; the statute of limitations (the time that may pass after an injury during which the patient may still bring suit); the nature of allowable evidence; and, in many states now, the size of damages that plaintiffs can recover for some forms of injury.[7] Naturally, these laws also affect the propensity to settle a case in advance of trial to some degree, as does the backlog of cases within the court system.

Another relevant body of the law provides regulation of insurance within each state. Hospitals, doctors, dentists, podiatrists, nurses, psychologists, and other providers of care all face financial risk associated with their attempts to heal people's injuries and illnesses. The tort laws within which providers must operate create financial risk for them. These providers of care come equipped—at no extra charge—with utility functions. If those utility functions make the individuals risk averse (as we would normally presume in economic analysis), then the risk created by the law leads them to seek insurance against those risks. The risks arise in at least two forms. First, all

---

[7]Many states now set limits, for example, on the size of awards for "pain and suffering" associated with an injury. Because of the highly subjective nature of pain and suffering and because of the occasional extremely large awards granted by courts for pain and suffering, these types of award became an obvious point of contention during the medical malpractice crises of the 1960s, 1970s, and 1980s, and many state legislatures chose to set limits for this area of damages in particular.

providers know that they have some chance of engaging in negligent behavior, either through mistaken knowledge, sloppiness, or fatigue.

Second, the imperfection of the court system creates additional risks; sometimes the patient may suffer an adverse outcome, but not through negligent behavior of the provider. Even so, patients cannot always distinguish an injury caused by negligence from one caused by something else, and they may sue because of the injury itself. An imperfect court system allows awards to some of those patients, even though negligence did not occur in some "pure" sense. This aspect of risk (the whimsical court system) bears heavily in the minds of many care providers. Every reader of this book has probably read about or personally encountered some medical malpractice lawsuit that appeared to be "without merit" by many standards. Providers fear this risk considerably—indeed, perhaps pathologically—and it forms a strong incentive for them to purchase medical malpractice insurance.

Several studies have attempted to measure the rates at which actual negligence and nonnegligent cases find their way into the legal system. Bovjberg (1995), using data from one large malpractice insurance carrier, estimates that the current rate of 15 malpractice *claims* per 100 physicians per year, down from a peak of 17 per 100 physicians per year in 1986. (The reduction is widely assumed to flow from various tort reforms in states' malpractice laws.) Because the U.S. economy has about 360 patients per physician, this implies about 1 of every 2,400 patients in the United States files a malpractice claim each year.

What's the mix of truly negligent injuries, non-negligent adverse events, and unharmed patients among these? Farber and White (1991) used independent reviewers to evaluate a series of claims from a sample of hospitals and concluded that negligence was present in 35 percent of the claims, no negligence was present in 42 percent, and that they could not make a determination from the medical records in the remaining 23 percent. These were claims *filed* by plaintiffs. The court system responded differently to negligent versus nonnegligent events. In events classified by Farber and White as negligent, two-thirds (66 percent) of plaintiffs received compensation, averaging a bit more than $200,000 per claim. For non-negligent cases, the courts awarded compensation in only 16 percent of the cases with an average award of just under $42,000.

As with tort law, the federal government has no control over the provision of insurance, so each of the 50 states defines the rules by which medical malpractice insurance can be provided. Some states actually enter the business of providing such insurance to doctors and hospitals, and others regulate the premiums that insurers can charge for such insurance. The various rules adopted by the different states have provided another "laboratory" to study the effects of insurance regulation on insurance rates, malpractice itself, and the effects of insurance costs on providers' participation in the market.

Finally, we can note in passing the small role played by criminal law in medical malpractice. Criminal cases differ from civil cases in two important respects. First, guilty defendants can be sentenced to prison in addition to having to pay monetary fines; civil cases cannot lead to this outcome. Second, only the government can bring criminal charges against an individual, a role served by district attorneys and their counterparts at various levels of government. In medical events, the most common source of a criminal charge involves financial matters (fraud), commonly perpetrated against a government provider of insurance, such as Medicare or Medicaid. For true medical issues, a doctor's behavior sometimes becomes so bad that the state files a charge of *criminal negligence* against the doctor. Cases sporadically reach the courts under charges of homicide when doctors terminate life support for individuals or assist patients in committing suicide.[8]

THE ECONOMIC LOGIC OF NEGLIGENCE LAW

> We have done those things we ought not to have done, and we have left undone those things we ought to have done. [Prayer of Confession]

Why do we have a law of negligence? Laws defining negligence (and responsibility to pay for damage) have two obvious purposes: to compensate victims ("fairness") and in an efficient way to deter people from harming others (Danzon, 1985b). Note the important condition—in an efficient way. One could think about trying to deter *all* damage that one person might inflict upon another, but (as we shall see) the costs of doing that would become prohibitive. Because of the costs of preventing every possible harm, a zero-damage world is not optimal. However, in any overall analysis of the negligence law, these goals stand out. If we cannot accomplish either one of them well

---

[8]The most prominent figure in this legal area was Dr. Jack Kevorkian, who assisted in the suicides of 130 terminally ill patients around the country. He had been tried and found not guilty of murder (or manslaughter) on numerous occasions. He was finally convicted of second degree murder in Michigan in 1999 in a case in which (unlike his previous interventions) he actually moved the controls sending the lethal injection to a patient with Lou Gehrig's disease whose own strength failed him as he tried to end his life. Kevorkian sought the trial, having taken a videotape of the event to national television media (*60 Minutes*) some 4 months earlier, with an estimated audience of 15 million viewers watching Kevorkian himself control the device that ended the patient's life.

with the negligence system, then consideration of alternative legal systems seems desirable.[9]

We can now turn to an analysis of negligence law and its application in medical malpractice. Negligence occurs when a provider of care causes harm to a patient that could reasonably have been prevented. In classic negligence cases, in order to gain compensation from the defendant, the plaintiff must prove not only that she was harmed, but also that the actions of some provider of care ("doctor" hereafter, for simplicity) was responsible for the harm. Furthermore, the plaintiff must show that the doctor's behavior did not meet "reasonable" standards of care.

In many cases, the relevant standard of care derives from "local custom," so in many malpractice cases, the testimony of other doctors is required to establish the relevant local custom of care. Put simply, a doctor's behavior that deviated importantly from local custom allows the inference of negligence. This standard of care has fallen by the wayside, giving way to a more "national" standard, reflecting the widespread dissemination of medical information through journals, continuing medical education seminars, national and regional medical meetings, and even a specialized cable television channel devoted in part to providing doctors with "current" information about modern methods of diagnosis and treatment. Interestingly, the old "local" standard of practice accurately captured the reality of widespread differences in "culture" about the correct ways to use various medical interventions, as documented well in the past several decades in the "medical variations" literature. (See the discussion in Chapter 3 about variations in medical practice to refresh your memory about this phenomenon.) Given the widespread variations in practice that we can readily observe, it would appear relatively easy to find a doctor from *some* locale who would testify (correctly) that the custom of care in his own community differed from the choices made by a doctor in some other community. Reliance on "local" custom eliminates that as a possible strategy by plaintiff's attorneys. The converse also appears to be true. Requiring that experts come only from the local community inhibits the ability of plaintiffs to establish an act of malpractice because it would require doctors to testify, in effect, against their personal acquaintances and friends.[10]

---

[9]The alternatives include a "no-fault" insurance system, as some states have adopted for auto insurance, and a "strict liability" system in which the provider of care pays for any harm, whether negligent or not. Workers' compensation for on-the-job injuries offers an example of the latter system.

[10]Kessel (1958) argued that the unwillingness of doctors to testify against one another was part of a widespread strategy of members of the medical profession to feather their own economic nests at the expense of patients.

The particular ways in which medical malpractice law has defined negligence (e.g., comparison with local custom) have been only a proxy for the more general approach. Negligence law in its most general structure offers a standard that has compelling economic logic. This standard, first set forth by Judge Learned Hand,[11] forms the "classic" basis for defining negligence. According to the Learned Hand Rule, negligence occurs when doctors fail to take some action to prevent harm and when it would on average cost less to prevent that harm than the costs of the harm itself. This definition closely matches the economist's prescriptions in cost–benefit analysis. More formally, suppose p = probability of some harm's occurring without any intervention by the doctor, D = the amount of damages incurred if the harm takes place, and C = the cost of preventing the harm. Then the Learned Hand Rule says that negligence has occurred if $C < p \times D$.

This rule, written as a mathematical inequality, suggests that the doctor has yes/no choices (either do or don't do some preventive activity). The logic of the rule also holds up when the choice involves "how much" or "how often" to do something. One interprets the rule in such cases in terms of incremental costs and incremental effect on the probability of harm, the extent of damage, or both.[12] Negligence occurs whenever a doctor doesn't undertake "enough" activity to prevent harm, with "enough" defined specifically in terms of incremental costs versus incremental benefits.

This formulation of the law has a powerful economic logic to support it; it places the burden of behavior on the person with the greatest knowledge about the appropriate technology—the doctor. In effect, it tells the doctor, "If you behave in a way that would minimize social costs of harm, you will never harm a patient negligently." Rationally behaving doctors would always advise their patients to do things in a way that corresponds exactly to economists' prescriptions for efficient use of resources. Likewise, rational patients would also always accept such advice for obvious reasons.

---

[11]It may be hard to imagine a person with a name more fitting for a judge. One can just visualize the "learned" hand writing "correct" opinions of law.

[12]Using calculus, consider a "social cost" function $SC = (p \times D) + C$, with these terms defined as in the text. The problem is how to minimize social cost. If both p and D fall as C rises (i.e., the "preventive" or "safety" activities actually have some effect), then we could find the point of minimum social cost by taking the derivative of SC with respect to C and setting the result equal to zero. This would occur if $D dp/dC + p dD/dC + 1 = 0$, or, equivalently, $-(D dp/dC + p dD/dC) = 1$. (Remember that these derivatives are negative if prevention "works.") If one stopped doing preventive activities at some point before the optimum, then social costs would still fall as preventive effort increased, that is, $dSC/dC < 0$. Under the logic of Judge Hand, stopping "too early" in the application of preventive activity would constitute negligence.

[margin note: More doctors responsible for some effects of after surgery]

Notice also that *in concept*, the Learned Hand Rule deters doctors from doing "useless" procedures and, indeed, from doing "too much" medical intervention. Broadly interpreted, the Learned Hand Rule would say that a procedure was unwarranted if the costs exceeded the benefits. However, in practice, the rule seldom if ever is applied in this way. Patients almost never sue doctors for doing (for example) useless surgery. The reasons why such cases seldom appear are complex, but they depend at least partly on the notion that the patient agreed to have the doctor do the procedure ("consent"). Thus, cases such as this would usually rest on the question of whether the consent was really "informed" or not. In addition, the patient would have to show harm; courts have proven reluctant to award damages unless the procedure turned out badly. They will not award damages for the cost of the procedure itself, except in very rare cases.

JUDICIAL ERROR, DEFENSIVE MEDICINE, AND "TOUGH GUYS"

In a world with perfectly functioning courts, doctors behaving according to the Learned Hand Rule would never lose a medical malpractice suit. Alas, the legal system does not perform perfectly.[13] Courts make errors of omission and commission, just as doctors do. Doctors often feel that courts find for plaintiffs just because a bad outcome has occurred rather than only when negligence has occurred.

Farber and White (1991) illuminate the issue of judicial error in an interesting way. They estimate that courts awarded damages to 66 percent of those negligently injured and only 16 percent of those injured without negligence. Combining these data with information on the mix of negligent and non-negligent injuries (see footnote 13) allows us to estimate that 77 percent of all malpractice awards are to people for whom negligence actually occurred. Similarly, given the disparity in awards ($205,000 per negligent injury, $42,000 per non-negligent injury), approximately 94 percent of the dollars awarded went to persons negligently injured, and only 6 percent to those injured without negligence.

Despite the evidence that decisions and dollars awarded tip heavily toward patients actually injured negligently, many doctors assert that they undertake "defensive medicine" to protect against this risk. That is, they carry out medical

---

[13]Recall the data from Farber and White (1991): Of claims filed (where negligence could be determined by the researchers), 35 percent showed negligence, 42 percent showed no negligence, and 23 percent could not be classified. Thus, of those for which the researchers could classify the case, 45 percent were negligent and 55 percent were non-negligent.

procedures for the purpose of preventing lawsuits rather than for purposes they believe will improve the patient's well-being.

"Defensive medicine" is difficult, perhaps impossible, to measure. Given the widespread variations in behavior of doctors' use of various interventions, it may well be that a considerable percentage of doctors believe that something is "medically inappropriate" when in fact, by a careful application of the Learned Hand Rule, it would be appropriate. In this case, negligence law would actually increase patients' well-being by "forcing" doctors to do things (such as carry out diagnostic tests) that they would not normally do. If one conducted a survey, those doctors would describe such activities as "defensive medicine," and they would bemoan the added costs to patients of such activities. However, under the logic of the Learned Hand Rule, total costs will fall with the use of such interventions, so patients have actually been made better off. Thus, negligence law can *in concept* serve to offset untoward variations in the use of medical care.

Danzon (1990) studied how patterns of medical care differ across regions with different rates of malpractice claims filings. (Recall that we have 50 distinct malpractice environments, creating somewhat of a natural experiment for studies such as this.) She found that rates of use of standard "defensive medicine" activities such as X-rays and laboratory tests were generally unrelated to measures of patients' propensity to sue.

In an interesting test of the role of defensive medicine on health care costs and outcomes, Kessler and McClellan (1996) used the various state tort reforms as the basis for their analysis. They looked at Medicare patients treated for heart attacks (acute myocardial infarction, or AMI) and chest pain due to poor blood supply to the heart (ischemic heart disease) for the period 1984–1990, when many of the states enacted tort reform. They look at total hospital expense for the year after the initial event as a measure of treatment intensity and measured mortality and rehospitalization rates as outcome measures. (Rehospitalization often signals incomplete treatment on the first hospitalization.) Their result? They found that treatment intensity fell after tort reform but no measurable changes in either outcome studied.[14] They conclude that the pressure of malpractice law caused doctors to expend resources (defensive medicine) that did not improve patient outcomes.

In a large review of available evidence, the Office of Technology Assessment (OTA) of the U.S. Congress sought to determine the extent of defensive medicine through four separate approaches (OTA, 1994). These approaches included (1) physician surveys, (2) "paper patient" clinical scenario studies, (i.e., studies

---

[14]Their research design is excellent. They looked at the changes in the states with tort reform in any year and compared those with comparable-year changes in states that had no tort reform, thus controlling for possible changes in medical technology.

that present physicians with a description of a specific patient's condition, test values, etc., and ask what those physicians would recommend for treatment), (3) statistical analyses linking medical procedure choices to malpractice liability risk, and (4) case studies. The OTA also explored the role of medical education in creating attitudes of doctors in training about defensive medicine.

After carefully reviewing the available literature (dozens of physician surveys and case studies, conducting its own clinical scenario study—to augment the one found in the literature—and the available statistical study—Harvard Medical Malpractice Study, 1990, to be discussed further in a later section), the OTA concluded " . . . a relatively small proportion of diagnostic procedures—certainly less than 8 percent—is performed with a conscious concern about medical liability risk" (OTA, 1994, p. 74).

A Game Theoretic Issue about Lawsuits

Doctors commonly complain that medical malpractice trials represent an expensive form of Russian roulette in which plaintiffs make outrageous claims, seek a settlement for a relatively small percentage of the claim, and occasionally go to trial and win a large verdict by convincing a sympathetic jury to help them, even when no negligence has actually occurred. In the view of many doctors, the medical malpractice system is worse than an "imperfect" system because it allows legal "blackmail" of doctors who have done no wrong.

The essence of the "blackmail" idea comes from a game-theoretic analysis of the problem. Individual doctors facing a medical malpractice suit confront the costs of defending the case, not only in financial outlay to lawyers but also in their own time in preparation for the case and in court. Most doctors carry malpractice insurance that covers not only payments to plaintiffs but also the legal costs of a defense. However, their own time and effort (and the mental anguish associated with the event) are not insured. As a result, each individual doctor faces some incentives to settle a case before trial, if for nothing else than to avoid the legal costs of a trial.

In game theory, when an individual repeatedly plays the same "game," it often pays off for the person to establish a reputation as a "tough" player. If a plaintiff's attorneys know that doctors (and hospitals) have such reputations, the attorneys will have less interest in filing frivolous suits. However, no single doctor has much incentive to spend the time and effort to establish such a reputation because the chances of their being able to take advantage of the investment are small. In this sort of game, particularly when the courts occasionally err in awarding verdicts to plaintiffs when negligence has not occurred, settlement often seems the wiser choice for each individual doctor.

Thus, the effort spent in establishing a "tough" image has many aspects of a public good with regard to the medical community; every doctor would benefit from a "hard line" stance relative to frivolous lawsuits, but no individual doctor has the incentive to help establish such a reputation.

One important party in the "lawsuit game" does have an incentive to establish such a reputation, however—the insurance company that provides the medical malpractice insurance to doctors. These companies often guide (or at least advise) the defense of a medical malpractice claim, and they sometimes have the contractual right to determine when a settlement will take place. The ability of an insurer to establish a "tough" reputation may be one of the reasons why medical malpractice insurance sales are typically quite heavily concentrated (few companies in a single region). If any single insurer can establish a "tough" reputation in bargaining with plaintiffs' attorneys, it will have created a competitive advantage that will allow it to dominate a market.

MEDICAL MALPRACTICE INSURANCE

Almost all doctors and hospitals carry medical malpractice insurance. This insurance pays for the costs of defending medical malpractice cases and for any awards against the provider. For individual doctors, the amount of insurance varies, but commonly doctors carry something in the neighborhood of $1 million and $3 million in "basic" coverage, meaning that the coverage will pay up to $1 million for a single judgment, and $3 million total during the life of the contract. (Despite the occasional news story to the contrary, very few medical malpractice judgments exceed $1 million, and those that do often have multiple defendants—a hospital and several doctors—to share the cost.) A 1989 survey showed that nearly half of the doctors carried this type of insurance (Paxton, 1989). This same survey showed that about half the doctors carried a second "excess coverage" policy that most commonly added another $1 million to $2 million in coverage. Doctors carry such insurance for precisely the same reason that individual persons carry health insurance—to reduce the uncertainty associated with a financial risk. Hospitals also commonly carry liability insurance because they too can be held accountable for harm to patients, even if caused by a doctor's negligence rather than that of any person employed by the hospital.[15]

---

[15]Recall here the usual relationship doctors and hospitals have. Hospitals do not usually employ doctors but rather grant them "attending privileges." However, courts of law have commonly held hospitals liable for harm created by doctors on their staffs, in part because the hospital's own staff (e.g., nurses, pharmacists) sometimes participates in the negligence and, if for no other reason, because the hospital's board of directors has the ultimate legal responsibility for ensuring the quality of the doctors.

The most recent available survey of physician practice expenses (AMA, 2003) gathered data on medical malpractice insurance costs as part of its assessment of physician practice costs. Overall, the reported premium costs were $18,000, ranging from $12,000 in pediatrics to $39,000 in OB-Gynecology. These costs represented about 4 percent of practice revenues overall, ranging from 2 percent in pediatrics to about 7 percent in OB-Gynecology.

EVIDENCE ON ACTUAL DETERRENCE

Does the medical malpractice system actually deter negligent behavior? This question sits centrally in the debate over medical malpractice reform. If we achieve no deterrence from this system, then reform seems more desirable, for we could certainly accomplish the goals of compensation of harmed persons more cheaply with alternative systems, such as a no-fault system or a social insurance system.

For deterrence actually to occur, several things must take place. First, injured patients must bring suit against providers. If the patients do not sue doctors, then no deterrence can possibly occur. Second, the doctors must bear the financial brunt of their mistakes. Insurance may undo any incentive effects that the legal system generates, depending on how the insurance policies are priced to doctors.

Do Injured People Bring Lawsuits?

The question of whether injured people actually bring lawsuits turns out to be fairly difficult to answer in practice. To do that, one must first find a set of people who have been injured by negligent behavior and then determine whether they filed lawsuits. Alternatively, one must accomplish some comparable method to estimate the numbers of negligently injured patients and the number of suits filed. Two separate studies have now undertaken that task, using similar methods and reaching quite similar conclusions.

The first of these studies took place in California (a hotbed of medical malpractice cases and precedents). The study (Mills et al., 1977) looked at hospital care in 1974. The California Medical Association (CMA) and the California Hospital Association (CHA) hired experts to study medical records in 23 hospitals scattered throughout California, and the medical–legal experts looked for *documented* evidence of injury due to negligence. They concluded that approximately 1 in every 125 patients was negligently injured during a hospital stay. From this sample, they estimated how many injuries occurred for the entire state in 1974, and then they compared this estimate with the number of lawsuits actually filed relating to that care. (The lawsuits could have been filed immediately or any time in the succeeding 4 years to be counted in the survey.)

The results proved somewhat disheartening for those seeking important deterrence from the medical malpractice system. The California study estimated that less than 1 injured person in 10 files a lawsuit. Of those who did (remember, these were people that the CMA and CHA experts thought had been injured), less than one-half actually received compensation. Using the experts' judgment as a "gold standard," this suggests substantial court error in favor of hospitals and doctors. Only 1 out of 25 injured patients received compensation! This probably overstates things because there were almost certainly other injured patients for whom hospital personnel did not record the event in the medical record, thus escaping detection by the CMA/CHA experts. It also completely ignores malpractice events occurring in doctors' offices rather than in hospitals (although suits arising from such events would have been counted).

Since this study was conducted, the rate of malpractice suits has dramatically increased. By 1985 the rate of malpractice suits doubled compared with that in 1978, the period of this CMA study (Danzon, 1985a). Even so, this says that at maximum only about one in five injured patients brings suit.

A study conducted in 1989 using 1984 hospital data from New York State produced quite similar results (Harvard Medical Malpractice Study, 1990; Brennan et al., 1991). The researchers sampled more than 30,000 medical records from 51 hospitals throughout New York State. They found (as in the earlier California study) that only a small fraction of negligent injuries led to patients' filing claims.

Specifically, the researchers estimated the rate of malpractice events per patient in one part of their study and malpractice legal claims per patient in a separate analysis. They estimated that 3.7 percent of hospitalized patients had an adverse event, and of those a little more than a quarter were due to negligence (as defined by their experts' review of records). Most of the adverse events caused problems lasting less than 6 months, but 13.6 percent led to death and another 2.6 percent to permanent disability. The rate of negligence grew rapidly with age of the patient and with the severity of the adverse event. For example, less than a quarter of the "low-severity" events were due to negligence, but a third of those with permanent disability and half of those adverse events leading to death were due to negligent treatment. Finally, the researchers found important differences both in the rates

TABLE 13.1 RATES OF ADVERSE EVENTS AND NEGLIGENCE AMONG CLINICAL-SPECIALTY GROUPS

Specialty	Rate of Adverse Events (%)	Proportion Negligent (%)	Rate of Negligence[a] (%)
Orthopedics	4.1	22.4	0.9
Urology	4.9	19.4	1.0
Neurosurgery	9.9	35.6	3.5
Thoracic and cardiac surgery	10.8	23.0	2.5
Vascular surgery	16.1	18.0	2.9
Obstetrics	1.5	38.3	0.6
Neonatology	0.6	25.8	0.2
General surgery	7.0	28.0	2.0
General medicine	3.6	30.9	1.1
Other	3.0	19.7	0.6

[a]Product of rate of adverse events and proportion negligent.
Source: Brennan et al. (1991, Table 4).

of adverse events and negligence across medical specialities. Table 13.1 shows their results.[16]

Combining the two sources of evidence allows an estimate of the rate of claims per incident. Using a variety of estimates of the number of claims filed (a fact not readily determined, due to the dispersed nature of the legal process and the fact that only cases ending in trial are "counted" for sure), the study concluded that about 8 times as many people were injured as filed suits and that about 15 times as many people were injured as received compensation. (The step from a ratio of 8 to 1 to a ratio of 15 to 1 occurs because not all injured patients win their cases or receive settlements.)

The New York State study also attempted to learn what sorts of injuries did not end up in litigation. The researchers took all cases with "strong" evidence of negligence and classified the degree of injury from one (not serious) to five (disability resulting in at least 50 percent decrease in social function)

---

[16]The most recent of such studies examined adverse events and negligence in Utah and Colorado in 1992 (Thomas et al., 2000). Using methods similar to those adopted in the earlier California and New York studies, this study examined the records of 15,000 hospitalized patients, a random sample of nonpsychiatric hospital discharges. They found a rate of adverse events of 2.9 percent of cases in both states, and negligence rates among those of 27.4 percent in Colorado and 32.6 percent in Utah. Death occurred in 6.6 percent of the adverse events and 8.8 percent of the negligent adverse events. Just under half of the adverse events (45 percent) was operative, and one-fifth was drug related. Although the rates of adverse events found in this study of 1992 hospitalizations are similar to those found in New York and California (modestly lower in each successive study using more recent data), the authors did not take the next step and compare these rates with propensity to sue.

to six (death). They concluded that those not filing claims tended to have less serious injury (usually self-healing in less than 6 months) or were very elderly persons with limited life expectancy.

Why do patients bring so few lawsuits? The economics of the problem dictate the answer in part. If an injury has small consequences, any court award will presumably also be small. If the activity of bringing lawsuits to court has any important fixed costs (such as shopping around to find an attorney), then small claims will tend to get filtered out. Indeed, the Harvard study classified 80 percent of the injuries as having only temporary consequences, perhaps a better testimony to the healing power of the body than to the efficacy of medical care. The propensity to sue seems to increase with the severity of injury, consistent with this "fixed cost" idea. For minor injuries, roughly 1 of 13 patients brought suit, while for permanent injuries, 1 of 6 sued.

A common complaint by doctors and providers is that patients bring lawsuits whenever *any* poor outcome occurs during medical treatment, whether due to negligence or not. The CMA/CHA study refutes this strongly. For each negligent event identified in the 23-hospital sample, the researchers found more than five more non-negligent "incidents" that should not count as malpractice. If any significant proportion of those nonnegligent injuries had filed suit, such suits would have swamped the suits filed for negligent injury.

Of course, due to the design in the California study, we have no way to determine how many of these non-negligently injured patients also brought lawsuits (and possibly won them, through a different type of court error). The actual mix of lawsuits observed in California relating to the care delivered in 1974 surely contained some "false positive" suits—those with people who were not negligently injured but did bring suits.

White (1994), reviewing these and other studies, concludes that overall, 2.6 percent of all persons negligently injured actually file claims, 1.0 percent of persons injured non-negligently file claims, and a very small 0.1 percent of noninjured patients file claims.

We still have no conclusive evidence on the central question of the extent of deterrence. We do know (from the California and New York studies) that a relatively small fraction of injured patients brings suit, and this logically tells us that any incentives for deterrence have been seriously blunted as a result. However, direct evidence on the extent of deterrence remains elusive.

Malpractice Insurance and Deterrence

Malpractice insurance presents an interesting and important dilemma for those trying to assess the role of liability in deterring injury. The incentives for individual providers (particularly doctors, but also hospitals) to purchase malpractice insurance seem quite clear. Because of risk aversion, when the courts allow plaintiffs to bring lawsuits against defendants, the financial risk creates obvious incentives to seek insurance. However, just as health insurance creates incentives for patients to increase medical care use, malpractice insurance *may* dull physicians' incentives to treat patients with proper caution. The importance of this effect hinges on the way insurance companies do business, including how they select their "customers" (i.e., which doctors they will insure), the information that they use about doctors in setting insurance premiums, and the amount of "risk-reduction" activity they undertake.

To begin, suppose that only two types of doctors exist in terms of their propensity to injure patients negligently. Call the probabilities of injury p_L and p_H (L and H for low and high risk, respectively), and suppose for greatest simplicity that when doctors harm patients, they create the same level of damage (D). Thus, the expected damage they could create would be $p_L D$ and $p_H D$ for low- and high-risk doctors, respectively. Finally, suppose that some effort to prevent harm, costing C, is sufficient to make any high-risk doctor a low-risk doctor (this makes doctors equal except for their efforts at risk prevention) and that the Learned Hand Rule would make it negligent not to use this level of effort (see previous discussion defining *negligence*).

We can now see the effects of insurance companies' pricing practices. If insurers could identify high- and low-risk doctors in advance and charge them insurance premiums reflecting their expected damage, then every doctor would decide to undertake the risk-prevention activity, thereby both reducing malpractice insurance premiums and minimizing the amount of harm created. In such a case, malpractice insurance would not blur the incentives of the legal system at all.

Now suppose in contrast that the insurance company charges all doctors the same premium, no matter what their risk. If some share of the doctors (s) decides to spend the money to become low-risk doctors, the insurance premium each doctor paid would be $R = [sp_L + (1 - s)p_H]D$. It turns out that under a remarkably wide range of circumstances, this "community rating" form of insurance blurs and may nearly completely eliminate at least the most direct and obvious economic incentives to undertake any damage-preventing activity. (Box 13.2 shows why this happens.) Thus, although negligence law makes doctors liable for harm in the case we have constructed, community-rated insurance may well lead all doctors to choose not to prevent the risk, driving s to zero and causing the insurance premium to rise from $p_L D$ to $p_H D$ for everybody.

Premiums do vary considerably by specialty, a characteristic of physicians that insurance companies can readily observe. Every insurer rates doctors by their type of practice, a specific form of experience rating. Table B in Box 13.3 shows typical premiums paid by specialty across the country.

Another way to look at the effect of specialty examines the premiums within a specific region. This "holds constant" the legal structure and provides a clearer picture of the specific effect of specialty on malpractice premiums and (by inference) costs of malpractice claims.

The data in Box 13.3 on premium levels, when combined with the Harvard study of the rate of negligent events occurring in New York State, provide an interesting insight into the world of malpractice liability. These two data sources are combined in Figure 13.2 for the specialties that are the same in the two data sources. As one can see, for four of these specialties (internal medicine, general surgery, cardiovascular surgery, and neurosurgery), the relationship between average malpractice premiums and the estimated rate of *negligent* hospital activity is nearly perfect. (These data suggest that premiums increased at a rate of $1.5 million per expected negligent event in 1988.) For these specialties, the malpractice insurance pricing seems precisely as one would expect in a competitive market, so long as the cost per claim is the same.

For the other three specialties shown (obstetrics, urology, and orthopedic surgery), premiums are much higher than the "systematic" relationship would suggest. This may in part explain why obstetricians, in particular, seem

FIGURE 13.2 Relationship between rates of negligent events and average medical malpractice premiums.

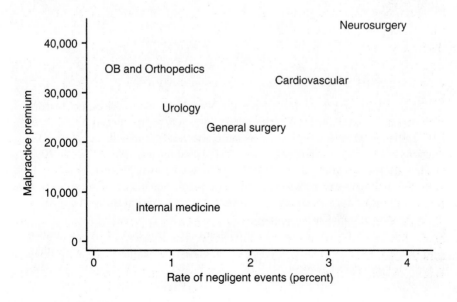

BOX 13.2 SHOULD DOCTORS BOTHER TO PREVENT RISKS?
AN APPLICATION OF GAME THEORY

A simple game theory model shows that when the pool of doctors becomes large enough and all doctors pay the same malpractice insurance premium ("community rating"), nobody would rationally take any costly steps to prevent injuries to patients. To see how this economic game works, we can define the payoffs to a doctor taking steps to reduce negligent harm and then show that for a sufficiently large pool of doctors (or sufficiently costly harm-prevention activity), the strategy of undertaking no prevention activity *dominates* the other choice, no matter what other doctors do. In such a case, rational behavior by doctors will lead to no harm prevention being undertaken.

Suppose first that the insurance pool contains 20 otherwise identical doctors, each of whom will create $100 in damage if they take proper injury-prevention steps (costing C each). Without the injury prevention, each doctor will create $200 in damage. Thus, the Learned Hand Rule requires them to spend C each, so long as C is less than $100 per doctor.

Now consider the payoffs to spending money on prevention if the doctors all pay the same malpractice insurance premium. Figure A shows these outcomes; the first number shown in each pair shows Doctor A's outcome (total costs of malpractice insurance plus prevention costs), and the second number of each pair shows the outcome for all other doctors.

FIGURE A

		All Other Doctors	
		Prevent	Do not prevent
Dr. A	Prevent	$100 + C$, $100 + C$	$195 + C$, 195
	Do not Prevent	105, $105 + C$	200, 200

Think about the problem from Dr. A's perspective. If all other doctors undertake prevention, Dr. A's lowest cost choice is to "not prevent" if $C > 5$. (Compare $100 + C$ with 105.) The same also holds true if all other doctors choose "Do not prevent" as their strategy (compare $195 + C$ with 200). Thus, no matter what other doctors do, Dr. A will select "Prevent" if and only if $C < 5$. It's easy to prove that the same result holds if some intermediate share of other doctors choose to prevent. For an empirical study of the issue, see Kessler and McClellan (1996).

Obviously, this presents a very different incentive than the no-insurance case. In effect, the incentive has been cut so that doctors will undertake prevention not at a cost of $100 or less but only at $5 or less. The fact that

$100 ÷ 20 = $5 is no accident. The 20 doctors in the pool blur each other's incentives by a factor of 20. It is also easy to see that if we make the pool contain 100 doctors rather than 20, the incentive gets worse. In that case, doctors would individually choose to prevent harm only if $C < 1$. As the pool becomes very large, the incentive to undertake costly injury prevention activities vanishes to zero.

This problem is a classic "noncooperative game" problem. If everybody could collude (cooperate), everyone would be better off; if everybody can't collude, each takes individual actions that make everybody worse off. Here, "patients" and "society" are also made worse off by the uncooperative game solution because doctors rationally choose (individually) not to undertake economically desirable prevention activities. In settings such as this, regulation sometimes helps.

concerned about the "validity" of the medical malpractice system. The high visibility of injuries to babies and the strong emotional content of such injuries seem to make obstetricians "stand out" as targets for malpractice suits and awards more than other doctors. This is almost certainly true of the insurance cost as well. This is quite consistent with the findings of Sloan et al. (1993) in a study of malpractice suits in Florida. They found that plaintiffs in cases with obstetric injuries were often motivated by a desire to "find out what happened, seek revenge, or prevent the doctor from harming others," rather than to seek compensation.[17]

In one important study of medical malpractice events, Rolph (1981) showed that insurance companies have at their disposal (but seldom use) information equally as useful in predicting future medical malpractice costs as the information they do use (medical specialty). This study showed that, holding specialty constant, previous claims experience explained as much of the variability in awards against doctors as did the information about specialty. For example, the average claims experience against Class VII doctors (e.g., neurosurgeons) is about seven times larger than the average for Class I doctors (e.g., family practitioners). Premiums paid by doctors in Class VII reflect these costs. However, it is also true that the average claims experience from those with the highest costs in the past 4 years (holding specialty

---

[17]It is also easy to understand the unusually high risk for urologists because an outcome from adverse events and negligence in their surgery commonly results in incontinence and/or impotence, events sure to capture the attention of the injured patient. The situation for orthopedic surgeons is less explicable.

BOX 13.3 COSTS OF MALPRACTICE INSURANCE

What is the cost of medical malpractice premiums? The answer is about as diverse as the profession of medicine itself, with premiums varying hugely by specialty, region, and year. Premiums have increased greatly during the past 15 years, explosively during periods of medical malpractice "crisis" as the data in Table A, a (sporadic) time series, reveal.

TABLE A

	Average Premium ($)	Average Annual Growth During Interval (%)
1974	1,300	—
1976	3,000	52.0
1981	3,650	4.0
1983	4,170	7.0
1986	8,040	25.0
1987	9,630	20.0
1988	10,950	14.0
1992	13,425	5.2
2000	18,000	3.7

Premiums differ hugely across specialty. For example, in 2000, doctors reported the average premiums shown in Table B; the last column compares each specialty's median premium with the overall average. These relative premium amounts remain fairly stable through time.

TABLE B PHYSICIAN MALPRACTICE PREMIUMS (THOUSANDS OF $)

Specialty	Medical Liability Premiums per Physician	Ratio to All Physicians
All practices	18	1
General/Family	14	0.78
Internal medicine	14	0.78
Surgery	24	1.33
Pediatrics	12	0.67
Radiology	19	1.06
OB/Gyn	39	2.17
Other	12	0.67

Source: AMA, 2003.
Note: Data reflect 2000 premium levels.

These median premium figures mask a large variability, some of which is explained by cross-state differences and urban-rural differences. Consider, for example, the distributions of claims for two extreme specialties in terms of median premiums costs—neurosurgery and pediatrics, shown in Table C (1988 data). Obviously, neurosurgeons' premiums center at the high end of the distribution while pediatricians' premiums are at the low end. Both distributions are quite wide, but they barely overlap.

TABLE C PERCENT OF DOCTORS PAYING PREMIUM

Premium	Neurosurgery (%)	Pediatrics (%)
More than $50,000	34	1
$40,000–$50,000	25	—
$30,000–$40,000	20	1
$20,000–$30,000	9	2
$15,000–$20,000	4	4
$10,000–$15,000	5	11
$8,000–$10,000	—	13
$6,000–$8,000	2	13
$4,000–$6,000	1	29
$2,000–$4,000	—	20
Less than $2,000	—	6

constant!) was about seven times larger than those in the lowest cost group over the past 4 years. Perhaps even more remarkable, insurance companies typically do not use previous claims history to set premiums for doctors within their specialty groups. Within specialty groups, the companies practice something akin to "community rating," whereby everybody in "the community" pays the same premium, even if the costs will differ predictably in the future.

Why insurance companies typically choose not to use previous experience by doctors in setting malpractice insurance premiums remains something of a mystery. It certainly has the effect of reducing incentives for doctors to choose appropriately safe care (see Box 13.2).

Even if individual insurance companies do not use "experience rating" (i.e., charging according to past risk, on the presumption that this predicts future risk), another common industry practice could lead to a similar result. Some insurance companies specialize in "good-risk" doctors only, while others accept any applicant. (See Box 13.4, which discusses this phenomenon.) However, some states negate this market-based experience rating by operating a state-owned malpractice insurance plan that sells insurance to any doctor. Obviously, if the lowest-risk doctors can all get malpractice insurance through private firms, the state-operated plan will have an unusually large concentration of poorer risks. Unless the state-operated plan prices the insurance appropriately, the overall distribution of insurance costs will not reflect risks appropriately, and the incentives for careful practice of medicine will get blurred or eliminated.

Why do states operate such plans? One reason is to try to keep doctors from leaving a practice within the state on the grounds that a "doctor shortage" exists and the state needs to do everything it can to retain doctors. Ironically, getting a few doctors out of practice may be the best thing that could happen to malpractice insurance premiums, as we shall see momentarily.

BOX 13.4 INSURANCE COMPANIES SPECIALIZE IN VARIOUS TYPES OF RISK (MARKETS PRODUCE "EXPERIENCE RATING" EVEN WHEN FIRMS DON'T)

Even if individual insurance firms don't use experience rating to price their insurance, the market may produce an equivalent result. That is, every firm might charge each of its customers the same price, yet each firm may accept different classes of risk. This can readily lead to high-risk customers paying higher rates and low-risk customers paying low rates, even if no single firm charges different rates to different risk classes. All that it takes is for the "good-risk" customers to shop around and find the best rates. The "bad-risk" customers will end up in a pool containing mostly bad risks, and the rates will necessarily reflect this sorting in the marketplace.

This phenomenon occurs commonly in automobile insurance. Look in the Yellow Pages of your telephone directory, and you will find good evidence of this. For example, in the Rochester, New York, directory, one advertisement appears with the following message:

> UNLIMITED INSURANCE SERVICES
> No one refused
> Drivers of any age
> We can help:
> DWI/DUI
> Accidents
> Cancelled policy
> Moving violations

By contrast, consider this advertisement from the same Yellow Pages:

> ARE YOU PAYING TOO MUCH?
> Business and Personal Insurance
> Preferred   Financial
> Driver rates   Planning

To which firm would you turn for insurance if you were 40 years old and had never had a moving violation or accident? What if you were 18 years old and had a DWI accident last month? If you need to get collision insurance for a 2008 Chevrolet sedan, with a deductible of $250.00, which firm do you think would have the lowest premium?

Some states even *require* that auto insurance companies charge the same premium to every customer. If a company wishes to evade that regulation, it establishes a portfolio of four or five companies with similar names but different rates. When a potential customer comes to one of its agents, the agent determines which risk class the customer belongs in and then makes an "assignment" to the corresponding insurance company from the portfolio available. Of course, "independent" insurance agents (those selling the insurance of many companies rather than working for a single insurer) have the same opportunity available even if no single company establishes a portfolio such as the one just described.

MALPRACTICE AWARDS: "LIGHTNING" OR A "BROOM SWEEPING CLEAN"?

The belief held by many doctors, some patients, and probably even some attorneys is that malpractice claims are completely whimsical, striking providers at random (much as lightning bolts from the sky), unrelated to the quality of care provided. A senior official of the American Medical Association summarized this view, asserting:

> The physician who gets sued is not the incompetent one, but rather the physician at the height of his career who is using frontier medicine on very sick patients, where the uncertainty of outcome is very high. All the doctor-owned insurance companies have documented this: they do not have large numbers of repeaters in terms of physicians being sued. [J. S. Todd, M.D., quoted in Holzman, 1988.]

[handwritten margin note: Doctors don't know what to do.]

The alternative view—indeed, the one embedded in the theory of deterrence—is that tort awards punish doctors for economically inappropriate behavior (as defined by the Learned Hand Rule) and that if a doctor persists in such behavior, we should expect to see multiple awards against that doctor.

Several studies have now produced strong evidence on this issue. The awards do not appear at random but rather concentrate heavily within a few doctors. One analysis of claims in southern California showed that doctors who had previous claims stood a much larger chance of having successful claims against them subsequently. More precisely, of more than 8,000 insured physicians, 46 (0.6 percent of the total) with four or more lost claims each accounted for 10 percent of all claims, and 30 percent of all awards. The chances of this occurring randomly if all doctors had equal probability of getting "struck by lightning" are vanishingly small, refuting the idea that the awards really are unrelated through time (Rolph, 1981). Note also that the assertion by Dr. Todd, which was just quoted, does not conflict with these results; indeed, it supports them in many ways—that is, very few "repeat offenders" exist in this southern California study, but they account for a disproportionately large fraction of total costs!

The awards may be related through time, but does this imply that the doctors with multiple awards against them provide a poorer quality of care? A more recent study (Sloan et al., 1989) analyzed insurance claims against doctors in Florida and found few relationships with usual markers of quality. Board-certified doctors had worse, not better, claims experience than their uncertified counterparts. The researchers found no consistent effect of medical school rankings, foreign versus U.S. medical schools,[18] or solo versus group practices. They *did* find that doctors with more frequent claims against them were more likely to have had complaints filed with the state medical examiners board.

The overall evidence is thus somewhat scattered but leaves several clear impressions. First, if malpractice awards are similar to "lightning," it clearly strikes a small handful of doctors with a much-higher-than-normal frequency, even after accounting for the effects of their specialty choice. We can conclude either that they practice unusually poor medicine or that they have a manner of dealing with their patients that invites lawsuits, independent of the quality of medicine they practice. It would also appear that many of the usual markers for quality, such as board certification, do not help detect such doctors.

TORT REFORM

Beginning with the malpractice "crises" of the 1970s, state legislators have been under common, if not constant, pressure to reform medical malpractice law. Part of the pressure obviously comes from doctors' footing the bills. (They have incentives to do this so long as they cannot pass along all of the costs to patients in the form of higher fees.) Tort reforms have steadily eroded the opportunity for extremely large plaintiff awards. A common change capped the award for "noneconomic" damages (e.g., "pain and suffering" awards) to $250,000 or some comparable amount. Many states have done this in recent years. As cases come to trial where such laws are now in effect, such

---

[18]Many people believe that foreign medical schools produce a lower quality doctor than U.S. schools.

caps can (and have been) challenged as unconstitutional by plaintiffs and their attorneys. State appeals and supreme courts have split on this issue. Some states, including California, Louisiana, and Nebraska, have upheld the constitutionality of caps so long as the state government can show a rational basis for the law. Others, nine in total, including Florida, Texas, Illinois, Ohio, and New Hampshire, have struck down such caps. Most of them were in the range of $250,000 to $500,000 maximum award for pain and suffering. The New Hampshire law, struck down in 1991, was notable for having an $875,000 cap (*The Wall Street Journal,* March 14, 1991).

Other changes aim more at the plaintiffs' lawyers. Common practices in the legal profession have plaintiff lawyers essentially becoming equity partners in a claim, taking the case on for a share of all awards rather than for per hour fees. From a purely economic standpoint, this "contingent fee" system has some positive features. First, it should prevent the filing of frivolous claims because the attorney confronts substantial fixed costs even to file a claim and would receive no compensation if no award materialized.

The contingent fee system also has the effect of reducing the incentive to take on cases for patients with lower income because many medical malpractice awards use lost wages as a basis for computing awards. For example, in a study of wrongful death awards, one study found a strong relationship between lost earnings and actual awards from the court (Perkins, Phelps, and Parente, 1990). Thus, some people have expressed concerns that the current malpractice system, coupled with a contingent-fee system, "shuts out" people with low-incomes from receiving compensation.

Highly visible awards to plaintiffs—shared commonly on a one-to-two basis with attorneys (one-third to attorneys, two-thirds to plaintiffs)—created a strong public sentiment against the common structure of awards for plaintiff's attorneys. For example, the landmark California malpractice reform of 1975 limited attorney fees to 40 percent of the first $50,000 of award, descending down to 15 percent of incremental awards at higher levels. Thus, plaintiff's attorneys in California and elsewhere now face a declining marginal revenue schedule with the size of the award, both reducing the incentive to file for large cases and the incentive to gather evidence that would increase the magnitude of awards.

Another approach has particular importance in a few select cases: namely, the requirement of "structured settlements" for persons permanently injured. Under previous approaches, awards for, for example, a child brain injured at birth might reflect the expected lifetime costs of care for the person. Under a structured settlement, the award would continue only so long as the child remained alive. Because such infants commonly die quite young, sometimes after a few years of life, the structured settlement ceases payments, which are far smaller in amount than would occur with many lump-sum awards. This approach has been mandated into law for some patients in recent tort reform in Virginia.

The effects of these various tort reforms on medical malpractice insurance premiums and awards have been documented only recently, in part because only by now has enough statistical evidence accumulated to measure the effects of these changes. However, the evidence seems to point toward substantial effects of at least some of these approaches. Table 13.2 displays the available data on malpractice awards over time. In the volatile period of the 1980s when tort reform was most active, one can readily see the effects of the reforms on median awards, maximum awards, and the number of awards exceeding $1 million.

Unfortunately, the available data (as released sporadically by Jury Verdict Research, the company that collects these data and sells them to interested parties) do not include the time period between 1988 and 1996. Despite the 8-year hiatus, the median awards (all that were reported in 2004) appear not to have climbed much ($473,000 in 1996 versus $400,000 in 1988). However, beginning in 1998, another abrupt increase took place, doubling the median awards to $1 million for three consecutive years (the last data reported). Although the dollar value of the median awards thus exceeded $1 million, we should remember that the CPI increased by 65 percent between 1986 (the year of the peak in median awards) and 2002, so the "real" median award remains at about three-quarters of the peak 1986 value in 2002. Only more future data will help us understand the extent to which the tort reforms of the 1980s and 1990s had lasting effects.

TABLE 13.2 JURY VERDICT AWARDS IN MALPRACTICE CASES

Year	Average $1,000	Median $1,000	Largest $1,000	Number Exceeding $1 million
1983	888	260	25,000	69
1984	649	200	27,000	71
1985	1,179	400	12,700	79
1986	1,428	803	15,800	92
1987	924	610	13,000	62
1988	732	400	8,100	54
1996		473		
1997		500		
1998		700		
1999		713		
2000		1,000		
2001		1,000		
2002		1,011		

Sources: 1983 to 1988 data: Jury Verdict Research as quoted in The Wall Street Journal; 1996 to 2002 data: Jury Verdict Research News Release, April 1, 2004.

To assess the overall effects of these changes, one can look as well at the effects on medical malpractice premiums because these should ultimately reflect changes in insurers' risks. One study (Zuckerman, Bovbjerg, and Sloan, 1990) used multiple regression analysis to study malpractice insurance premiums with data from 1974 through 1986. (Note that the study data do not include the years of dramatic drop in awards shown in Table 13.2.) This study used data from all 50 states, thus taking advantage of the substantial differences of the phasing in of tort reform across different states. In effect, the researchers let the various state legislators carry out experiments for them. The researchers analyzed effects not only of tort reform but also of other factors such as the number of trial lawyers in the region per capita. The most important changes in the tort law, they found, were those that capped physician liability (such as limitations on pain and suffering awards) and those that placed limits on how many years plaintiffs had to file a claim after an injury occurred (statute of limitations or limitations on the "discovery period"). The malpractice insurance premiums were unrelated to the number of attorneys per 1,000 persons, deflating the idea that plaintiffs' lawyers are the engine driving the malpractice cost explosion. Interestingly, insurance premiums were strongly and negatively related to the number of physicians per capita. This fact may reflect specialization effects. We know in general that as physicians per 1,000 population increase, specialization increases. (See discussion in Chapter 7 relating to physicians' location decisions.) If so, the negative correlation between malpractice insurance premiums and physician-per-capita measures provides indirect evidence this provides indirect evidence that specialty training reduces injuries, although direct studies on this question have shown no effects on the propensity of doctors to be sued (Sloan et al., 1989, using data from Florida).

These substantial reductions in premiums and awards seem to reduce the ability of "malpractice bashers" to claim that the medical–legal system is responsible for "all of" the increase in medical care costs that has taken place during the past several decades. In many ways, such an assertion seems obviously incorrect, given the clearly important roles of increased insurance coverage, increased per capita income (see Chapter 16 for further details), and increased availability of medical technologies. However, these data provide an important direct test. In a time when malpractice awards and premiums fell considerably (see Table 13.2 in particular), we did not see a corresponding reduction in medical care costs. As the legal phrase might suggest, *res ipsa loquitur.*

The major societal concern over medical malpractice insurance costs and other forms of liability (tort) insurance costs led the Congress, newly composed in 1995 with a Republican majority, to consider and pass major federal restrictions on state malpractice and tort laws. The combined effect of those changes, which passed the House of Representatives as part of the Republican's "contract with America," never passed the Senate and hence did not become public law. Whether President Bill Clinton would have signed such a bill if it had come to him remains unknown.

TORT REFORM WRIT LARGE

The most radical type of tort reform, considered sporadically, would completely scrap the current tort system in favor of a "no-fault" insurance plan to compensate persons injured in medical misadventures. The common model, workers' compensation, has functioned for most of this century with apparently favorable response from both workers and industry. Under the Workers' Compensation approach, no determination of fault is made. Rather, "the system" makes a determination of the magnitude of injury, on which basis insurers make payments. While this system does not completely eliminate "duels of experts" (there is still considerable dispute about the magnitude of loss in some of these cases), issues of fault do not exist, and the "overhead" borne by the system to determine fault is much lower than would otherwise occur (see Shavell, 1980).

Obviously, no-fault systems completely eliminate any direct economic incentive to undertake loss-preventing activities. The incentives are the same as those under an insurance scheme in which every doctor pays the same premium (see Box 13.2). The economic loss from such a plan, however, may be only very small if the current system produces little or no deterrence of negligent behavior.

Danzon (1985a) has made some calculations to suggest that even with all of its apparent problems, the medical malpractice system "pays its way" in a social cost framework if it can deter as few as 20 percent of the injuries that would occur in its absence. Alas, we have no good evidence yet (and never may, given the research problems associated with the issue) on just how much injury reduction actually takes place due to the risk of malpractice claims.

HMO LIABILITY: A NEW DOMAIN FOR MALPRACTICE LAW

As managed care has established a strong market presence, a new domain for negligence suits has arisen—claims against insurance carriers for denying benefit payments to insured individuals. The carriers now face liability on several legal fronts.

In the pressure to control costs (and hence insurance premiums), managed care plans often review and sometimes deny payment for certain types of treatment (often treatment they describe as "experimental" or "inappropriate"). Perhaps the most prominent of these was an $89 million award ($77 million of which was punitive damages) in 1995 to a patient denied coverage for a bone marrow transplant for breast cancer.[19] Even more dramatically, a 1999 award of $120 million ($116 million of which was punitive damages) was handed down in trial court against a managed care plan because its review processes allegedly delayed access to treatment.[20] Danzon (1997) argues that such cases should be considered as breach of contract disputes, not negligence.

A separate legal problem arises when the managed care organization restricts access of its enrolled population to a subset of all available providers (PPOs and related plans often use this strategy to control costs). The argument in favor of imposing liability on the insurer is that it has the best information about the doctors' histories, and it has mechanisms to control the doctors' behavior (Havighurst, 1997). The contrasting argument (Danzon, 1997) says that although such information and control mechanisms may exist, they are in fact very weak, and hence that liability should continue to reside with the provider of care directly.

The legal situation for these and related lawsuits has now been clarified. In 1974, the U.S. Congress passed legislation controlling employee benefit plans (Employee Retirement Income Security Act, known as ERISA) that (as federal legislation) supercedes state laws regulating employee benefits. It had been widely assumed that ERISA preempted state legislation as well in the arena of managed care and its potential for liability, particularly when the insurance came through employment groups.

Legal clarification came in June 2004 in a U.S. Supreme Court decision striking down the right to sue managed care plans.[21] In a unanimous decision, the Court ruled that the ERISA federal law completely preempted state law in this area despite the earlier ruling (in the fifth circuit court in Texas) that the issue was tort law, not contract law. This ruling appears to negate the laws in states that had established "right-to-sue" laws within their own states and provides strong protection to HMOs and related managed care organizations in terms of harms brought about by denial of benefits to enrollees (unless new legislation is passed that determines otherwise).

---

[19]*Fox v. Healthnet,* in California. Before an appeal was actually launched, the parties settled for a drastically reduced award, suggesting that the plaintiff's attorney felt that the appeals court would likely have eliminated much of the award.

[20]*Goodrich v. Aetna,* 1999. This case settled in April 2001 for the traditional "undisclosed amount."

[21]The case is known as *Aetna Healthcare v. Davila.*

SUMMARY

Negligence law is designed to serve two functions: to deter negligent behavior and to compensate victims of negligence. Formal definitions of negligence closely approximate a cost–benefit analysis, defining a provider's behavior as negligent if harm occurs to a patient and it would have cost less to prevent that harm than the expected amount of damage (in a statistical sense).

The current system of negligence law makes sense to operate if and only if an important amount of deterrence actually occurs because the system compensates injured persons poorly with estimates that only 1 in 15 to 1 in 25 negligently injured persons actually receive compensation.

Several strong forces work against successful deterrence within the current tort system. Few patients bring suit when injured, and medical malpractice insurance blunts the incentives of providers to exercise due caution because insurance premiums do not closely reflect individuals' propensities to be sued. Nevertheless, no clear evidence exists yet on the amount of deterrence produced by the tort system, and the case for moving to an alternative system has not yet been persuasively made.

RELATED CHAPTER IN *HANDBOOK OF HEALTH ECONOMICS*

Chapter 26, "Liability for Medical Malpractice" by Patricia M. Danzon

PROBLEMS

1. "There are not enough lawsuits in the current medical malpractice system." Discuss.
2. "The major purpose of medical malpractice insurance is to provide financial relief for people who are injured by medical care gone awry, and it does this very well." Discuss.
3. Describe the Learned Hand Rule, and discuss the economic logic underlying it.
4. What is the major role of the federal court system in medical malpractice law?
5. What role does malpractice insurance have (if any) on the rate of malpractice injuries to patients? Does it matter how that malpractice insurance is priced?
6. Many doctors claim that the malpractice insurance system is purely random, striking good doctors and bad doctors with equal propensity. What evidence do you know that supports or refutes this assertion?

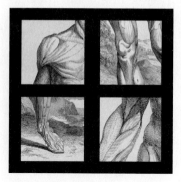

CHAPTER 14

Externalities in Health and Medical Care

This chapter discusses externalities involving health and the medical care system, both positive and negative. We can define *externalities* as events in which one person's actions impose costs on (or create benefits for) other persons. Every day of our lives we encounter externalities, such as traffic jams, cigar smoke drifting across the room in a restaurant, and a boom box blasting obnoxious music across the beach. All create externalities. Some people may consider an "event" a cost, and others may think it a benefit. The boom box provides an obvious example. One person may greatly enjoy Beethoven's Ninth Symphony coming from a nearby boom box, and another may hate it, but their positions may reverse if the boom box owner switches to Madonna's "Material Girl." Most externalities don't have such distinctions, however; they either uniformly provide benefits for or uniformly impose costs on others.

LEARNING GOALS

- Know the basic meaning of an externality and recognize its link to the definition and enforcement of property rights and the role of transaction costs in this problem.
- Discover the multiple externalities arising from contagious diseases:

  herd immunity
  vaccine demand
  vaccine supply

- Assess the externalities arising from tobacco use.
- Learn how information creates external benefits.
- Assess the importance of basic research as a positive externality.
- Understand external costs arising from the nation's blood supply.

Much of the latter part of this book deals, at least in part, with externalities and ways of dealing with them. Chapter 15 on regulation and Chapter 13 on the legal system discuss ways in which our society confronts and attempts to control some externalities. Chapter 15 also discusses the production and distribution of knowledge (biomedical research) and the production of knowledge about intelligent ways to use known medical interventions. This production of knowledge has at least some characteristics of externalities as well. *Externalities usually exist when property rights are not evenly assigned.*

EXTERNALITIES, PROPERTY RIGHTS, AND THE CONTROL OF EXTERNALITIES

A fruitful discussion of externalities must begin with a discussion of property rights because in many ways, externalities cannot occur when property rights are fully defined, and (conversely) when property rights are not fully defined or enforceable, externalities occur commonly, if not inevitably.

Property rights, at least as considered in English-based legal systems such as ours, define the conditions under which a person may own, use, and transfer an "object." The object may be a parcel of land (the traditional topic of property law), a personal object (a hat, an automobile), or a series of ideas (such as the manuscript for this book) or musical notes (such as Beethoven's Ninth Symphony). Important distinctions arise when we deal with existing objects (such as an automobile) or the *invention* or creation of a new class of ideas or objects. The branches of law that deal with invention (patent law and copyright law) have considerable importance in health and medical care.

From an economic perspective, the most important parts of property law include those that define the following:

- The ability of the owner to use the object.
- The ability of the owner to exclude others from using the object.
- The ability to transfer the object's ownership.
- Responsibilities of the owner toward others who use the object and to third parties involved in its use.

The simple example of an automobile shows the importance of these characteristics of property. If Henry and Marsha Ford own an automobile, it has little value to them if they cannot use it for their own transportation. It also has little value if they cannot legally exclude other people from using it because otherwise, it will never be available when they want to use it themselves. It has less value to them if they cannot sell it to another person. For example, the

Fords may wish to move to Manhattan, where a personal car is an expensive millstone around the owner's neck.

Liability law also determines the responsibilities that Henry and Marsha have if they let somebody else drive their car. If the brakes fail while their friend is driving it, are they responsible for the friend's injury? If the friend drives it negligently and injures or kills somebody else, do the Fords have any liability? If so, they will exercise more caution and prudence in their decisions about letting other people use the car, and possibly they will even take extra steps to prevent unauthorized use (if they would be liable for damage created by an unauthorized user).[1]

The same issues surround the invention of a new idea or device, and patent and copyright law protect the inventor's rights similarly. A patent or copyright provides the creator the right to use the idea and, most important, to exclude others from using the idea without permission. The inventor can also sell the patent, or "lease" it to others—that is, give them permission to use it in exchange for money. The legal system defines these rights, but the owners of property must often exert considerable effort to enforce them. An automobile parked on the streets of New York City may have the legal protection of exclusion, but in reality it stands a high chance of having an unauthorized user break and enter it, possibly to drive it, possibly to dismantle it and sell the parts. Alarm systems and garages provide some private enforcement of the property right, and police and the criminal justice system provide some public enforcement of it.

Particularly in the case of the rights surrounding inventions (patents and copyrights), the exclusion of illicit users presents a difficult problem. Industrial theft of an invention occurs commonly. Illicit copies of products ranging from Apple computers to Calvin Klein jeans to Chanel No. 5 perfume abound, and the manufacturers of such products spend considerable resources trying to detect and stop such illicit copies, often with private lawsuits to collect damages from the illicit user. Illicit copying of some copyrighted items seems impossible to stop. Probably few students and professors have not at some time violated copyright laws by illegally photocopying a journal article or sections of a book. Fewer still modern Americans have not illegally duplicated a recorded musical performance. In this

---

[1]This idea is not without substance. Swimming pool owners, for example, are sometimes held liable for drowning accidents, even if their pool is enclosed by a fence. Such pools have been held as an "attractive nuisance," and special standards of protection apply to the owners of such property.

case, although the law defines the property right, its enforcement is so costly to the copyright holder that illegal copying cannot be meaningfully stopped.

With this background of ideas about property, we can now begin our discussion of externalities in health and medical care with a bold assertion: Externalities occur if and only if the system of property rights fails to define ownership and/or liability surrounding an event or object. As we shall see through repeated example, the failure of property rights and/or liability law seems an essential part of every type of externality in the health care system and in other things that affect our health. This does not imply that "the solution" to such problems always rests in the legal system's defining property and liability. Regulation often serves as a better tool to control externalities, as Chapter 15 discusses. Economists often consider tax and/or subsidy schemes to control externalities as well, and these concepts also help convey the nature of externalities, even if "the solution" to the problem does not involve a tax or subsidy. Nevertheless, focus on the property rights idea helps us examine externalities more fruitfully.

EXTERNALITIES OF CONTAGION

Contagious diseases and their control provide perhaps the classic example of externalities in health and medical care. One person's action (sneezing) imposes costs on others (increased risk of getting a cold) that are not fully accounted for in the first person's actions. Those actions range from the most simple (carrying a handkerchief) to more costly (buying and using decongestant medicines that reduce sneezing) and even to more costly still (staying home from work and losing a day's pay).

The common cold provides a ludicrous but revealing example of the failure of property rights and liability law. If you sneeze into the air (which nobody owns), you create extra risks for others. The law also might make you liable for health damage you impose on others, so they could sue you for lost work time if they catch a cold from you.

If property rights and liability were perfectly defined *and enforcement costs were trivially small,* people's behavior regarding sneezing would change. For example, suppose that by law (and similarly for all others), you owned the air space within 2 feet of you. Then, not only would we all stay at least 4 feet apart unless given permission to trespass, but if you sneezed into other people's air space, they could claim damages.

In a remarkable analysis, Coase (1960) showed that the same behavior regarding sneezing would occur whether we each owned 2 feet of air space or

someone else owned it all, *so long as transactions costs were trivially small.*[2]
Alas, transactions costs in cases such as this overwhelm all other considerations. If you had to sue everybody who sneezed in your vicinity, you would have no time remaining for any other activity.

In the case of sneezing, social customs and "manners" create society's best control mechanism. These work reasonably well because most people whom you might infect with a cold see you repeatedly, and you select your behavior knowing that they can retaliate if you repeatedly impose costs on them. This sort of retaliation might include cutting you out socially, deliberately infecting you when they have a cold, or even reducing your pay at work (if you give your boss a cold too many times). The famous Golden Rule prescribes appropriate behavior in such settings. Amazingly, this sort of rule even seems to have good "survival" characteristics in a biological sense.[3]

Sometimes these sorts of social controls fail. For example, you have less incentive to control your sneezing on a crowded public bus than you do in a classroom or office, even though you are more likely to inflict a cold on somebody else. The obvious reason is that you have almost no chance of seeing any of those people again, so they have no chance to retaliate. In some

---

[2]Coase's landmark article, "The Problem of Social Cost," revolutionized economic and legal thinking about externalities. Coase won the Nobel Prize in Economics in 1991 for this work. The main idea, known as *the Coase theorem,* says that if transactions costs are very small, there will be the same amount of "externality" costs in a society no matter how property rights are assigned. He used the example of farmers' fields and a train throwing off sparks. If you assign the property rights to the farmers, their ability to sue the railroad will cause its owners to install the correct amount of spark arresters, that is, the amount whereby the marginal expected damage equals the marginal cost of prevention. If you assign property rights to the railroad, then the farmers will "bribe" the railroad owner to install spark arresters, again, just to the point at which marginal benefit equals marginal cost.

Many readers erroneously interpret Coase as saying that the assignment of property rights "doesn't matter" in efficiency considerations. The main thrusts of Coase's work are (1) that one should carefully attend to transactions costs when considering the allocation of property rights and (2) when transactions costs are large, the problem won't go away, even with full property rights.

[3]More precisely, experiments using computers have shown that a strategy of cooperation, coupled with a tit-for-tat punishment strategy for defectors, dominates almost any other known strategy in games of repeated interaction. In this type of strategy, you "cooperate" until your partner "defects" from the cooperative strategy on one play of the game. You immediately punish your partner by defecting for one play and then return to a cooperative strategy until your partner defects again. In cooperation games in which players with various strategies compete against one another, this tit-for-tat strategy outperforms almost all others, including some that have been designed specifically to defeat a tit-for-tat strategy. For an excellent discussion of these ideas, see Axelrod (1984).

societies, such as Japan, social custom then takes precedent. There, people wear surgical masks when they have a cold to cut down on the contagious effects of sneezing. The emergence of such a custom in a crowded society such as Japan probably makes more sense than, for example, in Wyoming, which has an average population density of about three persons and six cows per square mile.

More Serious Contagious Diseases

Some diseases have more serious consequences than the common cold, and we take more expensive steps to respond to them. These types of disease also highlight the importance of property and enforcement costs. (Box 14.1 discusses a contemporaneous contagious disease.)

Some diseases (such as dysentery) are transmitted readily through water systems. The famous case of "Aspenitis" involved the vacation town of Aspen, Colorado, where tourists and natives alike suffered common and serious intestinal illness. Research into the causes of the disease finally determined that the town's water lines and sewer lines, which ran parallel to each other through much of the town, had both broken and cross-contaminated each other. The contamination in one direction (from sewers to water system) had more serious consequences than in the other direction (from water system to

BOX 14.1 *EBOLA* VIRUS

One highly visible contagious disease has created its own "stir" in the minds of the public and the government. A virus that had previously broken out sporadically in Africa, the ebola virus, appeared again in a virulently contagious form in 1995. This disease spreads with ease with the most incidental person-to-person contact because it can spread airborne, for example, from a person's sneeze. Although the number of deaths due to the disease has been small, the very high fatality rate from the disease (75 to 90 percent of people who contract the disease die) and the extraordinary ease of transmission have caused two notable public events to take place. First, the 1995 movie *Outbreak* was loosely based on events related to this disease. Second (and perhaps related to the first), during a 1996 congressional deadlock over funding the federal government, a flareup of *ebola* in Africa led, within 24 hours, to passage of a special appropriation to bring the Centers for Disease Control back to full operation. Few political events have come to such swift conclusion as that to ensure funding for our country's best protection against a virulent, highly contagious, and highly fatal disease!

sewers). However, the potential liability of the owners of the water system (the town, in this case) caused them to find and repair the break rapidly.[4]

The threat of poliomyelitis in the 1950s caused dramatic changes in behavior. Before the Salk and Sabin vaccines became available, and even before people understood fully that a virus caused polio, they did understand that person-to-person communication of the disease was possible, although the exact vector was not known. A common response during the height of the polio epidemic of the 1950s was to close public swimming pools. Some of this occurred by regulation (i.e., by order of county health department officials) but some as a "voluntary" action by owners of swimming pools who might have been held liable for transmission of the disease.

Vaccines and Vaccination Policy

For some contagious diseases, scientists have discovered vaccines that make people much less susceptible to the diseases, often totally eliminating the risk for the vaccinated person. (The discovery of such vaccines represents a separate problem of externalities, as a later section in this chapter explores.) The nature of vaccines and contagious diseases offers a useful study of externalities.

Consider a society of, for example, 1,000 inhabitants on an island confronting the risk of a contagious disease, perhaps carried to the island from elsewhere by a vacationing person. Call this person Patient Zero.[5] Each Person j who comes in contact with Patient Zero has some probability π_{j0} of contracting the disease from Zero, depending on the virulence of the disease and the nature of their contact. Each Person j getting the disease also has a subsequent probability of transmitting it to some other Person i, which we can call π_{ji}. Some people may be "naturally immune" to the disease (e.g., because of previous exposure and hence a well-developed antibody system), so their probability of catching and spreading the disease is zero.[6] Suppose that we call the economic cost of getting the disease C (treatment costs, lost work, pain, etc.). Then Person i's expected cost is $C\Sigma_{j\neq i} \pi_{ij} = C\pi_i$, where π_i is Person i's probability of getting the disease—that is, $\pi_i = \Sigma_{j\neq i} \pi_{ji}$. This

---

[4]Berton Roueche's book *Eleven Blue Men* (1965) describes a number of fascinating episodes of detection of contagious diseases.

[5]The transmission of HIV in North America follows a clear path from a single person whom public health authorities call Patient Zero.

[6]Most viral diseases have this characteristic. Sometimes, we know with high likelihood whether we have had a specific disease. Mumps offers a good case in point. In other cases, we may not know whether we've had a disease. Many people became infected with the polio virus, for example, and recovered completely after a minor illness much like the flu, but they received natural immunity thereafter.

cost avoidance creates each person's private willingness to pay (WTP) for the vaccination. If people's private costs differ from each other, then a graph of the WTP for the vaccination will create what looks just like (and is) a downward-sloping demand curve at the societal level for the vaccine—that is, the demand curve one gets by adding each individual's demand curves. (See the discussion with Figure 4.7 in Chapter 4 to remind yourself how this "horizonal aggregation" works.)

Each person will rationally be vaccinated if the expected costs of the illness exceed those of getting the vaccine (including time, travel, fees, the pain of the vaccination process, and the expected side effects of the vaccine), which we can call C_v.

Two things appear immediately in this problem. The first is the concept of *herd immunity*. If any other persons in the society are immune—for example, if they have already become vaccinated—then Person i's chances of getting the disease from any vaccinated Person k fall to $\pi_{ki} = 0$. At the extreme, if everybody else in society had already become vaccinated, then that last person would never bother because Person i's chances of getting the disease (π_i) would fall to zero. In the language of externalities, herd immunity creates a positive externality for Person i.

Second, we can turn the question around and ask what private and social benefits occur if Person i is vaccinated. Holding constant the number of other people who are vaccinated, Person i will decide to be vaccinated if $C_v < C\pi_i$. However, the social benefit extends past Person i because, once vaccinated, Person i will contribute to the herd immunity for everybody else. To be precise, the net benefit for the entire society is $C\pi_i$ *plus* $C\Sigma_{j \neq i}\, \pi_{ij}$ because each Person j's chances of contracting the disease from Person i fall from π_{ij} to zero. Each person's *private* willingness to pay (WTP) for the vaccine is $C\pi_i$, and the *social WTP* is $C\pi_i$ plus the contribution to the herd immunity. The difference, $C\Sigma_{j \neq i}\, \pi_{ij}$, is the externality benefit. Figure 14.1 shows both the private and social *aggregate WTP* curves that vary with the proportion of the society vaccinated. The vaccine cost C_v appears as a flat line in this diagram because (by assumption) the costs per vaccination do not vary with the proportion of people vaccinated.[7]

Private decisions will lead to N_1 persons becoming vaccinated, the number at which WTP^p equals C_v. If the number vaccinated exceeds N_2, then the cost C_v exceeds even the social benefit, WTP^s, for the vaccine, and getting Person i vaccinated makes no sense from either a private or social standpoint.

---

[7] If economies of scale in vaccination exist, for example, through school vaccine programs, then the C_v line would fall. Similarly, if diseconomies of scale existed, for example, due to a fixed supply of some input necessary to make the vaccine, then the C_v line would rise.

FIGURE 14.1 Private and social aggregate willingness to pay.

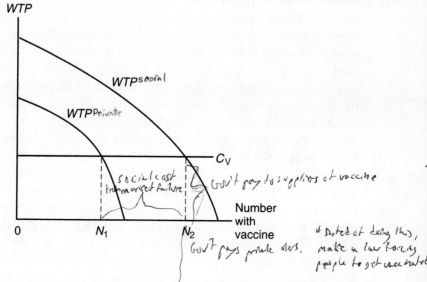

Between N_1 and N_2 of the population vaccinated, a conflict arises between the private and social decisions to be vaccinated. The private decision says, "Forget it!" The social decision says it is worthwhile. The public policy problem is how to induce enough people to be vaccinated in order to reach the proportion N_2 because private decisions will lead to only N_1 percent of the people being vaccinated.

Economists usually think about such problems in terms of an optimal tax or subsidy. Looking at Figure 14.1, to reach N_2 percent vaccinated using a subsidy, one would have to extrapolate the WTP^P demand curve down below the N axis and to the right until it reached N_2 and then pay a subsidy amounting to the difference between that curve and C_V. As the figure is drawn, merely giving away the vaccine (so $C_V = 0$ to the individual) wouldn't suffice because the WTP^P curve crosses the N axis at a smaller value than N_2.

Although the idea of an "optimal subsidy" has clear meaning to economists, this almost never turns out to be the actual *vehicle* that public policy uses to increase vaccination rates. Sometimes vaccines are provided free and at convenient locations (the mass polio vaccinations of the 1950s and 1960s provide a good example), but commonly compulsion also enters the picture. Schools, for example, often require that students have some set of vaccinations before they are admitted. Every inductee into the armed forces goes through a standard series of vaccinations. Overseas travelers (who may be exposed to a whole array of unusual diseases not prevalent at home) must present proof of vaccination against certain diseases before their government will issue a passport to travel. The government takes these steps in part to protect the traveler but, more important, to prevent the spread of disease to others—that is, in the name of "public health."

As with every compulsory act of government, some individuals may be harmed when such methods are used. Some people's religious beliefs, for example, prohibit their use of medicines. When the government imposes the requirement of vaccination on such people, it inflicts a real cost. Some vaccines also have side effects that occasionally strike the vaccinated person. On occasion, these side effects prove fatal, as with the infamous swine flu vaccine involved in an influenza vaccine program personally promoted by the President of the United States (he received his flu shot on national television). Unfortunately, the vaccine turned out to have some bad side effects for some people.[8] One of the advantages of a "subsidy" program is that it induces those people who bear the smallest costs to be vaccinated because only those people who derive a net positive benefit (including the subsidy) from getting the vaccine will respond to the subsidy.[9] However, subsidies increase the "on budget" costs of the government, whereas compulsion creates only "off budget" private costs. This distinction apparently drives many political decisions.

Vaccines Supply as an Externality

It is easy to outline the reasons why the demand for vaccines creates an issue concerning the public good. Each person who is vaccinated against a contagious disease also confers a benefit on others with whom they come in contact by reducing the risk that the others will become infected (herd immunity). Concern for the public good, as well as the cost, potential pain (in some cases), and risk if adverse side effects occur (rare, but nevertheless real) add to the case for intervention to correct the demand-side externality regarding vaccines.

In recent years, we have come to understand that vaccine supply also has aspects of a public good and hence deserves attention equal to or more than the demand-side issues. The supply-side issues include at least the following:

- special financial risk because of mutating target organisms
- medical-legal liability confounded by mass vaccination strategies
- production line failures or insufficient supply (à la military stockpile)

Each of these issues offers some assistance in dealing with the underlying concerns about vaccine supply. Let's treat each of them in turn.

---

[8]Because of the problems of this program, one wag asserted that the public health officials had sold a "pig in a poke" to the American people.

[9]The ideas behind an "all-volunteer" military force versus a compulsory draft rest on the same logic.

Financial Risk ~ *prices keep starting, so it gets expensive*

As Chapter 15 will discuss in more detail, the drug development process is expensive, time consuming, highly regulated, and risky. Many drugs fail the development process at various stages with an ultimate success rate of only 8 percent overall (Woodcock, 2006, p. 606). The world of vaccine development has several risks. One most prominently represented by the human immun-odeficiency virus (HIV) is the risk of mutation of the target organism, but this risk occurs with any drug (vaccine or antibiotic) that works against a living organism. Darwin explained this to us more than a century ago: Survivors in a harsh environment are better suited to propagate, and survival traits tend to accumulate through generations. Because microorganisms (viruses and bacteria) have very short life spans, this Darwinian mutation can occur rapidly. With HIV, mutation has thwarted almost all attempts at both treatment and prevention to date. Even if a vaccine succeeds against one generation of the target species, it might not succeed against later generations. This mutation creates a drug development risk that does not exist with most drugs.

Finally, demand is uncertain, particularly with (pardon the expression) "one-shot" vaccines for a seasonal influenza virus for which the target organism changes every year. If early reports suggest that the seasonal flu will not be very aggressive, some people will choose to avoid vaccination, thus reducing sales that provide the vaccine manufacturer's financial return on its research and development investments.

Medical-Legal Risk

Vaccines have several characteristics that make them particularly susceptible to medical-legal risk. First, by definition, the vaccine somehow is developed from the original target organism, which by definition is dangerous to human health. One of the great biological "tricks" in vaccine development is to find a way either to alter the target organism so it is no longer dangerous (but still elicits the immune response in the human body) or to find substitute biological components that trigger the immune response by "looking like" the virus or bacterium to the human immune system.[10]

Second, the optimal vaccination strategy for diseases that are highly contagious and can result in epidemics often requires mass vaccination in a very short time period. The benefit of such a strategy is obvious. One cost of the short time period is the loss of possible information about adverse side

---

[10]The recently developed vaccine for human papilloma virus (HPV) that causes cervical cancer is a case following the latter strategy. A viruslike particle in the vaccine triggers the immune response even though it is not actually a part of the virus that causes the cancer.

effects. After most drugs are approved by the FDA for human use, an extended period of "postmarketing surveillance" takes place where adverse event reporting helps track down side effects that eluded researchers in the drug's clinical trials.[11] However, in the case of vaccines against highly contagious diseases, in an ideal world, everybody is vaccinated at almost the same time. This eliminates the chance to find adverse side effects over a more extended time period. Thus, when such effects do emerge, they become natural targets for a class-action lawsuit against the manufacturer. Understanding this risk, many companies have exited the world of vaccine production.[12]

Production Line Risk

Vaccine production often entails using "brews" of biological substances, often a fragile process. Periods of vaccine shortage for influenza vaccines in recent years often have occurred because something affects the vaccine production process in one of only a small number of manufacturing plants making it, causing a failure to elicit the desired immune response. Thus, distributing the vaccine production across multiple sites and even across multiple companies has real advantages, but as Danzon and Pereira (2005) pointed out, the natural economies of scale in vaccine development seem to favor sole-supplier markets. Thus, finding a way to distribute the production (and hence reduce societal risk of a supply failure) represents another form of supply side externality.

SOLUTIONS TO THE EXTERNALITY PROBLEMS

Vaccine Injury Compensation Program

The national Vaccine Injury Compensation Program (VICP) was created in 1986 to help encourage vaccine production and distribution in the United States by reducing the financial risk to vaccine manufacturers from fault-based personal injury lawsuits. The program began in October 1988 with two interrelated goals. First, VICP established a no-fault compensation system for

---

[11]This issue reminds us of the power of the law of large numbers. Even large clinical trials will never accumulate as many subjects as will eventually take the drug, often with actual patients exceeding the number of subjects in randomized trials by many orders of magnitude. Thus, the power to detect low-frequency adverse events is necessarily greater in postmarketing surveillance than in the clinical trial setting.

[12]Between 1967 and 2004, the number of vaccine supply companies in the United States fell from 26 to 5 (Igelhart, 2005).

people who receive specific vaccines and then exhibit specific injuries or illnesses. This system is designed to be less costly, less adversarial, and faster than the usual tort system (as discussed in Chapter 13). VICP also removes much of the cloud of litigation hanging over vaccine producers, thus (hopefully) leading to the second goal: stabilizing and enhancing vaccine supply.[13]

The VICP pays for all associated medical costs of a harmed person up to $250,000 for pain and suffering costs and up to $250,000 for a vaccine-associated death. People injured after the law took effect in October 1988 are required to file for compensation through the federal program, although they may turn down an offered compensation and then sue using regular legal processes. According to a Department of Justice (DOJ) statement, few people resort to the tort system after refusing an award (Division of Vaccine Injury Compensation, 2006).

A $0.75 charge on each dose of vaccine administered through VICP (i.e., those specific vaccines itemized in the law) funds it. These funds go into a special trust fund administered by the Department of Health and Human Services, and the DOJ manages the legal process for the government (to ensure against fraudulent claims). According to DOJ reports, the average award in the first decade of the program's operation was about $750,000 and provided $1.2 billion in awards to more than 1,500 individuals.

Permanent Demand Support

An Institute of Medicine (IOM) report (IOM, 2003) proposed six alternative plans (plus "keep doing the same thing").[14] Four of these relied on different approaches to expand and stabilize demand through various federal or federal/state programs, such as expanding the Vaccines for Children (VFC) program,[15] to include additional eligibility categories, vaccine-purchase vouchers for populations who are economically disadvantaged, or widespread federal purchase and supply of all recommended vaccines. The IOM report eventually recommended an approach that would mandate vaccine payment in all health insurance plans (both private and public) and added a voucher system for populations who are economically disadvantaged.

---

[13]Some tort risk remains, however, because individuals can refuse the settlement offer and sue the vaccine manufacturer.

[14]Albert Einstein has been quoted as saying "The definition of insanity is to keep doing the same thing and expecting a different result."

[15]This program uses government funds to purchase vaccines to provide them free to children who are uninsured or underinsured. The VFC program now purchases about half of the vaccines regularly used for young children.

These alternative proposals affect the supply of vaccines only indirectly by ensuring steady demand for the product. The most powerful of these—to mandate that health insurance cover vaccines—would provide the widest market and hence the strongest assurance to vaccine suppliers. Such proposals also help solve the demand-side externality problem, of course.

Other Options

The combination of the VICP and these IOM-recommended "demand supports" could go a long way toward stabilizing the vaccine supply, but several problems remain. As Grabowski (2005) has pointed out, the IOM proposals still leave an intertemporal risk to vaccine manufacturers because vaccine research and development (R&D) can take years before the product can be marketed. Grabowski also alludes to the political risk that a vaccine might not be included on the list of approved products or at least not completely.[16] The fundamental problem is that current governments cannot bind future governments to action. This problem has been solved in some cases (e.g., malaria vaccine) by establishing escrow arrangements or other "precommitment" strategies to credibly assure vaccine manufacturers of the future revenue stream they want in order to commit to the R&D.

The solution to the remaining supply-side externalities may require different mechanisms. Grabowski (2005) has proposed federal/private partnerships for drug development to help reduce the supplier risk. Project Bioshield (enacted in 2004) creates government stockpiles for anthrax vaccine (demand pull) and new National Institutes of Health (NIH) support for research on various bioterrorism-related risks (supply push) enhances vaccine production. Another important feature of Project Bioshield is its authorization for the government to prepurchase drugs up to 8 years before expected FDA approval. This solves the time inconsistency problem of the lag between R&D costs and eventual product sales.

The Orphan Drug Act (more about this in Chapter 15) also creates incentives for pharmaceutical manufacturers to pursue drug development for small-market drugs by offering tax incentives and streamlined clinical trial and approval processes. While the smaller clinical trial studies of an orphan drug world may not work well in the more widely used vaccine world, the tax

---

[16]The case of HPV vaccine for cervical cancer presents a case in which political risk became a serious issue. Because the cancer is caused by a virus, it can be spread by sexual contact. Hence, the disease transmission can be reduced by vaccinating males as well as females. The issue became politicized upon release of the vaccine in terms of (1) vaccination of young girls and (2) males because of issues relating to sexual promiscuity.

credits and other approval streamlining processes have the potential to enhance permanent vaccine supply reliability.

Finally, the risks of failure at a given manufacturing site for vaccines can be mitigated by requiring multiple-site production resources (either within one company or by obligatory licensing others) in exchange for such things as tax credits and/or R&D support.

INTERNATIONAL ISSUES—EXPANDING THE SCOPE OF THE EXTERNALITY

Although previously mentioned in passing, the problem of contagious diseases now has an international aspect, arising both through naturally occurring diseases and also through the risk of bio-terrorism.

International Disease Transmission

Rapid international transmission of contagious diseases has become an issue of concern in the modern jet age. Two separate outbreaks of highly virulent influenza have highlighted this risk: the severe acute respiratory syndrome (SARS) in 2003 and the ongoing concerns about bird-to-human virus transmission known generally as "Avian flu."

The SARS epidemic of 2003 shows some of the potential concerns and public responses to a highly contagious and lethal disease in the age of jet travel. At the peak, SARS had infected more than 8,000 people in 27 countries, and at least five cases of transmission by international aircraft travel have been documented (Hollingsworth, Ferguson, and Anderson, 2006). Contemporaneous estimates of the case-mortality rate ranged from 5 to 20 percent, a level of lethality seldom seen in infectious diseases such as this. Final estimates placed the case mortality rate at just under 10 percent.

The SARS arose in China, and midpoint in the epidemic cycle, that country hospitalized and quarantined all patients with disease symptoms. At the peak of the cycle, China closed primary and secondary schools for two weeks and then (a few days later) many public venues (theaters, discos, etc.). The World Health Organization issued travel advisories banning noncritical travel to and from "hot-spot" areas (mostly in the Far East but including Toronto). The epidemic peaked around graduation time at U.S. universities and colleges, and many of them grappled with whether to ban families of graduating students from attending graduation events as a private response to the epidemic. In May 2003, the University of California at Berkeley refused admission to 500 students from hot-spot areas because of the perceived risk.

Most major drug companies and the NIH immediately began developing vaccines against SARS, and the prototype was developed within a year of the disease outbreak (but after the transmission cycle had stopped.) It used a protein found on the coating of the SARS virus that triggered immune response in test animals. Clinical trials began in 2006, but as of this writing in 2008, no vaccine is yet commercially available despite massive international efforts to produce one. Thus, the only methods to combat the disease at this point are the same as those used in 2003: quarantine and travel restrictions.

Travel restrictions have the potential to limit the spread of diseases like SARS according to mathematical simulation models, but to be wholly effective (rather than merely delaying the spread of the disease), travel bans from affected areas not just at major hubs must be ubiquitous (Hollingsworth, Ferguson and Anderson, 2006).

The economic issue of a travel ban, of course, is to balance the value of forgone travel (as impeded by travel bans) to those prevented from traveling to and from hot-spot areas against the public good of preventing disease spread. The issue obviously involves many potentially conflicting values including (at least in free nations) the rights to travel freely and to avoid unreasonable search. No simple approach exists for balancing the protection of the public (on the one hand) versus the preservation of freedom to travel and to avoid search (on the other hand), but economics and medicine combine to set the basic parameters of such quarantine and travel policies. A good travel policy will be more stringent whenever (1) the virus exhibits high rates of transmission across humans (or other species to humans), (2) the lethality of the disease is high, and (3) the costs of treating affected individuals (even if the disease is not highly lethal) is high. All of these involve biological and biomedical issues that the field of economics does not inform very well, so intelligent planning on such matters will involve biomedical scientists, lawyers, ethicists, political scientists, sociologists, anthropologists, and, yes, economists.

Avian influenza ("bird flu") has some special characteristics that cause concern among public health officials and create economic issues other than those related to the SARS outbreak in 2003. Avian flu is *mostly* confined to bird populations; many wild birds carry the virus without harm, but it sometimes infects domesticated bird flocks (chickens and ducks most prominently) and occasionally transmits from there to humans.[17] Experts' greatest concern is the coexistence of human and avian flu viruses in which the

---

[17]That the major carriers include wild migratory birds exacerbates this problem. It seems uncommonly expensive to enforce a worldwide travel ban against migratory birds. The supply of 10 gauge shotguns (and the adept users thereof) would seem to be an important limiting factor.

exchange of genetic information between the viruses could create a new strain that is highly communicable and lethal to humans. Many experts use phrases such as "when, not whether" in describing the risk of such species crossover. While all extant cases of Avian flu in humans (at the date of this writing) have come from bird-to-human transmission, the concerns about creating a human-to-human viral transmission make Avian flu a top public health priority.

All previously discussed issues arise when considering mechanisms to deal with Avian Flu: basic research to find the basis for vaccines, drug development costs and timing, mechanisms to ensure an adequate vaccine supply, and finally (at time of an outbreak) policies to limit disease transmission through quarantine and travel bans.

EXTERNALITIES FROM TOBACCO

Another important externality affecting health arises from the widespread use of tobacco products, primarily cigarettes, throughout the world. Two types of externalities exist from tobacco use. First, the smoke itself is unpleasant to many people, possibly more than smokers themselves realize. For persons with hay fever and asthma, any irritant, including tobacco smoke, can set off allergic reactions that are at least unpleasant and at most, in the case of asthmatics, potentially fatal. However, for most persons "bothered" by cigarette, cigar, and pipe smoke, the unpleasant smell is the most obvious manifestation of an externality, and until recently it was thought to be the only one of importance.

Response to this externality forms an interesting study in the use of regulation instead of a reliance on property rights and markets. During the past decade, many cities and states have enacted regulations that limit the areas where smokers may smoke in "public" buildings (i.e., those open to common access by strangers) including office buildings, restaurants, airports, and so forth. Typically, these rules require that restaurants (for example) provide nonsmoking sections and offer every customer a choice of smoking versus nonsmoking seating. In areas with more strict rules, smoking cannot take place in office buildings, even in "private" offices, if such offices might be used by persons other than the primary occupant.[18] Some companies have privately gone beyond the requirements of the law, not only totally banning

---

[18]These rules have created an entirely new social network in some businesses, namely, employees who meet at office building entrances to go outside to smoke. They also create interesting euphemisms, such as people saying that they are "going outside to get a breath of fresh air" when they are in fact going outside to smoke a cigarette.

smoking on their premises but also offering to pay for smoking-cessation programs for their employees. Numerous hospitals have totally banned smoking by patients, staff, and visitors, not only within the hospital itself but also in surrounding areas.

The logic for a regulatory approach to control smoking in public buildings arises directly from the "random" nature of access to such buildings. Trying to use agreements (contracts) between people in a restaurant to determine whether smoking would take place would be the height of absurdity, and nobody would think seriously of a full "property rights" approach to such a problem. The transactions costs of reaching agreements would overwhelm the problem. Similarly, even if owners of restaurants for example, wish to establish smoking and nonsmoking sections in their restaurants, they may fear the loss of customers who wish to smoke. (This is another example of a noncooperative game problem as discussed in more detail in Chapter 13 on medical malpractice. You may wish to look at Box 13.2 in which this problem is discussed.) Regulation offers an alternative—albeit draconian from the point of view of smokers—to solve the problem. Notice that previous rules freely permitting smoking have an exactly parallel nature except they are viewed as draconian from the point of view of nonsmokers.

Similarly, the U.S. Congress instituted a ban on smoking during airline flights of less than 2 hours duration in 1984. Then in 1988, Congress extended that ban to all domestic flights except those scheduled to require more than 6 hours' flight time (which occurs only on flights to Hawaii and Alaska). In this case, the logic for universal application of a regulatory regime seems somewhat thinner because a market response to the question of whether smoking should occur on an airplane seems more likely to emerge. Indeed, before any regulations on the subject occurred at all, some airlines privately banned smoking on all flights, "specializing" in the market for those customers who preferred nonsmoking flights. In a city-pair market with many daily flights (such as between New York and Boston or Washington), one might well expect such specialization to emerge. It did not, however, take widespread hold, and the regulatory approach soon swept over the market. In June 2000, the U.S. Department of Transportation banned smoking on all flights entering and leaving the United States, for both U.S. and foreign carriers, thus extending the 1990s domestic smoking ban to international flights.

The second and more serious externality arising from cigarette smoke has now become more carefully understood—even nonsmokers' health risks increase when they spend considerable time in close proximity with smokers. A series of epidemiology studies has emerged over the past several years showing substantially heightened risks of lung cancer, heart disease, and other lung diseases (such as emphysema) from nonsmokers who live in a house with at least one smoker. Indeed, one study demonstrated that even the *dogs* of smokers had a 50 percent increased risk of dying from lung cancer compared with dogs whose owners did not smoke.

The magnitude of secondhand smoke morbidity and mortality is yet to be fully determined, but evidence continues to accumulate that this is a more serious externality than had previously been recognized. A 1989 study compared the health outcomes of nonsmokers who live with smokers with that of nonsmokers who live with nonsmokers (Sandler, Comstock, Helsing, and Shore, 1989). This 12-year study of nearly 28,000 individuals found that the age-adjusted risk of death was 15 to 17 percent higher for nonsmokers who lived with smokers than for those who lived with nonsmokers. Such a study necessarily understates the actual health consequences of secondhand smoke, however, because it ignores the exposure outside of the home, which tends to increase the risks of those living with smokers and nonsmokers similarly.[19]

More recently, a case-control study investigated the risks of lung cancer for those exposed to secondhand smoke in the household (Janerich et al., 1990). Household exposure to 25 or more "smoker years" during childhood and adolescence doubled the risk of a person's later contracting lung cancer. (If two parents smoke for 15 years, that creates 30 "smoker years" of exposure.) The study estimated that one of every six cases of lung cancer among nonsmokers was due to secondhand smoke exposure acquired during childhood from parents.

These and other studies continue to clarify the role of this particular type of externality. Even with incomplete information, it seems safe to say that tobacco consumption does create an important health externality, certainly for those within the household, and possibly in other surroundings as well (e.g., the workplace). We can analyze the consequences of this behavior as of any other externality.

Private Taxes on Externalities

Sometimes liability law (see Chapter 13) supplants legislative action as a way to control externalities. The case of the illnesses caused by tobacco provides a good example. With major public intervention for nearly half a century

---

[19]To see why this causes an understatement of the actual health effect, consider the following hypothetical case: Suppose that all nonsmokers had a 10 percent increase in risk due to secondhand smoke acquired at work, restaurants, and so forth, and that the true effect of living with a smoker was a 20 percent increase in risk, compared to no secondhand smoke exposure at all. Then the actual increase in risk due to smoke exposure would be 32 percent ($1.2 \times 1.1 = 1.32$), but the apparent effect would be only the 20 percent increase.

now, tobacco consumption has fallen substantially (see the later discussion surrounding Figure 14.3). Taxes on tobacco sales have increased steadily, and much advertising has promulgated information about the risks of smoking.

In the midst of this smokers, former smokers, or their families have brought a number of private lawsuits against tobacco companies. Most of these centered on a "defective product" approach to liabilty, but the legal setting in each case would come through the law of torts that we examined in relationship to medical malpractice in Chapter 13. These suits have generally failed in the courts or on appeal because of several common defenses by the tobacco companies, mostly hinging on the idea that the dangers of smoking were well known, particularly after the mandatory federal requirements for posting warning labels on tobacco products and advertisements.

The major shift in the legal environment came when state governments began to sue tobacco companies to recover the costs of treating Medicaid patients with tobacco-related diseases. Several consecutive successes in the courts led to a major settlement agreement in 1998 between every state in the country and the major cigarette manufacturers.[20] In the agreement, the states promised not to sue again for health-related costs. In exchange, the tobacco companies have promised a stream of payments of nearly $0.25 trillion to the various states. The costs of these payments will, of course, become part of the production cost of manufacturing cigarettes, which should in turn drive up the price of cigarettes, just as a legislatively created tax would do.[21]

INFORMATION AS AN EXTERNALITY

Topics such as alcohol and tobacco consumption raise an important issue about the economics of information. It is widely understood that the production of knowledge creates a beneficial externality because the marginal costs to disseminate the knowledge are small compared with the marginal costs to produce it. Once produced, the logic goes, knowledge should receive widespread distribution and be limited only when the marginal costs of dissemination finally match the incremental benefits. In addition, the production of knowledge itself is likely to be undertaken too little in a society with less than

---

[20]Forty-six states signed the original agreement for $206 billion; the remaining four states settled separately for an additional $40 billion.

[21]During the political debate over this settlement, several people pointed out that the promised revenues to the states exceeded the present value of the profit stream of the tobacco companies, based on their current profitability, and hence concluded that the settlement would drive the tobacco companies out of business. Problem 6 at the end of this chapter asks for analysis of this issue, and (if properly answered) should demonstrate the fallacy in this line of reasoning.

perfectly functioning property rights to knowledge, creating a government role for the subsidy and/or production of knowledge.

Another issue arises in the categorization of externalities from such things as alcohol and tobacco use. Should, for example, the deaths of persons drinking alcohol "count" as an externality, or should they count as a purely private cost, presumably considered *taken into account* by people when they decide to engage in behavior that harms their own health (such as smoking tobacco or drinking alcohol)?

The pure economic model views consumers as being fully informed about the risks and benefits of consuming any commodity and making their decisions accordingly. The person's demand curve for tobacco or alcohol automatically incorporates those risks. If this is true, the logic for government intervention to reduce smoking and drinking rests *solely* on the external damage produced by these activities.

Another way to think about the problem suggests that at least some of the so-called private costs of these activities represent an externality. Consider, for example, a hypothetical demand curve for tobacco or alcohol by a fully informed consumer. Now contrast that demand curve with that of a consumer who is the same except (to pose an extreme case) for having *no* knowledge of the risks of the activity. Obviously, the "uninformed" demand curve will exhibit (at every quantity) a higher willingness to pay—that is, the demand curve will be shifted outward. At any price, the uninformed consumer will consume more than a fully informed consumer with otherwise identical tastes and circumstances. Figure 14.2 shows this problem.

FIGURE 14.2   Informed versus uninformed demand.

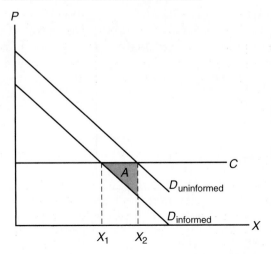

The welfare loss arising from the lack of information appears in Figure 14.2 as the triangular area A. The uninformed person consumes at a rate X_2 but would consume only X_1 if fully informed. The dotted area between the informed demand curve and the cost line C, bounded by X_1 and X_2, represents expenditures exceeding the optimal consumption. Adding up welfare triangles such as triangle A across the entire population represents the maximum possible value of the information necessary to move all persons from the uninformed to the informed demand curve. (Note that a similar logic arises when information causes the demand curve to shift outward rather than inward.)

In the example of tobacco, the case can be made that information arising from the past quarter of a century has produced just this sort of change in behavior. The precipitating event here was the publication of a major study in 1964 by the surgeon general of the United States (Luther Terry, M.D.) on the health risks of smoking (Surgeon General's Advisory Committee on Smoking and Health, 1964). Prior to that year, smoking rates had increased steadily from at least 1930 onward. Because of that initial study—"merely" the publication of new information—and the many subsequent changes in public policy and personal attitudes toward the use of tobacco, smoking rates began a steady decline that continues apace today. Figure 14.3 shows the actual per

FIGURE 14.3 Smoking behavior with and (projected) without information on risks.

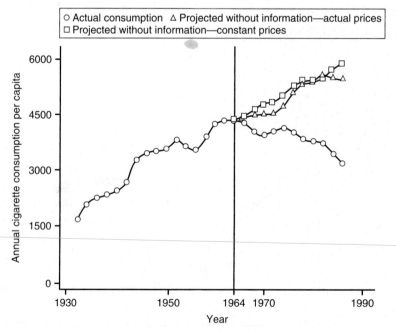

Source: Warner (1989).

capita cigarette consumption in the United States over time and projections of what the smoking rates would have been in the absence of the information campaign.

The projections shown in Figure 14.3 (Warner, 1989) stop at the time of the original research (1989), but history has shown that his projected trend downward continued. A few intervening data points demonstrate the continued decline in cigarette consumption (all in cigarettes per person over 18 years of age): 2,827 (in 1990), 2,525 (in 1995), 2,092 (in 2000), and 1,716 (in 2005) (Tobacco Outlook Report, 2007). Cigarette consumption by 2010 will have fallen below one-third of the peak levels in 1965 before the surgeon general's report. The reduction in tobacco use is now paying health dividends that are (in part) causing obesity to rise soon to the "top of the charts" as the leading true cause of death in the United States, quite likely overtaking tobacco within a few years (see Chapter 2 for discussion of the real causes of death).

To evaluate the economic gains from this information, one could readily apply the type of model portrayed in Figure 14.2 and estimate the annual gain from consumers' obtaining the information.

Note also that once produced, information creates a long stream of benefits, the present value of which must be offset by the cost of producing the information. If the information has a very long life, one can approximate the present value of the long stream of benefits by using a "perpetuity" calculation. To do this, one divides the annual benefit by the interest rate. Thus, for example, if the discount rate is 5 percent, the perpetuity value of information is 20 times the annual benefit.

RESEARCH AS AN EXTERNALITY

Most economists (and many others) recognize the production of "basic research" as a problem replete with externalities. The production of research is usually quite costly; its dissemination to other users usually carries relatively low cost, particularly compared with the costs of those other potential users of the research doing the same research again themselves. As noted at the beginning of the chapter, it is difficult to establish property rights to ideas unless they are embedded either in a specific product (which can be patented) or a manuscript (which can be copyrighted). Many other ideas have great economic benefit but cannot receive any legal protection. Because of this, the usual economic forces for invention and research are weakened in these cases.

An important example is the production of knowledge about how various medical interventions "work." As discussed in Chapter 3, we can find widespread patterns of variability in the use of many medical interventions, which create a significant welfare loss because of the variability alone (see Chapter 5). Another approach to studying the same phenomenon looks at the cost-effectiveness (CE) of investment in randomized clinical trials—research projects that study directly the production function that turns medical care into health—in the same way that one can measure the cost-effectiveness of various medical interventions themselves. Recall from previous discussions that CE studies analyze the number of healthy years (measured in QALYs) gained from using a medical intervention and the added cost of that intervention. The ratio of added costs divided by added QALYs describes the cost effectiveness of an intervention.

A physician/economist from Canada has analyzed whether the production of new knowledge, as accomplished through randomized clinical trials, is a good investment using CE criteria. In this work, Detsky (1989, 1990) modeled the likelihood that a study would show that a new therapy would work better than the old one (a combination of how much better it would work and the sample size in the study); the life years gained by using a new therapy, if it is indeed better; and the rate of implementation of the new therapy once it is demonstrated to be better. Detsky showed that a variety of large (and expensive) clinical trials has a wonderfully low cost per life year saved. Although many medical interventions themselves have CE ratios of tens or hundreds of thousands of dollars, Detsky showed that clinical studies showing the efficacy of various interventions have CE ratios as low as $2 to $3 per life year saved to a high (in the set he looked at) of $400 to $700 per life year saved. All of these CE ratios are much, much more favorable than almost all of the actual medical interventions undertaken in the United States (see Table 3.2 for some examples). This tells us, from a very different approach than that taken by Phelps and Parente (1990), that we continue to have a major underinvestment in research about the clinical effectiveness of various medical interventions.

REASONS FOR SO LITTLE RESEARCH ON MEDICAL EFFECTIVENESS

Both Detsky's studies of the CE ratios for clinical trials and the work of Phelps and Parente using medical practice variations data to study the expected gains from clinical studies provide strong support for greatly increasing the amount of clinical research undertaken in this country. This result raises the separate and important question of why this country (and indeed, most modern societies) has underinvested in this type of research. The answer appears to lie in the incentives and property rights issues associated with such research. (For a more complete discussion of these issues, see Phelps, 1992.)

Consider first the incentives for research into the effectiveness and safety of a pharmaceutical product. The drug company knows that if it can invent a new "wonder drug" that cures a previously incurable disease, it can patent and profitably sell the drug, recouping not only the costs of making the drug but also the costs of the research leading to its discovery. Thus, the legal protection of the patent system stands as a vital link in the production of new knowledge. (See also the discussion in Chapter 15 about how some regulation of the pharmaceutical industry has altered these incentives for research.)

By contrast, consider the economic gains to the study of effective ways to treat a disease that don't involve a specific product such as a drug or medical device. Prototypical "problems" such as this include learning whether one type of surgical intervention is better than another or whether one frequency of use/drug dose combination is better than another.[22] In these settings, because there is no "product" that can be patented, the economic gains from doing a study to learn which approach is better or worse are very small. In some cases, the *only* gains to doing studies such as this come from the prestige associated with publication of a study in a prominent medical journal for the doctors associated with the study. When the doctors are in a medical school where their promotion and tenure rest on their ability to carry out good research and have it published in prestigious journals, the economic incentives are somewhat higher but still not nearly as large as those associated with the successful invention of a patentable drug. Thus, the issue of underproduction of studies of medical effectiveness can be seen to relate directly to the economic incentives (or lack thereof) for producing such information.

---

[22]In surgical interventions, this dilemma is common, and almost invariably the issue has been decided on the basis of which intervention is "less invasive" rather than a careful study of actual costs and outcomes for the patient. Some examples of their dilemma include the choice of open versus transurethral resection of an enlarged prostate gland (in men), vaginal versus abdominal hysterectomy (in women), and the like. New surgical tools have allowed much less invasive surgery for many operations, including arthroscopic surgery in joints such as the knee and shoulder and laparoscopic surgery to remove the gallbladder. Sometimes the improved results of the less invasive surgery are so profoundly obvious that nobody ever takes the time to do a good randomized trial. However, such "obvious" improvements can sometimes be misleading, and it can take years or decades before careful studies eventually show how the "obvious" improvement was in fact none at all.

In nonsurgical interventions, the problem is often more subtle. For example, some doctors now advocate the use of very frequent, very small injections of insulin (carefully matched to blood-sugar tests drawn by the patient at frequent intervals during the day) versus the older routine of having several, larger doses of insulin injected daily by the patient.

TRANSFUSION-INDUCED AIDS AND HEPATITIS

Another important externality in the health care system arises from the transmission of dangerous and/or fatal diseases through transfused blood. Blood transfusion policy is complicated both in the biology and the public policy implications, but the problem remains of paramount importance even though (as has been true since April 1985) screening tests have been available to test donated blood for HIV antibodies, a sign that the person has acquired the viral infection that ultimately leads to AIDS. Problems of transfusion-induced disease persist because (1) the AIDS test is imperfect because some persons donate blood while infected but before their antibody levels reach detectable levels and (2) other diseases, notably hepatitis, continue to pass undetected into the blood supply system and create major health problems.

Analyses of the risks of AIDS infection have some intrinsic variability but suggest that the risks of acquiring AIDS through a single unit of blood lie somewhere between 1/300,000 and 1/100,000 (Cumming, Wallace, Schorr, and Dodd, 1989). The average transfusion recipient receives 5.4 units of blood, so the risks of acquiring AIDS from transfusion are approximately 1/20,000 to 1/60,000. If recent estimates of the value of reducing probabilities of death (consistent with "a value of life" of about $5 million) are correct (Moore and Viscusi, 1988a), then these risks from AIDS correspond to a cost of about $17 to $50 per unit of blood transfused.[23]

Thinking about blood supply policy in the context of property rights and liability has a long history, and the AIDS question has only served to remind us again of issues previously raised. An early and important work on this topic came from Richard Titmuss (1972), a British scholar who argued that the nature of a country's blood supply was in many ways a key indicator of its moral character. He strongly opposed using a commercial blood supply, at that time the main source of whole blood in the United States, and sought to promote a wholly voluntary (unpaid) donor supply. Many have argued for a voluntary supply on the grounds that it is allegedly safer; Titmuss made the argument as well on moral grounds.

Titmuss struck a raw nerve in the ranks of the economics profession in this country. A barrage of commentary on Titmuss's thesis emerged, including responses from Reuben Kessel (1974, of the "classic" Chicago school of thought), Armein Alchien (1973), and two subsequent Nobel laureates of

---

[23]This number comes from multiplying the $5 million figure by the incremental risk of 1/300,000 to 1/100,000.

substantially different political persuasion, Kenneth J. Arrow (1972) and Robert Solow (1971), the latter even before Titmuss's book was officially published.[24]

The essence of the argument appeared in Kessel's original blast at Titmuss. Kessel asserted that the *real* problem with blood supply in the United States was not that it was *over*commercialized but that it was *under*commercialized. The discussion turns closely on the question of the "liability" side of property rights law. In donated blood, the donor never acquires any liability for the blood's damage (if any), and, in fact, neither does the supplying agency (most predominantly, the American Red Cross and its affiliate agencies). Because of this failure to acquire liability, Kessel argued, agencies that collect and distribute blood have too small an incentive to worry about the safety of that blood, and hence we have too much infection through the blood supply.

The issue of blood safety shows precisely the relationship between the system of property rights and the creation of externalities. If, as Kessel and many others have argued, property rights were complete, suppliers of blood (as with manufacturers of stereos and cars) would have the strongest possible incentives to guarantee the quality of their product, to promote information about that quality, and (the other side of the coin) to take all necessary steps to prevent a legal liability suit if tainted blood were administered under their auspices.

The legal system has not conferred property rights (and liability) on the blood system, so the externality persists. Steps that would reduce the incidence of transfusion-related iatrogenic illness remain to be taken, yet the current legal and organizational incentives lead to their being ignored. Most prominently, tighter donor screening and exclusion provide potentially powerful tools to reduce transfusion-induced disease (Eckert, in Eckert and Wallace, 1985).

We should note here that the altruistic motives of blood-banking organizations are not under attack from this line of argument. Indeed, the complex issues associated with blood safety and supply provide a rich portrait of organizational purposes and show how such purposes must sometimes end in conflict. In the case of blood supply and safety, the conflict arises because blood-banking organizations wish both to encourage donors and to provide safe blood to patients. To satisfy the "donor encouragement" objective, blood banks are reluctant to exclude donors from donating blood, even if their

---

[24]An extended discussion of this topic appears in a written debate featuring Ross Eckert, an economist, on one side and management professor Edward Wallace on the other. See *Securing a Safer Blood Supply: Two Views* (Eckert and Wallace, 1985).

blood has been "implicated" in a previous illness.[25] Because of these conflicting objectives, even an altruistic organization will end up placing patients at risk; the question is one of balance. Altering the legal structure would, of course, alter the choices made by participants in this market. With the current legal incentives and structures, however, some blood donors create serious and potentially fatal health hazards for others and do not account fully for these costs in their own actions, thus creating another externality.

SUMMARY

Externalities occur when Person A's behavior imposes costs (or benefits) on other people (Persons B, C, ...) that Person A's private decision making does not account for. In almost all cases (perhaps all), these externalities arise because of the failure of our legal system to define property rights and hence legal liability fully. Health-affecting externalities arise in numerous ways, including (trivially) sneezing when you have a cold, (more importantly) giving vaccinations for infectious diseases, driving under the influence of alcohol, using tobacco, and donating of blood, among others. These examples serve to illustrate, but do not provide a complete catalog of, the types of health-affecting externalities that we might consider.

RELATED CHAPTERS IN *HANDBOOK OF HEALTH ECONOMICS*

Chapter 29, "The Economics of Smoking" by Frank J. Chaloupka and Kenneth E. Warner

Chapter 30, "Alcohol" by Philip J. Cook and Michael J. Moore

Chapter 31, "Prevention" by Donald S. Kenkel

PROBLEMS

1. What is the key economic characteristic of an externality? What legal issue is most likely to be present when externalities occur?

---

[25]Most transfusion recipients receive multiple units of blood. For example, if a patient becomes ill after receiving 10 units of blood (each from a different source), then each of those 10 donors has a 1/10 chance of being "contaminated." One blood-banking organization excludes donors only when the probability of implication reaches 0.3 to 0.4 (American Association of Blood Banks, no date, Chap. 18). Clearly, tighter restrictions are possible and would increase blood pool safety at a higher cost of obtaining blood.

2. Many people have criticized the U.S. blood supply system as being "too commercial" and prefer a more altruistic method of collecting and distributing blood for transfusions. The issue is whether donated blood contains viruses that might cause disease (such as hepatitis or AIDS) to the recipient. Reuben Kessel, an economist from Chicago, argued to the contrary that the problem with blood supply is that it was not sufficiently commercial. How might more commercialization improve the safety of blood supply in the United States? Are there risks to taking such an approach?

3. "Herd immunity" describes a beneficial externality arising from vaccination against contagious disease. Describe herd immunity precisely. What public policies might lead to the proper amount of vaccination? What might affect the ability of your proposed policies to achieve their goals? (*Hint:* Think about transactions costs.)

4. Many externalities have some aspect of "privateness." On a scale such that 0 = purely private to 1 = purely external, rank the following consequences of cigarette smoking in terms of how "external" they are, and discuss the logic underlying your answers. In your answers, think broadly about mechanisms of insurance and the possibility of "financial" externalities. (*Note:* There is no purely "correct" answer.)
   a. Lung disease to the smoker.
   b. Heart disease to spouses and children of smokers.
   c. Smoke emission into the air in a restaurant or commercial airplane.
   d. Smoke emission into the air in a private airplane or automobile.

5. Using Figures 14.2 and 14.3, estimate the annual per capita welfare gain in 1987 (the last year shown in Figure 14.3) assuming a demand elasticity of -0.5 for cigarettes and a price of $2 per pack (10¢ per cigarette). Assume actual consumption of 3,000, predicted (without information) of 6,000 per person.

6. For simplicity, assume that tobacco companies price as monopolists. Using standard monopoly pricing models, characterize the optimal monopoly price, quantity, and profits for a given demand curve and production cost. Now let the costs of production rise, as they would in response to the costs of the large settlements made by tobacco companies in the 1998 agreement with state governments.
   a. Show the new price, quantity, and profits of the tobacco company after incorporating the settlement payments into their costs.
   b. Does a settlement cost so large that it *would* drive the tobacco company out of business exist?

APPENDIX TO CHAPTER 14

Value of Life

The "value of life" turns out to importantly affect a number of questions in health economics and even, in some cases, health and safety regulation. The value of life is really a misnomer for two reasons. First, all of us eventually die, so value of preventing premature death would be a more proper phrase. Second, one seldom confronts the question of what any single individual's life is actually worth, or, at least, one can almost never measure that value.

Rather than attempting to measure the value of lives on a one-by-one basis, economists have turned to the related question of how much people are willing to pay for a small reduction in the probability of their dying (Viscusi, 1978). The idea then takes on a different slant. For example, if each of 1,000 people has something happen that decreases the chance of dying by 1/1000, then statistically we can say that 1 life has been saved (1,000 people of whom each has 1/1000 reduced chance of dying). Thus the *aggregate* willingness to pay by those 1,000 people for this risk reduction reflects the value of 1 statistical life saved.

Economists have turned to several sources to estimate the value of life following this approach. First, one can think of settings in the labor market in which some jobs are riskier than others, but otherwise the jobs have similar demands in terms of physical effort, mental skills, training, and so on. Economists use regression models to estimate wage rates in different occupations including explanatory variables such as age, education, and so forth, and as a measure of the on-job occupational risk. The relationship between on-job risk and wage rates provides a measure of how much extra compensation people require in order to accept the extra risk. For example, consider the work by Moore and Viscusi (1988a). The average hourly wage in the sample they studied was about $7, equivalent to an annual wage (assuming 2,000 hours of work per year) of $14,000. (The data came from a 1982 study of persons' income, occupation, education, and so forth.) To each person's occupation, they matched data from two sources, the U.S. Bureau of Labor Statistics (BLS) and the National Institute of Occupational Safety and Health (NIOSH), on occupational mortality rates. The average fatality rate in the NIOSH data was just under 8 per 100,000 full-time equivalent years, and in the BLS data, about 5 per 100,000. For a variety of reasons, Moore and Viscusi prefer the NIOSH data. Their estimates show that each increase of 1 death per 100,000 workers (e.g., from 8 to 9 per 100,000) increases the hourly wage by about 2.7 cents. This corresponds to $54 for a year's exposure to the risk, or correspondingly (adding up for 100,000 workers) $5,400,000 per statistical life in 1982.

Other approaches to the same problem yield quite different results. Merely shifting to the BLS measures causes the estimated value of life to fall by half, as Moore and Viscusi show. Alternative approaches have looked at quite different types of behavior to try to learn the same thing (e.g., how much people will pay for added safety in automobiles) and in some cases have turned completely away from market-related measures. One study, for example, looked at court cases for wrongful death to determine the magnitude of awards in civil trials when one person's behavior caused another person's death (Perkins, Phelps, and Parente, 1990). Others have looked at the implied value of life represented in government decisions to embark on various safety and regulatory programs (Graham and Vopel, 1981).

Even within a single type of study (such as the labor-market studies by Moore and Viscusi, 1988a, 1988b), wide variability exists in the estimated results. Moving across methods (for example, comparing labor market studies with court awards) gives an even wider dispersion of estimates. All that we can say at present is that the subject of placing a monetary value on "life" has some considerable importance, but that the estimates now available contain a wide degree of disagreement. One can easily find credible studies that disagree with one another by as much as a factor of 10 in their estimates of the value of life. As is true of many empirical problems in health economics, this one requires further work.

CHAPTER 15

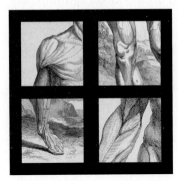

Managing the Market: Regulation and Technical Change in Health Care

This chapter considers two related facets of the health care market: the overall scope of regulation (including price, entry, and quality controls) and a separate discussion about a major issue in health care policy and regulation, the management of technical change. The first part of the chapter deals with various price-, quantity-, and quality-affecting regulations. The last part deals with the drug and device sectors of the economy as a special and important case.

In reviewing the scope of regulations that the U.S. health care system has experienced over the past half century, one can say readily that the myriad regulatory interventions come from one of two related purposes: to control the introduction of new products into the market (such as drugs and medical devices) or to manage somehow what the political system considers as important failures in the

LEARNING GOALS

- Understand the role of regulation in controlling market functions.

- Compare the economic gains from quality certification with the entry-restriction costs to license medical professionals.

- Grasp the economic logic for certificate of need laws and learn how they can either improve or distort a market's performance.

- Use economic models to illuminate the effects of price controls on quantity, quality, and price of health care service related to
  - Medicare pricing rules for hospitals and doctors.
  - Pay for performance (and associated issues of risk adjustment).

- Follow the various steps for introducing new medical technologies into the market:
  - Invention (and patent protection).
  - FDA-required testing and approval.
  - Inclusion by insurance plans as allowed benefit.
  - Adoption by providers and consumers (and advertising that encourages such adoption).

market functioning.[1] The "market failures" might fall in the realm of price controls to deal with escalating medical care costs (a consequence, some might say, of growing insurance coverage or even because of the not-for-profit nature of major health care providers). In response to such concerns, our society has experienced many forms of price controls and limitations on entry ("certificate of need laws").

Other areas in which market failure looms as a concern involve the quality of care and concerns that consumers of health care cannot judge quality effectively. Following such concerns, persistent regulation of quality has occurred through licensing of providers (doctors, dentists, nurses, therapists, pharmacists, etc.) and requiring large-scale testing of new drugs and medical devices before they can be marketed in this country.

These two areas of regulation come together in the following sense: When a new drug or medical device (or new treatment strategy using existing technology) is developed, the health care system must decide how and when to pay for such services (which almost invariably add to overall costs of treatment). These decisions now confront large government agencies (Medicare and Medicaid, the Veterans Administration, and military health care providers) and numerous private-sector insurance companies and individual plans, each of which must decide when and how to pay for new services.

A TAXONOMY OF REGULATION

Figure 15.1 includes the possible domains of regulation in the health care sector. It separates "input" from final product markets, and it isolates four separate areas in which regulation might apply: price, quantity, entry by new providers, and quality. Although this schematic is not exhaustive, it covers the major areas in which local, state, and federal regulation affect the U.S. health care system. As Figure 15.1 shows, some types of regulation actually have effects in more than one area. For example, licensure affects both entry into the market by various types of "labor" (each an input into the production of final products) and quality. Price control rules regulated by the Nixon administration's Economic Stabilization Program (ESP) during the 1970s were typical of the "price control" genre. A later section on price controls provides details. Certificate of need (CON) rules affect entry into the market by new providers and limit the quantities of inputs existing providers use. Thus,

---

[1] A standard view of traditional economic regulation (as espoused, for example, by Nobel Laureate George Stigler, 1968) holds that most regulations arise because the regulated industry prefers that to an unregulated market. However, much of the regulatory structure in health care seems to have different purposes and outcomes.

FIGURE 15.1 Domains of health care regulation.

	Price	Quantity	Entry	Quality
Input	Wage controls, antitrust	CON	Licensure, CON	Licensure, voluntary "boards"
Product	Medicare Antitrust law	—	FDA	Health department Tort law FPA Peer review

talking about each type of regulation separately rather than each of the "cells" in Figure 15.1 one at a time makes more sense. The set of regulations appearing in Figure 15.1 and the discussion that follows are not intended to be comprehensive but to review some of the main forms of regulation and the economic issues associated with them.

LICENSURE

Licensure of professionals has a long history, substantially preceding any other form of regulation. The idea of professional licensure probably arose originally from various guilds in Europe as they attempted to use the power of the state to their own advantage. Debates about licensure continue to carry the flavor that arises from this historical background. For example, proponents of licensure (usually existing practitioners in a field) praise it as a protection of citizens against fraudulent or unsafe providers of care. Opponents of licensure decry the entire idea as a tool to restrict entry and limit competition. As with the mythical "force" in the Star Wars movies, licensure has a "good side" (quality enhancement) and a "dark side" (limitation of entry and competition).

Licensure as we commonly think about it applies to *labor inputs* in the provision of health care but seldom to the organizations (firms) that produce the final products of health services.[2] In health care, virtually all licensure comes from the states rather than the federal government.[3] Licensure spans professionals ranging from physicians, dentists, and psychologists to

---

[2]An obvious exception is the licensure of hospitals and nursing homes. Such licensure is usually limited to obvious fire and safety questions and has little to do with the quality of care provided.

[3]The only important exception is the license to prescribe narcotic drugs, which comes from the federal government through federal control of those drugs.

nurses (R.N.s and L.P.N.s), pharmacists, physical therapists, social workers, and dental hygienists. Virtually all licensure of individuals is limited to areas of the economy in which the final product is a service rather than a good, suggesting that the consumer's inability to exchange the service is an important component in the logic of licensure.[4]

Presentation of licensure as a safety- and quality-enhancing regulation would contain the following premises:

- Important variation exists in the quality of individual inputs (e.g., doctors, nurses).
- Low-quality inputs translate, at least partly, into poor outcomes of the final product.
- Managers of the firms that produce the final product either cannot or do not wish to measure the quality of labor inputs they hire. (Tort liability makes firms liable for damage caused by their employees, so the idea that managers do not wish to measure quality of labor inputs could arise only because of a failure of the tort system to produce sufficient incentives for product quality and safety.)
- Consumers lack full information about product quality.
- The product cannot be readily exchanged (it is a "service" tailored to the individual), and/or use of a defective product or service would endanger the consumer.

The idea that consumers cannot perceive product quality accurately has a reasonable statistical basis because of the variability in outcomes that occurs even among "competent" providers. Health (H) is produced by medical care (m) with a random (v) outcome: that is, $H = g(m) + v$. In plain words, sometimes people get better even with minimal or poor medical care, and sometimes people get worse or die even with the best medical care. The term v captures these "random" outcomes, and the production function $g(m)$ captures the systematic effects of medical care. Medical care (m) is in turn produced by combinations of inputs, such as doctors (D) and capital (K), so $m = m(D, K)$. Finally, doctor quality can vary, so $D = D^* + u$, where D^* is average quality of doctors and u is the random doctor quality. Thus, the quality of m will vary according to u, and the final outcomes will vary according to the random component v in the production of health.

The consumer seeks to infer whether the doctor is "good" or not, but the inference problem is compounded by the various sources of "noise" in the system. Does a "good" health outcome guarantee that the doctor is "good"?

---

[4]We do not license farmers, although the food they produce is crucial to our survival, nor do we license the people who make automobiles. We do, however, license airline pilots, taxi drivers, and barbers.

(No; the doctor may merely have been lucky.) Does a "bad" health outcome guarantee that the doctor is "bad"? (No; it may have been a freak of nature despite the best care.) The consumer must try to draw information from a very limited number of events in some cases and may have almost no information available before making a choice. (For example, how many times can you sample a surgeon's ability to remove an appendix?) In statistical terms, the problem is that when one attempts to infer whether u is large or small (the doctor is "good" or "bad"), the noise sent up by the random component v may overwhelm the signal about u. If the variance in v is large compared with the variance in u, it may be almost impossible for a single patient to infer anything about the quality of a single doctor even after a series of encounters.[5]

Licensure can provide two types of information about quality, at least in concept. First, it can certify that the licensed person has sufficient command of the body of relevant knowledge to pass an examination on that material. (This does not test, for example, the manual dexterity of a surgeon, but it can test for knowledge about the indications for surgery and the proper procedures to follow if a surgical incision becomes infected.) Second, the licensure authorities are in a position to collect information about poor outcomes by an individual doctor (no matter what physician-firm the doctor works for or in what hospital that doctor practices). This gives the licensure authorities a much larger potential sample of events, which can in concept help identify an individual doctor's competence far faster than any single patient (or physician-firm) can.

Most state licensure authorities have relied almost exclusively on the first type of quality indicator; an examination passed when the doctor graduated from medical school may often suffice for an entire lifetime.[6] Licensure revocation turns out to be quite rare. It most commonly occurs for events that have little bearing on what we would normally consider "medical quality." Previous studies (e.g., Morrison and Wickersham, 1998; Clay and Conaster, 2003) found three reasons that dominate the list of actual revocations: (1) illegal drug use or prescribing by a physician, (2) fraudulent billing practices, and (3) sexual encounters between a doctor and his or her patients. Revocations for "bad quality" turn out to be rare.

---

[5]This explains why some doctors who lose their licenses can produce a list of patients who will testify about their marvelous qualities even in the midst of the licensure-revocation proceedings.

[6]Some states now have periodic relicensure examinations, but the idea of periodic reexamination is much more common in voluntary certification of quality as is discussed momentarily.

Voluntary Quality Certification

Most areas of medical care that have licensure requirements also have voluntary indicators of quality. For many providers, these are private quality-certifying groups, typically with the word *College* or *Board* in their titles. These organizations perform two functions. First, they designate certain training programs in their specialty as "approved," and, second, they administer written and oral examinations to applicants for their quality certification. Typically, before becoming eligible to take the examination (to "sit for the boards" in the usual jargon), the doctor must complete a certified training program, thus becoming "board eligible." These training programs are "residencies" in medicine, surgery, pediatrics, and so on, that "teaching" hospitals provide. Some of these subspecialty programs require additional specialized training beyond a residency. Thus, for example, one can become board eligible in pediatrics after a 3-year residency, but to subspecialize in neonatology (the care of sick newborn children) requires an additional 3-year "fellowship" in the subspecialty area, also at an approved site. Fellowship training usually takes place only at hospitals closely allied with medical schools; residency training is more diffusely provided, often at hospitals quite remote from medical schools both geographically and organizationally.

Voluntary quality certification has some distinct advantages over mandatory licensure. First, it is more difficult for a voluntary "board" to inhibit competition because it does not have the compulsion of the state at its disposal. Second, the boards have produced indicators of varying degrees of quality, providing more information to the market about quality than a single-quality license can provide. (Nothing, of course, prevents mandatory licensure from also providing more specific information about quality, but, in practice, one only knows that a provider is licensed.) Third, again in contrast to the usual practice of licensure, most medical specialty boards and many other quality-certifying private bodies have adopted requirements for repeat examinations periodically along with requirements for "continuing medical education" (CME) for the successful renewal of a board certification. This puts the specialty "boards" in one more line of business, namely the certification of the quality of producers of this CME activity.[7] Many states now have CME requirements for relicensure by physicians and other providers—for example, that a doctor acquire 100 hours of CME credit over a 3-year

---

[7]CME courses commonly take place at pleasant locations such as Aspen, Colorado; Kaanapali Beach, Hawaii; Carmel, California; and Naples, Florida. However, strict requirements about attendance at these events now are closely monitored, probably in response to early versions of CME courses that amounted to little more than tax-deductible vacations.

period—but few have adopted the reexamination rules that some specialty boards have.

Once an organization gains a market reputation for high quality, it has strong incentives to promote itself and its members. In other areas, franchises of businesses (such as McDonald's hamburgers, Midas mufflers, and Prudential realtors) provide quality certification and national advertising for their constituent firms. Specialty boards provide a comparable certification of quality that they promote widely such as enabling patients to call to determine whether an individual doctor is "board certified."[8]

Specialty boards and voluntary certification have their own problematic features just as mandatory licensure does. The first question that arises has to do with the quality of the certifier. That is, it may be quite difficult for individual patients to understand what a certification really means. For example, the American Board of Internal Medicine is a classic "specialty board," but the American College of Physicians (ACP) offers an alternative certification of quality, and to many patients, membership in the American Medical Association (AMA) has a similar connotation of quality. Which of these implies a higher standard of quality, if any?[9] This problem blurs into other areas as well. For example, voluntary certification of scuba instructors exists from at least four separate national organizations (National Association of Scuba Diving Schools, National Association of Underwater Instructors, Professional Association of Diving Instructors, and the YMCA), each of which proclaims its own certification as the best.

The second question that arises is the ability of a certifying body to restrict entry into the specialty de facto if not de jure. An organization that achieves a very strong market position in terms of quality certification can acquire a de facto ability to limit entry. Some of the various medical specialty boards may have achieved this position by limiting the number of approved residency positions throughout the country. (Recall that a trainee must complete a residency—approved by the specialty board—before sitting for the board exam itself.) Thus, limiting the number of approved residencies provides a convenient vehicle to limit the number of practitioners of a given specialty. The specialty boards, under scrutiny from the Federal Trade Commission, actively disavow any role in entry restriction, but when they limit the number of training positions, they automatically provide a de facto

---

[8]The American Board of Medical Specialties, a consortium of 23 specialty boards, has a toll-free telephone line (1-866-ASK ABMS) and a Web-based system allowing patients to determine whether a doctor is certified by any of those 23 boards or an additional 50 subspecialty boards operated by the 23 primary boards.

[9]The ACP has the most vigorous reexamination requirement of any of these bodies, requiring examinations every 5 years. The AMA requires only payment of a membership fee.

limit to entry, at least in settings in which the specialty board has achieved a sufficiently strong market reputation as "the" quality certifier.

Some evidence suggests that an effective restriction to entry has been achieved by a number of specialty boards, most notably those in surgical specialties and subspecialties and more recently in radiology, pathology, and anesthesiology. These specialties have two common markers. First, practitioners have unusually large economic returns to receiving the specialty certification. Evidence presented in Chapter 7 about returns to specialization provides the basis for this observation. It is of particular interest that the economic returns to surgical specialization persisted from the early 1960s (when Sloan, 1975, studied the market) through the 1980s (when Marder and Willke, 1991, made similar calculations).

Second, specialties in which de facto entry restriction exists have extensive queues of doctors trying to enter the specialty. The difficulties in obtaining residency positions and fellowships in these specialties and subspecialties match these economic returns; competition for these positions is notoriously fierce, and training positions are often committed 4 to 6 years in advance.

Quality Certification of Organizations

The previous discussion focused on the quality certification of individual providers of care: doctors, dentists, nurses, and the like. There are also important certifications of quality for hospitals, clinics, nursing homes, and even medical schools. Licensure plays a role here as well because every state licenses these organizations. This licensure commonly limits itself to fire safety, food preparation processes, and so on, seldom venturing into realms of "medical quality." In addition to State facilities license requirements, CMS maintains a regular quality control program for nursing homes and skilled nursing facilities that serve Medicaid and Medicare patients that includes regular (annual or more frequent) inspections. The inspections observe resident care processes, fire safety, food storage and preparation, and protection of residents from abuse. The inspection protocol includes interviews with a sample of residents of the institution. There are over 150 regulatory standards that nursing homes must meet at all times.[10] As with individual providers, voluntary certification has proven more of a degree of quality assurance.

The voluntary certification of hospitals comes through several groups. Any hospital may apply for certification from the Joint Commission on Accreditation of Health Care Facilities (commonly referred to as the *Joint*

---

[10]Source: http://www.medicare.gov/nursing/AboutInspections.asp

Commission), a cooperative body sponsored by the American Hospital Association and the American Medical Association (hence the term *joint* in its title).[11] This certification focuses on a wide variety of hospital activities resulting in specific reports given to hospitals regarding their on-site inspections that note specific "deficits" in performance. This process focuses on organizational structure and the process of operating the hospital but makes no attempt to measure outcomes (e.g., patient survival, infection rates, readmission rates). Accreditation from the Joint Commission is important to hospitals because many insurance plans limit their payments to accredited hospitals. Medicare allows approval from the Joint Commission as an alternative to a specific Medicare approval even though the Joint Commission approval is generally viewed as "easier" than Medicare approval.

Even medical schools have an accreditation program—the American Association of Medical Colleges (AAMC)—that serves the same role for them that the boards do for residency training. As with other certification bodies, the importance of accreditation depends in part on the externally perceived quality of the schools and partly on how other groups (including governments) include the private certification in their own quality-control mechanisms. For example, to receive a license from most states, a doctor must (as one precondition) graduate from an approved medical school, and the list of schools approved by various states almost universally reflects the approval list of the AAMC. Thus, just as Medicare delegates the certification process of hospitals to the Joint Commission, many state governments delegate the process of approving medical schools to the AAMC. This type of implicit or explicit delegation of regulatory authority obviously blurs the line between private voluntary certification and mandatory state licensure.

Quality Certification and Consumer Search

Another important issue arises when we consider quality certification in health care markets. How does certification affect consumers' incentives in searching for lower priced providers? In many markets, low price has a connotation (often correct) of low quality. When quality is intrinsically difficult to measure, sellers may be able to send a false "high-quality" signal by raising their prices, a strategy that will probably work only when the customer has relatively few encounters with the seller. (We would not expect this strategy to work as well for grocers and barbers as we would for vacation resorts and divorce lawyers.) Providing quality "assurance" about a provider of medical care may actually promote competition in the final product market (for medical services) even if it inhibits entry into the factor market (the market for

---

[11]See www.jointcommission.org to learn more about this organization.

physician labor). The models of market price and consumer search discussed in Chapter 7 show the importance of search in markets that are intrinsically monopolistically competitive, a model that seems to fit medical service markets (such as physicians, dentists) quite well. However, consumers may be quite reluctant to search for a lower priced provider if they cannot measure quality well. Thus, establishing a base floor for quality, as licensure does, or gradations of quality, as voluntary certification does, may move final product markets to a more competitive level.

"CERTIFICATE OF NEED" (CON) LAWS

A completely different type of regulation has been present in U.S. health care markets for decades—namely, limitation on construction of new "capital" facilities to try to limit total hospital use. These regulations prohibit the building of new hospital bed capacity (and often the addition of any "expensive" equipment in the hospital) without having government approval in advance. The architects of such laws attempt to determine how many hospital beds (and possibly how many MRI units, etc.) a given geographic area "needs" and then allow new construction only if available supply does not meet that "need." Because of this underlying logic, these rules are called *certificate of need* (CON) rules.[12]

CON-like programs have existed for many years, but until 1974 they had advisory capability (with only a few local exceptions). In 1974, the National Health Planning and Resources Development Act institutionalized the idea of health planning, provided federal funds to support planning agencies, and (to put some teeth into the law) limited Medicare capital payments to those facilities that the relevant planners had approved.

In 1986, President Ronald Reagan repealed the 1974 act that required states to use the CON process. Approximately one-quarter of all states have eliminated CON laws entirely since then although about three-quarters still maintain some form of them.[13] The most common type of regulation focuses on long-term care (nursing home) facilities (38 states) followed by acute hospital beds (28), ambulatory surgical centers (28), open heart surgery

---

[12]A book by economist Paul Joskow (1981) examines CON and other hospital regulations in detail. He offers a relatively complete history of CON laws and broadly reviews the literature on their effectiveness. His conceptual approach to CON laws differs somewhat from that discussed in this section, but much of the empirical evidence he summarized can be interpreted equally well in light of the models used in this book.

[13]www.ncsl.org/programs/health/cert-need.htm.

facilities (27), and cardiac catheterization labs. The list of regulated entitites includes behavioral health and birthing centers, for which only a single state regulates entry.

Basic Economic Issues with CON

CON rules attempt to estimate "need" for medical facilities and control entry as a way to eliminate excess capital investment and hence enable the industry to operate more efficiently. Perhaps it comes as no surprise that the areas of greatest attention for CON laws are nursing homes, in which every state has a significant financial interest through the state's share of Medicaid program costs.

Presumed overinvestment can be understood in the context of the monopolistic competition model regarding hospitals presented in Chapter 7. (The same would apply to nursing homes, ambulatory care facilities, and such hospital-base programs as open heart surgery, cath labs, and transplant centers.) For example, discussion of Figure 9.2 shows a hospital market in which the industry's entry is incomplete. In this situation, each individual hospital's demand curve for a specific quality cuts through the average cost curve for the same quality of care at two points.

If the industry experiences complete entry (as in unfettered monopolistic competition environments), every hospital's demand curve shifts to the left until it is tangent to the AC curve only at one point on the left side. Figure 15.2 shows this situation. In this figure, the EE curve labeled E_C represents this

FIGURE 15.2 Monopoly, competition, and ideal regulation to avoid excess capacity.

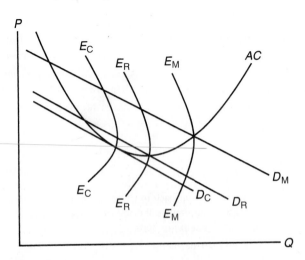

"full entry" position. The AC and demand curve tangency obviously occurs at a point above minimum AC. The EE curve labeled E_M shows the situation with no entry ("monopoly").

The hope and goal of CON regulation is to stop entry at some point at which production takes place at or near the minimum AC for each quality (the bottom of the U-shaped cost curve). If CON rules could succeed in this ambitious goal, they could indeed prevent "excess entry" and reduce costs of production. The EE curve labeled E_R shows this "holy grail" outcome.

Unfortunately, analysis of a CON's effects does not proceed so simply. If CON rules constrain the capital investment of a hospital that wishes to produce more services (e.g., hospital beds or cath labs) than the amount of capital resources would normally allow, the hospital has the option to use the same capital investment for other resources (e.g., more intensive nursing services) to treat more patients.

Figure 15.3 shows the consequences of this substitution in a simple world in which only two resources (hospital beds and nurses) are used to produce "treatments." If a CON rule restricts the number of beds the hospital can use to some fixed level (B_R in Figure 15.3) but the hospital wishes to produce Q_3 as the output level, the constraint actually causes costs to rise. (At output levels Q_1 and Q_2, the constraint is not binding because the hospital would use fewer beds than at B_R through their own cost minimization behavior. To produce Q_3, the hospital would prefer a mix of B^* beds and N^* nurses, but $B^* > B_R$, so it must substitute nurses for beds in an inefficient manner. The production function isoquant says that the hospital technically can produce

FIGURE 15.3 Cost minimization.

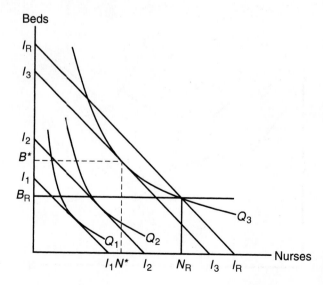

Q_3 using a combination of B_R beds and N_R nurses, but the total cost is higher (the budget line I_R) than the unconstrained budget would be (I_3).

Figure 15.4 shows how this affects the hospital's cost structure. For outputs that bind the bed constraint (such as Q_3 in Figure 15.3), the cost curve lies above the unconstrained AC curve. The dotted line cost curves in Figure 15.4 show the effects of a CON constraint in producing inefficient production choices.

The net effects of a CON law must therefore be ambiguous. Limiting entry into an environment of monopolistic competition has the possibility of reducing the industry's average costs of production as in Figure 15.2. The distortions caused in the productive process, however, necessarily raise production costs whenever the constraint is binding as it must be for the CON rules to inhibit entry.

Empirical Studies of CON Effects

A series of studies emerged shortly after the 1974 legislation requiring CONs to assess their actual effects on average cost of hospital care. Salkever and Bice (1976) used the different lengths of time that various states had employed CON laws to assess the effect on the rate of cost growth. This study found that bed increases had been constrained and "other costs" had increased faster than in unregulated markets (just as Figures 15.3 and 15.4 suggest) with a net result that states with long-active CON laws had costs increasing at slightly higher rates than those in other states.

FIGURE 15.4 Original and modified cost curves for several levels of quality.

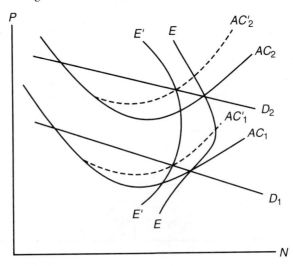

Sloan and Steinwald (1980a) conducted a similar study and (not surprisingly) found similar results. Their study also assessed the increases in nursing staff size specifically and found that nursing staff increase occurred in parallel with bed capacity constraint (again, as in Figures 15.3 and 15.4).

Price Controls

Every price is composed of a numerator (dollars) and a denominator ("quantity"): dollars per pound, dollars per hospital day, dollars per hospital stay, dollars per office visit, dollars per year of medical treatment. As simplistic as this notion might seem, each price specification leaves at least one dimension (often more) of the price unspecified and hence open for adjustment when a price control is established. The "dollars" part is relatively easy to measure.[14] Quantity is a different matter often because of the ability to adjust quality (and hence cost of production). As anybody who has watched the evolution of U.S. health policy knows, health care providers have an uncanny knack of adjusting things to deal with price controls.

Figure 15.5 shows the basic economic issues for a not for profit (NFP) provider when the provider can adjust quality and the regulator cannot fully

FIGURE 15.5 (a) Demand and cost curves for different qualities of output and (b) "decision maker's" preference function for various combinations of service intensity (S) and quantity of output (N).

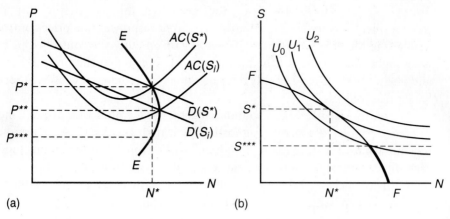

[14]But not always. Sometimes the price has "side payments" attached to it in real transactions. We can, however, generally ignore such issues in thinking about health care price controls in modern industrialized societies.

specify quality in the regulations.[15] Panel (a) shows the hospital's *EE* curve as seen in Chapter 9. Panel (b) shows the hospital decision makers' utility function, their market constraint—the *FF* curve, which is just the *EE* curve from Panel (a) in different form. The preferred output without a price control would have N^* units of service at a service intensity (quality) S^*.

Now suppose that the regulator specifies a maximum price of P^* or higher. This would not affect the hospital because it could continue to produce N^* at a price of P^*. In the language of regulation, the price control would not be "binding."

If the price control were set at P^{**}, the hospital would select the quantity-price point on the *EE* curve at that price, which would produce a lower quality of care (lower S) but higher output (N). If the price control were set at P^{***}, output would return along the *EE* curve to N^* but at a much lower quality.

The key idea is that when confronted by a binding price control, NFP hospitals will adjust quality of care to come within the constraint, moving along the *EE* curve to find the best solution given the constraint. The constraint removes some of the options on the *FF* curve in panel (b), leaving (for a control set at P^{***}, for example) only the bold section in the lower right hand of the *FF* curve as legal choices for the NFP hospital. The utility to the hospital decision makers falls from the original unconstrained U_1 to the lower level U_0.

A price control affects different hospitals in different ways. Figure 15.6 shows two hospitals with different cost structures. Hospital A, a relatively expensive hospital, will have to lower its price (and quality) to comply with the price control P_{DRG}. However, since Hospital B was already operating with price (P^*_B) that is lower than P_{DRG}, they need do nothing to comply with the pricing rule. Thus we can expect to see different responses to a price control such as the Medicare DRG rules, depending on whether the controlled price is set higher or lower than the price set by the hospital at the time. Thorpe and Phelps (1990) found exactly this phenomenon in their study of New York State price controls.

Sometimes a price control bundles together many otherwise distinct and discrete services. Medicare diagnostically related groups (DRGs) bundle together what were once many "line-item" services provided to patients (and each billed separately) into a single "hospital-stay" bundle. Capitation payments (as with classic HMOs) bundle together many possible medical interventions into a large aggregate: All of the medical care required by the

---

[15]Even with something as simple gasoline, quality cannot be readily specified. The octane rating is of course the most important factor, but other characteristics (detergents, antiknock additives, etc.) affect both the cost of production and the quality of the fuel. Think how much more difficult is would be to specify all of the relevant characteristics of a complex medical treatment.

FIGURE 15.6 Effects for two prototype hospitals, one high priced and the other low priced.

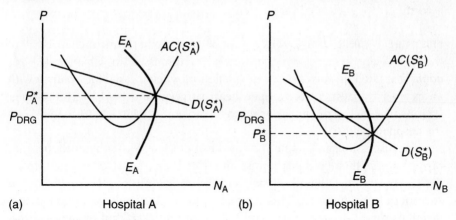

(a)   Hospital A   (b)   Hospital B

enrolled person for the coming month (or year). This bundling—often intended to create incentives for efficient production of health care—creates incentives to alter and distort behavior on other dimensions as well. The following sections discuss some specific Medicare pricing regulations and their consequences.

Medicare Hospital Pricing

Original Pricing Medicare's original pricing structure can be viewed as a price control because the Health Care Finance Administration (HCFA), the predecessor to the Centers for Medicare and Medicaid Services (CMS), specified the price that hospitals would receive for treating Medicare patients. Medicare at that time paid "à la carte" just as hospitals had been billing customers (and their insurance companies) for decades. Every discrete item used to treat a patient ended up on the patient's bill, and this price became the "charge" to a patient. Medicare calculated the price paid under a complicated system known as *ratio of cost to charges applied to charges* (RCCAC). It required each hospital to estimate the *overall* ratio of the charges for its services to the estimated costs of producing them.[16] This *ratio of costs to*

---

[16]In simple form, think of this as estimating the cost of running the hospital for a year in terms of the actual expenses it incurred. Now compare that total with the total charges listed on the bills of every patient who had been discharged from the hospital during the year. Although the payment mechanism was actually more complex than this, the ratio of the total costs to the total charges gives a sense of what the RCC would show. Typically, this amount was some number below 1.0 because the hospital charged more for its services than its cost to produce them.

charges (RCC) was then applied to every charge the hospital put on a hospital bill (hence, RCC applied to charges, or RCCAC). The hospital was paid accordingly for each Medicare patient.

Prospective Payment Changes The advent of prospective payment changed all of that. Medicare began paying hospitals (as discussed in Chapter 12) *per admission*. DRG protocols paid a hospital more when it cared for a patient with an expensive treatment (e.g., open heart surgery) and paid less for simpler treatments (e.g., hernia repair or setting a broken leg). On what "margins" did the hospitals adjust?

The discussions in Chapter 12 noted two of these. Most obviously, because hospitals were then paid per admission rather than à la carte, they had strong incentives to reduce length of stay and did so promptly (see Table 12.1 and surrounding discussion). This payment plan created related concerns that hospitals might discharge patients "sicker and quicker," but evidence shows that adverse health consequences (as measured by readmission rates and 90-day mortality rates) did not occur systematically.

Two other dimensions of adjustment occurred, both examples of what happens when sellers confront price controls. Both of these additional adjustments dealt with the "risk-adjustment" mechanism, in this case the DRG methods of classifying patients and hence specifying the DRG payment the hospital would receive for treating the patients.

First, the adjustment mechanism easiest to measure was dubbed "DRG creep." When Medicare divided the world of hospitalization into a set of discrete "bins" (separate DRGs), they confronted the obvious dilemma: too few (e.g., medical and surgical patients, at the extreme of two DRGs) would create too much within-group heterogeneity and therefore strong incentives for hospitals to screen out sickly patients and treat only the relatively low-cost ones. At the other extreme with many thousands of DRGs subclassifying every possible treatment into various stages of complexity depending on co-morbidities, the administrative complexity would have overwhelmed the hospital. Medicare settled on the actual number (recall it now has about 500) as a balance between complexity (a bad thing) and within-group heterogeneity (another bad thing, but for a different reason). Nevertheless, there will always be "near cousins" within the established DRGs from which the hospital might select one or the other as the "bin" into which to place the patient (and hence the DRG payment). Hospitals obviously had an incentive to pick the DRG (among those that might "fit") resulting in the highest payment from Medicare.

Not surprisingly, a software industry arose rapidly to help hospitals shift their DRG patterns favorably. Sometimes the distinction between two DRGs was the indication of a simple comorbidity such as fever or diabetes. The trick became to find any indication in the medical record that such comorbidities existed that would (if found) justify the higher-paying DRG.

After the implementation of the DRG system, many reports estimated the extent of DRG creep (Steinwald and Dummit, 1989; Carter, Newhouse and Relles, 1990; Carter 1991). On average, they showed about a 3% per year increase in the case mix index (CMI), the summary of the severity of all DRGs for all Medicare patients. Careful analysis (including reabstraction of the medical records of a large sample of patients) showed that about one-half of the annual change reflected true increases in patient severity and half primarily reflected better coding from the use of improved software (Carter, Newhouse, and Relles, 1990).

The second dimension arising from the new payment mechanism was the observation by many hospital leaders that (despite the overall precision of the DRG system), some DRGs paid relatively well (compared with the hospital's actual costs) while others paid relatively poorly. Astute hospital leaders (administration, medical staff, and trustees) found these opportunities and sought to shift the emphasis of their hospitalizations away from the less desirable DRGs to those with better revenue/cost implications. One consequence was a significant increase in medical center advertising to patients to attract those with specific illness conditions. Cardiac surgery seemed to be a general "winner" for many hospitals.[17]

Medicare Physician Pricing

Medicare's resource-based relative value system (RBRVS) pricing rule created in 1993 primarily increased the rates of compensation for various "cognitive" activities (talking and thinking) and reduced payments for "procedures." Because most doctors gain professional income from only one or the other (internal medicine doctors mostly engage in cognitive activities, surgeons mostly earn income from procedures), little short-run opportunity exists for many doctors to substitute cognitive for procedural activities.

As these compensation differentials set in (particularly as private health insurance plans also adopt them), the rate of return to cognitive specialties will rise and that of procedure-based specialties will fall. In the long run, this should shift the blend of specialties chosen by doctors coming out of training

---

[17]In a single local example, those flying into the Greater Rochester International Airport will be bombarded (as they exit the airport) with large illuminated advertisements for the two major hospitals in town seeking to attract cardiac surgery patients. These ads (and local TV, radio, and newspaper analogs) have existed and increased in intensity almost from the beginning of the DRG payment system.

with all of the attendant changes in markets that we would normally expect from a supply shift.

Medicaid Payments

As discussed briefly in Chapter 12, Medicaid is notorious among U.S. health care providers for underpaying relative either to the payments of other insurers or the costs of actually providing the care. Two emergent phenomena show the market response to these artificially low prices: quality of care changes and exit from the market.

The most obvious quality of care indicator in a simple physician visit is the duration of time the doctor spends with the patient. As it shrinks, the chance for meaningful information exchange between the doctor and the patient shrinks accordingly, hence increasing the chances for a missed diagnosis, decreasing the patient's understanding of her own medical condition, and satisfaction. For many patients, time spent with the doctor is the primary determinant of satisfaction.[18] Thus, Medicaid's inability to specify the quality of the office visit (specifically, time spent with patients) creates a way for doctors to circumvent the price control.

The other approach, taken by many physicians, is simply to refuse to treat Medicaid patients. In other words, they "exit" from the Medicaid market.

Capitation Payments

Capitation payments represent the extreme end of "bundling" services into a single payment. DRGs bundle hospital treatments into complete "hospitalization episodes." Capitation bundles medical treatment into units of time (typically one year). Just as DRGs cannot readily specify all possible complexity within a single hospitalization, capitation is even less able to specify the possible complexity of the various illness events that patients bring to the health care system.

Capitation models create two strong incentives: (1) to select relatively healthy patients and (2) to reduce treatment costs. Central to both incentives in many ways are the methods used to perform "risk adjustment" (i.e., adjust payments according to a calculation of the severity of illness for each enrolled patient).

---

[18]Recall in Chapter 6 the discussion of physician assistants (PAs) as primary care providers in the Air Force medical clinic experiment. The PA had less training than their physician counterparts, but they spent more time with patients, had equal patient satisfaction, and provided (by ranking from physician researchers) equal quality of care to their physician counterparts.

Numerous studies show that HMOs tend to select relatively healthy patients. Chapter 12 discussed this directly in Medicare HMO enrollment (Part C, or Medicare Advantge). This Part C experience also shows the importance of the risk-adjustment method. When done with age/gender (as originally), it overpaid because of selection. A subsequent approach underpaid, resulting in a massive exit from the program. A newer approach fixed that, resulting in rapid reentry by providers and large enrollment increases. All of this was providers' response to the fixed price and method of risk adjustment.

Capitation payments also create incentives to undertreat patients because the revenue for treating the patient for a year is fixed but expenses increase with treatment (Woodward and Warren-Boulton, 1984). The capitated provider, of course, must provide a higher overall level of utility to the patient with the combination of lower costs and lower treatment intensity than alternative (e.g., FFS) arrangements would allow, so this sets a lower boundary on the ability to restrict treatment intensity.

The randomized controlled trial in the pediatric clinic setting was discussed in Chapter 7 in the section on demand inducement (Hickson, Altmeier, and Perrin, 1987). In that setting, the experiment showed that physicians paid on a flat salary with a fixed set of patients to treat (equivalent in this case to capitation payments) not only provided less treatment than did doctors paid under a FFS arrangement but also well-child care below the standards published by the American Academy of Pediatrics.

Pay for Performance (P4P)

The most recent foray into health care pricing mechanisms comes from the world of business in seeking to create competition in health care along completely different dimensions than have existed to date. The goal of this approach (pay for performance, or P4P) is to create large regional (perhaps even national) centers of excellence for specialized medical procedures. Proponents of this approach argue that paying proportional to measurable outcomes (e.g., mortality rates for cardiac surgery) will lead to significant improvements in quality of care and lower prices to attain those quality improvements.

As has been seen in other controlled price environments, the key to P4P rests in the risk-adjustment methods used. "Outcomes" depend not only on the quality of the medical treatment but also on the condition of the patients treated at any medical center.

Using the language of medical production functions (from Chapter 3), assume that the definition of the quality of a medical outcome $QL = q(\text{Patient, Doctor}) + e$, where e is a random error term (factors beyond the control of either patient or doctor). Patients have random characteristics that are not observable to outsiders (comorbidities) but often are observable at least in part by doctors who might treat them. These can vary from skin palor to the level of concern expressed by a patient about a symptom. Doctors have random characteristics often not observable to patients but that can be estimated with sufficiently large samples (for each provider) and the patient's outcomes. Examples include the propensity to use expensive treatment or to refer patients to other medical facilities they own such as therapy or diagnostic imaging services.

The problem with trying to use statistical approaches to estimating the "doctor" component is the "noise" introduced by the patient component and "random luck" (the error term). Careful analysis of actual hospital data suggests that this process involves too much random variability to assess carefully the quality of individual hospitals (let alone doctors).

Two analyses exemplify the problem. In the first, Park et al. (1990) assessed the contributing effects of pure randomness, quality of care, and patient's severity of illness in deaths of patients with acute myocardial infarction (AMI—heart attacks) and congestive heart failure. They compared hospitals with high mortality rates for these conditions after adjusting for age, race and gender—the so-called targeted hospitals that had death rates in these conditions from 5 to 10.9 per hundred cases higher than the average in untargeted hospitals. The results do not bode well for the measures needed to make P4P work well. Park et al. found 56–82 percent of the differences due to pure randomness and concluded, "Identifying hospitals that provide poor-quality care based on administrative data and single-year death rates is unlikely; targeting based on time periods greater than 1 year may be better."

A second analysis (Hofer and Hayward, 1996) also considered mortality rates. The authors used hospital data at the level of individual DRGs and assumed (optimistically and counterfactually) that no intragroup heterogeneity exists within a DRG. They found that being an "outlier" (having bad mortality) in any two-year period (*outlier* referring to a hospital that had the worst 5 percent of case mortality rates) had little predictive power for their outcomes in future years. For acute myocardial infarction (AMI), for example, Hofer and Hayward found that only 24 percent of such outliers (less than one-fourth) would appear in later years as outliers. More than three-fourths of hospitals labeled as poor quality would really have had mortality rates not differing from the average in a statistically reliable way.

Better statistical analysis cannot solve such problems. They reflect the underlying variability in the world of medical treatment. Too much true random variability exists to allow good inferences about provider-specific quality for many medical and surgical treatments. Without the ability to measure more refined patient-illness characteristics, one simply cannot learn much from comparing case mortality rates even within the same DRG.

Further complicating this is the situation in which the quality of the outcome is less obvious. With cardiac care treatments (bypass surgery, heart attacks, congestive heart failure) and many cancers, the case mortality rate is both an obvious and important outcome.

Treatment of many chronic illnesses is complex. How, for example, could the quality of treatment of diabetes patients be rated? By using hospitalization rates? (These are rare events in the sense that relatively few diabetics are actually hospitalized in any given year but related data are available from insurance claims.) By using medical complication rates such as pressure sores, vision loss, or cardiac illness? (Again, these occur in a relatively small fraction of diabetic patients and are more difficult to measure from available data.) P4P proponents (Porter and Teisberg, 2006) assert that good risk-adjustment measures are available for some medical procedures (they cite seven in their book) and implementing them for many other important medical treatments is a simple matter. Unfortunately, assessments of the underlying statistical problems suggest otherwise.

An even more difficult problem arises if a true P4P pricing system were to be implemented by (say) Medicare or Medicaid, for example: Providers seeking good ratings in the P4P world would begin to screen out patients who were likely to have bad outcomes. (We know that providers can find ways to do this in general because of the known selection of healthy people into HMOs.) With heart disease, the patient's weight, smoking history, and comorbid conditions such as diabetes, family history (e.g., genetic makeup), physical condition, compliance with recommended therapy, and many other difficult-to-observe characteristics in addition to the underlying severity of the disease process contribute to patient survival. Similar factors affect cancer survival. None of these data can be measured easily without directly looking into medical charts of every patient whose outcome is being analyzed. Although data measurement can be done for research purposes, doing it regularly to assess the performance of every provider in a market (or in the nation) seems beyond possibility with current technology.[19] And if patients' contributions to the outcome are not measurable but adverse health outcomes count against the provider, selecting out those patients (doctors and hospitals finding ways to avoid treating them) seems inevitable.

---

[19]Widespread use of electronic medical records will eventually make this easier; see the section on electronic medical records later in this chapter.

Pay for Results (P4R)

A new payment approach has emerged in the British National Health Service (BNHS). It suggests an entirely new pathway for pricing such items as pharmaceutical drugs, but in concept the technique could be applied to other selected interventions as well (Garber and McClellan, 2007). The case in point was a new drug marketed by Johnson and Johnson (J&J) to treat a multiple myeloma cancer. The drug—very expensive per dose—works on only about 40 percent of patients, and the BNHS initially denied coverage for it. J&J responded by offering to forgo payment for patients who did not respond to the treatment—the ultimate in P4P. This 100 percent money-back guarantee creates quite different incentives than a commensurate reduction in price, particularly when the treatment itself is expensive on a per patient basis. Most of the cost of drugs is for R&D, and the cost to produce and sell a dose itself is often trivial. With a simple price reduction (in the case of this drug, an implicit 60 percent price reduction), the manufacturer still has incentives to maximize the drug's use. With a money-back guarantee for treatment failure, the manufacturer has strong incentives to educate physicians to avoid using the drug when treatment failure is imminent.

Administering this approach has important difficulties. First, the outcome must be clear, unambiguous, and easy for independent observers to determine. Patient survival in an otherwise fatal situation is just such an outcome. The determination of outcome cannot be subject to manipulation, and, as Garber and McClellan have noted, this approach will work best when patient characteristics and/or other treatments do not confound the results.

An Unresolved Externality Involving Hospital Rate Regulation

Having discussed competitive bidding in health care (Chapter 11), externalities in the production of information (Chapter 14), and now, hospital rate regulation (preceding sections), we can finally merge these ideas in a new and important topic in health policy. As competitive bidding comes to the hospital sector, it reveals a problem previously hidden in the innards of noncompetitive pricing: the support of graduate medical education (GME). As any teaching hospital CEO knows, the presence of residents and fellows in a GME program adds to its costs in several ways:

- directly from the costs related to their employment
- indirectly—more important—in the change not only in the nature of treatment (residents probably use more tests than more experienced physicians) but also in the mix of patients (quite predictably, teaching hospitals attract the sickest of all patients because physician coverage is available in the hospital 24 hours a day unlike in the typical nonteaching hospital.

The costs of GME have been absorbed by (1) extra Medicare payments to hospitals (which continues today) and (2) the higher prices charged by teaching hospitals (and paid by insurance plans and patients). In states with price controls, in particular, elaborate GME cost differentials also have worked their way into the rate formulae. As decontrol comes to hospital rate-setting practices, and, more important, as competitive bidding becomes more common, these previous mechanisms to fund GME seem at risk. In a purely competitive bidding setting, one would not expect buyers (insurers, etc.) to willingly pay fully for the extra costs of teaching. The benefits of that teaching (trained doctors) often flow out of the region where the doctors are trained.

Ultimately, the provision of GME appears to be a classic externality (see Chapter 14) in which the costs fall on some citizens and the benefits accrue to others. Whether the previous mechanisms to fund GME can persist in the new competitive and unregulated environment remains in doubt. Ultimately, what we know about the funding of beneficial externalities suggests that the federal government may have to step in ultimately to provide appropriate funding for this activity, perhaps through the Medicare program.

DRUGS AND DEVICES: THE NEW WAVE OF MEDICAL CARE

Looking back in Chapter 1, at the trends set forth in Tables 1.5 through 1.8 the relative fiscal importance of prescription drugs (and, although not shown in those tables, medical "devices") clearly has increased substantially in the past quarter century. Indeed, although one could state without fear of correction that the technology available to improve health increased greatly during that time, one could also conjecture (probably accurately, although only time will tell) that the changes coming in the next quarter century could far surpass them.

Although this may seem a crude generalization, the landmark inventions in medicine have been few and far between in general. The discovery of X-rays and their use in medical diagnosis surely stands as one of those landmarks, but in many ways, even the X-ray machine has been supplanted by other diagnostic devices (MRI imaging, PET imaging, and ultrasound). The most dramatic improvement in human longevity in the twentieth century probably came from the discovery and development of antibiotic drugs.

Before World War II, doctors had little available to combat infectious diseases, and (going back several centuries) it was not uncommon for infectious diseases to maim or kill large percentages of the population of entire nations.[20] The discovery of antibiotics (to treat bacterial infections) and vaccination (to stimulate humans' resistance to viral and other diseases) eliminated much of the threat of infectious diseases, but that aside, major medical advances have come more in the realm of surgery than medicines.

In surgery, perhaps the first major discovery was the ability to anesthetize patients (and support their vital functions during surgery) so that long and complicated surgeries became possible. (Before anesthetics, surgery was limited to a few interventions, including amputation of limbs, caesarian section deliveries, and limited abdominal surgery.) The combination of anesthesia and antibiotics opened the door to a continual growth in surgical intervention to cure or improve a wide array of maladies in every organ system in the body.

As the risk of infectious diseases declined, the causes of human illness and death shifted to other disease processes that had (in some sense) been masked by the infectious diseases' ravaging of human life. Increased longevity brought with it increased rates of heart disease, cancer, and stroke. Cancers have been treated by a variety of approaches, including surgery (to remove the primary tumor), radiation (to kill primary and secondary tumors), and chemotherapy, the latter a new and important class of drugs emerging mostly after World War II. Indeed, the National Cancer Institute's formation in 1955 led to the first systematic screening of chemical agents for effects on cancer cells. Chemotherapy to combat cancer thus stands (in addition to antibiotics and vaccines) as a second major therapeutic intervention in the twentieth century.

Until recently, however, drug invention has been more of a process of discovery than a systematic process. Indeed, most of the famous drug and device inventions have been the result of happenstance: The discoveries of X-rays and the powers of penicillin to prevent infections provide classic examples. Many of our modern drugs owe their discovery to "folk medicine" from around the world (by trial and error) whose healers had discovered the power of various substances to improve various medical conditions. The drug digitalis used for treatment of heart disease came directly from observations of the efficacy of the plant foxglove in treating "dropsy" (heart failure) as early as 1785.

---

[20]For example, the famous Black Plague (bubonic plague, spread by fleas carried by rats) killed 137 million people in total, sometimes as many as 2 million a year, and accounted for the deaths of one-third to one-half of many European nations in the fourteenth century. The famous children's nursery game "celebrates" these events: "Ring around the rosie, a pocket full of posie, ashes, ashes, we all fall down!" So many dead bodies littered the cities that people carried a pocket full of sweet-smelling "posie" to counteract the smell, and the burning of bodies created a perpetual haze of ashes. "We all fall down" foretells the ultimate death of many from the plague.

The advances in the scientific basis for drug discovery are well exemplified by the increased understanding of the role of foxglove in treating heart failure caused by the heart muscle's ineffective strength for pumping blood. The improvement from using foxglove most likely merely recorded the haphazard uses of various drugs tried to treat various illnesses. Modern biochemistry has now given insight into the mechanisms by which foxglove works. It alters the chemical exchange in the heart muscle involving sodium and potassium, increasing the concentration of calcium ions in the heart muscle (the desired outcome) and then its ability to function.

This discovery led to new classes of drugs that act on the body's control of the size and stiffness of arteries, factors in the cause of weak hearts, and hypertension (a cause of heart failure and stroke), and other illnesses and reduce the heart's workload.

The increased chemical armamentarium has many derivatives. First, it often lessens the need for surgery because the drugs can treat illnesses with the same or better efficacy but with fewer side effects and frequently lower cost. (This in turn leads to reduced use of the hospital, a trend also occurring in the past quarter century.) Some important results of drug therapy include the virtual elimination of surgery for (1) gastric ulcers (and gastro-esophageal reflux using the same or related medicines); (2) for stones in the bile duct or ureter by dissolving them; (3) enlarged thyroid glands; (4) dissolving blood clots; and (5) to remove coronary artery plaques.

Second, new drug discoveries have greatly expanded the range of diseases that can be treated *at all.* Conditions that were heretofore not treatable suddenly have become treatable, improving human health but also expand medical spending. Just in the last decade or so, for example, treatments (if not cures) have become available for such diseases as multiple sclerosis, many forms of cancer, heart disease, stroke and common and annoying illnesses such as "hay fever."[21]

The increase in the efficacy of therapeutic drugs has been matched by expenditures for them. Reasons for this include (1) expensive drug development and testing, (2) increases in the number of diseases and illnesses they treat, and (3) the needs of an aging population.

A parallel increase has come in medical devices, the most important of which is possibly magnetic resonance imaging (MRI), which uses powerful magnetic forces to cause cells, when captured by measurement devices in the MRI machines, to emit signals allowing reconstruction of three-dimensional

---

[21]Any person who has suffered serious hay fever or asthma has greatly benefited from the new class of antihistamine drugs that provide steady relief for 12–24 hours with significantly reduced side effects, most commonly drowsiness.

body images with extremely high clarity. Their use has resulted in great strides in not only the diagnosis of diseases and injuries but also improved medical knowledge by providing new insights into the relationship between observed physiological changes and medical symptoms. Other imaging devices include computed tomography (CT) scanners and the newly emerging positron emission tomography (PET) scanners that allow observation of physiological processes within the living body (metabolism, blood flow, etc.). Although until recently confined to research studies, PET scanners are now used in the diagnosis and staging of cancers (to give one example).[22]

What does the future for drug therapy and medical diagnosis portend? Many scientists claim that we are on the verge of many breakthroughs in drug therapy that will make past discoveries seem crude by comparison, just as the discovery of foxglove in the eighteenth century was supplanted by a better understanding of the drug's physiological mechanisms in the twentieth century. The primary source for this claim comes from the immense array of information accumulated in the Human Genome Project, which set out to sequence the entire structure of human genes (see Box 15.1). The project was accomplished far earlier than scheduled, with major work by the National Institutes of Health (NIH) directly, NIH-funded research laboratories and private companies carrying out their work independent of government funding.

The development of information about the roles and functions of individual genes has led to three major areas of possible drug therapy. First, by knowing the roles of various genes, scientists can learn more about disease processes, and hence "target" drug therapy more usefully. Second, by altering (for example) the genetic structure of viruses, scientists can "implant" new genes into humans that replace defective genes. Thus, "gene therapy" actually takes out defective genes throughout the human body and replaces them with "correct" copies. This could actually allow the cure of many diseases of an inherited nature (the list of which is too vast to even summarize here). Third, gene therapy can stimulate growth in specific types of cells in specific locations causing the body to self-heal various injuries. These possibilities lead to widespread optimism that we will soon have the ability to "cure" such things as major spinal cord injuries, restore the function of joints that have been damaged by athletic injury or disease processes, and reverse many of the symptoms once considered normal "aging."

---

[22]Because cancer cells grow and divide at a much faster rate than normal cells, they "burn" glucose at a high rate, and hence appear easily in PET scans studying normal human metabolism. Medicare began paying for PET scans for cancer diagnosis in 1998.

BOX 15.1   THE HUMAN GENOME PROJECT

What is the Human Genome Project (HGP) and why does it seem so important in the future of human health? The human genome—the genetic code that defines our very humanity—involves an enormously large number of genes, encoded information that tells every cell in each body what to do as well as when and under what circumstances. It is the "programming information" of the wonderfully complex human body. Understanding that code offers enormous promise for finding ways to cure disease and rebuild human bodies ravaged by injury, time, and disease.

The Human Genome project has met its stated goal—providing a "sequence" of the entire human gene structure.[*] Many scientists believe that *every* human disease has a genetic basis either directly or through modifying the body's response to an external stimulus (virus, bacteria, toxin, etc.). Thus, the genetic information from the HGP and subsequent research will allow new ways of diagnosing disease (or identifying those at higher risk of a disease) and—in many cases—creating gene-based therapies to cure disease.

Genetic tests currently cost hundreds to sometimes thousands of dollars per individual tested, but such tests will certainly decline in costs as scientists and engineers find ways to make the tests more routine and economies of scale enter the testing business.

Gene therapies actually change the genetic structure of an individual, either for that person alone ("somatic" therapy) or for his or her successor generations, by modifying the genetic content of human eggs and spermatazoa ("germ" therapy). The most common method for delivering the modified gene to a human now is to encapsulate the altered gene into a virus that "infects" the patient, causing the defective gene to be replaced with a correct gene. As the "infection" spreads, the entire body is "cured" of the genetic malformation and hence the genetic disease.

Another branch of genetic research—pharmacogenetics—studies how the genetic composition of individual humans alters the response to different drugs. The goals of pharmacogenetic research include the ability to tailor the dose of a drug to the individual, improve the safety and efficacy of vaccines, improve diagnostic capabilities,[†] and even tailor drugs specifically to match the genetic structure of individual patients. This type of research should also reduce greatly the number of drugs that fail to achieve their desired results and reduce or eliminate attempts to develop drugs that have major side effects, thus potentially lowering the overall cost of pharmaceutical drugs and health care in general.

[*]http://www.ornl.gov/TechResources/Human_Genome/home.html.

[†]Sometimes doctors can make a diagnosis based on a *nonresponse* to a given drug. When two alternative diagnoses exist, giving a drug that will cure one of them tells the doctors which disease the person has whether he is cured or not.

(continued)

BOX 15.1 THE HUMAN GENOME PROJECT (continued)

The public investment in the HGP has been funded mostly by the National Institutes of Health ($3.8 billion through 2003) and the Department of Energy ($1 billion through 2003 under its charter to study the effects of radiation on the human body). There has also been a large private investment in studying the human genome, most notably the Celera Genomics Corporation and Incyte.

Although the approach is wrapped in controversy, the U.S. patent system allows indivdual bits of genomic information to be patented, providing monopoly rights to the exploitation of that information for 20 years from the date the patent application is filed. (See related discussions in this chapter on patents and drug invention.) As of 2001, the U.S. Patent and Trade Office had received applications for more than 3 million fragments of genetic material and thousands of partial or complete genes. The ability to patent individual genes stems directly from the 1980 U.S. Supreme Court landmark case, *Diamond V. Chakrabarty,* that granted patent rights for the invention of a microbe that digests oil. Current patent law holds that genetic information may be patented in the same way that any other invention may be: It must meet the tests of being novel, useful, and not obvious, and described sufficiently for others to reproduce. (the last provision of the patent law leads some inventors *not* to patent their invention because the disclosure of the process allows others to pursue related work, and even without that, allows them to copy and use the work after the patent has expired.)

In addition to new drug development, information about an individual's genetic structure will also allow doctors to select specific drugs (when more than one drug is available to treat a given disease) by knowing how people with different genotypes react to different drugs. This "individualized medicine" can potentially improve cure rates for numerous diseases and at the same time point the way for development of new drugs that can cure individuals who are non-responders to existing drugs.

To provide a background for understanding how drug development has proceeded in the past and how it will proceed into the future, we can now turn to a description and analysis of the process of new drug invention and testing as well as the laws by which drug (and device) development occurs in the United States (and throughout the world).

How Pharmaceuticals Come to the Market

The development of a new pharmaceutical drug ("drug" hereafter, but not to be confused with hallucinogenic and illegal drugs) or medical device follows a long and complicated path in almost every case. The research often begins with some very basic scientific research carried out at a U.S. or foreign university, commonly using support (in the United States) from the NIH through a very competitive program to support basic research. In much of this work, the researchers propose to carry out a specific line of research, and the NIH funds it (or not) based entirely on its scientific merits. In this investigator-initiated work, the link between the science and the ultimate application is only sometimes apparent and often only distantly related to a specific drug. (The NIH also has programs of more targeted research, but most of the NIH-granted research funds come through the investigator-initiated program.) The NIH also conducts a large body of research in-house at its laboratories in the Washington, D.C. area and elsewhere.

As the research moves forward, a commercial application can become apparent, and, in such cases, the university where the work is carried out commonly seeks a patent on the research and then moves to commercialize it (invariably in a partnership with a pharmaceutical company). Several decades ago, the United States altered its rules about this patenting process and now strongly encourages universities to seek patent drug and related inventions and license the use of approved patents to industry.[23]

Drug companies conduct major research within their own proprietary laboratories, often more "applied" than NIH-funded research and often based on that earlier "basic" research. Estimates put the research costs of drug companies at about 20 percent of their total sales revenues. Some of this research is quite "basic," but is typically more "applied" with a clearer path between the research and the final product. Often drug companies acquire the rights to use basic research carried out in a university and continue the development to the point of having a marketable drug. Pharmaceutical manufacturing association reports indicate that drug companies evaluate about 1,000 compounds for every one that enters clinical trials. These early evaluations involve laboratory and animal studies.

---

[23]The history of this development is rather intriguing. Despite the enormous research expenditures through the NIH from the 1950s forward, very little commercial development of the knowledge thus gained had occurred. In the earlier rules, ideas developed with federal research grants were patented with the U.S. government holding the patent. By 1980, the government held more than 25,000 patents, and only 5 percent of them had been moved to commercial application.

The Bayh-Dole Act passed in 1980 authorizes universities to license patents and enables a sharing of the patent royalties between the university and the individual inventors. The only restriction on the use of such revenues within the university is that they be dedicated to "scientific research and education."

Once a drug emerges from this process that has great promise for healing human disease, it undergoes a rigorous clinical research process heavily regulated by the U.S. Food and Drug Administration (FDA). Its rules require testing that (in most cases) must demonstrate with a high degree of statistical reliability that the drug is both safe and efficacious (i.e., that it actually works).[24]

FDA Drug Testing

All new drugs entering the U.S. market must receive approval of the United States FDA. The basic time line of this approval process is shown in Figure 15.7.

Phase I Trials—Initial Safety Testing After successful animal testing, the first step in testing a new drug in human subjects is (not surprisingly) Phase I. Its primary goal is to ascertain the safety issues involved. In such studies, the

FIGURE 15.7 New drug development timeline. NDA, new drug application.

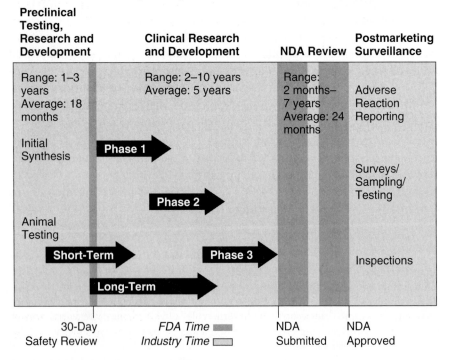

Preclinical Testing, Research and Development	Clinical Research and Development	NDA Review	Postmarketing Surveillance
Range: 1–3 years Average: 18 months	Range: 2–10 years Average: 5 years	Range: 2 months– 7 years Average: 24 months	Adverse Reaction Reporting
Initial Synthesis	Phase 1		Surveys/ Sampling/ Testing
Animal Testing	Phase 2		
Short-Term	Phase 3		Inspections
Long-Term			

30-Day Safety Review · FDA Time ▬ Industry Time ▭ · NDA Submitted · NDA Approved

Source: U.S. FDA (1995).

---

[24]For a detailed discussion of the FDA process, see the FDA's web site at http://www.fda.gov/.

drugs are administered in carefully controlled medical-laboratory conditions to volunteer patients, the primary goals being to ascertain the reaction of the human body to such drugs. These studies typically use 20 to 100 patients, take several months of time, and result in about 30 percent of the drugs so tested being discarded for reasons of safety. Those drugs passing the Phase I hurdle go on to the next step in human trials.

Phase II Trials—Initial Efficacy Testing

After drug safety has been demonstrated at least provisionally in Phase I trials, Phase II process begins; it usually involves many more patients, commonly several hundred, and (while assessing short-term safety considerations) primarily involves study of the drug's efficacy. These studies invariably involve a randomized controlled trial (see Box 3.1 for details of the design of such studies).

The requirement for demonstrating efficacy came after highly publicized and controversial U.S. Senate hearings (led by Senator Estes Kefauver) high-lighted that many drugs marketed (at that time) in the United States in fact did not have any effect on the diseases for which they were prescribed. Phase II trials usually center on patients with the disease for which the drug is intended and simply attempt to determine whether the disease responds favorably to the drug. Commonly, different doses are given at this point to find the lowest dose at which the disease responds well. Of those drugs passing from Phase I to Phase II, typically just under half will pass the Phase II tests. (Because about 70 percent of tested drugs pass Phase I and half of those pass Phase II, about one-third of originally tested drugs pass through Phase II and into Phase III.)

Phase III Trials—Extensive Efficacy and Safety Testing

After initial determination of efficacy in Phase II trials, additional tests of efficacy take place. These studies commonly involve many hundreds, often several thousands of patients normally recruited from hospitals, clinics, and doctors' practices. These studies allow researchers to further confirm the drug's effectiveness established in Phase II trials and provide a much larger sample to assess any possible side effects. Phase III testing eliminates some drugs that have passed Phase II, but the success rate is relatively high at this step, because drugs with obvious hazards were eliminated in Phase I and those with no significant effect on the disease were eliminated in Phase II. The FDA reports that about 25 to 30 percent of all drugs entering a testing protocol make it through Phase III.

Phase IV—Postmarketing Surveillance

Not all drugs that have passed Phase III clinical trials receive FDA approval for marketing; only about 20 percent of the original drugs brought for testing actually receive marketing approval.

After this comes years of "postmarketing surveillance" in which doctors and pharmacists are required to submit to the FDA any adverse events associated with taking the drug. The FDA analyzes these data and sometimes withdraws a drug from the market on the basis of information learned at this stage.[25]

Role of Insurance in Introducing New Technologies

In the world of modern medical care, new technologies have multiple hurdles to cross before they enter common use. As noted, a new medical drug or device typically begins its life in the laboratory, sometimes in industry and sometimes within a research university (the latter often funded by the NIH). Basic science results evolve to prototypes, which then enter the safety and efficacy testing phase discussed previously. If they succeed at that level, two hurdles between the new product and successful adoption by the medical community remain: obtaining insurance coverage and provider "acceptance."

Drug and device companies have myriad ways to create "acceptance" once a product has been approved for use (advertising to doctors and patients). Thus, the most important of these two "final" steps involves insurance coverage. Among the most important of those is Medicare because many private insurers turn to its process for advice about coverage decisions.

For drugs, the key to success comes with the inclusion in a drug insurance formulary—the list of drugs that the insurance plan will pay for. Among drugs that target the same basic disease, receiving a lower "tier" (less expensive) ranking is better because consumers will pay less out of pocket for it, but getting on the coverage list is the key. Once the drug obtains that status, insurance pays for it, and doctors can prescribe it.

The Centers for Medicare and Medicaid Services (CMS) have a Medicare coverage center—National Coverage Decisions (NCDs)[26]—that makes the crucial coverage determinations. To assist in that process, CMS regularly convenes

---

[25]A prominent example of drug withdrawal is the drug Seldane, the first of a now extensive crop of nonsedating antihistamines. Seldane was withdrawn from the market in 1992 when postmarketing data revealed a major (and previously unknown) risk to patients taking both Seldane and several antibiotic drugs including the commonly prescribed drug erythromycin. Patients with liver disease also had difficulties metabolizing Seldane and were at risk for serious complications. Neither of these drug–drug interactions would normally be encountered in Phase II or III trials because people with such complications would normally be excluded from participating in such studies. Introduced in 1985, the drug once held 80 percent of the U.S. market for antihistamine drugs.

[26]Medicare is administered by regional private contractors that can also make a local coverage determination if no NCD exists, but LCDs affect only the relevant region.

the Medicare Evidence Development and Coverage Advisory Committee (MEDCAC),[27] which oversees the gathering of scientific evidence of a product's efficacy and recommending its coverage (or not) to CMS.

The word *cost* does not enter Medicare coverage discussions formally. Observers of the coverage determination process report that cost enters discussions indirectly and that "big-ticket" items receive more scientific scrutiny than do lower-cost items, but cost has never been a formal criterion. Because of this, the NCDs do not employ formal cost-effectiveness (CE) analysis. The original 1965 Medicare act stated that treatments should be covered only when "reasonable and necessary" but gave no guidance to define these terms.[28]

The Medicare approach stands in sharp contrast to standard practices in Great Britain and much of Continental Europe where CE analysis formally enters coverage determinations. For example, in Great Britain, the National Institute for Health and Clinical Excellence (NICE) regularly makes recommendations to the British National Health Service regarding coverage determinations; while not binding, these suggestions have considerable force in the BNHS determinations. The implicit standard is that treatments costing less than £30,000 per quality-adjusted life year for a broad population will obtain favorable coverage determinations but more expensive ones often do not (Garber and McClellan, 2007).

Prescriptions

Law in the United States (more so than in almost any other country) prohibits consumers from *directly* purchasing many drugs. Rather, the patient must obtain a prescription from a doctor, literally a "permission slip from the doctor," that allows the pharmacist (the retail seller) to dispense the drug to the patient. A number of other drugs remain in the "over-the-counter" (OTC) market, which consumers may purchase directly. The distinction between prescription and OTC drugs is sometimes difficult to fathom. Many drugs are OTC because they had been on the market so long when the FTC was established that it probably would have been difficult to pull them back into prescription status (aspirin probably is the most prominent example). Others receive OTC status because all available evidence suggests that they have very few relevant side effects even if taken in very large doses, but some

---

[27]Formerly the Medicare Coverage Advisory Committee (MCAC). The title change reflects the growing urge by CMS to make these coverage decisions on strong scientific evidence.

[28]As with much of the early structure of Medicare, this language followed the private health insurance models available at the time. In particular, Aetna's insurance of federal employees used this same language in describing what services would be covered.

OTC drugs can be relatively dangerous if taken in greatly excessive quantities (including the ubiquitous aspirin). Some drugs pass from prescription to OTC status after an extended period of consumer use (many antihistamine drugs such as benadryl fit into this category). Some drugs are sold at two doses, the larger dose as a prescription drug and the lower dose as OTC.

The Legal Monopoly

Patents (for drugs and devices) establish a legal monopoly for the inventor for a period of 17 years. The purpose of this law is "to promote the progress of science and the useful arts by securing for limited times to inventors the exclusive right to their respective discoveries" (Article 1, Section 8 of the United States Constitution). Patents are particularly important for the pharmaceutical industry (Scherer, 2000) because the enormous investment in development and testing for drugs (estimated to average between $250 and $400 million per drug) can be readily undermined without patent protection because the chemical formula for the drug is well known after it is marketed (and indeed, the chemical content is required information in FDA rules). Thus, without patent protection, pharmaceutical companies would stand a large risk of losing the value of their investment by having other companies simply await the results of the FDA testing and then market the successful drugs without having undergone the development and testing costs.

The pricing of drugs during the patent-supported period varies depending (as one should expect) on the incremental value of the drugs in the market and their costs of production. In an analysis of drug pricing, Lu and Comanor (1998) looked at the pricing of 148 new drugs introduced during the decade beginning in 1978. More than 90 percent of these competed with an existing drug on the market that had similar therapeutic properties, so Lu and Comanor used FDA evaluations to characterize how much therapeutic gain each offered compared with existing drugs. New drugs with modest clinical improvements (about three-eighths of them) were priced (on average) just over twice the price of the extant competitors, those with important gains (about 10 percent of the new entrants) were priced over three times the prices of their competition (on average), and those characterized by the FDA as having little or no therapeutic gains were priced about the same as their competition.

Most drugs sold in the United States are also sold elsewhere in the world, and the market for manufacturing such drugs is truly international. Many observers note that the prices in the United States for new drugs exceed the price for the identical drug in other countries. Part of the difference comes from our very active tort system (see Chapter 13). Manning (1997) found that about half the difference between same-drug prices in the United States and Canada came from differences in costs attributable to the higher legal threat in the United States. The remaining differences come from a variety of sources, but probably the most notable high and increasing coverage of prescription drugs in health insurance (blurring the incentives for consumers to make price-sensitive comparisons) and the more centralized nature of the Canadian health care system, allowing for more central "bulk" buying.

Generic Drug Competition As noted, U.S. law provides a patent holder a legal monopoly for 17 years. After that, one would expect competition to emerge (because the patent provides precise information about the product, thus allowing competitors to produce it directly). The 17-year limit begins when a patent is filed, and (as detailed earlier) FDA drug testing requirements can add many years between filing a patent and the drug's actual marketing. Thus, in 1984, the Congress modified patent law to allow an extension of up to 5 years in the duration of a patent to allow for time lost in the FDA approval process.

This patenting process and prudent business practices have made drug companies among the nation's most profitable corporations. A study by *Fortune Magazine* put the median drug company profitability (profits as a percent of sales revenue) at 18 percent in 1999. But the legal monopoly of patenting does not ensure corporate success: Among the 12 drug companies in the *Fortune* survey (covering the 1,000 largest U.S. companies), profitability ranged from 33 percent to −9 percent. These differences hinge on the life cycle of a company's drug portfolio and the success of its drugs in the market.

Even with the ending of a legal monopoly at the end of the patent term, the value of a monopoly position can extend beyond the years of the patent. This may occur, for example, because patients and their doctors have become accustomed to the drug and its consequences and side effects, and hence may be reluctant to change to new "generic" drugs, even if chemically similar or even identical. However, multiple forces, both legal and private, stimulate the shift to generic drugs once they become available.

On the legal side, government programs such as Medicaid require the use of generic drugs when available. Many private insurance plans do the same thing. A common insurance arrangement for covered prescription drugs includes three tiers. For example, the consumer might pay a $5 per month copayment for generic drugs, a $20 per month copayment for "middle-tier" branded drugs, and $30 per month for more expensive branded drugs. The incentives for consumers and their doctors drive toward substitution of generic or middle-tier drugs whenever possible.

Even with the end of a legal monopoly (as the patent expires), patented drugs often retain a hefty price margin above generic versions of the same drug that enter the market. Figure 15.8 provides what Scherer (2000) describes

FIGURE 15.8 Keflex prices.

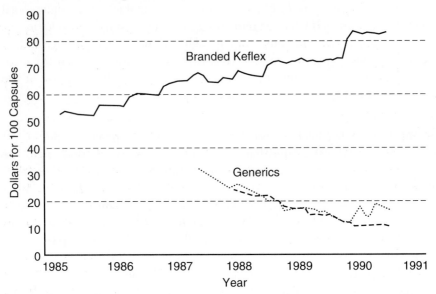

Note: For generics, dotted line shows price path for R&D-oriented firms and dashed line shows generic-specialist firms.

as a "not atypical" example of this issue, drawing on the work of Griliches and Cockburn (1995). Eli Lilly sold the drug—a powerful antibiotic of the cephalosporin class—through 1987 under the branded name Keflex. As Figure 15.8 shows, the price had crept up slowly for several years under patent protection from $55 to $65 per 100 capsules. That trend, perhaps remarkably, continued apace after the patent expired in April 1987, upon which time generic substitutes entered the market at prices initially about half that of Keflex, and then declining to about 20 percent of Keflex's (now higher) price. The price path of the generic substitutes behaved much as we might normally expect because up to 20 firms marketed generic equivalents to Keflex.

As the example of Keflex prices demonstrates, branded prescription drugs often continue to sell at relatively high prices even after the patent expires and generic competition enters the market. This can occur because (in part) of incomplete information on the part of doctors and their patients about the true degree of "equivalence" between the generic and branded versions of a drug and in part because (with generous insurance coverage) the choice may not matter to the patient or doctor. Doctors and patients may ignore the distinction if the patient's health insurance does not have multiple tiers, but health plans with multiple tiers often lead to doctors and patients discussing whether to use a branded drug (high-cost tier) or generic drug ("preferred" low-cost tier) and the differences (if any) that the doctor perceives in the quality of each choice.

The branded/generic arrangement will become increasingly common as more managed care plans develop tiered drug coverage. For example, a health plan might offer coverage for a set of generic prescription drugs (selling at a relatively low price) for $5 per month's dose as a copayment. They would offer coverage for higher priced branded drugs at (say) $20 or $25 per month's dose as the consumer's copayment. By producing both the branded and generic versions of the drug, the company is able to tap into both markets. Because other manufacturers can readily produce the generic drug after the patent has expired, it does the original branded manufacturer no good to sit on the sidelines in that market. By participating (with the generic drug), the branded drug maker can do better than by not participating, but in either case, profits will fall compared with the precompetition era when the patent provided a legal monopoly.

The branded/generic strategy does not pay off very often, however. A study by the Congressional Budget Office (1998) looked at 112 branded drugs that acquired generic competition at the end of the patent. Of those, only in 13 cases (about 10 percent of the drugs) did the original manufacturer gain more than 10 percent of the market share with its generic entrant. In the other 98 cases studied, new entrants effectively seized the market with their generic entrant. What seems to happen (see again the Keflex example in Figure 15.8) is that the original branded drug persists with a much smaller market share but sells at higher prices than the generic equivalents. Drug companies, of course, seek to reinforce this "brand loyalty" both with advertising and by promoting themselves using the descriptor "ethical" drug companies. We turn next to the question of advertising—to whom drug companies "pitch" their products and how they do it.

Drug Company Sales Efforts Advertising generally has the goal of increasing sales of a product. It does this by informing the consumer of the availability and characteristics (quality, price, etc.) of the product and often by creating a favorable association between the product and something the consumer already enjoys. For this reason, for example, famous actors and sports figures often appear in advertisements, or ads show consumers in settings sure to evoke pleasure (a happy party in a bar for a beer ad, an exhilarating ride through the country in an automobile, etc.). But the ways in which laws restrict access to prescription drugs make it more difficult for manufacturers to use common advertising techniques for their products. They commonly turn instead to the "agents" that consumers use as advisors for health care choices—their doctors.

Drug advertising for years has featured two approaches to convincing doctors about the value of prescription drug products: printed advertising in medical journals and direct face-to-face sales contacts either in doctors offices or in hospitals. More recently, drug companies have turned to direct-to-consumer advertising, either over broadcast and cable television or through the medium of the Internet. Annual drug advertising has been estimated at $15 billion a year for a market with overall sales of $357 billion.

Medical Journal Advertisements   Almost all medical journals contain large and detailed ads for drug products, normally focused on the illnesses treated by the medical specialty journal. Thus, for example, *Pediatrics* contains ads about drugs for children's diseases and for child doses of drugs. General interest journals such as *JAMA* and the *New England Journal of Medicine* contain a broad spectrum of ads covering drugs to treat hypertension, heart disease, depression, gastric disorders, allergies, and the like. Sampled issues of the *New England Journal of Medicine,* for example, contained about 120 pages of material, approximately one-third of which advertised prescription drugs. The largest ads appeared for Viagra (five pages), Reminyl (a drug to treat Alzheimer's disease, four pages) and Nexium (four pages of purple colored ads; see Box 15.2 for a discussion of this drug).

BOX 15.2 THOSE UNINFORMATIVE TV DRUG ADS

Anybody who watches television in the United States has probably encountered numerous "direct-to-consumer" (DTC) advertisements for drugs. This advertising strategy began in earnest in 1997 when the FTC relaxed restrictions on DTC ads. Very early came numerous ads for Rogaine, a drug designed to reverse "male pattern baldness" hair loss (which occurs much more often for men than women, but which can affect both). The other prominent advertising blitz that most Americans remember features Viagra, a drug designed to stimulate males' sexual responsiveness. The Viagra campaign featured former U.S. Senator (and defeated Presidential candidate) Robert Dole.* Other drugs with prominent DTC advertising campaigns now include antiallergy drugs, antidepressants, and drugs to combat the side effects of chemotherapy. This class of advertisements describes the drug's use and urges patients to talk to their doctor about obtaining a prescription if it is "right" for the patient; these ads also prominently list the potential side effects of the drug as required by FDA laws that regulate DTC ads.

*This is, of course, the same Dole of the Bayh-Dole Act that led to the major movement for universities to commercialize inventions deriving from federally sponsored research.

One potentially puzzling array of ads never says what the drug is intended to cure! These ads never mention any disease, cure, or anything. They simply show generic pictures (usually happy, healthy people of some defined age group), frequently repeat the name of the drug, and say "Ask your doctor if SuchAndSuch is right for you."

One example from a recent ad blitz: AstraZeneca recently launched an ad campaign to sell "the purple pill." What does this pill do? You could not find out from the ad content. Radio spots featured a pleasant female voice saying, "I didn't know there was a new purple pill until I asked my doctor." In the final pitch, a male voice said, "It's new, it's purple, and maybe you need to know about it!" When patients do "ask their doctor," they find out that the purple pill is Nexium, a drug, according to the original ads, that was intended to relieve heartburn.

Why didn't the ad identify the illnesses the drug can treat? The answer lies in the FDA rules for DTC ads: Once the ad mentions the drug's use, it must also list the possible side effects. However, if it does not claim a specific therapeutic benefit (i.e., a specific illness to be treated), the ad need not contain any information about side effects. The desired outcome (from the drug company's perspective) was to have an army of anxious patients ask their doctor "Is SuchAndSuch a good drug for me?" Of course, if they don't know the intended use of the drug, they have no way of knowing, but the drug company has achieved its goal: The patients become a quasi-sales-force repeatedly inquiring about the drug to their doctors.

These ads—essentially devoid of information content—exist only because of the specific structure of FDA rules about DTC advertising. The companies must make the trade-off between making the ad clearer and more focused (by naming the diseases that the drug treats) versus the problems associated with listing the side effects. Some companies choose the "no information-content" path, while others opt for more focused ads that go in the more specific direction.

Face-to-Face Sales Contacts with Doctors   A key advertising strategy for drug companies for years has involved face-to-face marketing with drug sales representatives—"detail" men and women—who travel to doctors' offices, hospitals, and medical meetings to convince doctors to prescribe *their* brand of drug to patients. Although precise estimates are difficult to find, recent studies (Gagnon and Lexchin, 2008) say that the value of drug samples given out by detail sales persons exceeds $15 billion per year about half of the annual advertising costs of drugs.

Gifts to doctors from drug companies often have a more durable nature, however. Many medical offices contain remnants of a visit from the detail salesperson: note pads, "sticky" notes, coffee mugs, pens and pencils, and the like, all of which provide the physician's implicit endorsement of the product. Drug companies also often sponsor receptions at medical conferences, and indeed sometimes may even sponsor elaborate research "retreats" (for "leaders" in a field) in vacationlike settings in which various combinations of real research presentations and drug company information dissemination take place.

Direct-to-Consumer Advertising The most recent wave of advertising for prescription drugs comes in the form of direct-to-consumer (DTC) ads, mostly over broadcast television. Although estimates vary, DTC advertising generally increased from a mere $55 million in 1991 to over $2 billion in 2000 and exceeding $4.2 billion in 2005 (Donohue et al., 2007). DTC ads take two forms: One specifies the drug, the disease that it treats, and a highly specific set of warnings about possible side effects. The FDA carefully monitors such ads and issued 30 orders in a recent year to have advertising content modified when it felt that the ads overstated the drug's efficacy and the range of diseases that it would treat or understated the side effects.

Other ads avoid completely information about the purposes of the drug or its side effects. They seek to gain consumer recognition and (hopefully) to have patients ask their doctor about the drug, seeking to stimulate a conversation between the doctor and patient that will lead to the use of the drug. See Box 15.2.

Electronic Medical Records

Electronic medical records (EMR) are distinct from other medical technologies but deserve discussion in terms of their effects on health care and their regulation. EMR technology does not involve treatment per se (and hence is exempt from regulation, for example, by the FDA), but its effects on patients can be significant.

The Institute of Medicine of the National Academy of Sciences produced a series of reports highlighting the frequency and nature of preventable medical errors in the U.S. health care system (IOM, 2000) followed by a study focusing on preventable drug errors (IOM 2007). The 2000 report ("To Err is Human") reported that 44,000 to 98,000 people die each year in hospitals due to iatrogenic disease or injury.

The 2007 report estimated that more than 1.5 million preventable adverse drug events occur annually in the United States, about half in the nursing home setting and the others divided between inpatient hospital care and ambulatory care.[29] The report identified electronic prescription ordering systems as a key tool available to reduce preventable ADEs resulting from such mechanisms as poorly legible handwriting on prescriptions,[30] drug-drug interactions, incorrect dosages, and incorrect time intervals for administering the drug.

A second possible benefit from widespread use of EMR technology comes in the realm of "medical practice guidelines" development (hence reduction in unwarranted variations in medical practice patterns). Most medical practice guidelines are developed using information contained in "transactions-based" medical claims data (Medicare, commercial insurance plans, etc.). These insurance claims records provide a rich source of data about treatments rendered to patients but are usually quite sparse in terms of identifying patient outcomes (a key in creating good guidelines) and comorbidities the patient might have that would interfere with successful treatment. The data in an EMR offer the possibility of greatly enriching the research data used for creating medical practice guidelines, thus creating a second benefit in addition to the direct benefits to patients (such as reducing drug errors).

Regulation of EMR Technology EMR regulation is an issue related to the information it contains. The content of medical records is protected as a result of the Health Insurance Portability and Accountability Act (HIPAA) of 1996. Title II sets standards for (paper and digital) medical record security and for electronic digital interchange (EDI) transactions between various organizations involved in health care (insurance carriers, providers, drug stores, etc.).

HIPAA's key privacy features for medical information require that health care providers give copies of medical records to the individual involved upon request and that errors identified by the individual be corrected. Its rules also strictly limit the ways in which medical information (records, test results, prescriptions, billing data) can be disseminated. Primarily, the rules forbid

---

[29]An adverse drug event (ADE) is any injury to the patient due to medication. Preventable ADEs include only those that would not have occurred with proper drug management (for example) allergic reactions to a drug to which the allergy was not previously known. An allergic reaction would be considered preventable, however, if the patient had previous allergic reactions to the drug.

[30]One wag alleged that medical schools require courses in handwriting obfuscation. If you believe that the idea has no basis in reality, try reading the next few prescriptions written by hand for you by a medical care provider.

dissemination of any record information that can be linked to a specific person without the individual's authorization. HIPAA rules also mandate very tight security measures for EMR to prevent unauthorized access by outsiders.

A "Nonevent" in Regulation

It seems worth noting at this point the considerably different treatment of drugs specifically (under the FDA law) and "medical interventions" in general. In contrast to the considerable regulation of drug safety and efficacy, no comparable regulation exists for the promulgation of new "treatments" or the assessment of previously used treatments. In this context, *treatments* refers to both surgical procedures and "strategies" for treating patients that do not involve surgery. This creates an odd schizophrenia in the production of knowledge and in the likelihood that a new treatment innovation will reach the market. Drug regulation in general, but particularly the pre-1984 rules, inhibits market entry. Nothing inhibits entry of a new surgical technique, however. This distorts the economic incentives regarding these alternative forms of therapy, probably tipping us toward "too much surgery" and not enough pharmaceutical treatment. This is a highly relevant comparison for many diseases that ranges across a wide spectrum of illnesses for which both surgical and nonsurgical approaches are feasible.

SUMMARY

Regulation pervades the health care sector; much of it is aimed at reducing costs in the industry. These regulations have attempted to limit entry and expansion in the industry (CON laws) and directly control prices (Medicare pricing rules). Empirical studies of these rules have found only that direct price controls work well, but not universally.

A number of regulations also directly attempt to improve quality of treatment. FDA rules to control safety and efficacy of drugs and medical devices provide an obvious example, as does licensure of various medical personnel (doctors, dentists, nurses, etc.). In both cases, private provision of information (advertising of drug quality, certification of provider quality by "boards") provides a nonmandatory alternative that coexists with mandatory licensure. In most (if not all) cases, private certification provides evidence of a higher standard of quality than the mandatory licensure requires.[31]

---

[31]Indeed, it would seem strange if this were not true because it would imply that the provider would be spending money and time to provide certification of quality that had no meaning to the consumer.

Many regulatory activities, whether aimed at controlling cost or enhancing quality, have the obvious side effect of changing the nature of competition, primarily because of the implicit or explicit effects on entry by competitors. CON laws directly attempted to control hospital entry. FDA rules (until the 1984 revisions) considerably restricted competition, especially in the entry of "generic" products.

Other regulations that attempt to control costs also have consequences for quality of care. The effect of price controls on quality of care seems obvious because not-for-profit hospitals can meaningfully respond to a binding price control only by reducing quality of care. (A for-profit hospital could reduce price and maintain quality simultaneously, although it would probably not choose to do so if confronted with a binding price control.)

Careful economic analysis of regulation in the health care sector remains an important realm of study; every regulation considered in this chapter has the *potential* for providing some social benefit, and none is unambiguously without merit. Each, in turn, has the *potential* for creating economic mischief, either through effects on competition or quality, or combinations thereof. Thus, we leave the discussion of regulation in the health care sector with the usual economist's two-handed evaluation: "On the one hand, they might be good, and on the other hand . . . ."

RELATED CHAPTERS IN *HANDBOOK OF HEALTH ECONOMICS*

Chapter 20, "The Industrial Organization of Health Care Markets" by David Dranove and Mark A. Satterthwaite

Chapter 25, "The Pharmaceutical Industry" by F. M. Scherer

Chapter 27, "Antitrust and Competition in Health Care Markets" by Martin Gaynor and William B. Vogt

Chapter 28, "Regulation of Prices and Investment in Hospitals in the U.S." by David S. Salkever

PROBLEMS

1. Calculate the present value of an annuity of 17 years' duration for an annual profit of $1 million from a new drug at discount rates of 5 percent and 10 percent. You can use "annuity" tables found in most business math texts, or you can generate them in a spreadsheet or statistical program.

   Now calculate the present value of the last 9 years of the annuity—that is, the present value of the 17-year annuity minus the present value of an 8-year annuity. The difference exemplifies the loss in profits due to the (average) 8-year testing imposed by FDA rules.

2. Calculate the present value of a "perpetuity" of monopoly profits at 5 percent and 10 percent. (*Hint:* The present value of a perpetuity of $1 is $1/r$, where r is the discount rate.) Now calculate the present value of a perpetuity after "discarding" the first 8 years of profits. Compare this with the present value of a 17-year annuity. Which provides greater incentive for invention—a perpetuity delayed by 8 years or a 17-year annuity? How does the answer change as you vary the discount rate from 5 percent to 10 percent?

3. The FDA regulates the sale of drugs in the United States by requiring evidence of safety and efficacy. What effects does this have that might improve the health of the U.S. population? What effects does this have that might harm the health of the U.S. population?

4. Discuss the possible benefits and costs (from a social perspective) of DTC advertising of drugs.

5. Regarding hospital regulation, the models of hospital behavior developed in Chapter 9 predict that the effects of DRG payments on hospital behavior will differ across hospitals because that system offers the same price to all hospitals. What types of hospitals will likely have to change their behavior when confronting the DRG system, and what will their changes do to hospital output and quality, if anything? What types of hospitals will likely do nothing?

6. "The free market has too much entry for hospitals, and regulators can potentially improve social well-being by restricting entry." Discuss.

7. "Licensure restricts entry into medical professions for such health care providers as doctors, pharmacists, and dentists. This can only benefit these professions and will always harm patients by making doctors, dentists, and so on, more expensive." Discuss.

8. What evidence do you know that shows whether price controls and CON laws really affect hospital prices?

9. If pharmaceutical companies have average profits (revenue in excess of costs) of 18 percent of sales, what does that (approximately) tell you about the elasticity of demand for these companies' products? (*Hint:* Go back to the markup formulas for a monopolist. You will have to make some assumptions about what part of drug companies' costs are fixed and what are variable. In thinking about this, the term *MC* in the formula might represent average variable costs in your thinking.)

CHAPTER 16

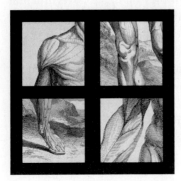

Universal Insurance Issues and International Comparisons of Health Care Systems

The preceding chapters have analyzed how the U.S. health care system works, emphasizing the interlocking roles of consumer demand, insurance coverage, tax policy, doctors, hospitals, and government regulation. It would probably be fair to state that, at least over the post-World War II era, U.S. health policy has emphasized a balancing of two concerns: access to care and control of costs. Massive increases in insurance coverage through employer-related access left two groups of concern: retired persons and low-income persons. In the 1950s and 1960s, access issues dominated, culminating in 1965 with the passage of laws creating Medicare and Medicaid. In the 1970s, issues of cost control began to emerge with the growth of CON laws, state hospital rate regulations, and increasingly strict payment mechanisms for both doctors and hospitals under Medicare and Medicaid. By the early 1980s, cost control had become *the* dominant issue in health policy. Shifts of the entire Medicare hospital payment system

LEARNING GOALS

- Apply the material throughout the textbook to focus on important issues relating to universal insurance choices:

  Why (if at all) should a country choose universal insurance?

  What medical services should be covered?

  How can universal insurance coverage balance protection against financial risk with welfare loss arising from excessive health care use?

  What mechanisms of financing governmentally provided insurance exist, and which cause the least economic distortion?

  What methods exist to control the introduction of new technologies into a nation's health system, and how do these affect health and economic welfare of the public?

- Draw from other nations' choices in these issues to help illuminate choices confronting the United States.

- Understand why the United States has the largest per capita health care spending among industrialized nations, yet worse health outcomes than nations spending less per capita for health care.

529

(Part A) from a fee-for-activity basis to the diagnosis-related prospective payment system in 1983 and to an alternative resource-based relative value system for physicians in 1992 provide good examples of these governmental concerns over unit costs and total spending within these programs.

As detailed in Chapter 1, growth in spending in the United States has proceeded almost without interruption, increasing the share of GNP devoted to health care from about 5 percent in 1960 to an estimated 17 percent by 2010. Per capita costs, even after adjusting for large changes in the overall consumer price index, have also increased steadily during this period. In constant dollars per capita, total spending is estimated to have increased more than 8-fold between 1960 and 2010, and the comparable spending increase for drugs is almost 10-fold for that period. (Review the data in and discussion surrounding Table 1.7 for details.)

At the same time, access issues continued to create concern. Despite the widespread increase in employer-related plans, the universal coverage of the Medicare population over the age of 65, the addition of more than 1 million disabled under Medicare, widespread coverage for the poor under Medicaid, and the increase of several million children insured via the SCHIP program, large groups of persons have no health insurance coverage. Current estimates of the number of persons who have no health insurance coverage at all now is about 47 million Americans, or almost one out of every six persons (see Box 16.1).

The dual concern about access to care and total spending increase has increasingly led health policy analysts and politicians to consider alternatives to the current health care system, including universal insurance, often looking to other nations for alternative models of organization.

As is commonly described in news and commentary on the U.S. health care system, the country simultaneously has among the highest spending per capita and the least comprehensive coverage of any major industrialized nation. We also have very high life expectancy and, by any objective standard, a broader and deeper set of medical technologies and interventions available than any other nation. Nevertheless, many people continue to call for a rethinking of how we organize our health care system. The Canadian health care system is a current "favorite" for comparison, but in previous years the British National Health Service (BNHS), the German system, the Swedish system, and others have been held up as desirable standards for the United States to emulate. Not surprisingly, careful examination of these alternative models indicates that they encompass a wide array of differences in cost growth, in ways to create "coverage," and in ways to pay providers. A subsequent section of this chapter describes a (partly representative) handful of the health care systems in various countries and seeks to draw from them any available lessons about the effects of the system on access, costs, and quality of care. First, however, it is desirable to step back and ask what one might

BOX 16.1   WHO DOES NOT HAVE HEALTH INSURANCE CURRENTLY?

Recent estimates put the number of Americans without insurance at about 47 million in 2006, representing 17% of people under 65. The rate of uninsurance climbs to 30% for the 18- to 24-year-old population. Uninsured people seem to be heavily (but not exclusively) concentrated among segments of society who are young and have lower education and lower income. Three-quarters of the uninsured are under the age of 35; nearly one-third of all young adults (aged 18–24) have no health insurance (Health 2007, Table 139).

Many of the uninsured persons in the U.S. are employed, often at small firms that do not offer health insurance coverage. For example (Kaiser Family Foundation 2008), 70 percent of uninsured adults have at least one full-time worker in the family. However, because of their employment income, most of these families will not be eligible for Medicaid, and for those with higher incomes, SCHIP is less useful as an insurance source for their children because of income limitations built into that program.

A recent report from the U.S. Bureau of the Census (DeNavis-Walt et al., 2006) shows the strong link between income and insurance coverage. For those with incomes under $25,000, 24.4 percent had no health insurance. For those between $25,000 to $50,000, the rate fell to 20.6 percent. For families with incomes between $50,000 and $75,000, the uninsured rate fell again to 14.1 percent, and for those with incomes at or above $75,000, only 8.1 percent lacked health insurance. These estimates of persons without insurance include coverage from government programs (Medicare, Medicaid, SCHIP and other federal and state programs).

consider to be the essential issues involved in the goal of a national health care policy or national health system and at least the options generally available to meet these goals in the U.S. context.

GENERAL CONSIDERATIONS FOR A NATIONAL HEALTH POLICY

The key issues national policy makers face include the following:

- Should the system have universal coverage, and, if so, how should it be accomplished?
- How should the government finance any parts of the system through governmental programs?
- What core benefits should be included (scope of benefits and cost sharing) in any universal plan?
- How will expenses be controlled?
- How will new technologies be introduced?

Universal Coverage Issues

Why Worry About Universal Insurance? The arguments for universal coverage center on several key ideas. One idea is that medical care is a "merit good," one for which access to all citizens should be assured (but see Hamilton and Hamilton, 1993 for a cautionary view). The economic logic behind this idea centers on the idea that each citizen might derive some utility from other citizens' ability to consume the merit good, thus making the collective demand for the good exceed the private demand.

A second idea says that those without insurance act as free riders on a health care system that has built into it (as a "safety net") many ways of providing health care to persons who "show up at the door" of health care providers, especially hospitals and most especially emergency rooms. Some individuals choose to be without insurance and then end up not paying for care when it is rendered—the proverbial "free ride." (See Box 16.2 for a discussion of how people get care without insurance.) One solution to this

---

BOX 16.2 WHAT DO PEOPLE WHO ARE UNINSURED DO WHEN THEY GET SICK?

A persistent theme in the discussion of people without insurance is the apparent mechanism for receiving medical care when they get sick. Commonly, these people appear either at a hospital clinic or a hospital emergency room, often leading to hospitalization. At that point, the hospital either transfers the patient to a public hospital (if available) or pays for the care as charity, writing off the expenses as a bad debt. (Hospitals seem to use either method interchangeably, so most people studying the problem lump together bad debt and charity care.) Thus, the argument goes, we are paying for this care anyway, either through taxes (to support public hospitals) or through higher hospital bills for those with insurance, so why not provide the insurance directly? Doing so would reduce the financial risk of those currently uninsured and would probably not add considerably to the total bill because hospital use is relatively insensitive to insurance coverage (see Chapter 5).

The ability of people who are uninsured to continue to rely on hospitals' charitable intentions to supply care appears tenuous. Particularly as competition increases in the hospital sector (due in large part to the actions of cost-conscious insurance plans), the ability of hospitals to cross-subsidize the care of the patients without insurance will decay.

Uncompensated care (an amalgam of charity and bad-debt care) represents about only 5 percent of all hospital bills (Sloan, Valvona, and Mullner, 1986), but the distribution of that 5 percent falls unevenly on public and teaching hospitals. The solution to this problem is not transparent. At a conference on the topic (See Sloan, Blumstein, and Perrin, 1986), several speakers offered various preferred strategies, but little consensus emerged. Each proposed solution (e.g., mandated worker coverage, expanding Medicaid) has its own drawbacks and political opponents. For the present, we can be sure only that the problem will continue to perplex policy analysts and legislators, but that will not make it go away. For better or worse, we will continue to confront the questions posed by people without insurance and by uncompensated hospital care for some time into the future. Only a universal health insurance plan will make the issue go away, and our country does not seem prepared to adopt such a strategy currently.

Of course, the other option for people without insurance is to avoid the expense of medical care entirely. In the Commonwealth Fund's 1999 National Survey of Workers' Health Insurance, a quarter of the overall population reported that they "did not see a doctor when needed or did not fill a prescription due to cost, or skipped a medical test or treatment due to cost"; that is, they did not get "needed" medical care in a specifically defined way. However, only 10 percent of the insured population "went without needed care," but 37 percent of the uninsured population did so.

problem, of course, is to eliminate all laws requiring hospitals (and others) to treat those in need but without the means to pay for care, but our society appears unwilling to do this (lending credence to the belief that health care is a merit good). Under current arrangements, hospitals (and others) must provide this care, and its costs are built into the prices charged to all paying customers. Creating universal insurance solves this problem because every citizen thereby is insured automatically, eliminating the free ride.

Perhaps the most substantial argument for universal insurance is the "market failure" argument set forth in Chapter 10. To the extent that this analysis is correct, a country creating universal insurance can improve at least the average well-being of its citizens and can possibly improve that of most citizens. The discussion surrounding Figure 10.9 shows how mandatory "community rating" can, at least in concept, do this. Mandatory universal insurance has many of the same properties and can help resolve market failures that may exist.

How Might a Society Accomplish Universal Insurance?

Three mechanisms are generally available to accomplish the goal of providing universal insurance. The first mechanism is direct government provision of health care (as in Britain) or health insurance (as in Canada, among others). The second is the requirement that all individuals purchase health insurance, supporting targeted groups with financial assistance. (Most states in the

United States adopt this approach for automobile liability insurance albeit with far less than 100 percent compliance.) Germany and Japan, for example, have these so-called individual mandates at the core of their systems as well, although mechanisms are typically available making it desirable for almost all citizens to acquire insurance without the force of the mandate. The third mechanism is the requirement that employers provide insurance for their workers. This approach has been the predominant focus of proposed universal insurance in the United States for administrations as diverse as those led by Presidents Richard Nixon, Jimmy Carter, and Bill Clinton, as well as some proposals from Senator Edward Kennedy, a spectrum of political thinking that is quite wide indeed! In the United States, these proposals are usually coupled with some governmental provision of insurance for those without strong labor force connections.

How Can Universal Insurance Be Financed?

Direct financing of government-provided programs (such as Medicare and Medicaid in the United States) is financed through taxation. Using instruments of taxation invariably means that the government chooses to redistribute wealth among its citizens as a part of the provision of universal insurance because the tax burden will, of necessity, fall on those who are not recipients of the insurance. The usual considerations of tax policy hold directly: Income tax financing will have a "progressive" redistribution. Wage taxes (such as FICA taxes in the United States) will have a "regressive" distribution. Consumption taxes (such as the value-added tax in Canada and most European countries) will have a close-to-neutral effect on income distribution, neither heavily regressive nor progressive.[1]

Mandating that all individuals purchase insurance (an alternative to providing insurance through governmental programs), at least without other financing mechanisms included in parallel, is probably a regressive program because the costs of the insurance (at least that of similar coverage) is similar

---

[1]In this context, the usual economists' definitions of *progressive* and *regressive* are adopted. A *progressive tax* is one that takes an increasing proportion of income from taxpayers as income increases. A *regressive tax* takes a higher proportion of income from lower-income taxpayers than from higher-income taxpayers. The U.S. income tax structure is generally progressive. The Social Security tax (FICA tax) is considered regressive because it taxes a fixed proportion of incomes up to a specified cutoff (6.2 percent on wage income up to $102,000 in 2008, for example, with no tax on wage income above that limit). The Medicare tax in the United States is more neutral, taxing incomes at 1.45 percent for all wage income (no cutoff). A value-added tax (VAT) taxes people as they consume goods and services, hence falling in close proportion to incomes.

for all individuals, no matter what their income. Recognizing this, many proponents of mandating individual insurance (e.g., Pauly, Danzon, Feldstein, and Hoff, 1991) also propose tax credits (direct dollars returned from the tax liabilities of citizens) to low-income families to assist them in purchasing insurance. Mandating community rating for private insurance (see discussion surrounding Figure 10.9) provides another basis for increasing the affordability of insurance for some populations, but it does not necessarily create a sufficient incentive on its own to create universal coverage through voluntary purchases.

Mandating insurance purchases by employers for their employees and families—a so-called *off-budget method* of financing universal insurance (because it is not "on" the government budget)—is widely described as equivalent to a "head tax" on the hiring of workers. However, most economic analyses of such requirements (including studies of Social Security taxes paid by firms for workers and mandated fringe benefits for workers) come to the conclusion that workers eventually pay much, if not nearly all, of the costs of such programs through reductions in wages that they would otherwise receive (Feldstein, 1974; Gruber, 1992). This creates concerns about the possible loss of jobs for workers at or near mandatory minimum wages because the ability to reduce their wages to offset the added costs of mandatory health insurance is eliminated and an employer's likely response to such a mandate is to eliminate the job entirely rather than pay the added costs of insurance (see Box 16.3).

No matter what mechanisms of financing are chosen—government programs, government subsidies for private insurance, mandated employer insurance, or combinations thereof—it seems virtually impossible to conceive of a program to finance universal insurance in the United States that does not impose additional tax burdens on the middle- and upper-income groups of the population because the groups without insurance currently (see Box 16.1) are those with low incomes, often working at minimum wage or part-time jobs, and government policy will almost invariably include subsidies to this group under any mandatory universal insurance plan.

Combinations of financing have been very popular in serious proposals for universal health insurance in the United States for the past quarter of a century over a wide political spectrum, as previously noted. The dominant strategy (albeit not successful in any attempts to date) has included (1) mandatory insurance for workers and their families, (2) continuation of Medicare for elderly people under federal financing, and (3) various mechanisms with government subsidies or programs (such as a federalized Medicaid) to provide insurance for those not covered through work-related plans or Medicare. The last group, in particular, would be the one receiving the large bulk of new tax money to support the extension of insurance to those remaining uncovered.

BOX 16.3 DEALING WITH WORKERS WITHOUT INSURANCE

The uninsured worker population represents the most inviting target of opportunity for lawmakers to address, and that invitation has not gone unheeded. In almost every proposal for national health insurance since the early 1970s, the keystone of the proposal would mandate that every employer provide some minimum standard insurance to employees and their families. This approach has been adopted by political leaders spanning the political spectrum from President Richard Nixon through President Jimmy Carter, and President Bill Clinton and Senator Edward Kennedy.

One problem with the mandated employer-provided coverage approach is highlighted in our understanding of the mix of people without coverage, a group in which workers with low income predominate. If the financial cost of such plans is eventually shifted back to workers (as would be expected in most labor markets; see Mitchell and Phelps, 1976; Gruber, 1992), the incomes of a group already with low income will fall even further. The other alternative, perhaps even less desirable, is that they will simply lose their jobs. This is particularly likely to occur for people working at or near the legally mandated minimum wage. For such people, the employers' costs of hiring them (inclusive of their insurance coverage) may be so high that firms find other ways to organize their production. Hiring fewer people and having them work more overtime hours offers one alternative because the insurance policy costs the same whether somebody works 20 or 60 hours a week. An earlier study of mandated national health insurance (Mitchell and Phelps, 1976) estimated that the unemployment problem could be considerable, particularly in some industries with low wages and little insurance coverage currently.

Play or Pay Programs

A recent system entrant in the policy debate carries the name "play or pay." This system (including the program the State of Massachusetts adopted in 2006 and a similar program mandated by the City of San Francisco, also in 2006) requires that employers either provide some minimum standard health insurance for workers and their families ("play") or contribute to a public fund that provides insurance for those left without employer-paid insurance ("pay.") Recent surveys suggest that perhaps a third of all states have proposed legislation following similar strategies.

The difficulty from such system arises from the federal 1974 ERISA law, which controls employee benefits federally and preempts state action that conflicts with it. Both the Massachusetts and San Francisco programs faced ERISA legal challenges at the date of this writing, and many legal observers expected the issue to be resolved only in the U.S. Supreme Court. Until and unless a higher court overturns these state and local laws, employers must comply with them as written.

Efficiency Costs of Financing No method of financing universal health insurance (or for that matter, any other government program) is free of costs. No matter how funds are raised (mandated employer-provided insurance, income tax, wage tax, VAT), people invariably respond by altering their behavior somehow to reduce their tax burden. Income taxes alter people's willingness to work in the market (labor supply). VATs alter the incentives to produce things "at home" versus buying market products, and they also increase the incentives for illegal tax evasion (that is, black markets). Mandated insurance alters firms' willingness to hire people, especially at low incomes, in the presence of minimum wage laws. Every financing mechanism distorts behavior and, hence, imposes costs on the economy.

In a study of the "general equilibrium" costs of financing universal health insurance, Ballard and Goddeeris (1999) found that universal insurance provided totally through the government, with tax increases necessary to finance the plan for all persons, created efficiency losses amounting to an additional 8 percent "efficiency cost" beyond the direct cost of the plan. For an individual mandate (requiring insurance) coupled with tax credits to support the finances of families with low-income, the increased tax burden created an efficiency loss of 5.4 percent of the total cost of the plan.

As will happen almost universally in such plans, the redistribution of income also created changes in well-being of identifiable groups in well-patterned ways. In the plans they modeled, the lowest income groups gained about $500 per household, while the highest income groups (those with incomes above $50,000) lost $1,300 to $3,100 per household in increased taxes, depending on the plan under consideration (all in 1991 dollars).

Single Payer Models

Many discussions of universal health insurance center around a particular aspect of "financing" that has many more ramifications: Should the system have a "single payer"? The U.S. health insurance market has long had many participants, ranging from for-profit (FP) insurance companies to not-for-profit (NFP) insurers and equally complex mixes of FP, NFP, HMOs, and other insurance and health care providers.

Proponents of a single payer system tout the large cost savings from having a uniform insurance claim process for all providers. In a series of studies beginning in 1983, Woolhandler and Himmelstein (and various colleagues) calculated differential administrative costs for the U.S. and Canadian health care system, concluding (in the most recent of the series), "In 1999, health administration costs totaled at least $294.3 billion in the United States, or $1,059 per capita, as compared with $307 per capita in Canada.... administration accounted for 31.0 percent of health care expenditures in the

United States and 16.7 percent of health care expenditures in Canada. Canada's national health insurance program had overhead of 1.3 percent" (Woolhandler, Campbell, and Himmelstein, 2003).

These administrative costs are not, of course, just "waste." Significant portions of them occur in both insurer and provider staffs as part of "managed care," which deals with the fundamental dilemma created by health insurance: how to reduce financial risk while minimizing the potential for increased use of health care to the point at which it provides little marginal value. Insurers hire staff to monitor doctors' treatment choices, and then doctors and hospitals hire staff to interact with the insurers' "managers."

The difficulty in asserting that the solution lies only in moving to a single payer system is that no analysis has yet identified the components of the administrative cost. On the insurance side, if the savings would come from economies of scale by dropping multiple insurers, mergers or single payer systems are the only solution. If the costs really represent "management" on both the insurer and provider sides in the world of managed care, then those costs provide some benefit. Eliminating them, however, would require either finding an alternative cost control system to replace managed care or simply deciding to bear the burden of increased medical spending (which, ironically, would not appear as administrative cost but would almost certainly exceed the costs of the managed care process). If the costs arise from the multiplicity of insurance plans (and the derivative costs for providers to understand each of them and bill accordingly), better computerization of the process is the only solution unless U.S. citizens suddenly decide they are collectively willing to give up the freedom of choosing among multiple insurance plans to gain lower administrative costs.

Finally, it is important to remember that single payer, government-run programs invariably involve large government spending (and hence taxation) to finance them. The efficiency cost of financing (see the previous section) details how and why this happens. These costs are never included in comparisons of administrative costs such as those by Woolhandler, Himmelstein, and colleagues, but they are nevertheless just as real and just as important as the administrative costs calculated by them. A full accounting of the "burden" should include both administrative costs and distortion costs arising from financing.

What Core Benefits Should Be Included in a Universal Plan?

In the U.S. context, most proposals for universal insurance use fairly standard definitions of covered services, typically those commonly covered in private health insurance (and Medicare) in the realm of "acute" medical services. This coverage typically includes all hospitalization and physician services for all illnesses except (issues under common dispute) psychiatric care, substance abuse care, family planning and abortion services (controversial for separate reasons), fertility treatments, and (under little dispute) elective cosmetic surgery.

Other types of treatment for which there is less unanimity regarding inclusion in universal health insurance include (1) long-term care (nursing home, home care, etc.), (2) out-of-hospital prescription drugs, and (3) dental services. The concerns in each case differ.

In the case of long-term care, the primary concern is the demand elasticity for care. As we saw in Chapter 10, the more elastic the demand for a service, the less desirable it is to bring that service into the umbrella of insured services because the welfare loss from including the service is higher in this case. The widespread availability of nonmarket substitutes for nursing home and agency-provided home health care (i.e., family and friends providing care) raises concerns that the demand elasticity for such services could be quite large, hence the concern for large welfare losses.

In the case of drugs and dental services, the question is more one of the logic of insuring the service when the underlying variance in risk (and hence expenditures) is low; for dental care, there are added concerns about the demand being quite price responsive, adding to the welfare loss from insuring such services. Partly in response to that concern, some private dental insurance plans use a 50 percent copayment rather than the more traditional 20 percent for medical services. (Again, review the logic of demand for insurance in Chapter 10.)

In addition to the question of what is covered, there is the question of the degree to which patients pay for services at the time of receiving care. This involves deductibles, copayments, and coinsurance choices. Medicare, for example, has a one-day-in-the-hospital deductible in Part A, and Part B has a 20 percent coinsurance after a fixed deductible (now $135 per person per year). The choice of copayments in general is mostly one of cost control, a topic to which we turn next. (Review the results in Chapters 4 and 5 regarding the effects of various deductibles and coinsurance rates on total use of care.)

Expenditure Controls

In any universal insurance plan, the first choice to be made for cost control is whether the insurance will rely on competition among competing private plans or on the force of government. In either case, the choice of consumer (patient) copayments can have important consequences for the cost of universal programs. Competitive forces can provide important mechanisms for cost control, as we have seen in recent years in California and other states (see discussion in Chapter 11).

Within the realm of mandatory government controls, the available mechanisms include price controls, entry restrictions on capital (see Chapter 15), or global payment caps (akin to universal capitation of the health care system; see the discussion of capitation in Chapter 11).

Less traditional approaches to cost control include emphasis on preventive care and mechanisms of review to eliminate "unnecessary" or "inappropriate" treatment. As appealing as these ideas seem on paper, they have not fulfilled their promises. While improving health, most preventive services fail to actually save money in the long run. They can and often do provide health improvements at relatively low cost per life year saved (Garber and Phelps 1997; Russell, 1990), but they seldom literally save money. As for identifying and eliminating unnecessary or inappropriate treatment, the estimates of the costs of such treatment are high, suggesting considerable opportunity to create savings without harming health outcomes, but the mechanisms for identifying such treatment and preventing it *in advance of treatment* have proven elusive.

Introduction of New Technologies

In many ways, the process by which health systems (either universal or pluralistic) introduce new technologies into the market stands as one of the most important issues for consideration, yet this issue seldom receives the same attention as do more obvious questions such as mechanisms for financing the plan, scope of benefits, and coverage limitations.

However, review of the time series data in Chapter 1 makes abundantly clear that technological change accounts for significant portions of the real per capita growth experienced in the United States in the last half century's health care spending. In a world with constant population and constant prices (see Table 1.7), U.S. health spending has increased by a factor of 8 in the last half century, a compound *real* growth rate of more than 4 percent per year. While some of this may be due to changes in relative prices (compare Tables 1.7 and 1.8), it is nevertheless clear that technical change drives medical spending—or more precisely, the rate at which new technologies are adopted drives medical spending changes. The demand for these new technologies has a strong positive link to income (see subsequent discussion related to Figure 16.1).

Policy makers tend to focus (perhaps obsess) on the increased medical spending, but careful economic analysis will also focus on the benefits of new technologies. The work by Hall and Jones (2007) discussed regarding Figure 3.1 and Table 3.1 strongly suggest that technological change in the U.S. health care system has had very strong payoffs in increased longevity.

Focusing only on the increasing costs of a health care system but not the commensurate benefits will certainly lead to bad decision making. The trick, of course, is matching the treatments available with patients who will benefit most from them, a task that the U.S. health care system has not done well. Comparison of the various "extensive margin" differences in the cost per QALY (see Table 3.2) show how careful matching of patients with treatments is essential to getting full value for medical dollars spent. Proper matching of patients with treatments, of course, requires proper incentives for patients (see Chapter 4 and 5), providers (see especially discussions of physicians in Chapter 7 and the various Medicare payment reforms in Chapter 12), and insurance plan involvement (see Chapter 11).

REVIEW OF HEALTH POLICY AND SYSTEMS IN SELECTED COUNTRIES

With the background of issues and ideas surrounding universal insurance, we quickly review some aspects of the universal insurance programs of several prominently cited countries. This review necessarily omits many nations whose systems could doubtless offer useful insights for the United States, and the description of those discussed will necessarily remain both brief and (to knowledgeable persons) simplistic. For persons interested in more detail on such comparisons, a number of recent publications (and citations therein) provide an expanded picture of other nations' systems.[2] The discussion in this chapter focuses on four countries: Canada, Germany, Japan, and the United Kingdom. Each country has substantial similarity to the United States in some important ways, although there are important differences in its health care system. All are major industrialized nations with large populations; two (Great Britain and Canada) have common legal heritage with the United States; two (Japan and Germany) rely heavily on employer-related insurance; three (all but Great Britain) primarily have private ownership of health care production. The key major difference between the United States and these countries is that all of them (and, indeed, almost all other industrialized countries) have universal insurance in one form or another. These discussions briefly explore the differences between these countries and the United States.

---

[2]Several sources seem particularly useful. First, John Igelhart (who edited *Health Affairs* for many years) has published a sporadic but extremely useful series of articles describing the health care systems of various countries in the *New England Journal of Medicine*. The countries he has discussed include Canada (1986a, 1986b, 1986c, and an update about "problems" in 1990), Japan (1988a, 1988b), and Germany (1991a, 1991b). One issue of *Health Care Financing Review* (1989 supplement) published by the Health Care Financing Administration of America (now CMS) was devoted entirely to international comparisons with extensive data and commentary; the author recommends this volume highly. Finally, a 1990 supplement to *Advances in Health Economics and Health Services Research* (Rosa, ed.) focused on international comparisons, with studies of 10 nations included. Full citations appear in the Bibliography.

SNAPSHOTS OF FOUR COUNTRIES

Canada

Many analysts use Canada's health care system as an important point of comparison to the U.S. health care system, in part because of Canada's obvious similarity to the United States in economic and political structure and in part because the health care cost behavior in the two countries, while once quite similar, has now diverged considerably; health care in Canada "costs less" than the United States, and cost increase is persistently lower there than in the United States. Before 1971, Canada spent 7.4 percent of its GNP on health care, and the United States spent 7.6 percent. Then the Canadians instituted the universal Medicare system coupled with strong and comprehensive controls on spending growth, and its share of GNP devoted to health care has increased only to about 10 percent, while the U.S. system now consumes about 16 percent of its GNP.

In preface to this discussion, we can point to the key issues surrounding universal insurance discussed earlier; details follow on some aspects of these choices. Canada has chosen universal insurance provided exclusively by the government and financed by a combination of VAT (fairly neutral in distribution) and income taxes (progressive). The scope of benefits includes almost all standard services, and charges for care range from nominal to none at the point of service. Hospitals are paid on negotiated budgets, and doctors on the basis of fees negotiated between the government and medical societies. These fee controls coupled with capacity constraints on the provision of care limit cost increases through time and provide a filter on the introduction of new technologies. Now for some details.

Canada's universal insurance plan is organized around its provinces (most analogous to states in the United States). Each province has its own Medicare system, with commonalities imposed by the federal government but with some regional differences. The Canadian system retains some similarities to that in the United States but has important differences. Before the Canadian Medicare system was enacted, Canadian and U.S. systems were similarly organized with employer-provided health insurance the most common vehicle for private insurance coverage, some governmental insurance programs, and both hospitals and doctors operating as private entities. Doctors' fees were determined quite similarly to those of U.S. doctors (i.e., market determination); hospital charges had evolved into a mixture of controls and bargaining, but hospitals were paid on a per service basis.

The introduction of Medicare changed three important features of the Canadian system. First, insurance coverage became universal provided by the provincial governments to all its citizens. Private insurance essentially vanished. Second, hospitals came under a central regulatory authority in each province with a total budget cap for all provincial hospitals established by governmental authority. Within that overall cap, each hospital in the province receives a direct budget. Third, physicians now receive fees according to a negotiated schedule within the province but generally continue to function as independent firms. Thus, Canada now has universal governmental insurance with mostly private production of medical care and a strong governmental regulatory control on prices paid to both hospitals and doctors. Health care cost increase in Canada is thus almost entirely a political decision because governments decide the rates of increase in spending in each province with virtually no role for markets to set prices.

The consequences of this difference appear readily in Canadian cost data. Since 1971, the proportion of GNP going to physicians in the United States has doubled, whereas in Canada it has increased by about 30 percent. Hospital spending has also increased at a lower rate than in the United States, although the comparison is not so dramatic. These differences depend primarily on payments for providers (doctors, hospitals) rather than on changes in utilization rates. The United States and Canada have maintained similar hospital admission rates (per capita) across the years. U.S. average lengths of stay have declined steadily over the past decade while Canadian average length of stay (ALOS) has remained steady.[3] Doctor office visits per capita have remained similar in both countries since 1971 when Canada adopted Medicare.

Payments to doctors have constituted one important difference as noted. Another important difference is the rate at which the health care system has adopted new technologies. Canadian hospitals cannot (by law) use private capital markets and must generally turn to provincial authorities for funds to support capital acquisitions such as more beds, MRI units, lithotripsy, and so on. The Canadian system has adopted new technologies at a notably slower pace than the U.S. system, accounting for an important part of the cost growth differential.

One consequence of the "rationing" within the Canadian health care system is that many patients seek care across their southern border into the United States, generally paying for treatment out of pocket, but they are ensured rapid treatment rather than the delays inherent in a rationed system such as Canada's. Many hospitals in the major cities in the United States that are proximate to major Canadian cities (e.g., Buffalo and Rochester for Toronto, Detroit for Windsor, Seattle for Vancouver) have thriving marketing activities focused on Canadian citizens.

---

[3]The Canadian system has seen a considerable increase in the number of elderly persons using the hospital in lieu of long-term care facilities, accounting for the failure of ALOS to decline in Canada as it has in the United States. These patients "clog up" the hospital system, creating a de facto constraint that prevents acute care hospitalizations from occurring.

Germany

Before presenting a more detailed discussion, we can again summarize answers to the key issues about universal insurance discussed earlier in this chapter. Germany creates universal insurance by mandating that all individuals belong to an approved plan with worker and union groups forming a backbone of the supply of such plans. Most commonly used services are included in coverage. Fees are negotiated with providers, the major cost control mechanism. Various government subsidies financed by income and wage taxes supply the governmental parts of these programs. Mandatory employer payments form an important part of the financing scheme, as well as individual contributions. Now for more details.

Germany is commonly touted as having the first "universal" health insurance plan, dating back to the social insurance plans of German Chancellor Otto von Bismarck in the 1880s. Bismarck's government established a spectrum of social insurance for workers and (partly) their dependents, apparently in response to labor unrest and the growing influence of labor unions. Initially, the sickness funds hired doctors directly, but in the pre-World War II era, the physicians gradually separated to "panels" that negotiated with the sickness funds to provide care for patients.

After an interim when Hitler's National Socialist (Nazi) party turned the health care system into a true socialist (government-owned and -operated) plan, the postwar German system returned to a sickness-fund-based system but with a large role for independent office-based (private practice) doctors. The sickness funds are now the prominent model, each operating as a not-for-profit entity (similar to Blue Cross and Blue Shield plans in the United States). Membership for workers and their families in some fund is compulsory, although the specific choice of which fund is free. In actual practice, choices are commonly based on occupation or geographic region (there are also numerous "local" funds independent of the regional or national funds with specific occupational connections). These plans account for seven of eight German citizens. Workers and firms both contribute to these funds, total contributions range from 8 to 16 percent of a worker's salary, averaging almost 13 percent. Unemployed persons have their premiums paid by the federal unemployment insurance fund. When a person retires, his or her pension plan pays mandatory insurance premiums, equaling (by law) a percent of his or her pension payment equaling the national average payroll contribution (now about 13 percent).

The link between the sickness funds and providers is much more formalized than comparable arrangements in the United States. To be eligible for payment from a sickness fund, a doctor must belong to a regional association of physicians. The sickness funds pay lump sums to the physicians' association, which in turn pays doctors for services provided. These regional associations function similarly to the physician groups with which IPAs and HMOs in the United States contract; the doctor belongs to the group practice, the insurance plan (HMO or IPA) pays the group itself, and the group pays doctors on a fee-for-service or salary basis, depending on the plan. The rates are negotiated between the sickness funds and the doctor associations.

Doctors in Germany almost always specialize in either hospital or ambu-latory treatment; very few of the ambulatory care doctors can admit patients to hospitals. In turn, hospital-based doctors are barred from practicing ambu-latory medicine and are paid an annual salary by the hospital, the amount commonly depending on specialty and seniority. Hospital-based physician salaries come from the overall operating costs of the hospital negotiated between the hospitals and the sickness funds. Thus, the financial incentives confronting doctors are quite different than those in the United States with a strong fee-for-service incentive in ambulatory care and an HMO-like incen-tive (straight salary) for hospital care.

Differences between the United States and Germany in medical care use correspond to these financial differences; with universal and virtually full-coverage insurance and with an active fee-for-service system in ambulatory care, German citizens consume about 7.3 patient visits per year. This com-pares with 3.9 in the United States and 6.1 in Canada (CRC, 2007, Figure 4). Doctor visits are also much shorter in Germany, the average being about 9 minutes in Germany for a primary care doctor versus 15 minutes in the United States.

One way the Germans achieve the high rates of service use while appar-ently not spending enormous sums of money on hospital care is through much lower staffing intensity in their hospitals than is typical in other coun-tries. German hospitals have about 2.0 employees per occupied bed currently, versus about 5.0 per occupied bed in the United States, about 4.2 in Canada, and 6.5 in the United Kingdom. (CRC, 2007, Figure 10.)

Japan

Japan's health care was deliberately modeled after Germany's in the pre-World War II era. Thus, Japan's "solutions" to the key issues confronting any universal insurance plan have considerable similarity to German solutions.

Japan's health care system has some elements familiar to those in the United States and some that differ remarkably. As in the United States and Germany, the large percentage of persons in Japan obtain their insurance via employer-related groups. In industries in which "insurance societies" or "mutual aid societies" are established, the society provides the insurance; in other industries, the national government sells it. These societies were formed as early as 1922 when a law enabled such insurance plans to organize. Both the structure of Japanese medicine and the reliance on industry-related insurance plans were specifically chosen to emulate the German system at the time, widely regarded as the world's best system during the early 1900s. A separate national health insurance plan is available for persons not eligible for some employer-related group. Participation in some kind of insurance group is mandatory following legislation that the Japanese Diet passed in 1961. Currently, the employment group plans insure about 75 million people, and the national health insurance plan insures the remaining 45 million. The employment groups contribute an average of 8.1 percent of an employee's pay (4.6 percent from the employer, 3.5 percent from the employee), although premium rates range from 6 to almost 10 percent of an employee's income. The governmental plans receive 8.9 percent of a person's monthly income, evenly split between employer and employee.

Most of the employer-group plans require copayments (e.g., 20 percent for inpatient care, 30 percent for ambulatory care) for dependents, with 10 percent copayments for workers. These plans also have a "catastrophic cap" feature that limits monthly out-of-pocket expenses. The community plans ("national health insurance") have premiums paid by the covered person with a *per household* cap and a 30 percent copayment, both of which are related to family income. On net, premiums pay for about half of the cost of these plans with the remainder coming from national and local government (tax) support. Retired persons are covered in the same plans with contributions from employment and community plans plus funds from both national and local governments with very small copayments for patients at the time of service (¥400 per hospital day, equal to about $3) and ¥800 *per month* for ambulatory care.

Despite the use of a highly pluralistic insurance system, the Japanese health care system has a rigid set of price controls known as the *national fee schedule.* Thus, no matter what the insurance plan, the payment to providers is the same (Ikegami and Campbell, 1995). Balance billing (charging patients more than covered by insurance) is strictly prohibited. This in part may explain the common Japanese practice of providing "gifts" to some doctors, estimated to be in the range of 3 or 4 percent of doctors' official fees. The regulated fees in Japan are substantially lower than those found in the United States, averaging about a quarter of Medicare's relative value fee schedule for comparable procedures. This difference in physician payments accounts for an important part of the gap between U.S. and Japanese spending on health care.

Most hospitals in Japan are private (many organized as not for profit, but with a substantial number owned by physicians), but the government operates some hospitals also. The mix between private and public hospitals is similar to that in the United States. Most of the large, complex hospitals in Japan are public, most with an affiliation to one of Japan's 80 medical schools.

Physicians primarily operate out of "clinics" rather than independently or in small-group practices. Many physicians own their own clinics (and hire other doctors to work in them), but particularly among younger doctors, the preference has shifted to salary arrangements with hospital clinics.

As in Germany, "clinic" doctors cannot follow their patients into the hospital, but (in contrast to the German setting) the presence of large ambulatory care clinics affiliated with the hospitals makes the freestanding clinic doctors very reluctant to refer their patients for hospitalization because they could well lose the patient to the hospital clinic. Japan's hospital admission rates are by far the lowest of any major country in the world (7.5 admissions per 100 persons), half of that of the U.S., Canadian, and British rates and a third of that found in Germany, Denmark, and Sweden (the countries with the highest hospital admission rates).[4] Doctors who work in private practice, unlike those in the United States, have much higher earnings than specialist's working in hospitals. In Japan, the specialists are salaried employees of the hospitals and are reported to earn about half of the annual income of their private practice (generalist) counterparts (Ikegami and Campbell, 1995).

The extremely low propensity to hospitalize patients in Japan is offset partly by extremely high rates of use of physician visits and prescription drugs, the two often going hand in hand. Japanese citizens see doctors on an average of 15 times per year, triple the U.S. rate. These visits are apparently extremely short in duration and almost always occur without an appointment. Hence, doctor visits are rationed by waiting time (about an hour's wait on average).

Ohnuki-Tierney (1984), an anthropologist studying the Japanese medical care system, reported typical workloads for physicians. Across several specialties, those physicians she studied commonly treated 40–50 patients in one 3-hour period, making the average visit length about 3.5–4.5 minutes in contrast to the average visit for primary care doctors in the United States of 15 minutes with longer visits for specialists. Thus, although the number of visits in Japan differs hugely from the U.S. rate, the number of minutes a typical patient spends annually with a physician is similar to if not less than in the United States.

---

[4]The Japanese rate, low as it is, represents a major increase over the past several decades. In 1960 the hospital admission rate in Japan was only 3.7 per 100 persons, half of the current rate. The increase is (as in other countries) due in part to the aging of the population, but it is also partly explicable with the shift to hospital-based clinics where hospital referrals are not as financially dangerous to the referring doctor.

Japanese citizens are also among the most heavily medicated in the world, a practice that corresponds closely to the economic incentives in Japanese society. In a recent study, Japanese citizens apparently were dispensed more than 20 prescriptions per persons per year compared with the U.S. average of about 6 prescriptions. This issue is of intrinsic economic interest because it both reflects the role of insurance on drug use and sheds some light on the question of "supplier-induced demand." U.S. visitors to Japan after World War II found it very surprising that Japanese doctors both prescribed and sold drugs, quite in contrast to the U.S. norm of separating prescribing and dispensing.[5] In 1955 the Japanese Diet passed a law requiring separation of prescribing and dispensing, but the law was apparently so riddled with exceptions that it had little effect. The law was supported by health insurance plans (which paid for the drugs) and the pharmacists' association, whose members would stand to benefit hugely from a change in the market structure, but strongly opposed by the Japanese Medical Association, whose members would, of course, lose by the change. Virtually all of the 27,000 freestanding "clinics" continue to dispense drugs, as, of course, do the hospital-clinics.

Insurance plan reimbursement for prescription drugs in 1980 constituted nearly 40 percent of all insurance benefits, although this had dropped to 28 percent by 1987 and to about 19 percent by 2004 (CRS, 2007 Figure 19). (By contrast, pharmaceutical expenses paid by all sources constitute 12 percent of the U.S. health care bill.) Most of the reduction in spending has been due to reductions in the government-decreed price list for drugs; during the 1980s, these regulated retail prices for drugs fell by more than 60 percent.[6] The rates of prescribing do not seem to have changed over this period, and the Japanese continue to consume prescription medications at a rate hugely above that in most modern societies.

The overall balance of these events has allowed Japan to operate its health care system with one of the lowest spending rates in the industrialized world. Per capita spending is well less than half of that in the United States,[7] and the Japanese spend only about 8 percent of their GNP on medical care. One obvious source of this difference is hospital spending; hospitalization rates in

---

[5]In earlier times, U.S. doctors functioned similarly; the "traveling" doctor in the 1800s both prescribed drugs and then sold them, often out of the wagon in which the doctor traveled.

[6]This creates an interesting issue of incidence. It appears in some discussions that the incidence of these reduced payments fell primarily on drug manufacturers and wholesalers rather than on the retailers (clinics and doctors).

[7]Remember that such calculations depend heavily on the exchange rate between currencies that is used to make such calculation. As the U.S. dollar declines against other nations' currencies, calculations of their spending will decline when converted to U.S. dollars.

Japan are very much lower than in the United States. When patients are hospitalized there, they remain for nearly 20 days, on average, but much of that care is more like hotel care than the intensive hospital care in the United States, so that overall spending for hospital services remains low. The combination of infrequent admissions and very long stays leads to a days-per-year use in Japan that is twice what it is in the United States. However, the intensity of hospital care is so low that overall Japanese costs remain much lower than U.S. costs. Hospital staffing ratios reflect this low intensity; in Japan, hospitals hire about 0.75–0.8 employees for each occupied bed; in the United States, staffing ratios are 3.5 times higher.

Physician costs are much more similar in the United States and Japan than one might expect. This results from the interaction of a very high rate of physician visits by the Japanese (a 15-visit per person rate in Japan versus the 5-visit U.S. rate) and the substantially lower fees per procedure as noted previously. The lower per visit payment rate for physicians leads to the much shorter time spent with a patient on each visit, making the total physician-contact time per year similar for patients in the two countries. Japanese doctors have gross revenues of about $350,000 per year—roughly twice the rates of doctors in Germany and Canada and 1.5 times those in the United States—but net incomes appear to be similar in Japan and the United States (Sandier, 1989, Figure 6). Finally, the relative supply of active physicians in Japan is lower than it is in the United States—one doctor for each 640 people in Japan and one doctor for each 425 people in the United States—so that total spending on doctors' services is quite similar for the two countries despite the higher per doctor gross income in Japan.[8] (*Gross income* reflects all payments to "physician-firms" and best represents the whole scope of services associated with "physician visits." Using net physician income would be analogous to trying to understand spending in hospitals by measuring nurses' incomes.)

The other remarkable feature of the Japanese system is that despite the substantially lower spending on medical services compared with that in the United States, Germany, or even Canada, the Japanese people appear to have among the best health outcomes of any major industrialized nation. Life expectancies at birth (82.1 years, overall) are the highest of any industrialized

---

[8]These aggregate data on physician supply and visit rates provide an independent confirmation of the very short time spent on each visit in Japan. On a per capita basis, the Japanese have about 80 percent of the physician supply that Americans do, but they use three times the number of physician visits. If doctors in Japan and the United States work about the same number of hours each year, then the typical Japanese doctor must see 3.75 times as many patients per hour as does the typical U.S. doctor ($3/0.8 = 3.75$). If the typical U.S. visit lasts 15 minutes, then the typical Japanese visit lasts exactly 4 minutes ($15/3.75 = 4$). Ohnuki-Tierney's estimate was 3.5–4.5 minutes.

country. The United States, by contrast, has a 77.5 year life expectancy. The contrast with earlier Japanese outcomes makes these results all the more remarkable: At the end of World War II, life expectancy in Japan was only 50 years for males and 54 years for females.

Japanese infant mortality is the lowest in the world—0.28 per 100 births, compared with about 0.53 in Canada, 0.41 in Germany, 0.51 in the United Kingdom, and 0.69 in the United States. (CRS, 2007, Figure 26.) In addition to the obvious effect of universal access to prenatal care, two factors account for these excellent results. First, the Japanese have an active maternal and child health program that includes issuing a handbook of information to every pregnant woman in Japan. Second, Japan has the highest abortion rate in the world (24 per 1,000 women of childbearing age). As has been shown in the United States (Joyce, Corman, and Grossman, 1988), increased accessibility of abortion reduces infant mortality, and we would expect a comparable result in Japan.

Nonmedical care factors probably play a very important role in these Japanese health outcomes. The traditional Japanese diet is almost devoid of fat, concentrating heavily on vegetables and fish. The role of diet in heart disease appears most prominently in the rates of heart surgery in Japan: 1 bypass surgery per 1,000 people per year compared with 26 per 1,000 in Canada and 61 per 1,000 in the United States. Rates of gallbladder removal (cholecystectomy) are even more remarkable, however—2 per 1,000 in Japan versus 219 per 1,000 in Canada and 203 per 1,000 in the United States—and the biomedical link between fat intake and gallbladder disease is well established.[9] The Japanese avoid surgery generally compared with Americans, but the coronary bypass surgery and cholecystectomy rates stand uniquely in their differences from other countries' rates. The difference seems due to Japanese persons' preferences to eschew the fat.

Great Britain

The British health care system diverges considerably from others already discussed in almost all aspects. In the United Kingdom, universal access is ensured through the provision of government-provided care that is available to all citizens. The system is financed almost entirely by progressive income taxes. The scope of benefits is "routine" by modern standards, but limitations on providers and supply provide de facto restrictions on use and are

---

[9]Gallstones, which clog up the gallbladder duct and lead to its surgical removal, are formed as a combination of bile salts (created by the gallbladder) and cholesterol.

important in the control of cost growth (Aaron and Schwartz, 1984). The British system emphasizes preventive care, especially for prenatal and maternity-related matters. Because virtually all doctors are on salary to the government, cost control is substantially easier than in more loosely organized market environments.

In the United States, the British health care system is the best known of any socialized system, although the health care systems of many other countries are also owned and operated by the state. The British National Health Service (BNHS) was formed in 1948 following a long evolution from voluntary and then mandatory social insurance programs that the British had developed during much of the twentieth century. The BNHS provides a pure model of a socialized health care system. Most hospitals are owned by the state, and, with few exceptions, all health care workers are employees of the state. A very small private insurance market exists in Great Britain, and a handful of hospitals provides service to persons with such insurance. The primary distinction between the Canadian, German, and Japanese systems (on the one hand) and the British system (on the other) is the ownership of the resources used to produce health services. In Great Britain, the state owns the resources of production; in the other nations, most of the resources are owned by private organizations, with some public ownership of hospitals and broad controls over prices and investment common in the hospital sector.

The direct control over resource investment provided by the BNHS has led to considerable differences in the British choices about the organization of health care compared with what has occurred in the United States or Canada, two societies with a similar cultural heritage. Part of the differences arise from income differences: Using purchasing power parity measures of the Organization for Economic Cooperation and Development (OECD), per capita income in Britain is only 70 percent of that in the United States, and systematic evidence across nations shows that aggregate spending closely relates to per capita income. As the next section shows, this income difference alone accounts for much (but not all) of the low per capita spending in Great Britain. Compared with the mix of services in the United States, that chosen by the BNHS is much more hospital and nurse intensive with a deemphasis on doctors.

Another feature in Great Britain is the relatively low density of doctors, reflecting a market force that not even a socialized health care system can control. British doctors emigrated to the United States and Canada in large numbers during the 1960s and 1970s, particularly after the economic returns to a medical license rose dramatically in the United States after Medicare was introduced in 1965. In 1960, the United States had 1.44 doctors per 1,000 population and the United Kingdom had 1.0 doctors per 1,000 population. Over the decades, physician supply increased greatly throughout the world, but the United States absorbed a disproportionate share of this increase. By 1987, the British supply of physicians had increased by a third to 1.36 doctors per 1,000, but the U.S. supply had nearly doubled to 2.33 per 1,000. Put differently, in 1960, Britain had a physician-to-population ratio that was about 70 percent of the U.S. figure, and by 1987 that ratio had slipped to 58 percent. (Review Chapter 7 about immigration of physicians to the United States in the post-Medicare era; many of those physicians came from Great Britain.)

AGGREGATE INTERNATIONAL COMPARISONS

Health Care Spending

This brief excursion through four nations' health care systems masks many important differences among the systems. Yet surprisingly, stepping back to an even higher level of aggregation suggests common behavioral patterns in health care spending among virtually every industrialized nation of the Western world: Aggregate per capita spending on health care turns out to be strongly related to per capita income. The relationship is so strong, in fact, that some analysts have suggested that little else remains to be explained by other factors such as the ownership of resources, cost controls, or the nature of the health insurance system in the various countries.

Kleimann (1974) and Newhouse (1977) first showed this strong relationship using data from industrialized countries in the early 1960s (Kleimann) and the early 1970s (Newhouse). They converted other countries' expenditures to U.S. dollars using currency exchange rates from the same period and estimated a simple linear model of the form Expenditures = constant + β (per capita income). Several subsequent studies have expanded the data set to include more than 20 countries (Culyer, 1989; Parkin, McGuire, and Yule, 1987; Gerdtham et al., 1988). Some important differences emerge when one uses currency exchange rates versus an alternative measure called "purchasing power parity" developed recently by the OECD. Box 16.4 discusses these issues in more detail.

A recent publication of a rich data set on 24 OECD countries (Poullier, 1989; Sandier, 1989; Schieber, 1990; Schieber, Poullier, and Greenwald, 1992) gives us the opportunity to explore some of these issues directly. Figure 16.1 shows the relationship between per capita income (measured as gross domestic product per person) and per capita health care spending. The size of the bubbles in Figure 16.1 shows the relative sizes of the countries, with the

BOX 16.4 INTERNATIONAL FINANCIAL COMPARISONS

A difficulty when making international spending comparisons arises when selecting the exchange rate with which to convert other currencies to dollars (or some other common unit). For example, between 1971 and 1999 (the year Germany converted to the Euro), the exchange rate between German marks and US dollars varied between 3.64 and 1.43. Within a single country, the exchange rate doesn't matter, but when we seek to learn whether the Germans spent "more" than Americans on medical care, we must convert deutsche marks (or since 1999, Euros) to dollars, and changes in the exchange rate alter our perception of how much Germans spend on health care. For example, suppose the average German spent 5,000 deutsche marks on medical care in a year. At an exchange rate of 3.64 deutsche marks to the dollar, we would describe that as $1,374. If the exchange rate is 1.43 deutsche marks per dollar, we would describe that as $3,497.

An alternative system uses "purchasing power parity" rates, a system designed to standardize each country's currency by comparing its prices to the OECD average for a fixed basket of goods. This system provides a much more stable picture of international spending. Between 1960 and 1987, the purchasing power parity conversion rate between the United States and Germany varied only between 3.37 and 2.47 deutsche marks per dollar, much less than the variation in the currency exchange rate.

The exchange rate problem accounts for differences in various writers' perceptions about where the United States "stands" in per capita spending. Maxwell (1981) reported that the United States was third in 1977 per capita medical care spending in the world ($769), behind Germany ($774) and Sweden ($928), based on average exchange rates for calendar year 1977. Comparable calculations using the OECD purchasing power parity index would place the 1977 German spending at slightly less than $600 per person and the Swedish spending at $625. By these calculations, the United States is an easy first-place winner in the per capita medical spending race.

Most analysts now prefer to use the purchasing power parity index when assessing international spending differences because it more closely resembles the kind of price index that economists commonly prefer to use for adjusting spending data across time and space. All of the data shown in this text comparing various countries use the OECD purchasing power parity index.

United States the largest (at the upper right) and tiny Luxembourg and Iceland showing as unlabeled small dots.[10]

---

[10]CRS (2007) shows very similar graphs using OECD (2004) data. See Figure 2. Their math does not provide the statistical analysis that follows using the earlier data.

FIGURE 16.1 Per capita income and per capita health care spending.

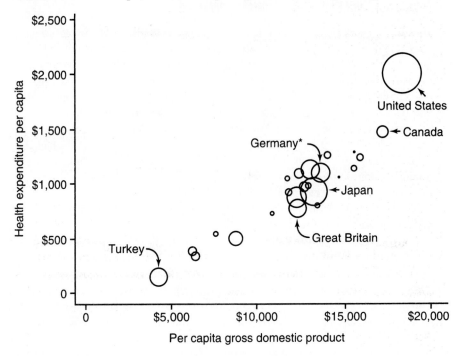

Formerly West Germany

Figure 16.1 shows an obvious nearly linear relationship between income and health care spending across a wide array of nations of different sizes, health care delivery systems, forms of government, geographic and climatic features, and ethnic basis of the population. A regression line through these points shows a very tight fit indeed. The exact model depends in part on whether one weights the data by each country's population (the preferred approach) and whether one ignores or includes "outliers,"[11] but the main idea persists broadly: Per capita income explains most of the international

---

[11]Outliers are identified as those single observations that create significant differences in the estimated regression parameters. In the regression of health care spending versus per capita income, the United States is an outlier, pulling the regression line up to itself. In a regression using logarithmic forms (see the following discussion), Turkey is an outlier that pulls the regression line down to itself. In both cases, eliminating the outliers reduces slightly the apparent relationship between income and health care spending.

differences in health care spending across countries, with the following as a typical estimated equation:

Health care expenditure

$$\text{per capita} = \quad -290 \quad\quad + 0.1(\text{per capita income})$$
$$\quad\quad (t = 3.5) \quad\quad (t = 14.3)$$
$$\quad\quad N = 24 \quad\quad R^2 = 0.91$$

If one calculates the income elasticity of demand from this regression (review Box 4.1 on elasticities if you need to), the estimated income elasticity is 1.35, a result very similar to that found by the earlier studies cited.

In Figure 16.1 (and statistically in the model), the United States has the appearance of having abnormally large health care spending because of the way that it is positioned above the regression line fitted to the data. This is particularly true if one fits a line to all of the data other than the United States and "predicts" what U.S. spending would be from that line. With that approach, U.S. spending is three-eighths larger than would be predicted.

Alas, in seeking to learn from these international income and spending patterns, nothing tells us that we should necessarily see a straight-line relationship to show how income relates to health care spending. For example, the relationship might just as well be linear in the logarithms of the data rather than using "natural" data. Figure 16.2 shows this relationship, again with the countries shown proportional to their population size.

The logarithmic regression with these data shows an even higher estimated income elasticity:[12]

Log (per capita

$$\text{medical spending}) = \quad -10.2 \quad\quad + 1.8\,[\log\,(\text{per capita income})]$$
$$\quad\quad (t = 10.0) \quad\quad (t = 17.0)$$
$$\quad\quad N = 24 \quad\quad R^2 = 0.93$$

In this case, income elasticity is estimated at 1.8, and the United States is not nearly as meaningful an "outlier." If we fit the same model to all other countries except the United States, however, the United States continues to appear unusually large in health care spending.

To know which model is correct, we need to conduct a very expensive experiment. We need to increase other countries' incomes so that some of

---

[12]In logarithmic data, the estimated coefficient on income is the income elasticity itself.

FIGURE 16.2 Per capita income and per capita health care spending (logarithmic relationship).

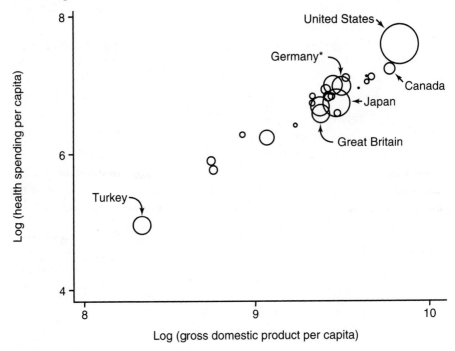

*Formerly West Germany

them reach the per capita income of the United States. Then we can see how they behave. In these times of restricted research budgets, this experiment is not likely to become funded. An alternative approach seeks to use the relationships in the data to tell which is the "best" model; in this approach, the logarithmic data appear to have a slightly better fit.[13] The dominant statistical question is whether one should include the United States in the equation used to predict spending of a country with U.S. per capita income but health care systems characteristic of the other countries in the data set. In that regard, other countries' systems are so diverse that there seems no

---

[13]One cannot just compare the R^2 in these models because the dependent variables differ. The proper approach uses a Box-Cox power transform to test whether the log or linear model is best. In these data, the logarithmic data have a somewhat better fit. Consult any recent econometrics textbook for further details.

particular reason to exclude the United States from the data set. When one includes the United States in the data set, only Turkey appears abnormal in a statistical sense, and the United States appears quite within the bounds of "normality."

Statistics cannot tell us whether the United States has abnormally large spending for health care, given its income, although many people look at data such as those in Figure 16.1 and assert that U.S. spending is abnormally large. Other perfectly reasonable models of health care spending (such as the logarithmic data model) place the United States right "on trend," in effect predicting that other countries, if given U.S. income levels, would behave similarly.

Looking at the nations in this data set, one finds few common features that might help explain why one country has abnormally large or small spending on medical care. Socialized medical care systems seem to have little effect. Great Britain has unusually small spending (below the regression line), but Sweden has abnormally large spending. Japan's spending is abnormally small, but not by much, despite the apparently large effects of diet on the use of at least some surgical procedures (coronary bypass and cholecystectomy, in particular). As Newhouse (1977) pointed out, the information on per capita income explains so much of the data that little else remains for other variables to affect systematically. Despite the obviously major differences in health care systems, nothing emerges at least from this type of comparison to suggest how one approach to organizing a health care system might dominate another.

Health Outcomes

The other major question confronting health analysts is how these differences in health care spending affect health outcomes. This turns out to be a question that we cannot answer cleanly with available data, but we can see some suggestive patterns in the data. The question is of obvious interest because if we could answer it, we would know more than we do now about the marginal productivity of medical care. The difficulty that analysts confront when attempting to judge such matters is the high correlation between income and medical care spending that the previous section displayed. We suspect that medical care affects health outcomes (favorably), but we also suspect that income, a second variable, by itself affects health outcomes—for example, by affecting the amount of good (and bad) consumption items that people consume. A third variable, education, probably affects both income and health outcomes favorably, lending further confusion to things.

Finally, if we compare current medical care use (or income) in various countries with the life expectancy of their adult populations, we might find very little relationship because life expectancy is affected by both current and past income, consumption patterns, and medical care use. A more sensitive indicator (because it happens "now") is the infant mortality rate or (correspondingly) the perinatal mortality rate.[14]

Because of the high correlation between per capita income and per capita medical spending, one can look at the effect of either variable on life expectancy or infant mortality and see essentially the same thing. Figure 16.3a shows the relationship between per capita income and male life expectancy, and Figure 16.3b shows per capita medical spending and male life expectancy. (Data for female life expectancy show a very similar pattern, but females generally live longer.) The statistical relationships are very weak in both cases, whether or not one includes the U.S. data point in the estimates.

The relationships between income (and medical spending) and perinatal mortality, as expected, are stronger than we see for life expectancy. Figure 16.4a shows the relationships for perinatal mortality rate and per capita income, and Figure 16.4b shows perinatal mortality and medical spending per capita. The statistical relationship is modestly tight if one excludes the U.S. data point from the estimation. Excluding the United States, the estimated equation for perinatal mortality is[15]

$$\text{Perinatal mortality} = 1.90 \qquad - 0.0000755(\text{per capita income})$$
$$(t = 6.53) \qquad (t = 3.28)$$
$$N = 21 \qquad R^2 = 0.35$$

The United States, Portugal, and Italy appear to have unusually large perinatal mortality rates compared with their income levels. Put differently, these countries seem to lie above the regression line.

The data relating perinatal mortality rates to per capita health expenditure show a somewhat weaker relationship. As Figure 16.4b shows, the United

---

[14]Infant mortality measures the proportion of all live-born children who die early in their lives. Perinatal mortality measures all stillborns plus infant mortality relative to all live births plus stillborns. The reporting practices of nations differ regarding the definition of a live birth; some count only infants weighing more than, for example, 0.5 or 1 kilogram, while other countries count births of all weights. The perinatal mortality rate provides a more uniform measure of outcomes.

[15]In this case, the statistical models say that the "natural" data are a better fit than the logarithmic data.

FIGURE 16.3 (a) Male life expectancy and per capita income. (b) Male life expectancy and per capita medical spending, by country.

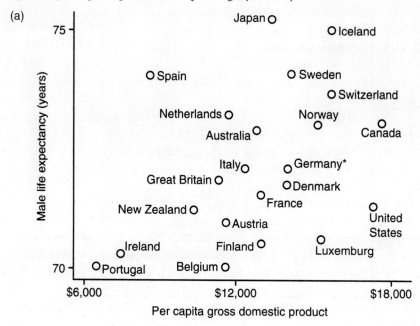

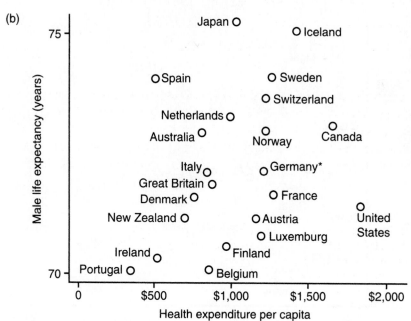

*Formerly West Germany

FIGURE 16.4 (a) Perinatal mortality rate and per capita income. (b) Perinatal mortality rate and per capita medical spending, by country.

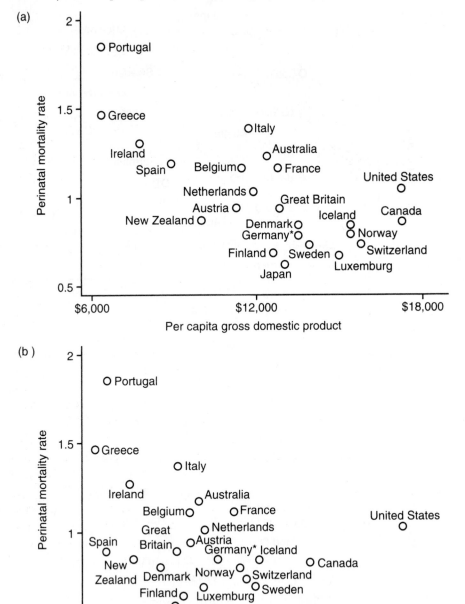

*Formerly West Germany

States "sticks out" even more in this graph than in the other. The estimated relationship (omitting the U.S. data) is

$$\text{Perinatal mortality} = 1.43 \qquad -0.000517 \text{ (per capita}$$
$$\text{health care spending)}$$
$$(t = 6.74) \quad (t = 2.30)$$
$$N = 21 \qquad R^2 = 0.21$$

The elasticity of perinatal mortality with respect to income is -0.98; the elasticity with respect to medical spending is -0.49, just half of the effect of income. (In both cases, if one includes the United States, the statistical relationship vanishes.) Although the relationship is not nearly as strong as that between income and medical care spending itself, it is clear that, at least for countries other than the United States, a strong statistical relationship exists between infant mortality and either medical spending or income.

Both of these relationships show "effectiveness" in reducing perinatal mortality, but we cannot tell whether it is "just" income or medical care, or a combination of the two.[16] We have every reason to believe that the things that income buys will improve health outcomes, but we also have good evidence at the level of individuals that, even holding income constant, prenatal care improves health outcomes as measured by perinatal mortality.

In any case, these data clearly show the United States as a statistical outlier, with substantially higher perinatal mortality than one would expect given the per capita income and the relationship between the two that exists in other countries. The causes of this discrepancy in outcome remain unresolved at this point. Critics of the health care system point to such data as evidence of the inferiority of the health care financing arrangements in the United States, noting that almost all other industrialized countries have universal health insurance and apparently achieve better outcomes than does the United States while spending less of their income on medical care. Others respond that the U.S. health care system must deal with a wide heterogeneity of persons that other systems do not, with persons of different ethnic backgrounds who speak diverse languages, and—in many cases of infant deaths—with immigrants (both legal and illegal), and so on. As one writer notes, "The

---

[16]In econometric terms, because we believe that income affects both the health outcome and medical care use, we cannot identify the separate relationship between medical care use and infant mortality. An attempt to estimate an equation including both income and medical care at the same time would be underidentified. Indeed, in pure econometric terms, the equation estimating health outcomes as a function of medical care is not "legitimate" because medical care is jointly determined with illness levels, which we cannot observe.

U.S. population, often referred to as a 'melting pot,' cannot be readily compared with those of Iceland or Japan, with their much more homogeneous populations.... The degree to which poor health outcomes reflect social causes vs. the inadequacy of the health system ... is hard to quantify" (Davis, 1989, pp. 105–106).

INCREASE IN COSTS AND HEALTH OUTCOMES

The final question we can address with these international comparison data is whether or not the U.S. health care system has experienced abnormally large cost growth and/or different changes in health outcomes through time. This is a different question than the ones posed in the previous section. It asks whether the *change* in costs and the *change* in health outcomes over time seem unusual in an international perspective.

A provocative article by Evans, Lomas, Barer, et al. (1989) laid down the gauntlet. They argued that the U.S. and Canadian health care systems were very similar in 1971 when Canada adopted universal health insurance and budget controls through its Medicare system, and that in the interim, U.S. health care spending has increased at a much faster pace than has Canadian spending. These spending comparisons were discussed in the earlier section on the Canadian system. Evans and colleagues did not discuss health outcomes. This section briefly (and certainly not definitively!) addresses the question of both cost growth and health outcomes in various nations.

Table 16.1 describes the annual per capita spending on health care in each of the five countries previously discussed, and Table 16.2 (top) shows the annual rates of in spending in these countries over available time periods. Table 16.2 (bottom) converts these data to annual rates in increased spending after correcting for the internal inflation rate in each country, so that each of its components shows real rates of spending increase. Note that these increases could reflect changes in productivity in the medical care sector,

TABLE 16.1 PER CAPITA SPENDING ON MEDICAL CARE (U.S. DOLLARS)

	1960	1970	1980	1990	2004
Canada	109	253	743	1,811	3,185
Germany	98	216	811	1,522	3,043
Japan	27	127	517	1,175	2,249
Great Britain	80	144	456	988	2,508
United States	143	346	1,063	2,600	6,102

Source: Program of the Organization for Economic Cooperation and Development Health Data (1993–1990); CRS (2007) for later data.

TABLE 16.2 ANNUAL RATES OF INCREASE IN NOMINAL PER CAPITA SPENDING (PERCENT)

	1960–1970	1970–1980	1980–1990	1990–2004
Canada	8.80	11.38	9.32	4.1
Germany	8.25	14.14	6.49	5.1
Japan	16.85	15.05	8.55	4.7
United Kingdom	6.01	12.21	8.05	6.9
United States	9.26	11.88	9.35	6.3
Corrected for Internal Inflation Rate in Each Country (Percent)				
Canada	5.89	3.64	3.58	2.0
Germany	5.33	8.71	3.71	3.1
Japan	10.55	5.83	6.57	4.1
United Kingdom	2.01	−0.93	1.92	4.3
United States	6.35	4.47	4.53	3.6

Source: Program of the Organization for Economic Cooperation AND Development HEALTH Data (1993).

changes in payment associated with changes in market power of factors (doctors, nurses, etc.), or both.

The data in the second part of Table 16.2 seem—at least in part—to refute the general thrust of Evans and colleagues, but the data do show a systematic trend. In every decade since 1960, Canada's postinflation medical spending increases have been smaller than those of the United States, although not by a great deal. The average annual difference in increase is about 1 percent. However, even small differences when compounded can lead to important changes through time. Had the Canadian rate matched the U.S. rate, it would have about half again higher annual per capita spending in 2010 for health care than it actually did.

We can also extend the comparison to other countries. Increases in Germany were much higher than in the United States in the 1970s but comparable or lower in other decades. Increase in Great Britain is commonly lower than that of other countries, and in Japan is commonly higher, although declining rapidly through time. The relatively low U.S. increase in medical spending in the 1970s is in no small part due to the U.S. price controls instituted in 1971 to 1974 and subsequent price controls in Medicare.

One area in which the United States differs distinctly from other developed nations is the relatively high rate at which we compensate physicians. Zaccagnino (1994) used OECD data to compare a set of industrialized nations that had similar private-practice physician markets but with varying payment mechanisms. He showed not only (see Figure 16.5) that the United States began with the highest physician payments per patient per year (in 1975) but also that U.S. compensation increased faster than in other countries. Fuchs and Hahn (1990) have also forcefully made the point that provider compensation is an essential component of both the levels and increased rates in spending.

FIGURE 16.5 Annual physician payments per capita, inflation adjusted.

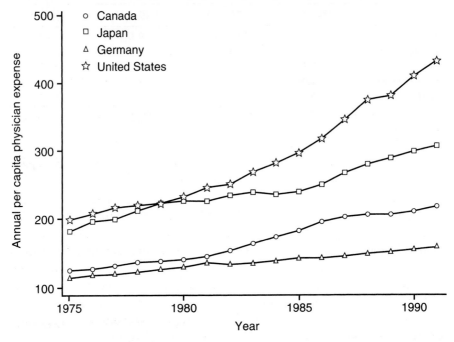

Source: Zaccagnino, 1994.

A more recent analysis (again using OECD data) shows a similar pattern (CRS, 2007). The CRS study calculated the average annual compensation of specialist physicians to per capita gross domestic product (GDP). Among 21 nations on the list, the United States was fourth on the list with a ratio of 5.7,[17] and the average in their sample was 3.6. Germany had a very low ratio of 2.7, while the UK and Canadian ratios were near that of the United States at 4.9 and 5.1, respectively. The United States was the highest for compensating general practice doctors (4.1 ratio versus an overall average of 2.9).

Data in Table 16.3 show perinatal mortality rates in the corresponding periods (1960–2000), and Table 16.4 shows the annual decline in perinatal death rates in each decade (1960–1990) of these data. The United States started out second to best in 1960 as the best among these countries and ended up as worst by 1989. Comparing Table 16.3 with recent data (OECD as cited in CRS, 2007) shows that the United States still has among the highest infant mortality rates among OECD nations (third among all reporting to the OECD with a rate of 6.9 per thousand, exceeded only by Turkey and Mexico)

---

[17]The highest nations were Australia, the Netherlands, and Belgium.

TABLE 16.3 PERINATAL MORTALITY RATES (PERCENT)

	1960	1970	1980	1989	2000
Canada	2.84	2.18	1.09	0.79	0.6
Germany	3.58	2.64	1.16	0.64	0.5
Japan	3.73	2.03	1.11	0.57	0.4
United Kingdom	3.36	2.38	1.34	0.90	0.8
United States	2.86	2.30	1.32	0.96	0.7

Source: Scheiber, Poullier, and Greenwald (1992, Table 26). Data for 2000 extrapolated from various international data for the 1990s.

versus an average of 4.0. As international observers have come to expect, Japan has the lowest with a rate of 2.8 per 1,000.

By taking data from various international sources, one can estimate the 2000 perinatal mortality rates as shown in the last column in Table 16.3. These data show that the United States has now probably moved ahead of United Kingdom in perinatal mortality outcomes. Improvements in medical care technology (notably newborn intensive care), access to abortion, and (especially in the United States) reduced maternal smoking account for the steady improvement in this key health outcome over the past four decades.

The relationship between changes in spending and changes in the perinatal mortality rate within countries is very weak if it exists. Over the entire period shown in these tables, a modestly weak association exists between annual changes in spending and perinatal mortality rates, but the result is driven entirely by the Japanese experience, where there are both high growth rates in spending and large reductions in perinatal care. Given the large changes in per capita income in postwar Japan, it is difficult to know what to make of such data.

These data suggest the following hypothesis: The United States, with higher medical spending than any other country, is closer to the "flat of the curve" than other countries in the sense that additional spending on medical care is less likely to produce increases in health outcomes. Ignoring the Japanese data, the United States experienced modestly higher growth in health care

TABLE 16.4 ANNUAL CHANGES IN PERINATAL DEATH RATES(PERCENT)

	1960–1970	1970–1980	1980–1989	Overall
Canada	−2.6	−6.7	−3.5	−4.3
Germany	−3.0	−7.9	−6.4	−5.8
Japan	−6.0	−7.3	−7.1	−6.3
United Kingdom	−3.4	−5.8	−4.3	−4.4
United States	−2.2	−5.5	−3.5	−3.7

Source: Scheiber, Poullier, and Greenwald (1992).

spending in the postwar era but fewer decreases in perinatal mortality. Japan, by contrast, started with the lowest investment in health care per capita and had the largest increases in spending and the largest gains in perinatal mortality. We might well characterize Japan as having been on the "steep of the curve," if that forms a legitimate contrast to the "flat of the curve."

We still confront a puzzle in analyzing health care spending and outcomes: Does more spending increase health outcomes? Contrasting the U.S. and Japanese experiences suggests that the answer is "yes" if you begin with little health care and "not so much" if you begin with lots of health care. In all countries, spending increased and health improved, using both the perinatal death rate and overall life expectancy as measures of improved health. Alas, we still confront the added puzzle: Does the added health gain come from increased medical spending, increased income in general (which leads to added health spending), or increased educational spending, which fueled both the increased income and the improvements in health? We cannot answer such questions with the aggregate data provided by the OECD.

A FINAL CONUNDRUM

Every modern society faces a growing challenge as the populations age throughout the world: What is the proper care for elderly citizens in their final months of life? In the United States, a recent study has provided a provocative analysis, saying, in effect, that widespread variations in medical spending occur from region to region in the United States (using Medicare data as the basis of analysis) yet these differences have no observable effect on the longevity of the patients treated (Fisher et al., 2000). These results suggest that adding medical resources does not necessarily increase longevity hence further complicating analysis of how to best care for an aging population.

SUMMARY

International comparisons of health care systems can provide several types of useful information for those studying the U.S. health care system (and probably conversely). As comparisons of aggregate spending on medical care and its relationships to health outcomes show, many regularities exist across countries despite the very large differences in organization of health care systems in those countries. The relationship between per capita income and spending almost certainly shows that, at the level of societies, medical care is a luxury good. (This stands in large contradistinction to cross-sectional results for individuals within the United States where income elasticities are very small. Health insurance should produce that kind of income-related equality within a country, but it has nothing to do with cross-national comparisons.) Although the United States has much larger health care spending per capita than any other nation, much of it (nearly all, if one looks at the logarithmic relationships between health care spending and income) is quite "in line" with what one would expect when looking at choices made by other nations. The very strong relationship between per capita medical care spending and per capita income is all the more remarkable given the wide diversity of health care systems that various countries have chosen.

Either higher income or additional medical care spending (or both) seems to improve health outcomes both for infant mortality and for adult life expectancy. On these comparisons, however, outcomes in the United States look particularly unfavorable because U.S. mortality and life expectancy results are notably worse than one would expect for a country with its income and medical care spending.

Careful study of the health care delivery systems also reveals many other ways to achieve the same goals that U.S. institutions have sought to achieve: for example, broad access to care, cost control, and so forth. The roles of incentives in the use and provision of care are especially open to study across nations because the diversity of choice makes a far richer field of study than one could find within any single country.

RELATED CHAPTERS IN *HANDBOOK OF HEALTH ECONOMICS*

Chapter 1, "International Comparisons of Health Expenditures" by Ulf G. Gerdtham and Bengt Jönsson

Chapter 19, "Child Health Care in Developed Countries" by Janet Currie

Chapter 34, "Equity in Health Care Financing and Delivery" by Adam Wagstaff and Eddy van Doorslaer

Chaper 35, "Equity in Health" by Alan Williams and Richard Cookson

PROBLEMS

1. Describe the "typical" person in the United States without insurance, and discuss how that person's uninsured state is quite predictable.

2. Chapter 10 discussed a problem of "market failure" in health insurance resulting from the inability of insurers to classify correctly the "types" of individuals seeking to buy insurance from them and their response. Does mandating "universal insurance" (i.e., requiring every individual to have a health insurance policy from some source) solve this problem completely, or is some other step (e.g., requiring community rating) necessary?

3. Why do you think that some proposals for universal health insurance have either not included dental services or have limited them in scope and then only with copayments higher than proposed for doctor and hospital care?

4. Explain in terms your parents would understand how mandating employer-paid insurance is likely to lead to a permanent loss of jobs for low-paid workers.

5. The Japanese health care system has two unusual features compared with many other nations' systems: (a) hospitalization rates are very low, but once a patient is admitted to the hospital, lengths of stay are very high; and (b) the population seems to receive prescription drugs at a very high rate. What organizational features of the Japanese system are distinct to it, and which of them could plausibly lead to these two features?

6. "The United States has higher medical care expenses per person than any other country, and this proves that the U.S. system is wasteful." Discuss.

7. What evidence do you know about from international comparisons of hospital use that points dramatically to the role of lifestyle (e.g., dietary composition) on illness rates and hospital use? (*Hint:* Think about demand for specific hospitalizations for which diet might have an effect, for example, heart disease.)

8. The U.S. health care system costs more per person than that in other countries. How much of the difference is explained by higher incomes in the United States than in other countries?

Author's Postscript _____

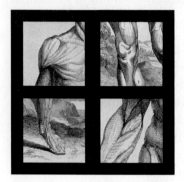

Finishing this book completes many readers' formal study of health economics. For a few, it may represent only the beginning of a long excursion into the subject. Economists everywhere are now finding that the study of subjects in the domain of health economics offers a fascinating opportunity to pursue and expand other specialized economic tools and interests. Persons with separate interests in the economics of uncertainty, game theory, cost function estimation, demand theory and modeling, labor economics, industrial organization and regulation, econometrics, public finance and taxation policy, and other traditional fields in economics are now turning to the vast array of unsolved problems in health economics for new and interesting applications in their own special fields. Indeed, no health economist can hope to master all of the areas of expertise that one might bring to bear on the subject of health economics. As knowledge expands, specialization invariably increases. (Remember Adam Smith's dictum: "Division of labor is limited by the extent of the market." The market is growing larger!) This trend is quite natural and desirable, for very little in the study of health economics is so "special" that others cannot enter the field and make important contributions. As will be painfully obvious to persons who have completed this textbook, a vast array of unsolved problems remains as fertile ground for future study. Yet, I hope that this textbook also points out the importance of carefully scrutinizing the special circumstances that often surround the study of health economics. Careful modeling of the novel institutional arrangements in health care will pay considerable dividends as will studies of why particular institutions emerge in some settings but not others. (International comparisons of institutions may

569

provide very fruitful paths for some studies.) As I noted in the Preface, I believe that careful attention to the role of uncertainty will often, if not always, yield considerable payoff in studying behavior and institutions in the area of health care.

I also believe that we will find increasingly that the fruitful study of health economics reaches further into the medical detail of problems than has been true in the past. Biology has moved from the broad classification of plants and animals to the study of organ systems, to the study of cells, and now to that of molecules. Physics has moved from the study of objects to the study of atoms, and now to that of subatomic particles. So also has the study of economics reached for increasing detail. Early studies in health economics used highly aggregated data—for instance, average spending by persons in the 48 (or 50) states per year. This work charted the way for studies with much finer data gathered at the level of individual annual spending on medical care, for example. Studies using household surveys and the RAND Health Insurance Study represent this class of work at its best. Studies of providers similarly shifted from aggregate data to data on hospitals, departments within hospitals, physician-firms, individual physicians, nurses, and so forth.

We can and should now turn to even more disaggregated data—for instance, patients' behavior within single clinical episodes and the corresponding behavior of providers. Work on medical practice variations, for example, has highlighted the importance of turning to specific clinical conditions to understand behavior more broadly. I believe that when we make this step in health economics, it will allow us to improve our understanding of much behavior that now remains puzzling and unresolved. As we successfully complete such studies, we will be able to build back up to a much better understanding of the macrobehavior in health care systems that we strive to understand. Both the data sets and the computational power now exist to make such studies feasible, but gathering new and highly detailed data on apparently "small" problems seems a prerequisite to making many important advances. It would seem that any new researcher in health economics should become highly adept in the methods of statistics and econometrics, including those skills necessary to study discrete choices. I also believe that collaboration with clinician-researchers will have a growing payoff for at least some economists because of their detailed knowledge of both clinical events and institutions involved in the production of health care.

For those readers who end their study of health economics at this point, I hope that what you have learned will assist you in your chosen work or study. For some, I also hope that this book will be only the beginning of an extended excursion into this fascinating realm.

APPENDIX

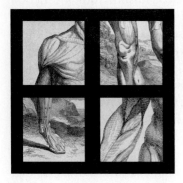

Introduction to Basic Economics Concepts

This appendix serves as a *very* brief overview of some of the main economics concepts used throughout this book. If the reader has had an introductory or intermediate economics course before this (and the book aims at such a student), this material should serve as a quick reminder of the basic concepts. For the student who has never encountered economic thinking before, please remember that entire books and one- to two-semester courses usually cover the material that follows, and judge the adequacy of the coverage of this material found here with mercy.

THE CONCEPT OF UTILITY AND DEMAND CURVES

Economists begin their study of human behavior by making what some would consider a rash assumption, namely that every consumer has a stable set of preferences that allows comparison of different "bundles" of goods (taken here very broadly to mean goods and services produced in the market or activities that might take place out of the market). These preferences are normally represented as a "utility function" showing how additional amounts of each good increase total "well-being" or (in the usual term) "utility." Economists normally presume that "goods" continue to add utility as more are consumed, so sometimes the "good" becomes the removal of a noxious substance. For example, garbage *removal* may be the good rather than garbage. The list of possible goods is very large. Think about how many bar codes exist for all the stores in the world; each one describes a different good and this still

571

misses items such as "watching a sunset" for which no bar code (yet) exists. To simplify the discussion, we usually abstract from the specific names of these goods and simply call them $X_1, X_2, \ldots$ etc. Thus, the utility function becomes Utility $= U(X_1, X_2, \ldots X_N)$ where N is the number of goods that one might possibly wish to consider. For reasons of simplicity—including our ability to diagram these concepts readily—economists often collapse the discussion to two goods (which can then be pictured on a two-dimensional graph, as you will see shortly). This actually does not cause a great loss of precision in thinking because these two goods can be one specific good (such as popcorn or peanuts) and the other a "composite bundle" of all other goods and services.

Economic thinking rests fundamentally on the premise that consumers make choices to maximize their utility, limited by the amounts of goods that the consumer's income can purchase. In more elaborate versions of this problem, income itself represents choices made by the consumer in the current period (how much to work versus how much to enjoy leisure) as well as the cumulative effects of many past decisions (how much education to seek, how hard to study in classes of health economics, how much to save for the future). We assume that consumers not only know their preferences but also how to act to maximize their own utility. Although few economists believe that this literally occurs in every human choice, a very fruitful study of human behavior emerges from this simple yet powerful paradigm.[1]

These types of decisions can be portrayed easily either in graphs or by using the branch of mathematics known *as calculus*. The basic "problem" of the consumer is to maximize utility subject to a budget constraint,[2] and this can be easily portrayed (in a simplified version) in a two-dimensional graph. In this graph, we focus on a specific good (say, X_1) and choices between that good and *all other* goods. Figure A.1 shows two key features about how goods affect utility. First, for any specified amount of X_{other}, adding more X_1 adds to total utility but at a decreasing rate. This conforms to the simple idea that we eventually become "sated" in our consumption of a specific good. The formal statement of this says that we have positive but diminishing *marginal* (or *incremental*) utility for any specific good such as X_1. (The same is said

---

[1]A classic discussion of these issues is found in Milton Friedman's *Essays in Positive Economics* (1966).

[2]This type of problem commonly uses an approach devised by mathematician Joseph-Louis Lagrange, known (not by coincidence) as *Lagrange multipliers*. Lagrange is usually considered to be French, but he was born in Turin, Italy, and wrote his famous essay on finding maxima and minima in 1755 in Italian at age 19, probably younger than almost every reader of this textbook! (What had *you* done by age 19?)

FIGURE A.I

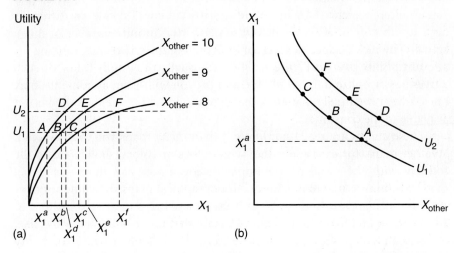

(a)

(b)

symmetrically for X_{other} because it represents a bundle of all other goods and services. Indeed, any one of those could be pulled out and treated similarly to X_1.) The other key feature of Figure A.1(a) shows that similarly shaped curves exist for each possible level of X_{other}, but utility is lower as the amount of X_{other} falls so that these curves "nest" one under another as the amount of X_{other} falls.

Now comes an important step: We take the information from the curves in Figure A.1(a) and transform the same information into a different graph, one using X_1 and X_{other} on the axes. (This is why we want to work only with two goods. Otherwise this becomes an n-dimensional graph that's difficult if not impossible to draw for $n \geq 3$.) To see how this works, pick a specific level of utility in Figure A.1(a) (say, U_1), and think about the combinations of X_1 and X_{other} that could create exactly U_1. Figure A.1(a) shows three possible levels of X_{other}, arbitrarily designated as 8, 9, and 10 (but they could be anything because we haven't said in what units X_{other} is measured). Points A, B, and C all have exactly the same level of utility (U_1), but each has a different combination of X_1 and X_{other}. The graph of those points (and all others like them if we'd drawn more curves in Figure A.1(a) for different amounts of X_{other}) creates an *isoutility* curve at utility level U_1 in Figure A.1(b).[3] More commonly, economists call these *indifference curves* because the consumer is literally indifferent to which of any combination of goods on each curve is

---

[3]These come from the Greek word *isos* meaning "equal."

best to consume.[4] Points D, E, and F from Figure A.1(a) translate into a separate indifference curve U_2 in Figure A.1(b). We could create an extremely large number of such curves in Figure A.1(b) (an infinite number of them, actually) by picking specific levels of utility in Figure A.1(a) and graphing the relevant points over to Figure A.1(b). We usually draw only a few of such curves to symbolize the overall idea, and (as you will see in a moment), only one of them eventually matters—the highest one achievable with the budget available to the consumer.

These curves are really no different than many maps you've often read. Weather maps, for example, either with curves or colors, show areas of the country with the same temperature. Meteorologists call these *isothermal* maps, meaning "same temperature." Topographical maps show lines of constant altitude, and anybody who's ever used these maps soon becomes able to look at them and figure out what the terrain that the map depicts looks like.

The next step allows us to move from the ephemeral world of utility (which we can't really see or measure) to the concrete world of prices and quantities. Begin with (and slightly generalize) the graph in Figure A.1(b) and then think about how to add information about the consumer's buying power, the "budget" available to buy goods and services. In the simplest model, the consumer's income (I) is fixed at a specific level (say, I_1). In Figure A.2(a), this income appears as a downward-sloping straight line with a slope determined by the relative prices of X_1 and X_{other}.[5] The trick is to find the highest possible level of utility (remember that the consumer is trying to maximize utility within the constraint of the budget available), and it's easy

---

[4]A personal note: The word *indifferent* has a specific meaning to economists not universally shared by others. It refers to combinations of things that create the same utility. Early in my marriage, my wife would sometimes ask me, "Do you want peas or corn with the meat loaf tonight?" Because I'd just learned the concept of indifference in an economics class, I would respond "I'm indifferent," meaning "either would be fine." Before I explained this concept clearly, she heard instead "I don't want either" as my message, and this came close to ruining our marriage until I explained the underlying economic idea to her. I can now say "I'm indifferent" without having to call a marriage counselor.

[5]To show why the budget line is a straight and downward-sloping line in this graph, begin with the notion that all available income is spent on goods X_1 and X_{other} purchased at prices of p_1 (for X_1) and (arbitrarily) a price of 1 for other goods. Thus $I = p_1 X_1 + X_{\text{other}}$. Now we ask what combinations of goods could exactly consume the total budget I. To do this, increase X_1 by a little bit and ask how much X_{other} has to fall to keep within the budget. Adding one unit of X_1 causes spending to increase by p_1, so the amount of X_{other} has to fall by exactly $1/p_1$ to keep total spending the same. The constant-budget line in the graph with X_1 and X_{other} on the axes thus has a slope of $-1/p_1$. More generally, in a graph of X_i versus X_j, the budget line will have a slope of $-p_j/p_i$.

to see that one does this by finding the highest possible indifference curve that just touches the budget constraint at one point. This is called a *tangent point*,[6] and it's easy to show that the consumer can't do any better than to pick the bundle of goods where the budget line is exactly tangent to one of the indifference curves. (To see this, think about trying to achieve any higher level of utility; it would require using more income than is in the budget. Going in the other direction, any feasible point on the budget constraint except the tangent must lie on a lower indifference curve, and, hence, must create lower utility.)

Figure A.2(a), on the following page, shows two incomes (I_1 and I_2) that were picked because they are just tangent to the indifference curves U_1 and U_2. The optimal consumption for the consumer with these tastes (that is to say, with this utility function) and a budget of I_1 is the combination (X_1^*, X_{other}^*). If the consumer's income were to rise to I_2, the optimal combination would shift to $(X_1^{**}, X_{other}^{**})$.

Now comes the final step of creating demand curves from the indifference curve map. The "thought experiment" here is to ask what happens if income remains the same and the price of X_{other} remains at 1, but the price p_1 goes up or down. Because the slope of the income line is the ratio $1/p_1$, raising p_1 causes the budget line to flatten out and vice versa. Figure A.2(b) shows three different prices for p_1, labeled p_1^*, p_1^{**}, and p_1^{***}, but it should be clear that we can pick as many different prices as we wish and just add complexity to the graph.

When p_1 is lowest among these three values (at p_1^*), the buying power is highest, so the top of these three income lines is the one that matters. The optimal choice leads to consumption of the pair (X_1^*, X_{other}^*) in Figure A.2(a). If the price goes up to p_1^{**}, the budget line rotates downward around the lower right intersection (it must flatten out, as described before, but if all the budget were spent on X_{other}, the same amount would be available no matter what the price p_1, which is why it rotates around that specific point). For a price p_1^{**}, the optimal consumption is the pair $(X_1^{**}, X_{other}^{**})$. Similarly, if the price rises again to p_1^{***}, we get a new tangency at quantity X_1^{***} and so on. We could make as many such points as we wanted by making very small changes in the price p_1 and filling in lots and lots of budget lines in Figure A.2(a) (but it would get very messy). Figure A.2(c) simply takes these tangency points and graphs them in a new way, showing combinations of p_1 and X_1 that follow directly from the consumer's utility-maximizing choices for the given budget I.

---

[6]This comes from the Latin word *tangens*, meaning "touching."

FIGURE A.2

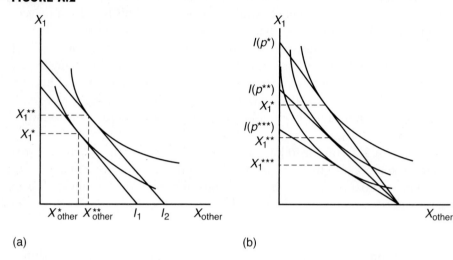

(a)

(b)

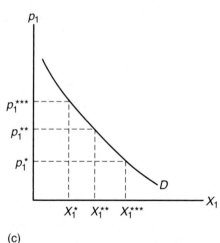

(c)

THE DEMAND CURVE BY A SOCIETY: ADDING UP INDIVIDUAL DEMANDS

All of the discussion thus far really centers on a single individual, but the transition from the individual to a larger group (society) is quite simple. The aggregate demand curve simply totals at each price the quantities on each individual demand curve for every member of the society.[7] Figure A.3 shows

[7]This is called *horizontal aggregation* because of the common penchant for drawing demand curves with price on the vertical axis and quantity on the horizontal axis of the diagram. Adding things "horizontally" in such a diagram produces the correct aggregate demand curve by showing the quantity consumed at any price by all of the consumers in the market.

FIGURE A.3

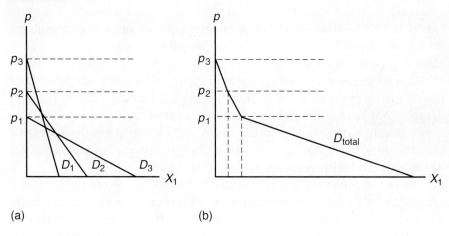

(a)   (b)

such an aggregation for a three-person society, but it should be clear that the process can continue for as many members of society as are relevant with the demand curve for each of the three persons shown and labeled as D_1, D_2, and D_3. The aggregate demand curve [Figure A.3(b)] D_{total} adds up, at each possible price, the total quantities demanded. D_{total} coincides with D_1 at higher prices because only person 1 has any positive demand for X_1 at prices above p_2. There is a kink in D_{total} at p_2 where person 2's demands begin to add in, and again at p_1, where person 3's demands begin to add in.

USING DEMAND CURVES TO MEASURE VALUE

The previous discussion speaks as if the quantity of medical care that people demand is affected (for example) by price. Demand curves show this relationship, describing quantity as a function of price. They can also be "inverted" to describe the incremental (marginal) value consumers attach to additional consumption of medical care at any level of consumption observed. This approach uses the "willingness-to-pay" interpretation of a demand curve. The only thing that is done here is to read the demand curve in a direction other than is normally done. Rather than saying that the quantity demanded depends on price (the interpretation given above), we can say equally well that the incremental value of consuming more X_1 is equivalent to the consumer's willingness to pay for a bit more X_1. Just as the quantity demanded falls as the price increases (the first interpretation of the demand curve), we can also see that the marginal value to consumers (incremental willingness to pay) falls as the amount consumed rises. We call these curves *inverse demand curves* or *value curves*.

Inverse demand curves (willingness to pay curves) slope downward generically because consumers have declining marginal utility for any good (see Figure A.1), expressing the more common idea of satiation. Ten wonderful restaurant meals a year is terrific. Ten a month would be fine too, but in most cities, one would tend to have worn out the novelty of restaurant visits. Thus, the tenth restaurant visit per month creates less added (marginal) value than the tenth per year. Ten restaurant meals a day would be downright burdensome not to mention unhealthy and would probably have negative marginal value for most people (the value curve would drop below the horizontal axis). No intelligent consumer would go to this extreme, of course, unless bribed to do so (negative prices for restaurant visits).

We can extend the same idea one step further by noting that the total value of using a certain amount consumed to consumers is the area under the demand curve out to the quantity consumed. If we subtract the cost of acquiring the good (or service), we have the unusual but important concept of "consumer surplus," the amount of value received above and beyond the amount paid to acquire the good. As an example (using discrete quantities of consumption), suppose the first restaurant visit each month created $100 in value to the consumer. If the meal cost $30, the consumer would get $70 in consumer surplus out of that visit. A second meal per month might create an additional $75 in value, again costing $30, and creating $45 in consumer surplus. A third restaurant meal per month might create a marginal value of $35 and a consumer surplus of only $5. A fourth meal would create only $20 in marginal value and would cost $30.[8] Table A.1 summarizes these data.

Two ideas appear in this discussion. First, demand curves can predict quantities consumed: Intelligent decision making will continue to expand the amount consumed until the marginal value received just equals the marginal cost of the service. (In the case of the restaurant meals, we don't quite achieve "equality" because we described the incremental value of restaurant meals as a lumpy step function, dropping from $100 to $75 to $35 to $20, and the cost was described as $30.)

The second concept is that of total consumer surplus to the consumer from having a specific number of restaurant meals each month. As noted, intelligent planning would stop after the third meal each month. Total consumer surplus sums up all of the extra value to consumers (above the costs paid) for each restaurant meal consumed.

---

[8]Note that we have to carefully specify the unit of time in demand curves. The quantity consumed is described as a rate per unit of time. Thus, the same ideas as discussed here on a "per month" basis would apply to 12 meals per year, 24 meals per year, and so on because the incremental utility of 1 meal a month ought to equate exactly to 12 meals a year.

TABLE A.I CONSUMER SURPLUS IN RESTAURANT MEAL EXAMPLE

Meal	Value Created ($)	Price Paid ($)	Consumer Surplus ($)	Total Consumer Surplus ($)
I	100	30	70	70
2	75	30	45	115
3	35	30	5	120
4	20	30	−10	110

It is easy to prove that consumer surplus is maximized by a simple rule: Expand the amount consumed until the marginal benefit has just fallen to match the marginal cost. In this case, at the third restaurant meal per year, the marginal benefit has fallen to $35, the marginal cost is $30 per visit, and stopping at that rate of meals per year maximizes consumer surplus as the last column of Table A.1 shows. Of course, the type of "incremental value" data shown in Table A.1 is just a lumpy version of a demand curve. One could easily create a bar graph of the data in Table A.1 and then draw a smooth line through the midpoints of the tops of each of the bars in and call it a demand curve; adding up such curves across many individuals would smooth things out even more.

The concept of "consumer surplus" is one of the most powerful used by economists, often phrased as "consumer welfare" rather than "consumer surplus." Many problems studied by economists seek ways to increase (or, best of all, maximize) consumer surplus for individuals or an entire society.[9] These concepts appear in Chapter 4, in which you study some novel problems arising as the step is taken from the general ideas in this appendix to the specific problems associated with demand for medical care.

THE PROBLEM OF SUPPLY OF GOODS

Having gone through the concepts of consumer demand, we can now turn to the problem of how goods and services are supplied to the market. The concepts are actually quite similar. The idea of a "utility function" has a close

---

[9]Aggregating consumer surplus from individuals to the level of an entire society requires a decision about how one person's welfare adds to another's. One way to do it (the most common in economics) says "the welfare created by $1 is the same, no matter whom you give it to." See, for example, Harberger (1971). Others would use some societal "weighting function" in which the value of improving a person's well-being differs from person to person. For a detailed analysis of this concept, see Bator (1957) in an article with a very misleading title (it says "simple" but it's not!). The work of Rawls (1971) delves into these concepts of "economic justice" in great detail, and his work has spawned an enormous literature of commentary best found in your library. All of this analysis comes under the field of "welfare economics."

match in a "production function" (showing how inputs combine to create the final product).

For a first pass at the concepts of production theory, we can step back for a moment and reflect on our own experiences in "producing" things: More effort leads to more output. In most productive processes, that relationship between "more in" and "more out" doesn't follow a straight path but one that includes dips and hills. In a discussion of production functions, we can speak about areas in which returns to scale are different—increasing, constant, and decreasing.

Figure A.4 illustrates these concepts for one of several possible inputs (which we'll call A_1). On the top portion, we see the production function graphed showing total output as input A_1 increases. Initially (in region a),

FIGURE A.4

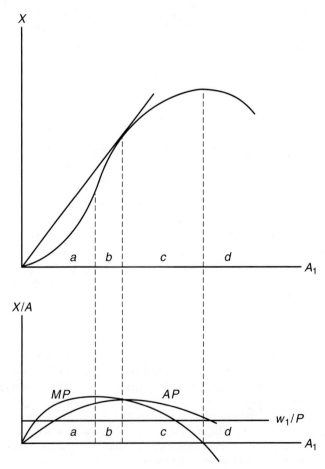

output rises faster than the input. This is the realm of "increasing returns to scale." Then come realms *b* and *c*, where output rises with more use of input A_1, but at a decreasing rate. This is the realm of decreasing returns to scale. Finally, at the boundary between regions *c* and *d*, output reaches a maximum and then begins to fall. Region *d* is irrelevant for any rational productive process because it requires additional resources (more A_1) but yields less output *X*.

On the bottom of Figure A.4, the same production function is shown, but here the vertical axis scale has become the ratio of *X/A* rather than the total amount of *X* produced (as on the top). The upper and lower portions of Figure A.4 relate in the following way: If you draw a ray from the origin in the top portion to any point on the curve, it shows the ratio *X/A*. If you plot that ratio in the bottom (i.e., the slope of the ray in the top), you get the average product (*AP*) of A_1 (X/A_1). The *AP* peaks at the point dividing regions *b* and *c* in the top (where the slope of the ray is as large as it can get).

The bottom portion of Figure A.4 also shows the *marginal product of A_1*, defined as the rate at which *X* changes for a tiny change in the amount of A_1 used, *holding constant all other inputs*.[10] The marginal product *MP* rises faster and then falls faster than the average product *AP*.

Now comes a bit of calculus sleight of hand: It's easy to prove that the optimal use of input A_1 comes at the point at which the marginal product of A_1 just equals the ratio of w_1/P, where *P* is the price of the final product and w_1 is the price of A_1, or slightly recast, $P \times MP = w_1$.[11, 12] The idea makes intuitive sense: It says to expand the use of input A_1 just to the point at which the "value of the marginal product" (price times the *MP*) just equals the cost of adding another unit of A_1.

We can now see that rational production processes always operate in the realm in which the *MP* is positive but declining (region *c* in Figure A.4). The optimum—the best that the firm can do—comes at one of the two points at which the *MP* curve intersects the line w_1/P in the bottom of Figure A.4. One of those intersections occurs in region *a* and the other in region *c*. But to stop in region *a* means not using a very productive input A_1 through the entire

---

[10]In the notation of calculus, the marginal product is defined as $\partial X/\partial A_1$.

[11]Economists commonly use the symbol *w* for prices of inputs (sometimes called "factor prices") because one of the inputs is always "labor" with a "wage" attached to it. Thus, the letter *w* generally indicates the price in an input market. The letter *W* took on a new meaning in the U.S. presidential election of 2000.

[12]*Proof:* The firm seeks to maximize profits, defined as $\Pi = PX - C(X)$ where *X* is a function of A_1, A_2, etc. Also, the cost of production is $C = w_1A_1 + w_2A_2 + \cdots + w_NA_N$. Thus, to find the optimum, differentiate the profit function with respect to A_1, giving $P\,\partial X/\partial A_1 - w_1 = 0$. This solves for the expression $\partial X/\partial A_1 = w_1/P$. QED.

range at which the value of the marginal product exceeds the cost of adding more input. Thus, the second of the intersections is the relevant one—in region c—and shows the rule for optimizing the firm's profit. (This also works for not-for-profit firms that seek to minimize costs of a given amount of production, an issue that arises in Chapters 8 and 9 in considering not-for-profit hospitals.)

The same process can be shown in another (now familiar) way: We can show the production function (and how it relates to several inputs at once) using Figure A.5 (similar to the "indifference curve" maps showing consumer utility in Figure A.1).

To keep things notationally correct, we can talk about the production of a specific good (say, X), with inputs we'll call A_1, A_2, etc., available to the company producing X at prices w_1, w_2, etc. The producer's production function is "given" the same way that the consumer's utility function is "given" for the analysis.[13] The inputs in the production function combine (as defined by the function itself) to produce the output X. We'll use the generic function $g(\cdot)$ to describe production functions here, so $X = g(A_1, A_2, \dots A_M)$ where there are M inputs in the production function. We can readily graph the production function with the same techniques as we used to graph the utility function, using any two of the inputs (A_1 and A_2 if we wish) on the axes of the graph,

FIGURE A.5

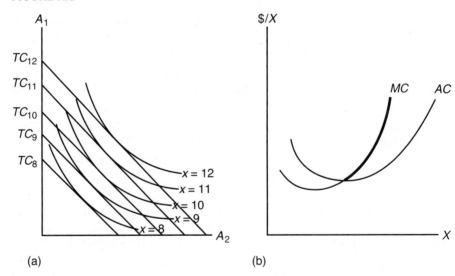

(a)

(b)

---

[13]This simple introduction ignores the problem of optimal investment in R&D to improve the production function.

and now drawing "isoquants" showing combinations of the various inputs that produce the same level of output (some specific quantity of X such as $X = 10, X = 11$, etc.). Figure A.5 shows such a figure.[14]

Because the quantities of X have specific (and observable) values (unlike the utilities of the previous discussion), we can say something specific about the spacing between the isoquants. Think about the space between the isoquants for $X = 10, X = 11$, and $X = 12$. If they are the same distance apart (being somewhat loose for the moment about what "the same distance" means), then we have a production that has "constant returns to scale" in the sense that (for example) adding $k\%$ to all of the inputs will add $k\%$ the output. If we get less than an $k\%$ increase in the output for an $k\%$ increase in the inputs, we have "decreasing returns to scale," and in this case, the isoquant curves will get further and further apart as we move to higher levels of X. Conversely, if we get more than an $k\%$ increase in output when we add $k\%$ to all the inputs, we have "increasing returns to scale," and the isoquants will be spaced closer and closer together.

Just as in the problem of consumer demand, we can talk about the total costs of the firm as the adding up of all the costs of its inputs. Thus, total cost (TC) is defined as $TC = w_1A_1 + w_2A_2 + \cdots + w_MA_N$. Again to keep the figures manageable, we can (without loss of generality) restrict ourselves to two inputs, so $TC = w_1A_1 + w_2A_2$ (where A_2 can be "other inputs besides A_1"). The TC line has a downward slope for the same reasons that the budget line of the individual consumer has a downward slope, and the slope of that line is given by the ratio of the relative prices of the two inputs (in this case, the slope is $-w_2/w_1$ because we have graphed A_1 on the vertical axis and A_2 on the horizontal axis. The firm wishes to find the lowest possible total cost for any level of output (say, $X = 10$). It does so by finding the TC line just tangent to the isoquant for an output of $X = 10$. Any lower TC line would bring a combination of inputs not sufficient to produce an output of $X = 10$, and any higher cost would, by definition, be higher than necessary. The lowest possible cost occurs at the tangency of an isoquant and a TC line. Figure A.5(a) shows such tangent lines for output quantities $X = 9, X = 10$, and so forth, labeled as TC_9, TC_{10}, and so on.

Two more concepts—those of marginal cost and average cost—become useful in a bit. Marginal cost asks the following simple question: "If I move from $X = 10$ to $X = 11$ in output, how much does the TC change?" Of course, the amount it changes can differ as you move from $X = 1$ to $X = 2$ and then again from $X = 10$ to $X = 11$, and similarly for $X = 21$ to $X = 22$, and so on. Thus, the marginal cost (MC) in Figure A.5(b) will

---

[14]Just as in the consumer demand case, we really are talking about rates of production for a given amount of time (e.g., a day, a month, or a year).

vary depending on the level of production, so we need to think about the marginal cost at $X = 10, X = 11, \ldots$ and so forth, which we could describe as $MC(X = 10)$, $MC(X = 11)$, and so on, or in more general form, $MC(X)$.

The average cost (AC) is an easier concept: It indicates what the total cost is per unit of output, found by simple division of TC/X. Of course, AC can also vary with the level of output, so we really need to think about the AC also varying with the level of output, hence, $AC(X = 10)$, $AC(X = 11)$, and so on, or more generally, $AC(X)$.

We can readily graph $TC(X)$ versus X as well as $MC(X)$ versus X and $AC(X)$ versus X.[15] Figure A.5(b) converts the information in Figure A.5(a) to a new graph showing quantity produced (X) on the horizontal axis and both $MC(X)$ and $AC(X)$ on the vertical axis. This shift really just shows the spacing between the TC curves that are tangent to each isoquant. To calculate the AC, we just compute the ratio of the TC line associated with a given X by the amount of X itself. To calculate the MC for a given value of X, we take the difference between TC for that amount of X and for the next smaller amount of X.[16]

Returning for the moment to the ideas of increasing, constant, or decreasing returns to scale, it can easily be shown (play with the figures if you wish) that when we have constant returns to scale, we have an $AC(X)$ curve that's a straight, flat line. When we have increasing returns to scale, we have a downward-sloping AC curve. Conversely, when we have decreasing returns to scale, we have an upward-sloping AC curve. *Most production functions exhibit initially increasing returns to scale and then as output expands, decreasing returns to scale. This turns into the "typical" AC curve with a U shape as characteristically shown in economics texts and here.*

The MC curve has typically more of a J-shaped appearance, turning up faster than the AC curve. "Standard" production functions also have the characteristic that $MC = AC$ (i.e., the MC and AC curves intersect) at the point at which AC is at the lowest possible point. The "traditional" shapes of MC and AC curves follow directly from the same assumptions about "returns to scale" shown in Figure A.4, with initially increasing, then decreasing returns to scale, corresponding directly to the concepts of declining and then increasing AC.

---

[15]The Appendix to Chapter 3 develops these ideas more fully for the specific case of medical care.

[16]If we think of units of X as being discrete (such as tons of steel), then the MC curve will be a little kinky, but if we were to think about the MC curve for pounds, ounces, or grams of steel, it would get much smoother. Calculus simply works out the problem assuming that we can make very, very small changes in X and then calculate the change in TC associated with that change. In other words, we get a completely smooth curve by assuming that X can be produced in continuously divisible units.

We are now in a position to describe the supply curve for a competitive firm if we assume that it wishes to maximize profits (the normal assumption for normal firms, but one we diverged from in studying not-for-profit hospitals in later chapters). It is easy to prove (but we won't do so here) that the profit-maximizing competitive firm will expand output up to the point— we'll call it X^*—at which the price in the market (a "given" for a competitive firm) just matches the $MC(X^*)$. Thus, as the price increases, the competitive firm will expand output by "marching up" its MC curve. In other words, the MC curve *is* the supply curve of a competitive firm. Again, this makes good intuitive sense: The profit-maximizing firm will decide to increase output by one more unit if (and only if) the price it receives from selling that one added unit of output at least covers the added costs (MC) of producing it. Limiting production to any amount below the point at which $MC = P$ means that the firm was forgoing some potential profits, and expanding output above that point means that the firm spent more to produce the added units of production than it received in revenue when selling them. Thus, the profit-maximizing rule says "produce up to the point at which $MC = $ price."

This rule requires another caveat: If the price is below AC of production, the firm will stop producing because it would lose money compared to quitting business. Thus, the relevant supply curve of a competitive firm is the segment of the MC curve lying at or above the AC curve. Figure A.5(b) shows the relevant segment of the MC curve as a heavier line.

Finally, we can add all of the supply curves of all the firms willing to participate in the market (i.e., those that can at least cover their average costs), adding "horizontally" the same way we can add demand curves of consumers. This gives us the market supply curve in aggregate. This aggregation takes place in exactly the same way that consumers' demand curves are aggregated to form a market-level demand curve (horizontal aggregation).

MARKET EQUILIBRIUM

The preceding two sections have shown how economists think about consumers' demands for various products and how those add up to a market-level demand curve. Similarly, we can see how production theory leads us to using the MC curve of each firm (in the segment above AC) as its supply curve, and we can add up those curves for each firm participating in the market to create the market-level supply curve. With the concepts of demand and supply in hand, we're now in position to determine the equilibrium output and price in a competitive market. To do this, we simply place the market-level demand and supply curves into the same figure (Figure A.6) and find

FIGURE A.6

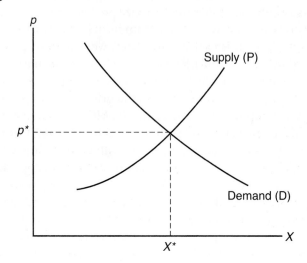

the intersection point. That intersection determines the equilibrium market-level quantity X^* and price p^*.

To see why the point (X^*, p^*) determines the equilibrium, think about moving away from that point with quantity either rising or falling. If quantity "tried" to be higher (for example, if producers tried to push more output into the market), consumer's willingness to pay would fall below the equilibrium price p^* for any output larger than X^*, but the added (marginal) costs of producers would rise (because they would be marching up the upward-sloping portions of the MC curve), and all producers would lose money on every amount sold. This would hold true for any quantity where $X > X^*$ in Figure A.6.

Similarly, if something tried to hold back the amount produced below X^*, then consumers in aggregate (represented by the aggregate demand curve) would willingly pay a price above p^* and it would cost less than p^* to produce a bit more output (because the producers would be on the upward-sloping segment of their MC curves). Such a situation would produce an opportunity for profits enough to make any profit-maximizing entrepreneur drool—price higher than incremental cost!—and every producer would try to expand output. Producers could do so successfully, but the price would fall to induce consumers to buy the added production (as they march down the aggregate demand curve). This eventually leads back to the point at which the demand curve and the supply curve intersect. At that point, the quantity supplied by producers and the quantity consumed by consumers just equal each other, and the consumer's willingness to pay (the height of the demand curve) just matches the incremental costs of producers (the *MC* curve). These are the essential features of a competitive equilibrium.[17]

This means that at the level of the individual firm, the competitive equilibrium story is really quite simple: Each firm faces a demand curve that is flat (horizontal), and in fact, the height of that demand curve must be exactly the point at which the *AC* curve reaches its minimum. The reason why this remarkable result occurs is because of search and entry. Consumers are presumed to search for lower prices and flee from any seller charging a price higher than can be found elsewhere in the market. Similarly, producers are presumed to be willing and able to enter the market when opportunities arise to make unusually large profits. Such profits occur whenever price exceeds average costs of production. Since producers all sell along their *MC* curves, the only point that meets all of these criteria is where $P = MC = AC$, which occurs at the very point where *AC* reaches a minimum.[18]

A separate branch of economic analysis studies the demand for various "input factors" in their own markets, creating demand curves for these inputs from the producers of the "final products" that can then be matched (in their own markets) with supply curves for those inputs. This creates (in a very similar way) market equilibria for inputs, showing the quantities demanded and the prices for those input factors (described earlier as w_1, w_2, etc.). These "factor demand curves" ultimately "derive" from the demands consumers have for the final products, as mediated by the production processes available to producers, hence the common name of *derived demand curves* for input factors. The essential point here for this level of review of economic theory is that we

---

[17]Another interesting feature relates to the concept of welfare economics: Total consumer surplus is maximized in a competitive market, and nothing—no social planner, no genius producer, no government—can improve on the competitive market equilibrium in terms of adding consumer surplus. The original proof of this concept came from Italian economist V. Pareto, who (ironically) spent most of his life as an economic planner for the Italian Nazi (state socialist) party trying to do as a planner something he'd proved impossible as an economist.

To be clear, in many situations, a competitive market will *not* lead to the best social outcome. Most prominent among these settings are cases in which externalities of production or consumption exist. Air pollution from automobiles or smokestacks, traffic congestion on freeways, and the spread of infectious diseases are classic examples of externalities. Chapter 14 is devoted in its entirety to a discussion of externalities. Anybody interested in these topics must absolutely read (as a beginning step) "The Problem of Social Cost," by Nobel Laureate Ronald Coase (Coase, 1960).

[18]The proof is fairly simple, again using calculus. Define $AC = TC(X)/X$ and find the point at which it reaches a minimum by taking the derivative and setting it to zero. Thus [recalling that $MC = d(TC)/dx$], $d(AC)/dX = [X*MC(X) - TC(X)]/X^2$. Setting this equal to zero and rearranging terms gives the solution that $MC = TC(X)/X$, and, hence, $MC = AC$. This proves that when *AC* reaches a minimum, $MC = AC$. This is why economists always draw *MC* and *AC* curves with the *MC* curve passing through the *AC* curve at its minimum.

can use the concepts of supply and demand equally well for final product markets and input markets, and the analysis of market behavior in either case.

MONOPOLY PRICING

All of the analysis to date presumes a "large" number of buyers and sellers in the market, each behaving independently (no collusion), with consumers seeking to maximize utility and producers seeking to maximize profits. This situation changes in some important ways when the number of sellers is small and (in the extreme case) when the number of sellers in a market is exactly one, we have a "monopoly." If the monopolist has the same motives as other producers (maximizing profits), the market will function differently than in a competitive market.

The key distinction between "monopoly" markets and competitive markets is the concept of "price taker." In a purely competitive market, enough buyers and sellers are participating in the market so that each one of these "economic agents" acts as if its own behavior did not affect the final market price. On the buyers' side, it means that nobody's purchases of X have enough impact on the market to alter the equilibrium price. On the sellers' side, it means that nobody's output decisions have an effect on the equilibrium price.

One way to state this same idea is that the supply curve to any consumer is a flat line (in the usual price-quantity diagram of supply and demand curves), suggesting that—in effect—the market can produce all of the product the consumer wishes to buy at the same price. Similarly, it says that sellers *individually* confront a demand curve that is flat (a constant price received for their product) in the sense that if they tried to raise their price above that market-equilibrium price, all of their potential buyers would migrate to some other seller who kept the price at p^*. Thus, in either the case of buyers or sellers, a competitive market means that both face a constant price in all of their decision making; hence, we can view both buyers and sellers in a competitive market as *price takers*. In other words, they "take" the price as a given fixed amount in their own decision making.

In monopoly markets, just the reverse situation occurs: The seller *must* recognize that when the amount produced changes, the price will change accordingly because the seller confronts a demand curve that matches the market demand curve. Thus, if the seller wishes to expand output, the price in the market must fall (along the demand curve) to induce consumers to actually buy the additional amount produced. So long as the seller can't set different prices for different buyers, this means that the monopoly seller's profit-maximizing decision must account for consumer preferences for their product (as expressed in the market-level demand curve).

Figure A.7 shows the essential features of the monopolist's problem. The new and essential feature in this diagram is the "marginal revenue" curve, a curve showing how much new total revenue the producer will receive by expanding output by one unit. Think about a situation in which the producer sold 100 units at a price of $4 per unit. Now suppose that to expand to 101 units of output, the price would have to fall to $3.99 per unit to increase total buying by consumers to 101 units. (*Somebody* has to decide to increase the quantity demanded by 1 unit, and in this example, the reduction from $4 to $3.99 causes just one person to increase his or her demand by 1 unit.) Revenue at 100 units is $4 × 100 = $400. Revenue at 101 units is $3.99 × 101 = $402.99. Thus, the marginal revenue at 101 units is $2.99—*not* the $3.99 received for the 101st unit of sales. The difference is that the producer had to give up $0.01 on 100 other units of sale ($1.00 loss) to induce consumers collectively to buy one more unit. Conveniently, when the demand curve is drawn as a straight line (as in Figure A.7(a)) the marginal revenue (*MR*) curve is also a straight line, beginning at the same point on the vertical (price) axis of the figure, but dropping at twice the rate of the demand curve.[19]

The monopolist's goal of maximizing profits has a simple logic: Keep expanding output until the *MR* received just matches the *MC* of adding the next unit of output and then stop. In other words, expand production until *MR* = *MC*. In Figure A.7, this occurs at an output level of X_m. Then the monopolist sets the price (using the demand curve) to clear the market by

FIGURE A.7

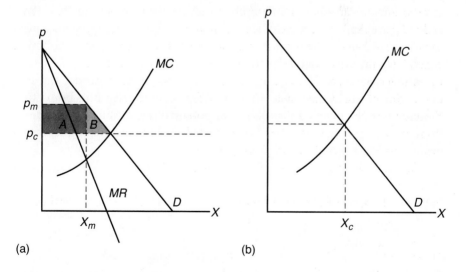

(a)

(b)

---

[19]Thus, for example, if the demand curve is of the form $p = a - bX$, then the *MR* curve has the form *MR* − a − $2bX$.

setting price at p_m. At that price, consumers wish to buy exactly X_m units, thus "clearing the market." The profits captured by the monopolist can't be any larger at any other output.[20]

Several important features distinguish monopoly from competitive markets. First, and most obviously, the price is higher and the total amount produced (and hence consumed) is smaller in the monopoly market than a corresponding competitive market would produce with the same demand curves of consumers and similar production characteristics on the part of suppliers. The other point—and the reason economists usually express a distaste for monopolies—is that the monopoly market produces less consumer surplus than a competitive market would produce. (More formally, it produces less economic surplus defined as the sum of consumer surplus and an equivalent concept of producer surplus that we'll not delve into here.) To see this briefly, look at Figure A.7(b), reproducing Figure A.7(a) but adding the equivalent price and quantity (p_c and X_c, respectively) that a competitive market would produce if the same MC curve were present in a competitive market. If somehow the competitive market outcome could be achieved, output (and consumption) would expand from X_m to X_c, and the price would fall from p_m to p_c. Consumer surplus would rise because consumers would get to both consume more and pay less for what they consumed. The rectangle A in Figure A.7(a) represents the transfer of profits gained through monopoly pricing from the monopolist to the consumers. The triangle B represents the gain in consumer surplus created by expanding output to X_c. Those who own part of the company achieving the monopoly profits shown in rectangle A probably feel differently about the virtues of shifting to a competitive price than consumers of the product. But triangle B represents a pure social waste because consumers gain the consumer surplus at nobody's expense (in the sense that the monopolist isn't losing triangle B).

The other feature about monopolies is that they tend to attract entrants into their (unusually profitable) markets. Abnormally large profits by existing producers imply profit opportunities for potential rivals. Thus, unless something stands in the way of entry, economists usually expect to see monopoly profits erode.

---

[20]The proof requires a bit of calculus: Define profits as $\Pi = p(X)X - TC(X)$, where $p(X)$ is the demand curve (expressed with price as a function of quantity) and $TC(X)$ is the total cost of producing X. To find the maximum profit, take the derivative with respect to X, set it to zero, and solve the resulting equation. Thus, $d\Pi/dX = X(dp/dX) + p - d[TC(X)]/dX = X(dp/dX) + p - MC(X) = 0$. Reshuffling these terms slightly gives $MC = p + X(dp/dX)$. The latter term is just the marginal revenue function—the price (from the demand curve) adjusted by the amount that price falls as you change $X(dp/dX)$. Because the demand curve is downward sloping, dp/dX is negative, and MR is less than price.

What types of things can stand in the way of entry? Often the answer is government interference in the market. Many countries have long had industrial policies designed to protect the profits of incumbent producers. (Another distinct literature studies the reasons for this, known as *political economy*.) Governments requiring licenses for producers is a common example, and in the United States, governments require licenses not only for physicians, nurses, and pharmacists but also for barbers, lawyers, taxicabs, ice cream vendors, and an amazingly large additional array of classes of sellers.

Sometimes the nature of production creates a "natural monopoly." For example, if the market is so small that a single firm can produce all of the desired output while still experiencing declining average costs, then the market usually sustains only one seller. Classic examples of such markets are the distribution of natural gas and electricity and (formerly) telephone service. But as commonly happens in a world with technical progress, new techniques can evolve to allow competition in what was once a "natural monopoly." The entrance of cellular telephones to compete with land-line telephone systems provides a useful case study of the effects of new technologies on the way a market functions. Often the government steps in when the market has a true natural monopoly to control the prices charged; examples include gas, electricity, and (formerly) telephone distribution.

Something else that can get in the way of competitive pricing is simple collusion between sellers. If sellers get together and agree on output, they can act "as one" and hence achieve monopoly prices even when many firms participate in the market. OPEC is one prominent international organization that deliberately tries to control the output of crude oil in world markets. Within individual countries, government policy can either aid and abet collusion (a common outcome in many countries), or it can vigorously work to oppose collusion. In the United States, major laws passed early in the twentieth century (most notable the Sherman Anti-Trust Act and the Robinson-Patman Act) make collusion illegal, and the U.S. Department of Justice and the Federal Trade Commission act as major "watchdogs" to prevent collusion in U.S. markets. In other countries (and sometimes in the United States in the past and at present), the government actively works to support collusion among producers. One way to support such activities comes when the government restricts entry into a market (such as with licenses for taxicabs).

MONOPOLISTIC COMPETITION

Some markets behave neither as competitive markets nor monopolistic markets. A huge volume of literature has evolved to attempt to understand how markets work when they fit neither the competitive nor the monopolistic paradigm, a branch of economic analysis known as *industrial organization* (or more succinctly, *IO*). This literature seeks to understand how producers interact with one another in their behavior in these "in-between" situations. Possible outcomes in price and quantity commonly range between the competitive and monopoly equilibria, but the market's actual characteristics and the nature of interaction between producers determine just where the equilibrium will end up. The analysis of all of these potential markets lies far beyond the scope of this appendix and, indeed, for the analysis in the main text in general. However, one particular type of market equilibrium appears useful in studying many health care markets—the outcome known as *monopolistic competition*—so we will provide a brief overview of that market here.[21]

Monopolistic competition (as the phrase suggests) combines elements of both monopoly and competitive markets. Most usefully, we can think about them as emerging in situations in which one of the key elements of a competitive market—consumer search—breaks down. Thus, we can add one more item to the list of things at the end of the previous section that leads to monopoly pricing: failure of consumer search.

Think for a moment about a market with many buyers and a large handful of sellers, none of whom colludes on output or price, and into which market entry is perfectly free. If entry is truly unrestricted, then unusually large profits will induce entry, ultimately to the point of eroding away those extra profit opportunities. In monopolistic competition, we presume that such free entry can occur readily.

Now continue for a moment with the thought experiment of how the market would behave if *nobody* looked around for a low price when going out to purchase some good or service, and suppose that all of the sellers knew that all of the consumers behaved in this way. Each seller would then logically behave as a monopolist, knowing that whatever fraction of all buyers decided to buy from each seller would represent an opportunity for price setting just as a true monopolist would have. Each seller would, in effect, have a mini-monopoly, his or her own share of the total market, without fear that charging a higher price would cause consumers to flee to other sellers. (They wouldn't flee, of course, if they never shopped for a better price than the first one they found.)

In this extreme-form case (absolutely no comparison shopping), the market equilibrium would look like a series of monopoly markets. Now let's

---

[21]The discussion that follows paraphrases work by Schwartz and Wilde (1979), Schwartz and Wilde (1982a,b), and Sadanand and Wilde (1982).

alter the story a bit, having *some* but not all consumers in the market engaging in a search for lower prices. Now each seller faces a different pricing problem: If each one keeps its price high, each will make more money from the nonshoppers but runs the risk of losing the sale to the shoppers (who might find a lower price from another seller in their search for a better price). Thus, each seller will set prices in a way that trades off higher profits from nonshoppers in return for attracting more business from shoppers.

It doesn't take a lot of mathematics to understand the way such markets will work: The higher the percentage of consumers who shop (and the more they shop before buying), the closer the market will move toward the competitive equilibrium. The less people shop, the more it will move toward the monopoly equilibrium. Thus, the nature of the monopolistically competitive equilibrium will hinge greatly on the costs of search that consumers encounter.

Another way to phrase this story is based on the nature of the demand curve facing each seller. In a purely competitive case, the demand curve is completely flat in the usual price-quantity diagram, and we describe each seller as a price taker. Each seller has no control over the price it receives. In the other extreme—the monopoly market—the demand curve facing the seller is downward sloped, and in fact is the same (by definition) as the market demand curve (derived by adding all of the demand curves of all of the consumers in the market). In the monopolistic competition model, the demand curve facing each seller is a mix of those two cases, the mix being determined by the extent of consumer shopping taking place. With much shopping occurring, the mix mostly contains the competitive model (a flat demand curve). With little shopping occurring, the mix mostly reflects the monopoly model (a downward-sloping demand curve reflecting the market demand curve). Thus, the slope of the demand curve facing each firm in a monopolistically competitive market must lie somewhere between the slope of the market demand curve and a slope of zero (a horizontal, flat demand curve).

Figure A.8 shows the final equilibrium picture for each firm in the market. The demand curve still slopes downward (because incomplete shopping mixes in some of the slope of the market demand curve with the flat demand curve of pure competition). However, profits must fall to zero because of the presumption of completely free (unfettered) entry. The latter condition occurs when the average costs of production just match the price received by the firm. Thus, to understand the monopolistically competitive equilibrium, we need to know the average cost curve of the firm (but not its marginal cost as in the case of purely competitive markets or monopoly markets). Entry by competitors spreads the available customers around to different firms, which we portray by showing that as entry occurs, the demand curve for the firm shifts inward (while still retaining a nonzero slope because of incomplete shopping). The

FIGURE A.8

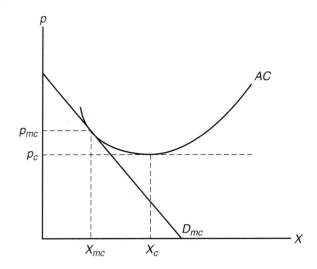

shift inward can and must continue only to the point at which revenue from sales just covers costs of production. This takes place when the demand curve for each firm has shifted in to the point at which it just touches the *AC* curve of the firm at one point (on the left-hand branch of the *AC* curve). This defines the monopolistically competitive equilibrium: Each firm's demand curve is tangent to its *AC* curve, so each firm makes no unusually large profits, and each firm faces a downward sloping demand curve.

The equilibrium price charged by this firm will be p_{mc} and its output will be X_{mc}. Obviously, the price will be higher than the competitive case [where $P_c = \min(AC)$], and each firm's output will be lower than would occur in a competitive market. As a final observation, we might note that if the extent of comparison shopping increased sufficiently, the demand curves facing each firm would rotate more and more toward the flat demand curves facing a competitive firm, and when enough shopping takes place (it turns out not to require 100% of the buyers to carry out comparison shopping), the market "collapses" to the competitive equilibrium.

BIBLIOGRAPHY

Aaron, H. J., and Schwartz, W. B., *The Painful Prescription: Rationing Hospital Care*, Washington, DC: The Brookings Institution, 1984.

Aber, M., and McCormick, C., "Risk Adjustment and the Health of the Medicare HMO Population," *Health Care Financing Review* 2000, Spring.

Alchien, A. A., *The Economics of Charity: Essays on the Comparative Economics of Giving and Selling, with Applications to Blood*, London: Institute of Economic Affairs, 1973.

AMA, Center for Health Policy Research, "Physician Socioeconomic Statistics 2003 Edition: Profiles for Detailed Specialties, Selected States and Practice Arrangements," in J.D. Wassenaar and S.L. Thran, eds., Chicago: AMA Press, 2003.

American Hospital Association, *Trendwatch Chartbook 2008*, Chicago: American Hospital Association 2008.

American Medical Association, *Current Procedural Terminology (CPT)*, 4th ed., Chicago: The American Medical Association, 1990.

American Medical Association, *Physician Socioeconomic Statistics*, Chicago: American Medical Association, 1994.

Anderson, O. W., *Blue Cross Since 1929: Accountability and the Public Trust*, Cambridge, MA: Ballinger Publishing Company, 1975.

Arrow, K. J., "Gifts and Exchanges," *Philosophy and Public Affairs* 1972; 1:343–362.

Arrow, K. J., "Uncertainty and the Welfare Economics of Medical Care," *American Economic Review* 1963; 53(5):941–973.

Association of American Medical Colleges, "Rising Medical Students Indebtedness," *Contemporary Issues in Medical Education* December 1999; 2(5):1–2.

Association of American Medical Colleges, *Trends: US Medical School Applicants, Matriculants, Graduates, 1994*, Washington, DC: AAMC, April 1995.

Auster, R., and Oaxaca, R., "Identification of Supplier-Induced Demand in the Health Care Sector," *Journal of Human Resources* 1981; 16:124–133.

Axelrod, R. C., *The Evolution of Cooperation*, New York: Basic Books, 1984.

Ballard, C. L., and Goddeeris, J. H., "Financing Universal Health Care in the United States: A General Equilibrium Analysis of Efficiency and Distributional Effects," *National Tax Journal*, March 1999; 52(3):31–51.

Bator, F., "The Simple Analytics of Welfare Maximization," *American Economic Review* March 1957; 47:22–59.

Becker, E. C., Dunn, D., and Hsiao, W. C., "Relative Cost Differences Among Physicians' Specialty Practices," *Journal of the American Medical Association* 1988; 260(16):2397–2402.

Becker, E. R., and Sloan, F. A., "Hospital Ownership and Performance," *Economic Inquiry* 1985; 23(1):21–36.

Becker, G. S., "Theory of the Allocation of Time," *Economic Journal* 1965; 75:493–517.

Becker, G. S., Grossman, M., and Murphy, K. M., "Rational Addiction and the Effect of Price on Consumption," *American Economic Review* 1991; 81(2):237–224.

Benham, L., "The Effect of Advertising on the Price of Eyeglasses," *Journal of Law and Economics* 1972; 15(2):337–352.

Benham, L., and Benham, A., "Regulating Through the Professions: A Perspective on Information Control," *Journal of Law and Economics* 1975; 18:421–447.

Benham, L., Maurizi, A., and Reder, M., "Migration, Location and Remuneration of Medical Personnel: Physicians and Dentists," *Review of Economics and Statistics* 1968; 50(3):332–347.

Blumberg, L. J., Dubay, L., and Norton, S. A., "Did the Medicaid Expansions for Children Displace Private Insurance? An Analysis Using the SIPP," *Journal of Health Economics* 2000; 19(1):33–60.

Boardman, A. E., Dowd, B., Eisenberg, J. M., and Williams, S., "A Model of Physicians' Practice Attributes Determination," *Journal of Health Economics* 1983; 2(3):259–268.

Booten, L. A., and Lane, J. I., "Hospital Market Structure and the Return to Nursing Education," *Journal of Human Resources* 1985; 20(2):184–196.

Bovjberg, R. R., *Medical Malpractice: Problems and Reforms,* Washington, DC: The Urban Institute, 1995.

Brennan, T. A., Leape, L. L., Laird, N. M., Hebert, L., Localio, A. R., Lawthers, A. G., Newhouse, J. P., Weiler, P. C., and Hyatt, H. H., "Incidence of Adverse Events and Negligence in Hospitalized Patients," *New England Journal of Medicine* 1991; 324(6):370–376.

Brook, R. H., Ware, J. E., Rogers, W. H., et al., "Does Free Care Improve Adults' Health? Results from a Randomized Controlled Trial," *New England Journal of Medicine* 1983; 309(24):1426–1434.

Buchanan, J., and Cretin, S., "Fee-for-Service Health Care Expenditures: Evidence of Selection Effects Among Subscribers Who Choose HMOs," *Medical Care* 1986; 24(1):39–51.

Buchanan, J., and Hosek, S., "Costs, Productivity, and the Utilization of Physician Extenders in Air Force Primary Medicine Clinics," Santa Monica, CA: The RAND Corporation Report R-2896-AF, June 1983.

Bunker, J. P., and Brown, B. W., "The Physician-Patient as Informed Consumer of Surgical Services," *New England Journal of Medicine* 1974; 290(19):1051–1055.

Bureau of Health Professions, *Physician Supply and Demand: Projections to 2020*, US Department of Health and Human Services, HRSA, October 2006.

Burstein, P. L., and Cromwell, J., "Relative Incomes and Rates of Return for U.S. Physicians," *Journal of Health Economics* 1985; 4:63–78.

Business Wire, "Striking Price Differences Persist in Medigap," 2005.

Cady, J. F., "An Estimate of the Price Effects of Restrictions on Drug Price Advertising," *Economic Inquiry* 1976; 14:493–510.

Calle, E. E., Thun, M. J., Petrelli, J. M., et al., "Body-Mass Index and Mortality in a Prospective Cohort of US Adults," *New England Journal of Medicine* 1999; 341:1097–1105.

Carter, G. M., Newhouse, J. P., and Relles, D. A., "How Much Change in the Case Mix Index Is DRG Creep?" *Journal of Health Economics* 1990; 9(4):411–428.

CBO (Congressional Budget Office), "Effective Marginal Tax Rates on Labor Income," Washington, DC: Government Printing Office, 2005.

Chamberlin, E. H., *The Theory of Monopolistic Competition*, 8th ed., Cambridge: Harvard University Press, 1962.

Chassin, M. R., Brook, R. H., Park, R. E., et al., "Variations in Use of Medical and Surgical Services by the Medicare Population," *New England Journal of Medicine* 1986; 314(5):285–290.

Chou, S. Y., Grossman, M., and Saffer, H., "An Economic Analysis of Adult Obesity: Results from the Behavioral Risk Factor Surveillance System," *Journal of Health Economics* 2004; 23(3):565–587.

Clay, S. W., and Conaster, R. R., "Characteristics of Physicians Disciplined by the State Medical Board of Ohio," *Journal of the American Osteopathic Association* 2003; 108(2):81–88.

Coase, R., "The Nature of the Firm," *Economica* 1937, New Series; 4:386–405.

Coase, R., "The Problem of Social Cost," *Journal of Law and Economics* 1960; 3:1–45.

Coffey, R. M., "The Effect of Time Prices on the Demand for Medical Services," *Journal of Human Resources* 1983; 18:407–444.

Coggon, D., Reading, I., Croft, P., et al, "Knee Osteoarthritis and Obesity," *International Journal of Obesity* 2001; 25(5):622–627.

Cohen, J. W., "Medicaid Physician Fees and Use of Physician and Hospital Services," *Inquiry* 1993; 30(3):281–292.

Connor, R. A., Feldman, R. D., and Dowd, B. E., "The Effects of Market Concentration and Horizontal Mergers on Hospital Costs and Prices," *International Journal of the Economics of Business* 1998; 5(2):159–180.

Cook, P., Moore, M. J., "Alcohol" in *Handbook of Health Economics,* in Culyer A. J. and Newhouse, J. P., eds, pp. 1629–1673, Amsterdam: Elsevier Science BV, 2000.

Cook, P. J., and Graham, D. A., "The Demand for Insurance and Protection: The Case of Irreplaceable Commodities," *Quarterly Journal of Economics* 1977; 91(1):143–156.

Cook, P. J., and Tauchen G., "The Effect of Liquor Taxes on Heavy Drinking," *Bell Journal of Economics* 1982; 13(Autumn):379–390.

Corder R., *The Red Wine Diet,* New York: The Penguin Group, 2007.

Cordingly, D., *Under the Black Flag,* New York: Harcourt Brace, 1997.

Courtemanche, C. A., "Silver Lining? The Connection Between Gasoline Prices and Obesity," *Social Science Research Network,* 2007 December.

Cowing, T. G., Holtman, A. G., and Powers, S., "Hospital Cost Analysis: A Survey and Evaluation of Recent Studies," *Advances in Health Economics and Health Services Research* 1983; 4.

Cromwell, J., and Mitchell, J. B., "Physician-Induced Demand for Surgery," *Journal of Health Economics* 1986; 5:293–313.

CRS, "CRS Report to the Congress: U.S. Health Care Spending: Comparison with Other OECD Countries," Congressional Research Service of the United States Congress, September 17, 2007.

Cullen, T. J., Hart, L. G., Whitcomb, M. E., Lishner, D. M., and Rosenblatt, R. A., *The National Health Service Corps: Rural Physician Service and Retention,* Seattle: WAMI Rural Health Research Center, 1994, pp. 1–21.

Cullis, J. G., Jones P. R., and Propper, C., "Waiting Lists and Medical Treatment," in A. J. Culyer and J. P. Newhouse, eds., *Handbook of Health Economics,* Amsterdam: Elsevier Science BV, 2000.

Culyer, A. J., "Cost Containment in Europe," *Health Care Financing Review* December 1989, Annual Supplement; 21–32.

Cumming, P. D., Wallace, E. L., Schorr, J. B., and Dodd, R. Y., "Exposure of Patients to Human Immunodeficiency Virus Through the Transfusion of Blood Components That Test Antibody Negative," *New England Journal of Medicine* 1989; 321(14):941–946.

Cutler, D. M., and Gruber, J., "Does Public Health Insurance Crowd Out Private Insurance?" *Quarterly Journal of Economics* 1996; 111(2):391–430.

Cutler, D. M., and McClellan, M., "Is Technological Change in Medicine Worth It?" *Health Affairs* 2001; 20(5):11–29.

Cutler, D. M., and Meara, E., "The Technology of Birth: It is Worth It?" in A.M. Garber, ed., *Frontiers in Health Policy Research,* Cambridge, MA: MIT Press, 2000.

Cutler, D. M., McClellan, M., and Newhouse, J.P., "How Does Managed Care Do It?" *RAND Journal of Economics* 2000; 31(3):526–548.

Cutler, D. M., McClellan, M. B., Newhouse, J. P., and Remler, D., "Are Medical Prices Declining? Evidence from Heart Attack Treatments," *Quarterly Journal of Economics* 1998; 113(4):991–1024.

Danzon, P. M., "An Economic Analysis of the Medical Malpractice System," *Behavioral Sciences and the Law* 1983; 1(1):39–54.

Danzon, P. M., "Liability and Liability Insurance for Medical Malpractice," *Journal of Health Economics* 1985a; 4:309–331.

Danzon, P. M., "Liability for Medical Malpractice: Incidence and Incentive Effects," University of Pennsylvania, Working Paper, 1990.

Danzon, P. M., "Tort Liability: A Minefield for Managed Care," *Journal of Legal Studies* 1997; 26(2):491–519.

Danzon, P. M., *Medical Malpractice: Theory, Evidence and Public Policy,* Cambridge, MA: Harvard University Press, 1985b.

Danzon, P. M., and Lillard, L. A., "Settlement Out of Court: The Disposition of Medical Malpractice Claims," *Journal of Legal Studies* 1982; 12(2):345–377.

Danzon, P., and Pereira, N. S., "Why Sole-Supplier Vaccine Markets May Be Here To Stay," *Health Affairs* 2005; 24(3):694–696.

Darby, M. R., and Karni, E., "Free Competition and the Optimal Amount of Fraud," *Journal of Law and Economics* 1973; 16(1):67–88.

Davidson, S. M., Singer, J. D., Davidson, H. S., Fairchild, P., and Graham, S., "Physician Retention in Community Health Centers," Report to the Agency for Health Care Policy and Research, Report Number HS07053, Boston: John Snow Inc., 1996.

Davis, K., "Comment on 'What Can Americans Learn from Europeans?'" *Health Care Financing Review* December 1989, annual supplement; 104–107.

Davis, K., and Russell, L. B., "The Substitution of Hospital Outpatient Care for Inpatient Care," *Review of Economics and Statistics* 1972; 54(1):109–120.

Decker, S. L., "Medicaid physician fees and the quality of medical care of Medicaid patients in the USA," *Review of Economics of the Household* 2007; 5(1): 95–112.

DeNavas-Walt, C., Proctor, B. D., and Lee, C. H., "Income, Poverty and Health Insurance Coverage in the United States, 2005," US Census Bureau Current Population Reports P60-231 Washington, DC: U.S. Government Printing Office, 2006.

Department of Health and Human Services, *International Classification of Diseases (ICD-9-CM),* 2nd ed., Washington, DC: U.S. Government Printing Office (PHS)-80-1260, September 1980.

Detsky, A. S., "Are Clinical Trials a Cost-Effective Investment?", *JAMA* October 6, 1989; 262:13(1795–1800).

Detsky, A. S., "Using Cost-Effectiveness Analysis to Improve the Efficiency of Allocating Funds to Clinical Trials," *Statistics in Medicine* 1990; 9:173–183.

DeVany, A. S., House, D. R., and Saving, T. R., "The Role of Patient Time in the Pricing of Dental Services: The Fee-Provider Density Relation Explained," *Southern Economic Journal* 1983; 49(3):669–680.

Diehr, P., Cain, K. C., Kreuter, W., and Rosenkranz, S., "Can Small Area Analysis Detect Variation in Surgery Rates? The Power of Small Area Variations Analysis," *Medical Care* June 1992; 30(6):484–502.

Dionne, G., "Search and Insurance," *International Economic Review* 1984; 25(2):357–367.

Division of Vaccine Injury Compensation, "National Vaccine Compensation Program Strategic Plan," Department of Health and Human Services, Health Services and Resource Administration, 2006.

Donohue, J. M., Cevasco, M., and Rosenthal, M. B., "A Decade of Direct-to-Consumer Advertising of Prescription Drugs," *New England Journal of Medicine* 2007; 357(7):673–681.

Dranove, D., "Demand Inducement and the Physician/Patient Relationship," *Economic Inquiry* 1988a; 26(2):281–298.

Dranove, D., "Pricing by Non-Profit Institutions," *Journal of Health Economics* 1988b; 7(1):47–57.

Dranove, D., and Satterthwaite, M. A., "The Industrial Organization of Health Care Markets," in A. J. Culyer and J. P. Newhouse, eds., *Handbook of Health Economics,* Amsterdam: Elsevier, Inc., 2000.

Dranove, D., and Wehner, P., "Physician-Induced Demand for Childbirths," *Journal of Health Economics* 1994; 13:61–73.

Dranove, D., and White, W. D., "Agency and the Organization of Health Care Delivery," *Inquiry* 1987; 24:405–415.

Dranove, D., Shanley, M., and White, W., "Price and Concentration in Hospital Markets: The Switch from Patient-Driven to Payer-Driven Competition," *Journal of Law and Economics* 1993; 34:179–204.

Dudley, R. A., and Luft, H. S., "Managed Care in Transition," *The New England Journal of Medicine,* 2001; 344(14):1087–1092.

Eckert, R. D., and Wallace, E. L., *Securing a Safer Blood Supply,* Washington, DC: American Enterprise Institute, 1985.

Economic Research Service, *Tobacco Outlook Report,* U.S. Dept. of Agriculture, Washington, DC: U.S. Government Printing Office, 2007.

Ehrlich, I., and Becker, G., "Market Insurance, Self Insurance and Self-Protection," *Journal of Political Economy* 1973; 80(4):623–648.

Ellis, R. P., and McGuire, T. G., "Cost Sharing and the Use of Ambulatory Mental Health Services," *American Psychologist* 39:1195–1199, 1984.

Emanuel, E. J., and Emanuel, L. L., "Four Models of the Physician-Patient Relationship," *JAMA* 1992; 267:2221–2226.

Employee Benefits Research Institute, EBRI Databook on Employee Benefits, Washington, DC, 1992.

Epstein, A. A., Stem, R. S., and Weissman, J. S., "Do the Poor Cost More? A Multihospital Study of Patients' Socioeconomic Status and Use of Hospital Resources," *New England Journal of Medicine* 1990; 322(16): 1122–1128.

Epstein, R. A., and Sykes, A. O., "The Assault on Managed Care: Vicarious Liability, Class Actions and the Patients' Bill of Rights," University of Chicago Law School Working Paper No. 112, December 8, 2000.

Epstein, R. M., Shields, C. G., Franks, P. et al. "Exploring and Validating Patient Concerns: Relation to Prescribing for Depression" *Annals of Family Medicine* 2007; 5(1):21–28.

Escarce, J. J., Polsky, D., Wozniak, G. D., Pauly, M., and Kletke, P. R., "Health Maintenance Organization Penetration and the Practice Location Choices of New Physicians," *Medical Care* 1998; 36:1555–1566.

Evans, R. G., "Supplier-Induced Demand," in M. Perlman, ed., *The Economics of Health and Medical Care,* London: Macmillan, 1974, pp. 162–173.

Evans, R. G., Lomas, J., Barer, M. L., et al., "Controlling Health Expenditures— The Canadian Reality," *New England Journal of Medicine* 1989; 320(9):571–577.

Evans, R. G., Parish, E. M. A., and Scully, F., "Medical Productivity, Scale Effects, and Demand Generation," *Canadian Journal of Economics* 1973; 6:376–393.

Farber, H. S., and White, M. J., "Medical Malpractice: An Empirical Examination of the Litigation Process," *RAND Journal of Economics* 1991; 22(2):199–217.

Farley, P. J., "Theories of the Price and Quantity of Physician Services: A Synthesis and Critique," *Journal of Health Economics* 1986; 5:315–333.

Feenberg, D., and Coutts, E., "An Introduction to the TaxSim Model," *Journal of Policy Analysis and Management* 1993; 12(1):189–194.

Feldman, R., "Price and Quality Differences in the Physicians' Services Market," *Southern Economic Journal* 1979; 45:885–891.

Feldman, R., and Begun, J. W., "The Effect of Advertising: Lessons from Optometry," *Journal of Human Resources* 1978; 13(Supplement):253–262.

Feldman, R., and Dowd, B., "Is There a Competitive Market for Hospital Services?" *Journal of Health Economics* 1986; 5:277–292.

Feldstein, M. S., "Hospital Cost Inflation: A Study of Nonprofit Price Dynamics," *American Economic Review* 1971; 61:853–872.

Feldstein, M. S., "Tax Incidence in a Growing Economy with Variable Factor Supply," *Quarterly Journal of Economics* 1974; 88:551–573.

Fisher, E. S., Wennberg, J. E., Stukel, T. A., et al., "Associations Among Hospital Capacity, Utilization, and Mortality of US Medicare Beneficiaries,

Controlling for Sociodemographic Factors," *Health Services Research* 2000; 34(6):1351–1362.

Fox v. Health Net of California. California Superior Court, Riverside County, No. 219692.

Frank, R. G., Berndt, E. R., Busch, S. H., and Triplett, J. E., "Measuring the Prices of Medical Treatments," Washington, DC: Brookings Institution, 1999.

Frayling, T. M., Timpson, N. J., Weedon, N., et al., "A Common Variant in the FTO Gene Is Associated with Body Mass Index and Predisposes to Childhood and Adult Obesity," *Science* 2007; 316:889–894.

Friedman, B., and Pauly, M. V., "Cost Functions for a Service Firm with Variable Quality and Stochastic Demand," *Review of Economics and Statistics* 1981; 63(4):620–624.

Friedman, M., *Capitalism and Freedom,* Chicago: University of Chicago Press, 1962.

Friedman, M., *Essays in Positive Economics,* Chicago: University of Chicago Press, 1966.

Friedman, M., and Kuznets, S., "Income from Independent Professional Practice," New York: National Bureau of Economic Research General Series No. 45, 1945.

Frymoyer, J. W., "Back Pain and Sciatica," *New England Journal of Medicine* 1988; 318(5):291–300.

Fuchs, V., "Time Preference and Health: An Exploratory Study," in V. Fuchs, ed., *Economic Aspects of Health,* Chicago: University of Chicago Press for NBER, 1982.

Fuchs, V. R., "Comment," *Journal of Health Economics* 1986; 5(3):367.

Fuchs, V. R., "The Supply of Surgeons and the Demand for Operations," *Journal of Human Resources* 1978; 13(Supplement):35–56.

Fuchs, V. R., and Hahn, J. S., "How Does Canada Do It? A Comparison of Expenditure for Physicians' Services in the United States and Canada," *New England Journal of Medicine* 1990; 323(13):884–890.

Fuchs, V. R., and Kramer, M., "Determinants of Expenditures for Physicians' Services," Washington, DC: U.S. Dept. of Health, Education and Welfare, 1972.

Gagnon, M. A., and Lexchin, J., "The Cost of Pushing Pills: A New Estimate of Pharmaceutical Promotion Expenditures in the United States," 2008; 5(1).

Garber, A. M., and McClellan, M. B. "Satisfaction Guaranteed—'Payment by Results' for Biologic Agents," *New England Journal of Medicine* 2007; 357(16):1575–1577.

Garber, A. M., and Phelps, C. E., "Economic Foundations of Cost-Effectiveness Analysis, Journal of Health Economics," 1997; 16(1):1–31.

Gaynor, M., and Gertler, P., "Moral Hazard and Risk Spreading in Partnerships," *RAND Journal of Economics* Winter 1995; 26(4):591–613.

Gaynor, M., Li, J., and Vogt, W. B., "Substitution, Spending Offsets, and Prescription Drug Benefit Design," *Forum for Health Economics & Policy* 2007; 10(2):1–31.

Gerdtham, U., Anderson, F., Sogaard, J., and Jonsson, B., "Economic Analysis of Health Care Expenditures: A Cross-Sectional Study of the OECD Countries," CMT Rapport 1988: Linkoping, Sweden: Centre for Medical Technology Assessment, 1988.

Ginsberg, P., "Altering the Tax Treatment of Employment-Based Health Plans," *Milbank Memorial Fund Quarterly* 1981; 59(2):224–255.

Glied, S., "Managed Care," in A. J. Culyer, and J. P. Newhouse, eds., *Handbook of Health Economics,* Amsterdam: Elsevier Science BV, 2000.

Glover, J. A., "The Incidence of Tonsillectomy in School Children," *Proceedings of the Royal Society of Medicine* 1938; 31:1219–1236.

Goldberg, G. A., Maxwell-Jolly, D., Hosek, S., and Chu, D. S. C., "Physician's Extenders' Performance in Air Force Clinics," *Medical Care* 1981; 19:951–965.

Goldstein, G. S., and Pauly, M. V., "Group Health Insurance as a Local Public Good," in R. N. Rosett, ed., *The Role of Health Insurance in the Health Services Sector,* New York: National Bureau for Economic Research, 1976, pp. 73–110.

Goodrich v. Aetna U.S. Healthcare, Inc., No. RCV020499 (Cal. App. Dept. Super. Ct. Jan. 20, 1999).

Gould, J., "The Economics of Legal Conflicts," *Journal of Legal Studies* 1973; 2(2):279–300.

Grabowski, H., "Encouraging the Development of New Vaccines," *Health Affairs* 2005; 24(3):697–700.

Graham, J. D., and Vopel, J. W., "Value of a Life: What Difference Does It Make?" *Risk Analysis* 1981; 1(1):89–95.

Grannemann, T. W., "Reforming National Health Insurance for the Poor," in M. V. Pauly, ed., *National Health Insurance: What Now, What Later, What Never?* Washington, DC: American Enterprise Institute, 1980.

Grannemann, T. W., Brown, R. S., and Pauly, M. V., "Estimating Hospital Costs—A Multiple-Output Analysis," *Journal of Health Economics* 1986; 5(2):107–127.

Green, J., "Physician-Induced Demand for Medical Care," *Journal of Human Resources* 1978; 13(Supplement):21–33.

Greenlick, M. R., and Darsky, B. J., "A Comparison of General Drug Utilization in a Metropolitan Community with Utilization Under a Drug Prepayment Plan," *American Journal of Public Health* 1968; 58(11):2121–2136.

Gronbaek, M., Becker, U., Johanson, D., et al., "Type of Alcohol Consumed and Mortality From All Causes, Coronary Heart Disease, and Cancer," *Annals of Internal Medicine* 2000; 133:411–419.

Grossman, M., "On the Concept of Health Capital and the Demand for Health," *Journal of Political Economy* 1972b; 80(2):223–255.

Grossman, M., *The Demand for Health: A Theoretical and Empirical Investigation,* New York: Columbia University Press (for the National Bureau for Economic Research), 1972a.

Grossman, M., "The Human Capital Model," in A. J. Culyer, and J. P. Newhouse, eds., *Handbook of Health Economics,* Amsterdam: Elsevier Science BV, 2000, Chapter 7.

Grossman, M., and Chaloupka, F., "The Demand for Cocaine by Young Adults: A Rational Addiction Approach," *Journal of Health Economics* 1998; 17(4):427–474.

Gruber, J., and Owings, M., "Physician Financial Incentives and Cesarean Section Delivery," *RAND Journal of Economics* 1996; 27:99–123.

Gruber, J., and Simon, K., "Crowd-Out Ten Years Later: Have Recent Public Expansions Crowded Out Private Health Insurance?" National Bureau of Economic Research, NBER Working Paper Series, January 2007.

Guterman, S., *Putting Medicare in Context: How Does the Balanced Budget Act Affect Hospitals?* Washington, DC: The Urban Institute, 2000.

Hadley, J., Holohan, J., and Scanlon, W., "Can Fee for Service Co-Exist with Demand Creation?" *Inquiry* 1979; 16(3):247–258.

Halbrook, H. G., Jay, S. J., Lohrman, R. G., et al., "The Learning Curve and the Cost of Heart Transplantation," *Health Services Research* 1992; 27(2):219–228.

Hall, R. E., and Jones, C. I., "The Value of Life and the Rise in Health Spending," *Quarterly Journal of Economics* 2007; 122(1): 39–72.

Hamilton, V., and Hamilton, B., *Does Universal Health Insurance Equalize Access to Care? A Canadian-U.S. Comparison,* McGill University, Working Paper, 1993.

Handy, B. M., Phelps, C. E., Mooney, C., Mushlin, A. I., and Perkins, N. A. K., "A Comparison of Three Methods of Case-Mix Adjustment in Physician Level Analysis of Practice Variations," Working Paper, Dept. of Community and Preventive Medicine, University of Rochester, July 1994.

Harberger, A. C., "Three Basic Postulates for Applied Welfare Economics: An Interpretive Essay," *Journal of Economic Literature* 1971; 9(3):785–797.

Harris, J., "The Internal Organization of Hospitals: Some Economic Implications," *Bell Journal of Economics* 1977; 8:467–482.

Harris, J. E., "Regulation and Internal Control in Hospitals," *Bulletin of the New York Academy of Medicine* 1979; 55(1):88–103.

Harvard Medical Malpractice Study, *Patient, Doctors, Lawyers: Medical Injury, Malpractice Litigation and Patient Compensation in New York,* Cambridge, MA: Harvard University, 1990.

Hay, J., and Leahy, M., "Physician-Induced Demand: An Empirical Analysis of the Consumer Information Gap," *Journal of Health Economics* 1982; 3:231–244.

Health Care Financing Review, International Comparison of Health Care Financing and Delivery: Data and Perspectives 1989; 7 (Annual Supplement).

Health Insurance Association of America, *Source Book of Health Insurance Data—1989,* Washington, DC: 1989.

Health Insurance Association of America, *Source Book of Health Insurance Data—1993,* Washington, DC: 1993.

Held, P., "Access to Medical Care in Designated Physician Shortage Areas: An Economic Analysis." Princeton: Mathematica Policy Research, June 1976.

Herfindahl, O. C., "Concentration in the US Steel Industry," Unpublished Doctoral Dissertation, Columbia University, 1950.

Hershey, J., Kunreuther, H., Schwartz, J. S., and Williams, S. V., "Health Insurance Under Competition: Would People Choose What Is Expected?" *Inquiry* 1984; 21(4):349–360.

Hickson, G. B., Altmeier, W. A., and Perrin, J. M., "Physician Reimbursement by Salary or Fee-for-Service: Effect on Physician Practice Behavior in a Randomized Prospective Study," *Pediatrics* 1987; 80(3):344–350.

Hillman, B. J., Joseph, C. A., Mabry, M. R., Sunshine, J. H., Kennedy, S. D., and Noether, M., "Frequency and Costs of Diagnostic Imaging in Office Practice: A Comparison of Self-Referring and Radiologist-Referring Physicians," *New England Journal of Medicine* 1990; 323:1604–1608.

Hirshman, A., *National Power and the Structure of Foreign Trade,* Berkeley: University of California Press, 1945.

Hodgkin, D., and McGuire, T. G., "Payment Levels and Hospital Response to Prospective Payment," *Journal of Health Economics* 1994; 13(1):1–29.

Hofer, T. P., and Hayward, R. A., "Identifying Poor-Quality Hospitals: Can Hospital Mortality Rates Detect Quality Problems for Medical Diagnoses?" *Medical Care* 1996; 34(8):737–753.

Hollingsworth, T. D., Ferguson, N. M., and Anderson, R. M., "Will Travel Restrictions Control the International Spread of Pandemic Influenza?" *Nature Medicine* 2006; 12:497–499.

Holmer, M., "Tax Policy and the Demand for Health Insurance," *Journal of Health Economics* 1984; 3:203–221.

Holzman, D., "Malpractice Crisis Therapies Vary," *Insight* December 12, 1988.

Hotelling, H., "Stability in Competition," *Economic Journal* 1929; 39:41–57.

Hsiao, W. C., Braun, P., Kelly, P. L., and Becker, E. C., "Results, Potential Effects and Implementation Issues of the Resource-Based Relative Value System," *Journal of the American Medical Association* 1988; 260(16): 2429–2438.

Hsiao, W., Braun, P., Yntema, D., and Becker, E., "Estimating Physicians' Work for a Resource-Based Relative Value System," *New England Journal of Medicine* 1988; 319(13):835–841.

Hughes, E. X. F., Fuchs, V. R., Jacoby, J. E., and Lewit, E. M., "Surgical Work Loads in a Community Practice," *Surgery* 1972; 71:315–327.

Iglehart, J. K., "Canada's Health Care System," *New England Journal of Medicine* 1986a; 315:202–208.

Iglehart, J. K., "Canada's Health Care System," *New England Journal of Medicine* 1986b; 315:778–784.

Iglehart, J. K., "Canada's Health Care System: Addressing the Problems of Physician Supply," *New England Journal of Medicine* 1986c; 315:1623–1628.

Iglehart, J. K., "Financing Vaccines: In Search Of Solutions That Work," *Health Affairs* 2005; 24(3):594–595.

Iglehart, J. K., "Health Policy Report: Canada's Health Care System Faces Its Problems," *New England Journal of Medicine* 1990; 322(8):562–568.

Iglehart, J. K., "Health Policy Report: Germany's Health Care System" (first of two parts), *New England Journal of Medicine* 1991a; 324(7):503–508.

Iglehart, J. K., "Health Policy Report: Germany's Health Care System" (second of two parts), *New England Journal of Medicine* 1991b; 324(24): 1750–1756.

Iglehart, J. K., "Health Policy Report: Japan's Medical Care System," *New England Journal of Medicine* 1988a; 319(12):807–812.

Iglehart, J. K., "Health Policy Report: Japan's Medical Care System—Part Two," *New England Journal of Medicine* 1988b; 319(17):1166–1171.

Iglehart, J. K., "The American Health Care System—Medicare," *New England Journal of Medicine* 1999; 340(4):317–332.

Ikegami, N., and Campbell, J. C., "Medical Care in Japan," *New England Journal of Medicine* 1995; 333(19):1295–1300.

Institute of Medicine, "Financing Vaccines in the 21st Century: Assuring Access and Availability," Washington, DC: National Academy Press, 2003.

Janerich, D. T., Thompson, W. D., Varela, L. R., et al., "Lung Cancer and Exposure to Tobacco Smoke in the Household," *New England Journal of Medicine* 1990; 323(10):632–636.

Joskow, P., *Controlling Hospital Costs: The Role of Government Regulation,* Cambridge: MIT Press, 1981.

Joyce, T., Corman, H., and Grossman, M., "A Cost-Effectiveness Analysis of Strategies to Reduce Infant Mortality," *Medical Care* 1988; 26(4):348–360.

Kahn, K. L., Draper, D., Keeler, E. B., et al., "The Effects of the DRG-Based Prospective Payment System on Quality of Care for Hospitalized Medicare Patients," Santa Monica, CA: The RAND Corporation, Report Number R-3931-HCFA, 1992.

Kahneman, D., and Tversky, A., "Prospect Theory: An Analysis of Decision Under Risk," *Econometrica* 1979; 47:263–289.

Kaiser Family Foundation, Data Source: Kaiser Commission on Medicaid and the Uninsured, statehealthfacts.org., 2008.

Kastler, J., Kane, R. L., Olsen, D. M., and Thetford, C., "Issues Underlying Prevalence of 'Doctor Shopping' Behavior," *Journal of Health and Social Behavior* 1976; 17:328–339.

Keeler, E. B., Buchanan, J. L., Rolph, J. E., et al., "The Demand for Episodes of Treatment in the Health Insurance Experiment," Santa Monica, CA: The RAND Corporation, Report R-3454-HHS, March 1988.

Keeler, E. B., Newhouse, J. P., and Phelps, C. E., "Deductibles and the Demand for Medical Care Services: The Theory of a Consumer Facing a Variable Price Schedule Under Uncertainty," *Econometrica* 1977; 45(3):641–655.

Keeler, E. B., Wells, K. B., Manning, W. G., Rumpel, J. D., and Hanley, J. M., *The Demand for Episodes of Mental Health Services*, RAND Corporation Report R-3432-NIMH, October 1986.

Kessel, R. A., "Price Discrimination in Medicine," *Journal of Law and Economics* 1958; 1(2):20–53.

Kessel, R. A., "Transfused Blood, Serum Hepatitis, and the Coase Theorem," *Journal of Law and Economics* 1974; 17:265–290.

Kessler, D., and McClellan, M., "Do Doctors Practice Defensive Medicine?", *Quarterly Journal of Economics* 1996; 111(2):353–390.

Kissick, W. L., Engstrom, P. F., Soper, K. A., and Peterson, O. L., "Comparison of Internist and Oncologist Evaluations of Cancer Patients' Need for Hospitalization," *Medical Care* 1984; 22(5):447–452.

Kitch, E. W., Isaac, M., and Kaspar, K., "The Regulation of Taxicabs in Chicago," *Journal of Law and Economics* 1971; 14(2):285–350.

Klatsky, A. L., Armstrong, M. A., and Kipp, H., "Correlates of Alcoholic Beverage Preference: Traits of Persons Who Choose Wine, Liquor or Beer," *Addiction* 1990; 85(10):1279–1289.

Kleimann, E., "The Determinants of National Outlay on Health," in M. Perlman, ed., *The Economics of Health and Medical Care*, London: Macmillan, 1974.

Kletke, P. R., Polsky, D., Wozniak, G. D., and Escarce, J. J., "The Effect of HMO Penetration on Physician Retirement, "*HSR: Health Services Research* 2000; 35(3):17–31.

Kwoka, J. E., "Advertising and the Price and Quality of Optometric Services," *American Economic Review* 1984; 74(1):211–216.

Lakdawalla, D., and Philipson, T., *The Growth of Obesity and Technological Change: A Theoretical and Empirical Examination,* Cambridge: National Bureau of Economic Research 2002, Working Paper 8926.

Lancaster, K., "A New Approach to Consumer Demand Theory," *Journal of Political Economy* 1966; 74(2):132–157.

Lave, J. R., and Lave, L. B., "Hospital Cost Functions," *American Economic Review* 1970; 58:379–395.

Lee, R. H., "Future Costs in Cost-Effectiveness Analysis," *Journal of Health Economics* 2008; 23(4):809–818.

Leffler, K., "Physician Licensure: Competition and Monopoly in American Medicine," *Journal of Law and Economics* 1978; 21(1):165.

Lerner, A. P., "The Concept of Monopoly and the Measurement of Monopoly Power," *Review of Economic Studies* 1934; 1:157–175.

Levy, M. A., Arnold, R. M., Fine, M. J., and Kapoor, W. N., "Professional Courtesy—Current Practices and Attitudes," *New England Journal of Medicine* 1993; 329(22):1627–1631.

Lewis, C. E., "Variations in the Incidence of Surgery," *New England Journal of Medicine* 1969; 281(16):880–884.

Liebowitz, A., Manning, W. G., and Newhouse, J. P., "The Demand for Prescription Drugs as a Function of Cost-Sharing," *Social Science and Medicine* 1985; 21:1063–1069.

Long, S. H., Settle, R. F., and Stuart, B. C., "Reimbursement and Access to Physicians' Services Under Medicaid," *Journal of Health Economics* 1986; 5:235–252.

Luft, H. S., "The Relationship Between Surgical Volume and Mortality: An Exploration of Causal Factors and Alternative Models," *Medical Care* 1980; 18:940–959.

Luft, H. S., *Health Maintenance Organizations: Dimensions of Performance,* New York: Wiley & Sons, 1981.

Luft, H. S., Bunker, J. P., and Enthoven, A. C., "Should Operations Be Regionalized? The Empirical Relation Between Surgical Volume and Mortality," *New England Journal of Medicine* 1979; 301:1364–1369.

Ma, C. A., and McGuire, T. G., "Optimal Health Insurance and Provider Payment," *American Economic Review* 1997; 87(4):685–704.

Magid, D. J., and Koepsell, T. D., et al. "Absence of Association Between Insurance Copayments and Delays on Seeking Emergency Care Among Patients with Myocardial Infarction," *New England Journal of Medicine* 1997; 336(24):1724–1729.

Manning, W. G., Benjamin, B., Bailit, H. L., and Newhouse, J. P., "The Demand for Dental Care: Evidence from a Randomized Trial in Health

Insurance," *Journal of the American Dental Association* 1985; 110: 895–902.

Manning, W. G., Keeler, E. B., Newhouse, J. P., Sloss, E. M., and Wasserman, J., "The Taxes of Sin: Do Smokers Pay Their Own Way?" *JAMA* 1989; 261(11):1604–1609.

Manning, W. G., Newhouse, J. P., Duan, N., et al., "Health Insurance and the Demand for Medical Care: Evidence from a Randomized Experiment," *American Economic Review* 1987; 77(3):251–277.

Manning, W. G., Wells, K. B., and Benjamin B., "Cost Sharing and the Use of Ambulatory Mental Health Services," *American Psychologist* 1984; 39:1077–1089.

Marder, W. D., and Willke, R. J., "Comparison of the Value of Physician Time by Specialty," in H. E. Frech III, ed., *Regulating Doctors' Fees: Competition, Benefits, and Controls Under Medicare*, Washington, DC: American Enterprise Institute, 1991, pp. 260–281.

Mark, D. B., Naylor, C. D., Hlatky, M. A., Califf, R. M., Topol, E. J., Granger, C. B., Knight, J. K., Nelson, C. L., Lee, K. L., Clapp-Channing, N. E. et al., "Use of Medical Resources and Quality of Life After Acute Myocardial Infarction in Canada and the United States," *New England Journal of Medicine* 1994; 331(17):1130–1135.

Marquis, M. S., "Cost Sharing and Provider Choice," *Journal of Health Economics* 1985; 4:137–157.

Marquis, M. S., and Holmer, M., "Choice Under Uncertainty and the Demand for Health Insurance," Santa Monica, CA: The RAND Corporation Note N-2516-HHS, September 1986.

Marquis, M. S., and Phelps, C. E., "Demand for Supplemental Health Insurance," *Economic Inquiry* 1987; 25(2):299–313.

Maxwell, R. J., *Health and Wealth: An International Study of Health-Care Spending*, Lexington, MA: Lexington Books, 1981.

McCarthy, T., "The Competitive Nature of the Primary-Care Physician Services Market," *Journal of Health Economics* 1985; 4(1):93–118.

McClellan, M., and Staiger, D., "Medical Care Quality in For-Profit and Not-for-Profit Organizations," in D. M. Cutler, ed., *The Changing Hospital Industry: Comparing Not-for-Profit and For-Profit Institutions*, Chicago: University of Chicago Press, 2000.

McCombs, J. S., "Physician Treatment Decisions in a Multiple Treatment Model," *Journal of Health Economics* 1984; 3(2):155–171.

McGinnis, J. M., and Foege, W. H., "Actual Causes of Death in the United States, *JAMA* November 10, 1993; 270(18):2207–2212.

McGuire, T. G., "Physician Agency" in Culyer, A. J., and Newhouse, J. P., eds, *Handbook of Health Economics*, Amsterdam: Elsevier Science BV, 2000.

McGuire, T. G., and Pauly, M. V., "Physician Response to Fee Changes with Multiple Payers," *Journal of Health Economics* 1991; 10(3):385–410.

McKenzie, G. W., *Measuring Economic Welfare: New Methods,* Cambridge: Cambridge University Press, 1983.

McKenzie, G., and Pearce, I., "Exact Measures of Welfare and the Cost of Living," *Review of Economic Studies* 1976; 43:465–468.

McLaughlin, C. G., Chernew, M., and Taylor, E. F., "Medigap Premiums and Medicare HMO Enrollment," *Health Services Research* 2002; 37(6):1445–1468.

McPherson, K., Strong, P. M., Epstein, A., and Jones, L., "Regional Variations in the Use of Common Surgical Procedures: Within and Between England and Wales, Canada, and the United States of America," *Social Science in Medicine* 1981; 15A:273–288.

McPherson, K., Wennberg, J. E., Hovind, O. B., and Clifford, P., "Small-Area Variations in the Use of Common Surgical Procedures: An International Comparison of New England, England, and Norway," *New England Journal of Medicine* 1982; 307(21):1310–1314.

Medicare Payment Advisory Commission, Report to the Congress: Medicare Payment Policy, Washington, DC: MedPac, 2003.

Melnick, G. A., and Zwanziger, J., "Hospital Behavior Under Competition and Cost-Containment Policies," *Journal of the American Medical Association* 1988; 260(18):2669–2675.

Mills, D. H., Boyden, J. S., Rubsamen, D. S., and Engle, H. L., *Report on Medical Insurance Feasibility Study,* San Francisco: California Medical Association, 1977.

Mitchell, B. M., and Phelps, C. E., "National Health Insurance: Some Costs and Effects of Mandated Employee Coverage," *Journal of Political Economy* 1976; 84(3):553–571.

Mitchell, J. M., and Scott, E., "New Evidence on the Prevalence and Scope of Physician Joint Ventures," *JAMA* 1992a; 268(1):80–84.

Mitchell, J. M., and Scott, E., "Physician Ownership of Physical Therapy Services: Effects on Charges, Utilization, Profits, and Service Characteristics," *JAMA* 1992b; 268(15):2055–2059.

Mobellia, P., "An Economic Analysis of Addictive Behavior: The Case of Gambling," City University of New York, Ph.D. Dissertation, 1991.

Mokdad, A. H., Marks, J. S., Stroup D. F., and Gerberding, J. L. "Actual Causes of Death in the United States, 2000," *JAMA* 2004; 291(10):1238–1245.

Moore, M. J., and Viscusi, W. K., "Doubling the Estimated Value of Life: Results Using New Occupational Fatality Data," *Journal of Policy Analysis and Management* 1988a; 7(3):476–490.

Moore, M. J., and Viscusi, W. K., "The Quantity-Adjusted Value of Life," *Economic Inquiry* 1988b; 31:369–388.

Moore, S. H., Martin, D. P., and Richardson, W. C., "Does the Primary-Care Gatekeeper Control the Costs of Health Care? Lessons from the SAFECO Experience," *New England Journal of Medicine* 1983, 309(22):1400–1404.

Morrison, J., and Wickersham, P., "Physicians Disciplined by a State Medical Board," *JAMA* 1998; 279:1889–1893.

Mukamel, D. B., and Mushlin, A. I., "Quality of Care Information Makes a Difference: An Analysis of Market Shares and Price Changes Following Publication of the New York State Cardiac Surgery Reports," *Medical Care* 1998; 36(7):945–954.

Mullahy, J., and Sindelar, J. L., "Alcoholism, Work, and Income," *Journal of Labor Economics* 1993; 11(3): 494–520.

Nelson, D. E., Giovino, G. A., Emont, S. L., et al., "Trends in Cigarette Smoking Among US Physicians and Nurses," *JAMA* 1994; 271(16):1273–1275.

Newhouse, J. P., "A Design for a Health Insurance Experiment," *Inquiry* 1974; 11(3):5–27.

Newhouse, J. P., "A Model of Physician Pricing," *Southern Economic Journal* 1970a; 37(2):174–183.

Newhouse, J. P., "Medical Care Expenditure: A Cross-National Survey," *Journal of Human Resources* 1977; 12:115–125.

Newhouse, J. P., "The Economics of Group Practice," *Journal of Human Resources* 1973; 8(1):37–56.

Newhouse, J. P., "Toward a Theory of Nonprofit Institutions: An Economic Model of a Hospital," *American Economic Review* 1970b; 60(1):64–74.

Newhouse, J. P., Phelps, C. E., and Marquis, M. S., "On Having Your Cake and Eating It Too: Econometric Problems in Estimating the Demand for Health Services," *Journal of Econometrics* 1980; 13(3):365–390.

Newhouse, J. P., Williams, A. P., Bennett, B. W., and Schwartz, W. B., "Does the Geographical Distribution of Physicians Reflect Market Failure?" *Bell Journal of Economics* 1982a; 13:493–505.

Newhouse, J. P., Williams, A. P., Bennett, B. W., and Schwartz, W. B., "Where Have All the Doctors Gone?" *Journal of the American Medical Association* 1982b; 247(17):2392–2396.

Nguyen, N. X., and Derrick, F. W., "Physician Behavioral Response to a Medicare Price Reduction," *Health Services Research,* August 1997; 32(3):283–298.

Noether, M., "The Effect of Government Policy Changes on the Supply of Physicians: Expansion of a Competitive Fringe," *Journal of Law and Economics* 1986; 29(2):231–262.

Office of Technology Assessment, U.S. Congress, *Defensive Medicine and Medical Malpractice,* Washington, DC: U.S. Government Printing Office, July 1994.

Ohnuki-Tierney, E., *Illness and Culture in Contemporary Japan: An Anthropological View,* Cambridge: Cambridge University Press, 1984.

Olsen, D. M., Kane, R. L., and Kastler, J., "Medical Care as a Commodity: An Exploration of the Shopping Behavior of Patients," *Journal of Community Health* 1976; 2(2):85–91.

Organization of Economic Cooperation and Development Health Data 2008: Statistics and Indicators for 30 Countries, Paris: OECD, 2008.

Park, R. E., Brook, R. H., Kosecoff, J, Keesey, et al., "Explaining Variations in Hospital Death Rates: Randomness, Severity of Illness, Quality of Care," *JAMA* 1990; 264(4):484–490.

Parkin, D., McGuire, A., and Yule, B., "Aggregate Health Care Expenditures and National Income: Is Health Care a Luxury Good?" *Journal of Health Economics* 1987; 6(2):109–128.

Pathman, D. E., Konrad, T. R., and Ricketts, T. C., "The Comparative Retention of National Health Service Corps and Other Rural Physicians: Results of a Nine-Year Follow-up Study." *JAMA* 1992; 268(12):1552–1558.

Pauker, S. G., and Kassirer, J. P., "The Threshold Approach to Clinical Decision Making," *New England Journal of Medicine* 1980; 302:1109–1117.

Pauly, M. V., "Medical Staff Characteristics and Hospital Costs," *Journal of Human Resources* 1978; 13(Supplement):77–111.

Pauly, M. V., "Taxation, Health Insurance, and Market Failure," *Journal of Economic Literature* 1986; 24(6):629–675.

Pauly, M. V., "The Economics of Moral Hazard," *American Economic Review* 1968; 58(3):531–537.

Pauly, M. V., "The Ethics and Economics of Kickbacks and Fee Splitting," *Bell Journal of Economics* 1979; 10(1):344–352.

Pauly, M. V., *Doctors and Their Workshops,* Chicago: University of Chicago Press, 1980.

Pauly, M. V., and Redisch, M., "The Not-for-Profit Hospital as a Physicians' Cooperative," *American Economic Review* 1973; 63(1):87–99.

Pauly, M. V., and Satterthwaite, M. A., "The Pricing of Primary Care Physicians' Services: A Test of the Role of Consumer Information," *Bell Journal of Economics* 1981; 12:488–506.

Pauly, M. V., Danzon, P., Feldstein, P., and Hoff, J., "A Plan for 'Responsible' National Health Insurance," *Health Affairs* Spring 1991; 10(1):5–25.

Perkins, N. K., Phelps, C. E., and Parente, S. T., "Age Discrimination in Resource Allocation Decisions: Evidence from Wrongful Death Awards," University of Rochester, Public Policy Analysis Program Working Paper, 1990.

Phelps, C. E., "Bug-Drug Resistance: Sometimes Less Is More," *Medical Care* 1989; 29(2):194–203.

Phelps, C. E., "Diffusion of Information in Medical Care," *Journal of Economic Perspectives* Summer 1992; 6(3):23–42.

Phelps, C. E., "Good Technologies Gone Bad: How and Why the Cost Effectiveness of Medical Interventions Changes for Different Populations," *Medical Decision Making* 1997; 17(1):107–112.

Phelps, C. E., "Induced Demand—Can We Ever Know Its Extent?" *Journal of Health Economics* 1986a; 5:355–365.

Phelps, C. E., "Information Diffusion and Best Practice Adoption," in A. J. Culyer, and J. P. Newhouse, eds., *Handbook of Health Economics,* Amsterdam: Elsevier Science BV, 2000.

Phelps, C. E., "Large-Scale Tax Reform: The Example of Employer-Paid Health Insurance Premiums," University of Rochester Working Paper No. 35, March 1986b.

Phelps, C. E., "The Demand for Health Insurance: A Theoretical and Empirical Investigation," Santa Monica, CA: The RAND Corporation Report R-1054-OEO, July 1973.

Phelps, C. E., "The Demand for Reimbursement Insurance," in R. N. Rosett, ed., *The Role of Health Insurance in the Health Services Sector,* New York: National Bureau for Economic Research, 1976.

Phelps, C. E., "The Origins and Purposes of Not for Profit Organizations," University of Rochester Working Paper, 2001.

Phelps, C. E., and Mooney, C., "Variations in Medical Practice Use: Causes and Consequences," in R. J. Arnould, R. F. Rich, and W. D. White, eds., *Competitive Approaches to Health Care Reform,* Washington, DC: The Urban Institute Press, 1993.

Phelps, C. E., and Newhouse, J. P., "Coinsurance, the Price of Time, and the Demand for Medical Services," *Review of Economics and Statistics* 1974; 56(3):334–342.

Phelps, C. E., and Newhouse, J. P., "Effects of Coinsurance: A Multivariate Analysis," *Social Security Bulletin* June 1972; 35(6):20–29.

Phelps, C. E., and Parente, S. T., "Priority Setting for Medical Technology and Medical Practice Assessment," *Medical Care* 1990; 28(8):703–723.

Phelps, C. E., and Sened, I., "Market Equilibrium with Not-for-Profit Firms," University of Rochester, Working Paper, 1990.

Phelps, C. E., Hosek, S., Buchanan, J., et al., "Health Care in the Military: Feasibility and Desirability of a Closed Enrollment System," Santa Monica, CA: The RAND Corporation Report R-3145-HA, April 1984.

Phelps, C. E., Mooney, C., Mushlin, A. I., et al., "Doctors Have Styles—And They Matter!" University of Rochester, Working Paper, 1994.

Polsky, D., Kletke, P., Wozniak, G., and Escarce, J., "HMO Penetration and the Geographic Mobility of Practicing Physicians," *Journal of Health Economics* 2000; 19(5):793–805.

Pope, G. C., Kautter, J., Ellis, R. P., et al., "Risk Adjustment of Medicare Capitation Payments Using the CMS-HCC Model," *Health Care Financing Review,* 2004 Summer.

Porter, M. E., and Teisberg, E. O., *Redefining Health Care,* Boston: Harvard Business School Press, 2006.

Poullier, J. P., "Health Data File: Overview and Methodology," *Health Care Financing Review* 1989, Annual Supplement; 111–118.

Pratt, J. W., Wise, D. A., and Zeckhauser, R., "Price Differences in Almost Competitive Markets," *Quarterly Journal of Economics* May 1979; 93:189– 211.

ProPAC (Prospective Payment Assessment Commission), *Medicare Prospective Payment and the American Health Care System: Report to the Congress,* Washington, DC: 1989.

Rawls, J., *A Theory of Justice.* Cambridge, MA: Harvard University Press, 1971.

Reinhardt, U., "A Production Function for Physician Services," *Review of Economics and Statistics* 1972; 54(1):55–66.

Reinhardt, U., "The Theory of Physician-Induced Demand: Reflections After a Decade," *Journal of Health Economics* 1985; 4(2):187–193.

Reinhardt, U. E., "Manpower Substitution and Productivity in Medical Practices: Review of Research," *Health Services Research* 1973; 8(3):200–227.

Reinhardt, U. E., *Physician Productivity and Demand for Health Manpower,* Cambridge, MA: Ballinger Publishing Company, 1975.

Rice, T. H., "Induced Demand—Can We Ever Know Its Extent?" *Journal of Health Economics* 1987; 6:375–376.

Rice, T. H., and Labelle, R. J., "Do Physicians Induce Demand for Medical Services?" *Journal of Health Politics, Policy and Law* 1989; 14(3):587–600.

Rodgers, J. F., and Muscaccio, R. A., "Physician Acceptance of Medicare Patients on Assignment," *Journal of Health Economics* 1983; 2(1):55–73.

Roemer, M. I., "Bed Supply and Hospital Utilization: A Natural Experiment," *Hospitals* 1961; 35:36–42.

Rogerson, W. P., "Choice of Treatment Intensitites by a Nonprofit Hospital Under Prospective Pricing," *Journal of Economics and Management Strategy,* 1994; 3(1):7–51.

Rolph, J. E., "Some Statistical Evidence on Merit Rating in Medical Malpractice Insurance," *Journal of Risk and Insurance* 1981; 48:247–260.

Rooks, J. P., Weatherby, N. L., Ernst, E. K. M., et al., "Outcomes of Care in Birth Centers: The National Birth Center Study," *New England Journal of Medicine* 1989; 321:1804–1811.

Roos, N. P., Flowerdew, G., Wajda, A., and Tate, R. B., "Variations in Physician Hospital Practices: A Population-Based Study in Manitoba, Canada," *American Journal of Public Health* 1986; 76(1):45–51.

Rosa, J. J., ed., *Advances in Health Economics and Health Services Research— Comparative Health Systems: The Future of National Health Care Systems and Economic Analysis,* Greenwich, CT: JAI Press, 1990 (Supplement).

Rosenthal, G., "Price Elasticity of Demand for General Hospital Services," in H. E. Klarman, ed., *Empirical Studies in Health Economics,* Baltimore: The Johns Hopkins University Press, 1970.

Rosett, R. N., and Huang, L. F., "The Effect of Health Insurance on the Demand for Medical Care," *Journal of Political Economy* 1973; 81:281–305.

Rossiter, L. F., and Wilensky, G. R., "A Reexamination of the Use of Physician Services: The Role of Physician-Initiated Demand," *Inquiry* 1983; 20: 231–244.

Roter, D. L., and Hall, J. A., *Doctors Talking to Patients/Patients Talking to Doctors: Improving Communication in Medical Visits.* Westport, CT: Auburn House, 1992.

Rothschild, M., and Stiglitz, J., "Equilibrium in Competitive Insurance Markets: An Essay on the Economics of Imperfect Information," *Quarterly Journal of Economics* 1976; 80:629–649.

Roueche, B., *Eleven Blue Men and Other Narratives of Medical Detection,* New York: Berkley Medallion Books, New Berkley Medallion Edition, 1965.

Russell, L. B., "The Cost Effectiveness of Preventive Services: Some Examples," in R. B. Goldbloom and R. S. Lawrence, eds., *Preventing Disease: Beyond the Rhetoric,* New York: Springer-Verlag, 1990.

Russell, L. B., and Manning, C. L., "The Effect of Prospective Payment on Medicare Expenditures," *New England Journal of Medicine* 1989; 320: 439–444.

Ruther, M., and Helbing, C., "Medicare Liability of Persons Using Reimbursed Physician Services: 1980," *Health Care Financing Notes,* December 1985.

Sadanand, A., and Wilde, L. L., "A Generalized Model of Pricing for Homogeneous Goods Under Imperfect Information," *Review of Economic Studies* 1982; 49:229–240.

Sandier, S., "Health Services Utilization and Income Trends," *Health Care Financing Review* December 1989, Annual Supplement: 33–48.

Sandler, D. P., Comstock, G. W., Helsing, K. J., and Shore, D. L., "Deaths from All Causes in Non-Smokers Who Lived with Smokers," *American Journal of Public Health* 1989; 79(2):163–167.

Satterthwaite, M. A., "Competition and Equilibrium as a Driving Force in the Health Services Sector," in R. P. Inman, ed., *Managing the Service Economy,* Cambridge: Cambridge University Press, 1985.

Satterthwaite, M. A., "Consumer Information, Equilibrium, Industry Price, and the Number of Sellers," *Bell Journal of Economics* 1979; 10(2):483– 502.

Scherer, F. C., "The Pharmaceutical Industry," in J. P. Newhouse and A. Culyer, eds., *Handbook of Health Economics,* Amsterdam: Elsevier, 2000.

Schieber, G. J., "Health Care Expenditures in Major Industrialized Countries, 1960–87," *Health Care Financing Review* 1990; 11(4):159–167.

Schieber, G. J., Poullier, J. P., and Greenwald, L. M., "US Health Expenditure Performance: An International Comparison and Data Update," *Health Care Financing Review* Summer 1992; 13(4):1–87.

Schwartz, A., and Wilde, L. L., "Competitive Equilibria in Markets for Heterogeneous Goods Under Imperfect Information: A Theoretical Analysis with Policy Implications," *Bell Journal of Economics* 1982a; 13(1):181–193.

Schwartz, A., and Wilde, L. L., "Imperfect Information, Monopolistic Competition, and Public Policy," *American Economic Review* May 1982b; 72(2):18–23.

Schwartz, A., and Wilde, L. L., "Intervening in Markets on the Basis of Imperfect Information," *Pennsylvania Law Review* 1979; 127:630–682.

Schwartz, W. B., Newhouse, J. P., Bennett, B. W., and Williams, A. P., "The Changing Geographic Distribution of Board-Certified Specialists," *New England Journal of Medicine* 1980; 303:1032–1038.

Scitovsky, A. A., "Changes in the Costs of Treatment of Selected Illnesses, 1951–1965," *American Economic Review* 1967; 57:1182–1195.

Scitovsky, A. A., and McCall, N. M., "Coinsurance and the Demand for Physician Services: Four Years Later," *Social Security Bulletin* 1977; 40:19–27.

Scitovsky, A. A., and Snyder, N. M., "Effect of Coinsurance on the Demand for Physician Services," *Social Security Bulletin* June, 1972; 35(6):3–19.

Seale, M. T., McGuire, T. G., and Zhang, W. "Time Allocation in Primary Care Office Visits" *Health Services Research* 2007; 20(9):1871–1894.

Shavell, S., "Strict Liability vs. Negligence," *Journal of Legal Studies* 1980; 9:1–25.

Shea, S., Stein, A. D., Basch, C. E., et al., "Independent Associations of Educational Attainment and Ethnicity with Behavioral Risk Factors for Cardiovascular Disease," *American Journal of Epidemiology* 1991; 134(6):567–582.

Shone, L. P., Lantz, P. M., Dick, A. W. et al, "Crowd-out in the State Children's Health Insurance Program (SCHIP): Incidence, Enrollee Characteristics and Experiences, and Potential Impact on New York's SCHIP," *Health Services Research* 2008, 43(1), Part II:419–434.

Showalter, M. H., "Physicians' cost shifting behavior: Medicaid versus other patients," *Contemporary Economic Policy* 1997; 15(2), 74–84.

Simon, C. J., Dranove, D., White, W. D., "The Effect of Managed Care on the Incomes of Primary and Specialty Physicians, *Health Services Research* 1998; 33(3):549–569.

Sloan, F. A., "Lifetime Earnings and Physicians' Choice of Specialty," *Industrial and Labor Relations Review* 1970; 24:47–56.

Sloan, F. A., and Feldman, R., "Competition Among Physicians," in W. Greenberg, ed., *Competition in the Health Care Sector: Past, Present, and Future.* Washington, DC: Federal Trade Commission, 1978.

Sloan, F. A., and Vraciu, R. A., "Investor-Owned and Not-for-Profit Hospitals: Addressing Some Issues," *Health Affairs* Spring 1983; 25–34.

Sloan, F. A., Blumstein, J. F., and Perrin, J. M., eds., *Uncompensated Hospital Care: Rights and Responsibilities,* Baltimore, The Johns Hopkins Press, 1986.

Sloan, F. A., Githens, P. B., Clayton, E. W., Hickson, G. B., Gentile, D. A., and Partlett, D. F., *Suing for Medical Malpractice,* Chicago: University of Chicago Press, 1993.

Sloan, F. A., Mergenhagen, P. M., Burfield, W. B., et al., "Medical Malpractice Experience of Physicians: Predictable or Haphazard?" *Journal of the American Medical Association* 1989; 262:3291–3297.

Sloan, F. A., Mitchell, J., and Cromwell, J., "Physician Participation in State Medicaid Programs," *Journal of Human Resources* 1978; 13(Supplement): 211–245.

Sloan, F. A., Valvona, J., and Mullner, R., "Identifying the Issues: A Statistical Profile," in F. A. Sloan, J. F. Blumstein, and J. M. Perrin, eds., *Uncompensated Hospital Care: Rights and Responsibilities,* Baltimore: The Johns Hopkins University Press, 1986, pp. 16–53.

Sloss, E. M., Keeler, E. B., Brook, R. H., et al., "Effect of a Health Maintenance Organization on Physiologic Health: Results from a Randomized Trial," *Annals of Internal Medicine* May 1987; 1–9.

Solow, R., "Blood and Thunder," *Yale Law Journal* 1971; 80:1711.

Stano, M., "A Clarification of Theories and Evidence on Supplier-Induced Demand for Physicians' Services," *Journal of Human Resources* 1987a; 22:611–620.

Stano, M., "A Further Analysis of the Physician Inducement Controversy," *Journal of Health Economics* 1987b; 6:227–238.

Stano, M., "An Analysis of the Evidence on Competition in the Physicians' Services Market," *Journal of Health Economics* 1985; 4:197–211.

Stano, M., and Folland, S., "Variations in the Use of Physician Services by Medicare Beneficiaries," *Health Care Financing Review* 1988; 9(3):51–57.

Stein, A. D., Shea, S., Basch, C. E., et al., "Independent Associations of Educational Attainment and Ethnicity with Behavioral Risk Factors for Cardiovascular Disease," *American Journal of Epidemiology* 1991; 134(12):1427–1437.

Steinwald, B., and Dummit, L. A., "Hospital Case Mix Change: Sicker Patients or DRG Creep?" *Health Affairs* 1988; 8(2):35–47.

Steinwald, B., and Neuhauser, D., "The Role of the Proprietary Hospital," *Law and Contemporary Problems* 1970; 35:818.

Steinwald, B., and Sloan, F. A., "Determinants of Physicians' Fees," *Journal of Business* 1974; 47(4):493–511.

Stigler, G. J., and Becker, G. S., "De Gustibus Non Est Disputandum," *American Economic Review* 1977; 67(92):76–90.

Surgeon General's Advisory Committee on Smoking and Health, *Smoking and Health,* Washington, DC: US Public Health Service, Office of the Surgeon General, 1964.

Swartz, K., "The Uninsured and Workers Without Employer-Group Health Insurance," Monograph, Washington, DC: The Urban Institute, 3789–02, August 1988.

Taylor, A. K., and Wilensky, G. R., "The Effect of Tax Policies on Expenditures for Private Health Insurance," in J. Meyer, ed., *Market Reforms in Health Care,* Washington, DC: American Enterprise Institute, 1983.

Testa-Wojtekczka, M., "Explaining Physician Responses to Patient Requests— A Mechanistic Approach with Application to Direct-to-Consumer Pharmaceuticals Advertising," Department of Community and Preventive Medicine, University of Rochester School of Medicine and Dentistry, 2008.

Thomas, E. J., Studdert, D. M., Burstein, H. R., et al., "Incidence and Types of Adverse Events and Negligent Care in Utah and Colorado," *Medical Care* 2000; 38(3):261–271.

Thorpe, K. E., and Florence, C., "Health Insurance Coverage Among Children: The Role of Expanded Medicaid Coverage," *Inquiry* 1998; 35(4):369–379.

Thorpe, K. E., and Phelps, C. E., "Regulatory Intensity and Hospital Cost Growth," *Journal of Health Economics* 1990; 9:143–166.

Titmuss, R. M., *The Gift Relationship: From Human Blood to Social Policy,* New York: Vintage Books, 1972.

Tobacco Outlook Report, Economic Research Service, U.S. Department of Agriculture, 2007.

Torrance, G. W., "Measurement of Health State Utilities for Economic Appraisal," *Journal of Health Economics* 1986; 5(1):1–30.

Torrance, G. W., "Utility Approach to Measuring Health-Related Quality of Life," *Journal of Chronic Diseases* 1987; 40(6):593–600.

Triplett, J. E., ed., *Measuring the Prices of Medical Treatments,* Washington, D.C.: The Brookings Institute, 1999.

Tversky, A., and Kahneman, D., "The Framing of Decisions and the Psychology of Choice," *Science* January 1981; 211(30):453–458.

Viscusi, W. K., "Labor Market Valuations of Life and Limb: Empirical Evidence and Policy Implications," *Public Policy* 1978; 26(3):359–386.

Vogel, R., "The Tax Treatment of Health Insurance Premiums as a Cause of Overinsurance," in M. V. Pauly, ed., *National Health Insurance: What Now, What Later, What Never?* Washington, D.C.: American Enterprise Institute, 1980.

Wall Street Journal, The "New Hampshire Top Court Strikes Down Limits on Pain-and-Suffering Awards," March 14, 1991, p. B7.

Walsh, T., McClellan, J. M., McCarthy, S. E. et al., "Rare Structural Variants Disrupt Multiple Genes in Neurodevelopmental Pathways in Schizophrenia," *Science* 2008;320(5875):539–543

Wang, S. J., Middleton, B., and Prosser, L. A., "A Cost-Benefit Analysis of Electronic Medical Records in Primary Care," *American Journal of Medicine* 2003; 114(5):397–403.

Warner, K. E., "Effects of the Antismoking Campaign: An Update," *American Journal of Public Health* 1989; 79(2):144–151.

Watt, J. M., Deizon, R. A., Renn, S. C., et al., "The Comparative Economic Performance of Investor-Owned Chain and Not-for-Profit Hospitals," *New England Journal of Medicine* 1986; 314(2):89–96.

Wedig, G. J., "Health Status and the Demand for Health," *Journal of Health Economics* 1988; 7:151–163.

Weeks, W. B., Wallace, A. E., Wallace, M. M., and Welch, H. G., "A Comparison of the Educational Costs and Incomes of Physicians and Other Professionals," *New England Journal of Medicine* 1994; 330(18):1280–1286.

Weiner, J. P., "Forecasting the Effects of Health Reform on U.S. Physician Workplace Requirement: Evidence from HMO Staffing Patterns," *JAMA* July 20, 1994; 272(3):222–230.

Welch, H. G., Miller, M. E., and Welch, W. P., "Physician Profiling: An Analysis of Inpatient Practice Patterns in Florida and Oregon," *New England Journal of Medicine* 1994; 330(9):607–612.

Wennberg, J. E., "Small Area Analysis and the Medical Care Outcome Problem," in L. Sechrest, E. Perrin, and J. Bunker, eds., *Research*

Methodology: Strengthening Causal Interpretation of Non-Experimental Data, Rockville, MD: Department of Health and Human Services, PHS90-3454, 1990, pp. 177–213.

Wennberg, J. E., and Gittelsohn, A., "Health Care Delivery in Maine I: Patterns of Use of Common Surgical Procedures," *Journal of the Maine Medical Association* 1975; 66:123–130, 149.

Wennberg, J. E., McPherson, K., and Caper, P., "Will Payment Based on Diagnosis-Related Groups Control Hospital Costs?" *New England Journal of Medicine* 1984; 311(5):295–330.

White, M. J., "The Value of Liability in Medical Malpractice," *Health Affairs* 1994; 13(4):75–87.

Winfree, P. L., and DeAngelo, G., "SCHIP and 'Crowd-Out': The High Cost of Expanding Eligibility," Washington, D.C: The Heritage Foundation Web Memo No. 1627, September 20, 2007.

Wolinsky, F. D., and Corry, B. A., "Organizational Structure and Medical Practice in Health Maintenance Organizations," in *Profile of Medical Practice 1981,* Chicago: American Medical Association, 1981.

Woodbury, S., "Substitution Between Wage and Nonwage Benefits," *American Economic Review* 1983; 73(1):166–182.

Woodcock, J., "Innovations for the Drug Development Pathway: What is Needed Now," in Charles G. Smith, ed., *The Process of New Drug Discovery And Development,* New York: Informa Health Care, 2006.

Woodward, R. S., and Warren-Boulton, F., "Considering the Effect of Financial Incentives and Professional Ethics on 'Appropriate' Medical Care," *Journal of Health Economics* 1984; 3(3):223–237.

Woolhandler, S., Campbell, T., and Himmelstein, D. U., "Costs of Health Care Administration in the United States and Canada," *New England Journal of Medicine* 2003; 349(8):768–775.

Yip, W., "Physician Responses to Medical Fee Reductions: Changes in the Volume and Intensity of Supply of Coronary Artery Bypass Graft (CABG) Surgeries in Medicare and the Private Sector," *Journal of Health Economics* 1998; 17:675–700.

Young, L. R., and Nestle, M., The Contribution of Expanding Portion Sizes to the U.S. Obesity Epidemic," *American Journal of Public Health* 2002; 92(2):246–249.

Zaccagnino, M. J., International Health Care and Physician Remuneration, Senior Honors Thesis, University of Rochester, 1994.

Zeckhauser, R. J., "Medical Insurance: A Case Study of the Trade-Off Between Risk Spreading and Appropriate Incentives," *Journal of Economic Theory* 1970; 2(1):10–26.

Zuckerman, S., Bovbjerg, R. R., and Sloan, F. A., "Effects of Tort Reforms and Other Factors on Medical Malpractice Insurance Premiums," *Inquiry* 1990; 27:167–182.

Zwanziger, J., Melnick, G. A., and Bamezai, A., "The Effect of Selective Contracting on Hospital Costs and Revenues," *Health Services Research* 2000; 35(4):849–868.

ACKNOWLEDGMENTS

Page 44, Table 2.6, reprinted with permission from the American Medical Association. **Page 69, Table 3.2** from "Economic Foundations of Cost-Effectiveness Analysis" by A. M. Garber and C. E. Phelps, *Journal of Health Economics* 16(1):1–31, 1997. Reprinted by permission of Elsevier Science. **Page 84, Figure 3.3** from "Physician Profiling: An Analysis of Inpatient Practice Patterns in Florida and Oregon" by H. G. Welch, M. E. Miller, and W. P. Welch, *New England Journal of Medicine* 330(9):607–612. Copyright © 1994 Massachusetts Medical Society. All rights reserved. **Page 130, Table 5.1; page 131, Table 5.2; page 133, Table 5.4** from "Health Insurance and the Demand for Medical Care: Evidence from a Randomized Experiment" by W. G. Manning, J. P. Newhouse, and N. Duan, *American Economic Review* 77(3):251–277, 1987. Reprinted by permission of the American Economic Association. **Page 131, Table 5.3; Page 136, Table 5.6** from Emmett B. Keeler, et. al., "The Demand for Episodes of Medical Treatment in the Health Insurance Experiment," RAND/ R-3454-HHS, Santa Monica, CA: RAND, 1988. Copyright© RAND 1988. Reprinted by permission. **Page 133, Table 5.5** from "The Demand for Dental Care: Evidence from a Randomized Trial on Health Insurance" by W. G. Manning, B. Benjamin, H. L. Bailit, and J. P. Newhouse, *Journal of the American Dental Association* 110:895–902. Copyright © 1985 American Dental Association. Adapted 2002 with permission of ADA Publishing, a Division of ADA Business Enterprises, Inc. **Page 173, Box 6.1 table** from AMA Center for Health Policy Research, "Physician Socioeconomic Statistics, 2003." Chicago: American Medical Association; 2003. **Pages 201–202, Table 7.2** from "Does the Geographical Distribution of Physicians Reflect Market Failure?" by J. P. Newhouse, A. P. Williams, B. W. Benentt, and W. B. Schwartz, *Bell Journal of Economics,* 13:493–505, 1982. Reprinted by permission of RAND. **Page 216, Table 7.3** from "Medical Care as a Commodity: An Exploration of the Shopping Behavior of Patients" by D. M. Olsen, R. L. Kane, and D. Kastler *Journal of Community Health* 2(2):85–91, 1976. Reprinted by permission of Kluwer Academic/Plenum Publishers. **Pages 288–291, Box 9.1** from "Statistical Summary" American Hospital Association, 1993. Reprinted by permission of the American Hospital Association. **Page 371, Table 11.5** from "Forecasting the Effects of Health Reform on U.S. Physician Workplace Requirement: Evidence from HMO Staffing Patterns" by J. P. Weiner, *JAMA* 272(3):222–230, July 20, 1994. Reprinted by permission of the American Medical Association. **Page 414, Figure 12.3**, reprinted with permission from the American Hospital Association. **Page 436, Table 13.1** from "Incidence of Adverse Events and Negligence Among Clinical-Specialty Groups" by T. A. Brennan, L. L. Leape, N. M. Laird, et al., *New England Journal of Medicine* 324(6):370–376. Copyright © 1994, Massachusetts Medical Society. All rights reserved. **Page 448, Table 13.2** from "Medical-Malpractice Insurance

Dates" by J. R. Schiffman, *Wall Street Journal*, April 28, 1989. Copyright © 1989 by Dow Jones & Company, Inc. Reproduced with permission of Dow Jones & Company Inc. via Copyright Clearance Center. Reprinted by permission of the Copyright Clearance Center. **Page 474, Figure 14.3** from "Effects of the Antismoking Campaign, An Update" by K. E. Warner, *American Journal of Public Health* 79(2): 144–151, 1989. Reprinted by permission of the American Public Health Association.

INDEX

salary *vs.* fee-for-service,
360–362
staffing patterns, 370–371
Hodgkin, D., 400, 401
Hofer, T. P., 504
Hoff, J., 535
Holdbacks, 363–364
Hollingsworth, T. D., 467, 468
Holmer, M., 333
Holohan, J., 226*n*
Holtman, A. G., 254*n*
Holzman, D., 445
Horizontal aggregation, 102*n*,
576*n*, 585, 585*n*
Hosek, S., 176
Hospice benefits, Medicare, 398
Hospital costs, 254–258
cost curve, 259–262
length of stay within DRGS,
variability in, 255–256
long-run *vs.* short-run costs,
258–259
quality of care, size, and
ownership, 260–262
Hospitals
board of trustees, 240, 241,
249, 251*n*
costs (*See* Hospital costs)
demand curve facing,
264–265, 288–291
learning goals, 238
in marketplace (*See* Hospitals
in marketplace)
organizational structure,
239–244
outpatient surgery, 262–264
performance of for-profit
vs. not-for-profit,
248–249
quality of care, size and
ownership, 260–262
relative value unit (RVU) per
admission, 85
residual claimants (*See*
Residual claimants)
utility-maximizing hospital
manager, 266
Hospitals in marketplace
competition for medical staff,
281–282
competition for patients,
282–283
equilibrium quality and price
model, 274–278

features providing general
attractiveness, 271
features that attract physicians
to, 270–271
for-profit hospitals, role of, 286
insurance and competition in
decision making, 278
insurance coverage changes,
280
labor markets, 286–287,
291–293
learning goals, 269
medical staff, market for,
270–272
nursing shortages, 292–294
"old style" *vs.* "new style,"
283–285
patients and, 272–274
quality and output changes,
278–280
quality and quantity decisions,
296–299
wage rates for specialized *vs.*
unspecialized hospital
workers, 291
Hotelling, H., 198
House (TV series), 170*n*
House, D. R., 216, 218, 226*n*, 227,
228
Hsiao, W. C., 172, 405
Huang, L. F., 127
Hughes, E. X. F., 224, 261
Human Genome Project (HGP),
510, 511–512
Human immunodeficiency virus
(HIV), 459*n*, 463, 478
Human papilloma virus (HPV),
463*n*, 467*n*
Hunt, S. S., 261

*ICD, the International
Classification of Diseases*
(WHO), 169*n*
Iglehart, J. K., 406, 464*n*, 541, 541*n*
Ikegami, N., 546, 547
Illness
from addiction, 143–144
demand, 142–145
effects, on demand for medical
care, 139
episode-of-illness analysis,
129–131
episode-of-illness-based payment plans, 379, 406–407

events, 100–101
levels of, and medical spending,
311
and pleasure, joint production
of, 143
severity of, interaction with
elasticities, 149
without insurance, 106–108,
112–113
Income. *See* Per capita income
(PCI)
Income elasticity, 112
Income tax subsidization for
health insurance, 4–5,
326–332, 335
Incremental productivity
(marginal productivity), 37,
57–59, 88–90
Indemnity insurance, 108, 113
Indifference curves, 35, 92–98,
573–574
Indifference map, 95
Indifferent, defined, 574*n*
Indirect standardization, 81
Induced demand
aggregate demand, exogenous
shifts in, 229–230
consumer information, role of,
232–233
economists' perspective on,
228
meaning of, 225–226
physician/agent making
referrals, 230–231
for physicians, 225–229
physicians as agent for the
patient, 230
physicians' referral to
self-owned facilities,
231–232
welfare loss created by, 310
Industrial organization (IO), 592
Infant mortality rates, 550, 558,
561*n*, 564, 567
Information, provision of, 144–145
Informed consent, 424
Institute of Medicine (IOM), 465,
466, 524
Insurance. *See* Health insurance
Insurance pool, 344
Intensive margin, 59–60, 70
International Classification of
Diseases, Version 9 (ICD-9),
38*n*